AF324034

Surgery of the Aorta and Its Body Branches

Mark D. Morasch, M.D.
Associate Professor of Surgery
Division of Vascular Surgery
Department of Surgery
Northwestern University
Feinberg School of Medicine
Chicago, IL

William H. Pearce, M.D.
Violet R. and Charles A. Baldwin
Professor of Vascular Surgery
Chief, Division of Vascular Surgery
Department of Surgery
Northwestern University
Feinberg School of Medicine
Chicago, IL

James S. T. Yao, M.D., Ph.D.
Professor Emeritus
Division of Vascular Surgery
Department of Surgery
Northwestern University
Feinberg School of Medicine
Chicago, IL

2010
PEOPLE'S MEDICAL PUBLISHING HOUSE—USA
SHELTON, CONNECTICUT

People's Medical Publishing House–USA
2 Enterprise Drive, Suite 509
Shelton, CT 06484
Tel: 203-402-0646
Fax: 203-402-0854
E-mail: info@pmph-usa.com

PMPH-USA

09 10 11 12 13/PMPH/9 8 7 6 5 4 3 2 1

13-digit ISBN: 978-1-60795-054-7
10-digit ISBN: 1-60795-054-5

Printed in China by People's Medical Publishing House of China
Copyeditor/Typesetter: Spearhead Global, Inc.; Cover Designer: Mary McKeon

Library of Congress Cataloging-in-Publication Data

Morash, Mark D.
  Surgery of the aorta and its body branches / Mark D. Morash, William H. Pearce, James S.T. Yao.
      p. ; cm. — (Modern trends in vascular surgery)
  Includes bibliographical references and index.
  ISBN 978-1-60795-054-7
  1. Aorta—Surgery. 2. Blood-vessels—Surgery 3. Aortic aneurysms—Surgery. I. Pearce, William H. II. Yao, James S. T. III.
Title. IV. Series: Modern trends in vascular surgery.
  [DNLM: 1. Aortic Aneurysm—surgery. 2. Aorta—surgery. 3. Postoperative Complications—prevention & control. 4. Randomized Controlled Trials as Topic. 5. Vascular Surgical Procedures—methods.
WG 410 M829s 2010]
  RD598.5.M67 2010
  617.4'13—dc22

2009047955

Contents

1 Operative Vascular Surgery in the Endovascular Era   3

K. Craig Kent, M.D., F.A.C.S.

2 How to Train Surgeons in Open Procedures in the Era of Endovascular Surgery   13

Christopher M. Chambers, M.D., Ph.D. Gregorio A. Sicard, M.D.

SECTION II Contemporary Open Techniques For Abdominal Aortic Aneurysms   31

SECTION XI New Findings In Thoracic Aortic Endovascular Technology   395

Preface

The Northwestern University Vascular Symposium is an educational event that has been in existence, uninterrupted, since 1976. Each year, 40 or so leading vascular surgeons from the US and from overseas serve as symposium faculty. They speak and take part in discussions regarding topics of special interest to vascular and cardiac surgeons and to those interested in the medicine of vascular disease. In addition, for many years now, the faculty have authored chapters that have been published as a compendium to the symposium. The compendium book is published as a permanent record of their contributions. This book has been widely successful and is a popular component of the meeting each year. Until recently, the book was made available to the public after the symposium and was always a sell-out.

Surgery of the Aorta and Its Body Branches is a compilation of updated chapters from the most recent symposia. Over the last five years the compendium was published privately and was not commercially marketed; it was distributed only to participants of the symposium. It has become apparent that the book has been missed by many who, for whatever reason, were unable to travel to Chicago for the annual event. We also recognized that the lack of worldwide circulation did an injustice to the faculty members whose chapters represent a real contribution to the medical literature. *Surgery of the Aorta and Its Body Branches* is the brainchild of Dr. James Yao and Dr. William Pearce. It highlights the advancement of diagnosis and management of aortic disease in recent years.

The book begins with a series of chapters that discuss current issues regarding volume and training for open surgery in this, the era of endovascular surgery. The next few sections touch upon contemporary open techniques used for the treatment of thoracic, thoracoabdominal, and abdominal aortic aneurysms, as well as a section on reoperative aortic surgery.

The subsequent sections focus on endovascular intervention and discuss broad topics including the use of endoprotheses for the treatment of not only straightforward aneurysms, but, amongst other topics of interest, the management of acute dissections, traumatic injury, and the most common complications seen with endografting. In addition, there is a section that reviews the contemporary clinical data underlying the decision making behind endovascular aortic repair. The book ends with sections that broach the topics of endovascular and open management of aortic branch pathology.

Treatment of vascular disease is changing and surgeons must make changes accordingly. The Northwestern Symposium strives to keep those involved in the management of vascular pathology on the cutting edge of techniques and technology. Our hope is that this textbook will open the expert discussions to a broader audience.

Mark D. Morasch, MD
William H. Pearce, MD
James S.T.Yao, MD, PhD

Acknowledgment

We thank the administrative staff of the Division of Vascular Surgery—Sara Minton and Jan Goldstein—for their support. Special thanks to Susan Parmentier of Greenwood Academic for reprocessing chapters of the last five Northwestern Symposia. We would also like to thank W.L. Gore & Associates for a generous education grant to support the Northwestern Vascular Symposium over the years. Finally, we thank Mr. Jason Malley of People's Medical Publishing House-USA and Mr. Harjeet Singh from Spearhead Global, Inc. for their expert assistance.

Mark D. Morasch
William H. Pearce
James S.T. Yao

Contributors

Paul A. Armstrong, M.D.
Division of Vascular and Endovascular
　Surgery
Universtiy of South Florida College of
　Medicine
Chief, Vascular Surgery
James A. Haley Veterans Hospitals
Tampa, Florida

Ali Azizzadeh, M.D.
Assistant Professor
Department of Cardiothoracic and Vascular
　Surgery
The University of Texas Medical School at
　Houston
Director, Endovascular Surgery
Memorial Hermann Heart & Vascular
　Institute, Texas Medical Center
Houston, Texas

Dennis F. Bandyk, M.D.
Professor of Surgery
University of South Florida
Director, Division of Vascular and
　Endovascular Surgery
Tampa General Hospital
Tampa, Florida

Marshall E. Benjamin, M.D.
Associate Professor of Surgery
University of Maryland Medical Center
Director, Maryland Vascular Center
Baltimore Washington Medical Center
Baltimore, Maryland

Ramon Berguer, M.D.
Frankel Professor of Vascular Surgery
Professor of Engineering
University of Michigan Medical School
University of Michigan Health System
Ann Arbor, Michigan

Kristen L. Biggs, M.D.
Assistant Professor of Surgery
Division of Vascular Surgery, Department
　of Surgery
University of New Mexico School of
　Medicine
Albuquerque, New Mexico

Susan A. Blackburn, R.N., M.B.A.
Divisions of Vascular and Cardiac
　Surgery
University of Michigan Medical School
University of Michigan Health System
Ann Arbor, Michigan

Jan D. Blankensteijn, M.D.
Associate Professor of Surgery
VU Medical Center
Amsterdam, The Netherlands

Thomas C. Bower, M.D.
Professor of Surgery
Vascluar Surgery
Gonda Vascular Center
Mayo Clinic
Rochester, Minnesota

Katharine E. Brown, D.O.
Associate Professor in Surgery
University of California at San Diego
San Diego, California

Erik Buskens, M.D.
Julius Center for Health Sciences & Primary
   Care
University Medical Center Utrecht
Utrecht, The Netherlands

Rabih A. Chaer, M.D.
Division of Vascular Surgery
University of Pittsburgh Physicians
University of Pittsburgh Medical Center
Pittsburgh, Pennsylvania

Elliot L. Chaikof, M.D.
Professor and John E. Skandalakis Chair of
   Surgery, Division of Vascular Surgery,
   Department of Surgery,
Emory University School of Medicine
Chief, Division of Vascular Surgery and
   Endovascular Therapy
Emory University
Atlanta, Georgia

Christopher M. Chambers, M.D.
Vascular Surgeon
Metropolital Hospital
Grand Rapids, Michigan

Kenneth J. Cherry, M.D.
Professor of Surgery
Department of Surgery, Division of
   Thoracic and Cardiovascular Surgery
University of Virginia Medical Center
Charlottesville, Virginia

Andy C. Chiou, M.D.
Assistant Professor of Clinical Surgery
Department of Surgery
Peoria, Illinois

Tuan-Hung B. Chu, M.D., R.V.T.
Endovascular, Interventional Vascular and
   Peripheral Vascular Surgery.
Surgical Assoicates of Dallas
Dallas, Texas

Daniel Clair, M.D.
Professor of Surgery
Cleveland Clinic Lerner College of
   Medicine at Case Western University
Chairman, Department of Vascular
   Surgery
Cleveland Clinic
Cleveland, Ohio

Sheila M. Coogan, M.D.
Assistant Professor, Department of
   Cardiothoracic and Vascular
   Surgery
The University of Texas Medical School at
   Houston
Director, Vascular Laboratory
Memorial Hermann Heart & Vascular
   Institute, Texas Medical Center
Houston, Texas

John A. Cowan, Jr., M.D.
Department of Surgery, Division of
   Vascular Surgery
University of Michigan Medical School
Ann Arbor, Michigan

Enrique Criado, M.D., FACS
Professor of Vascular Surgery
University of Michigan Medical School
University of Michigan Health System
Ann Arbor, Michigan

Michael D. Dake, M.D.
Professor of Cardiothoracic Surgery,
   Department of Cardiothoracic
   Surgery
Stanford University School of Medicine
Medical Director, Cath/Angio
   Laboratories
Stanford University Medical Center
Stanford, California

R. Clement Darling, M.D.
Professor of Surgery
Albany Medical College
Chief, Division of Vascular Surgery
The Vascular Group, PLLC
Albany, New York

G. Michael Deeb, M.D.
Professor, Department of Surgery
Herbert Sloan Collegiate Professor
University of Michigan Medical School
Director, Multidisciplinary Aortic Clinic
University of Michigan Health System
Ann Arbor, Michigan

Justin B. Dimick, M.D., M.P.H.
Assistant Professor of Surgery
University of Michigan Medical School
University of Michigan Health System
Ann Arbor, Michigan

Yves-Marie Dion, M.D.
Professor of Surgery in the Division of
    Vascular Surgery
Laval University
Québec City University Hospital Center
    (CHUQ)
St-François d'Assise Hospital
Redearcher, Québec Biomaterials Institute.
Quebec City, Quebec, Canada

Gary Dobson, M.D., FRCPC
Department of Anesthesiology
University of Calgary
Calgary, Alberta, Canada

Matthew J. Eagleton, M.D.
Assistant Professor of Surgery
Cleveland Clinic Lerner College of
    Medicine at Case Western Reserve
    University
Attending Surgeon
Cleveland Clinic
Cleveland, Ohio

Matthew S. Edwards, M.D.
Associate Professor, Surgery Vascular
Wake Forest University School of Medicine
Vascular Surgeon
North Carolina Baptist Hospital
Winston Salem, North Carolina

Jonathan L. Eliason, M.D.
Assistant Professor of Vascular Surgery
University of Michigan Health System
Ann Arbor, Michigan

Mark K. Eskandari, M.D.
Assoicate Professor in Surgery-
    Vascular
Northwestern University's Feinberg
    School of Medicine
Chicago, IL

Anthony L. Estrera, M.D.
Associate Professor, Department of
    Cardiothoracic and Vascular
    Surgery
The University of Texas Medical School at
    Houston
Chief of Cardiac Surgery
Cardiovascular Intensive Care Unit
Memorial Hermann Hospital - Texas
    Medical Center
Houston, Texas

Mark A. Farber, M.D.
Associate Professor of Vascular Surgery and
    Interventional Radiology
University of North Carolina
Director, UNC Endovascular Institute
UNC Hospitals
Chapel Hill, North Carolina

John D. Frusha, M.D.
Vascular Surgery Associates
Medical Director of Vascular Associates
    Laboratory
Baton Rouge, Louisiana

Nicholas J. Gargiulo, III, M.D.
Associate Professor of Surgery
Albert Einstein College of Medicine
Attending Vascular Surgeon
Montefiore Medical Center
New York, New York

Patrick J. Geraghty, M.D.
Associate Professor, Surgery and
    Radiology
Division of General Surgery,Vascular
    Surgery Section
Washington University
Barnes-Jewish St. Peters Hospital
St. Louis, Missouri

Kristina A. Giles, M.D.
Division of Vascular and Endovascular
  Surgery,
Beth Israel Deaconess Medical Center,
Boston, Massachusetts

Richard M. Green, M.D.
Vascular Surgeon
Lenox Hill Hospital
New York, NY

Roy K. Greenberg, M.D.
Associate Professor of Surgery
Cleveland Clinic Lerner College of
  Medicine at Case Western Reserve
  University
Director, Endovascular Research and
  Peripheral Vascular Core Laboratory
The Cleveland Clinic Foundation
Cleveland, Ohio

John P. Harris, M.D.
Department of Surgery
University of Sydney
Division of Surgery
Royal Prince Alfred Hospital
Sydney and Camperdown, New South
  Wales, Australia

Stephen M. Hass, M.D.
Division of Vascular Surgery,
University of Maryland
Baltimore, Maryland

Heitham T. Hassoun, M.D.
Assistant Professor of Vascular
  Surgery
The Johns Hopkins Hospital
Vascular and Endovascular Therapies
Methodist Cardiovascular Surgery
  Associates
Methodist Hospital System
Baltimore, Maryland and Houston,
  Texas

Stephen A. Hebert, R.N.
Vascular Surgery Associates
Baton Rouge, Louisiana

Peter K. Henke, M.D.
Associate Professor of Vascular Surgery
University of Michigan Medical School
University of Michigan Health System
Ann Arbor, Michigan

Tam T.T. Huynh, M.D., B.S.
Associate Professor of Surgery
Vascular Surgery Division
University of Texas Medical School
Texas Medical Center
Houston, Texas

Loay Kabbani, M.D.
Vascular Fellow
University of Michigan Medical School
Ann Arbor, Michigan

Blair Keagy, M.D.
George Johnson Distinguished Professor of
  Surgery
University of North Carolina
Chief, Division of Vascular Surgery
UNC Hospitals
Chapel Hill, North Carolina

K. Craig Kent, M.D.
A.R. Curreri Professor of Surgery
Chairman, Department of Surgery, Section
  of Vascular Surgery
University of Wisconsin School of Medicine
  and Public Health
University of Wisconsin Hospital
Madison, Wisconsin

Brian S. Knipp, M.D.
Resient, General Surgery
University of Michigan Medical School
Ann Arbor, Michigan

Michel Lacombe, M.D.
Department of Surgery
Hôpital Beaujon
Clichy, France

Frank A. Lederle, M.D.
Professor of Medicine
VA Medical Center
Minneapolis, Minnesota

Evan C. Lipsitz, M.D.
Associate Professor of Surgery
Albert Einstein College of Medicine
Interim Chief, Division of Vascular Surgery
  Medical Director
Vascular Diagnostic Laboratory
Montefiore Medical Center
New York, NY

Peter S. Liu, M.D.
Clinical Lecture, Department of
  Radiology
University of Michigan Medical School
University of Michigan Health System
Ann Arbor, Michigan

Graham W. Long, M.D.
Vascular Surgeon
Peripheral Vascular of NVA
Bloomfeild Hills, MI

Alan B. Lumsden, M.D.
Professor & Chairman
Methodist DeBakey Heart & Vascular
  Center
Medical Director
Methodist Hospital
Houston, Texas

Lindsay Machan, M.D.
Associate Professor
University of British Columbia
Interventional Radiologist
Vancouver Hospital and Health Sciences
  Center
Vancouver, British Columbia, Canada

Douglas P. MacMillan, M.D.
Asheville Radiology
Carolina Vascular
Asheville, North Carolina

Michel S. Makaroun, M.D.
Professor of Surgery
University of Pittsburgh
Chief, Division of Vascular Surgery
University of Pittsburgh Medical Center
Pittsburgh, Pennsylvania

Jon S. Matsumura, M.D.
Professor of Surgery, Chief, Vascular
  Surgery
University of Wisconsin School of Medicine
  and Public Health
University of Wisconsin Hospital
Madison, Wisconsin

James May, M.D., M.S., FRACS, FACS
Bosch Professor of Surgery & Associate
  Dean Surgical Sciences
University of Sydney
Vascular Surgeon
Royal Prince Alfred Hospital
Sydney and Camperdown, New South
  Wales, Australia

K. McCune, M.D., FRCS (Ed.)
University of Calgary
Calgary, Alberta, Canada

James W. McNeil, M.D.
Assistant Clinical Professor of Surgery
Louisiana State University, New Orleans
CVT Surgical Center
New Orleans and Baton Rouge, Louisiana

Robert R. Mendes, M.D.
Assistant Professor of Surgery
Division of Vascular Surgery
UNC Hospitals
Chapel Hill, North Carolina

Charles C. Miller, III, Ph.D.
Professor, Department of Cardiothoracic
  and Vascular Surgery
Center for Clinical Research & Evidence-
  Based Medicine
Center for Biotechnology
The University of Texas Medical School at
  Houston
Houston, Texas

Randy D. Moore, M.D., M.Sc., FRCSC
Assistant Professor
University of Calgary
Calgary Health Region
Calgary, Alberta, Canada

Mark D. Morasch, M.D.
Associate Professor in Surgery-Vascular
Practice Director
Northwestern University's Feinberg School
    of Medicine
Northwestern Memorial Hospital
Chicago, Illinois

Mona Motamedi, B.A. (Honours)
Research Coordinator/Database Manager
University of Calgary
Calgary Health Region
Calgary, Alberta, Canada

Andrew J. Olinde, M.D.
Clinical Instructor
Ochsner Clinic
Vascular Surgery Associates
Baton Rouge, Louisiana

Babak J. Orandi, M.D.
Department of Surgery, Division of
    Vascular Surgery
University of Michigan Medical School
Ann Arbor, Michigan

Himanshu J. Patel, M.D.
Assistant Professor of Surgery, Section of
    Cardiac Surgery
University of Michigan Medical School
University of Michigan Health System
Ann Arbor, Michigan

Philip S.K. Paty, M.D.
Associate Professor of Surgery
Albany Medical Center
The Institute for Vascular Health and
    Disease
The Vascular Group, PLLC
Albany, New York

William H. Pearce, M.D.
Violet R. and Charles A. Baldwin Professor
    in Vascular Surgery
Northwestern University's Feinberg School
    of Medicine
Chief, Division of Vascular Surgery
Northwestern Memorial Hospital
Chicago, Illinois

Eric K. Peden, M.D.
Assistant Professor of Surgery in the
    Department of Cardiovascular
    Surgery,
Chief of Vascular Surgery
Methodist DeBakey Heart and Vascular
    Center
Houston, Texas

Brian G. Peterson, M.D.
Vascular Surgeon
St. Louis University Hospital
St. Louis, Missouri

Kenneth T. Piercy, M.D.
Vascular Surgeon
Mid-South Surgeons
Columbia, Tennessee

Eyal E. Porat, M.D.
Adjunct Professor, Department of
    Cardiothoracic and Vascular
    Surgery
The University of Texas Medical
    School at Houston
Director, Cardiothoracic Surgery
Rabin Medical Center
Houston, Texas and Petah-Tikva,
    Israel

Monique Prinssen, M.D.
Division of Vascular Surgery
Department of Surgery
University Medical Center Utrecht
Utrecht, The Netherlands

Michael J. Reardon, M.D.
Thoracic Surgery
Methodist DeBakey Heart and
    Vascular Center
Houston, Texas

John E. Rectenwald, M.D.
Associate Professor of Vascular
    Surgery
University of Michigan Medical
    School
University of Michigan Health System
Ann Arbor, Michigan

Jean-Baptiste Ricco, M.D., Ph.D.
Professeur des Universités
Université de Poitiers
Praticien Hospitalier, Chef de
   Service
Centre Hospital
Poitiers, France

Heron E. Rodriguez, M.D.
Assistant Professor in Vascular
   Surgery
Northwestern University's Feinberg
   School of Medicine
Division of Vascluar Surgery
Northwestern Memorial Hospital
Chicago, IL

Hazim J. Safi, M.D.
Professor and Chairman
University of Texas Medical School
Chief, Memorial Hermann Heart &
   Vascular Institute
Texas Medical Center
Houston, Texas

Stephanie Saltzberg, M.D.
Assistant Professor of Surgery
Albany Medical Center
Vascular Surgeon
The Vascular Group, PLLC, Kingston
Albany and Kingston, New York

Albert D. Sam II, M.D.
Clinical Assistant Professor
Louisiana State University School of
   Medicine
Vascular Surgery Associates
Baton Rouge, Louisiana

Elliot B. Sambol, M.D.
Vascular Surgeon
Princeton Surgical Associates
Princeton, New Jersey

Layne Sandridge, M.D.
Vascular Surgeon
Arizona Heart Institute
Phoenix, Arizona

Marc L. Schermerhorn, M.D.
Assistant Professor
Harvard Medical School
Beth Israel Deaconess Medical Center,
Chief, Vascular surgery
Boston, Massachusetts

Charles J. Shanley, M.D.
Marion and David Handleman Research
   Professor of Vascular Surgery
University of Michigan Medical School,
Department of Surgery
William Beaumont Hospital,
Royal Oak, Michigan

Palma M. Shaw, M.D.
Assistant Professor of Surgery
Boston University School of Medicine
Co-Director, Endovascular Surgery
Boston Medical Center
Boston, Massachusetts

Gregorio A. Sicard, M.D.
Eugene M. Bricker Professor, Surgery
Division Head of General Surgery, Section
   Head of Vascular Surgery,
Vice Chairman, Department of Surgery
Washington University
Barnes-Jewish West County Hospital
St. Louis, Missouri

James C. Stanley, M.D.
Marion and David Handleman Research
Professor of Vascular Surgery
University of Michigan Medical School
University of Michigan Health System
Ann Arbor, Michigan

Gale L. Tang, M.D.
Associate Professor of Washington
   University
University of Washington
VA Puget Sound Health Care System
Seattle, Washington

Joep A.W. Teijink, M.D.
Department of Surgery
Atrium Medical Center
Heerlen, The Netherlands

William D. Turnipseed, M.D.
Professor, Division of General Surgery
Chief, Section of Vascular Surgery
University of Wisconsin Madison
Director, Vascular Noninvasive Diagnostic
  Lab
Madison, WI

Rudolf P. Tutein Nolthenius, M.D.
Department of Surgery
Albert Schweitzer Hospital
Dordrecht, The Netherlands

Gilbert R. Upchurch, Jr., M.D.
Leland Ira Doan Research Professor of
  Vascular Surgery
Professor of Vascular Surgery
University of Michigan Medical School
University of Michigan Health System
Ann Arbor, Michigan

R. James Valentine, M.D.
Professor, Surgery and Vascluar Sugery
University of Texas Southwest Medical
  Center
Dallas, Texas

Steven M.M. van Sterkenburg,
Department of Surgery
Rijnstate Hospital
Arnhem, The Netherlands

Frank J. Veith, M.D.
Professor of Surgery
The William J. von Liebig Chair in Vascular
  Surgery
The Cleveland Clinic and New York
  University
The Cleveland Clinic and New York
  University Medical Center
Cleveland, Ohio and New York, New York

Martin A. Villa, M.D.
Department of Surgery, Division of
  Vascular Surgery
University of Texas Medical School
Houston, Texas

J.C. Walkes, M.D.
Clinical Associate Professor, Department
  of Cardiothoracic and Vascular
  Surgery
The University of Texas Medical
  School at Houston
Director, Valve Program
Memorial Hermann Heart & Vascular
  Institute, Texas Medical Center
Houston, Texas

Margaret H. Walkup, M.D.
Resident
Vascular Surgery
University of North Carolina
Chapel Hill, North Carolina

David S. Wang, D.O.
Instructor of Radiology
Department of Radiology, Division of
  Musculoskeletal Radiology
University of Virginia Medical
  Center
Charlottesville, Virginia

Geoffrey H. White, M.D.
Associate Professor of Surgery
University of Sydney
Head, Department of Vascular
  Surgery
Royal Prince Alfred Hospital
Sydney and Camperdown, New South
  Wales, Australia

David M. Williams, M.D.
Professor, Department of Radiology
University of Michigan Medical
  School
University of Michigan Health System
Ann Arbor, Michigan

David B. Wilson, M.D.
Vascular Surgeon
Michigan Vascular Center
Flint, Michigan

Mark C. Wyers, M.D., FACS
Cardiovascular Institute's Division of
  Vascular Surgery
Beth Israel Deaconess Medical Center,
Boston, Massachusetts

Robert M. Zwolak, M.D., Ph.D.
Professor of Surgery, Vascular
Dartmouth Medical School
Dartmouth-Hitchcock Medical Center
Lebanon, NH

Current Issues of Open Surgery in The Era of Endovascular Surgery

Operative Vascular Surgery in the Endovascular Era

Elliot B. Sambol, M.D.
K. Craig Kent, M.D., F.A.C.S.

Of all areas of medicine, vascular surgery has perhaps undergone the greatest evolution over the past 15 years. A field that was once associated with complex and challenging open procedures is now dominated by minimally invasive endovascular technology. This change of venue has necessitated that practicing vascular surgeons retrain in minimally invasive techniques, and has produced a need to incorporate percutaneous intervention into fellowship training in vascular surgery.

There is little doubt that many of these advances have been beneficial to our patients. However, the move to minimally invasive techniques has led to a substantial drop-off in the number of traditional open vascular procedures that are performed. The "endovascular revolution," despite its clearly proven clinical advantages, has made traditional open surgical cases a rare commodity. This has a number of implications regarding the training of both current and future vascular surgeons, which we will address in the following chapter. We will attempt to answer the following questions:

1. How dramatically have minimally invasive approaches impacted the number of open vascular interventions?
2. How has the reduction in open cases impacted resident training for both general and vascular surgery programs?
3. How should future training programs in general and vascular surgery be constructed?
4. Who in the future should be performing complex open vascular reconstructions?

THE IMPACT OF ENDOVASCULAR TECHNIQUES ON THE NUMBER OF OPEN VASCULAR INTERVENTIONS

The first endovascular abdominal aortic aneurysm repair (EVAR) was performed in 1991 by Parodi et. al.[1] Prior to this, vascular surgeons were, for the most part, uninvolved in percutaneous intervention. At this point in time, catheter-based procedures constituted only approximately 10–20% of the total vascular case volume. In the late 1990s, however, the number of percutaneous interventions performed in the United States skyrocketed. Based on data from the National Hospital Discharge Survey (NHDS) data set, more than 200,000 endovascular procedures were performed in 2003 compared to only a few hundred performed in 1980. This almost exponential increase in the number of percutaneous procedures appears to be continuing and is related to a number of factors. First, as the U.S. population increases and becomes more aged, there is a higher prevalence of vascular disease, and hence, more patients requiring care. Second, minimally invasive techniques allow many patients that were previously too high risk for surgery the opportunity to undergo intervention. Finally, in many circumstances, persuasive data suggest that a minimally invasive approach is preferable to open surgery.[2,3]

In reviewing these trends, it becomes apparent that traditional open vascular procedures are rapidly diminishing in number, but they have not become extinct. As an example, approximately 20–30% of AAAs have anatomic constraints that prohibit endograft placement, thus necessitating open repair. Moreover, those AAAs requiring open repair are more complex and, therefore, mandate advanced surgical skills. A recent study evaluated the complexity of open AAA repair in both the pre- and post-EVAR era.[4] The authors found that the post-EVAR open repairs required more frequent suprarenal cross-clamping, and that these patients had a higher frequency of iliac aneurysmal and occlusive disease. In this particular study, despite the increased complexity of open cases in the post-EVAR era, morbidity and mortality rates were not statistically different from those in the pre-EVAR era. The authors' findings demonstrate that excellent outcomes can be achieved in complex cases by experienced surgeons who trained during a time when endovascular interventions were less common. However, vascular surgeons of the future will likely have substantially less experience with open aneurysm repair, yet be faced with complex interventions when open surgery becomes necessary. A similar paradigm could be predicted for lower extremity occlusive disease. Only patients with the most complex anatomy will require surgical bypass. This may also be true as well for carotid, renal, and mesenteric occlusive disease.

HOW HAS THE REDUCTION IN OPEN CASE NUMBERS IMPACTED RESIDENT TRAINING FOR BOTH GENERAL AND VASCULAR SURGERY PROGRAMS?

With the transformation in the treatment algorithm for vascular disease, the training of vascular surgeons has become complex. Vascular surgery fellows (VSF) completing their training in 2007 do so with an overwhelming number of endovascular procedures that far exceed the minimum requirements set forth by the Residency Review Committee (RRC). Conversely, VSFs at many programs are now in danger of finishing their two years of training with only the minimum number of open vascular reconstructions. The drop-off in the use of traditional open surgical skills has caused the tide to shift. Whereas the strength and reputation of vascular fellowship programs was once based on endovascular caseloads and exposure to cutting edge interventional procedural skills, now the opposite is true. The most coveted fellowships seem to be those that have the highest volume of open cases. Moreover, as the open caseload has declined for VSFs, there has been a concomitant decrease in the exposure of general surgery residents (GSR) to open vascular surgery.

Grabo et. al. recently performed an up-to-date analysis of the effect of endovascular interventions on the training of GSRs.[5] They used data from the Accreditation Council for Graduate Medical Education (ACGME) website to determine trends in procedures for both GSRs and VSFs over the last decade. They found that general surgery training has suffered with respect to open vascular cases. The total number of major vascular cases logged by finishing GSRs has decreased from a mean of 190 in 1998 to 130 in 2006 (Figure 1–1). In reviewing specific subsets of vascular cases, there were, over the past 10 years, 22%, 23%, and 47% decreases in case volume in the major areas of peripheral-obstructive, cerebrovascular, and aneurysm repair, respectively, for GSRs (Figure 1–2). This diminution in open cases, however, has not been replaced by a substantial reciprocal rise in the endovascular experience (Figure 1–2). The mean number of endovascular cases performed in 2006 for general surgical residents was only 10 with an average of only four endovascular procedures performed during the chief year.

In contrast, for VSFs, there has been a steep upward trend in total case numbers with a mean of 280 in 1998 to 516 in 2006 (Figure 1–1). It should be noted that this near doubling of cases, at least in part, is reflective of the fact that most vascular fellowships increased from one to two ACGME approved years during this period of time. Also contributing to this increase was a durable rise in endovascular procedures with more than a three-fold increase in the mean number of therapeutic interventions performed by VSFs from 2001 (mean = 42) to 2006 (mean = 150). Despite the significant increase in endovascular procedures, open case volume has diminished. Over the last decade, fellows have experienced a decrease in the mean number of open cases in the following categories: peripheral-obstructive (75 to 70, 6% change, not significant), cerebrovascular (61 to 50, 19% change, p<.0001), and aneurysms (41 to 33, 19% change, p<.0001) (Figure 1–3).

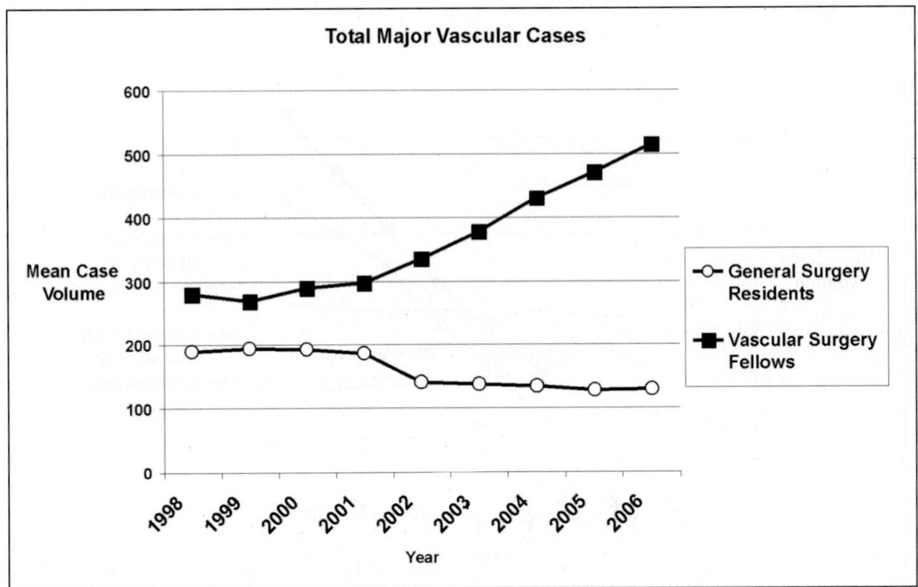

Figure 1-1. Trends in the mean number of major vascular procedures performed by vascular surgery fellows (VSF) and general surgery residents (GSR). (Data acquired from the ACGME at www.acgme.org)

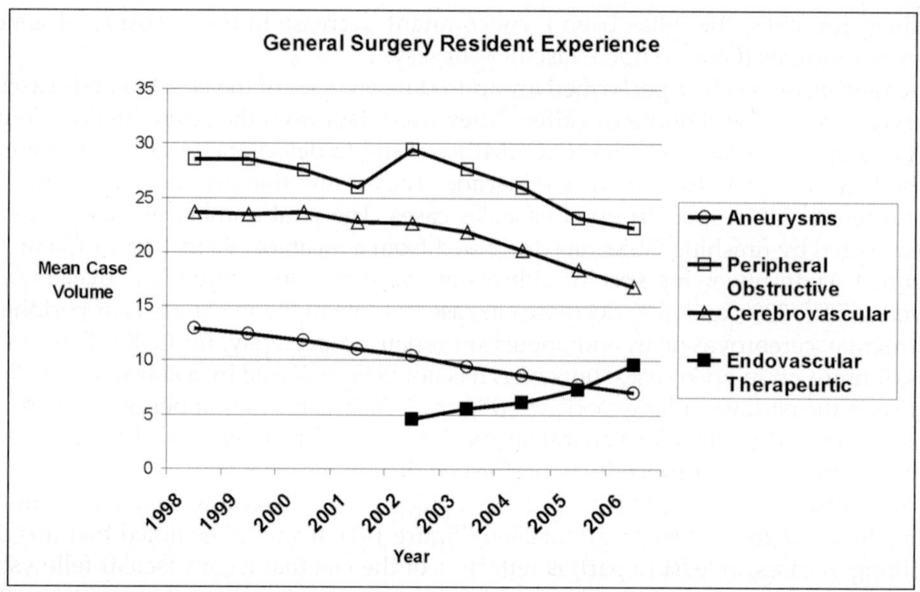

Figure 1-2. Mean number of cases performed by general surgery residents by year in the major vascular categories listed. (Data acquired from the ACGME at www.acgme.org)

Many groups have looked specifically at AAA repair and its impact on the training of both VSFs as well as GSRs. At Emory, with the adoption of EVAR, there was an overall increase in the total number of AAA procedures performed per year that had a positive impact on the total VSF caseload.[6] Subgroup analysis of the open repairs

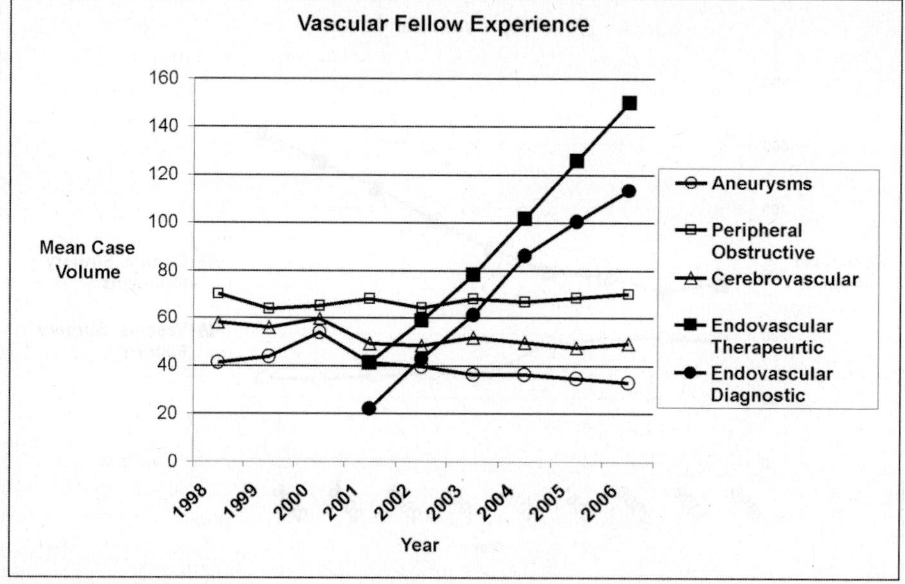

Figure 1-3. Mean number of cases performed by general surgery residents by year in the major vascular categories listed. (Data acquired from the ACGME at www.acgme.org)

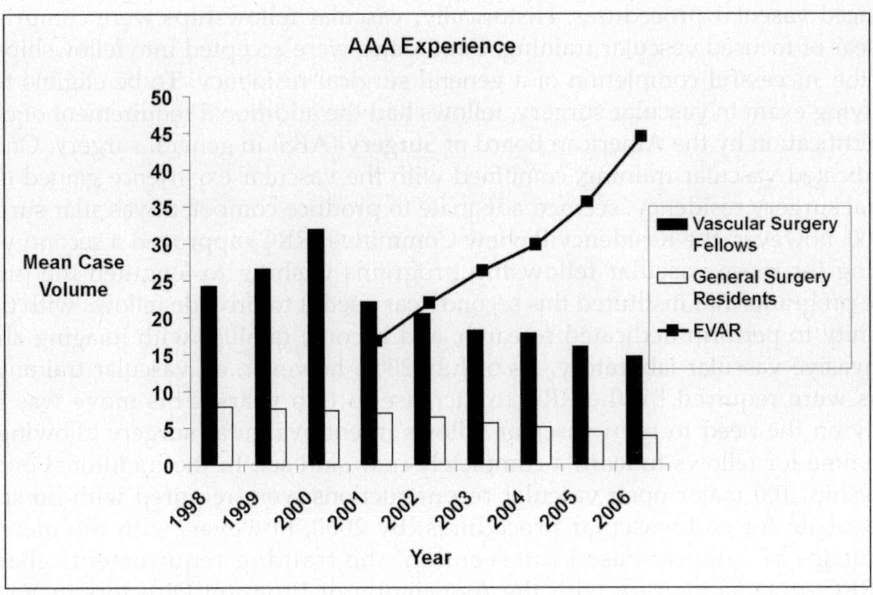

Figure 1-4. Bars represent the mean number of open AAA repairs performed by VSFs and GSRs. Line graph depicts EVARs performed by VSFs.

revealed that fellows were continuing to perform complex AAA repairs in the post-EVAR era without a significant reduction in volume. Infrarenal AAA experience, however, dropped significantly after introduction of EVAR with an annual mean pre-EVAR case volume of 40 versus post-EVAR of 19. The authors concluded that despite a decline in open volume, the higher number of total patients treated with the introduction of EVAR enhanced familiarity with the disease process. In this same study, evaluation of the GSR experience with AAA from 1993–2001 showed a 50% reduction in the number of open repairs, from eight to four. This trend had also been identified at the Ochsner Clinic in New Orleans as well as Washington University in St. Louis, both very active academic vascular centers, where GSRs experienced significant reductions in their exposure to open AAA repairs with the increasing use of EVAR.[7,8] Using the ACGME data collection system (www.ACGME.org), the national trend in AAA experience for both VSFs and GSRs is illustrated in Figure 1–4. On a national level, there is a decreasing number of open AAA repairs performed by VSFs and GSRs, but alternatively, VSFs are exposed to an increasing volume of EVARs. This diminished exposure of VSFs to open procedures could impact the comfort level of these surgeons in performing open repair of complex aneurysms in the future.

HISTORY OF TRAINING VASCULAR SURGEONS

There is value in understanding the history of training in vascular surgery. For many years, the predominance of vascular surgery in this country was performed by general or cardiac surgeons. In fact, the very first vascular fellowship in the United States was not begun until 1982. Until the early 1990s, fellowship training in vascular surgery was infrequent, and those who completed training performed the more advanced vascular procedures. Historically, vascular fellowships were comprised of one year of focused vascular training. Candidates were accepted into fellowships only after the successful completion of a general surgical residency. To be eligible for the qualifying exam in vascular surgery, fellows had the additional requirement of obtaining certification by the American Board of Surgery (ABS) in general surgery. One year of dedicated vascular training, combined with the vascular experience gained during general surgery residency, seemed adequate to produce competent vascular surgeons. In 2000, however, the Residency Review Committee (RRC) approved a second year of training for those vascular fellowship programs wishing to lengthen the process. Those programs that instituted this second year used it to provide fellows with the opportunity to perform dedicated research, and become familiar with imaging and the noninvasive vascular laboratory. As of July 2006, however, all vascular training programs were required by the RRC to increase to two years. This move was based largely on the need to train vascular fellows in endovascular surgery allowing adequate time for fellows to learn a completely new skill set. In the traditional one-year fellowship, 100 major open vascular reconstructions were required with no specific prerequisite for endovascular procedures. By 2000, however, with the increasing prevalence of catheter-based intervention, the training requirements changed. The RRC, in collaboration with the Association of Program Directors in Vascular Surgery (APDVS) and the Vascular Surgery Board (VSB) of the ABS, established new standards for vascular competency. Credentialing recommendations were formulated based on the American Heart Association's (AHA) 1992 multidisciplinary document that set forth the requisite numbers of endovascular interventions for nonsurgical interventionalist training.[9] Today's vascular residents must, therefore, perform a minimum of 100 diagnostic arteriograms, 50 endovascular interventions, and an additional five EVARs. In parallel with these changes in training, there has been a dramatic expansion of the number of vascular fellowships. From 1983 to 2007, the number of vascular fellowship programs in this country has gone from one to 92 with 119 available positions.

Training in vascular surgery has again changed dramatically with the recent approval of a primary certificate in vascular surgery. The primary certificate allows trainees the opportunity to complete vascular surgery training without prior certification in general surgery. There are four types of training programs now available.[10] First is the standard program that consists of two years of vascular training after the completion of a five-year general surgery program. The second pathway is referred to as the Early Specialization Project (ESP), which is a "4+2" model. Residents skip the chief residency year in general surgery and move directly to a two-year vascular fellowship. Trainees completing this paradigm can sit for both the general surgery and vascular surgery boards. An additional pathway requires six years of training divided into three years of general surgery plus three years of vascular surgery. This system is similar to the current plastic surgery training model. Finally, an integrated program is now available that consists of a "2+3" arrangement whereby a resident completes two years of core general surgery training before shifting to a focused three-year vascular surgery curriculum . It is too early to tell how these new training models will impact vascular education. It is anticipated that by exposing trainees to vascular surgery at an earlier point, they will gain greater exposure to open vascular techniques as well as a versatile armamentarium of endovascular skills.

HOW SHOULD FUTURE TRAINING PROGRAMS IN GENERAL AND VASCULAR SURGERY BE CONSTRUCTED?

The substantial decrease in the number of available open vascular procedures has raised questions as to whether GSRs or VSFs should have priority. There still remain institutions without vascular fellows where general surgeons have a robust exposure to open vascular procedures. Moreover, there are other institutions with vascular fellowships where the open case numbers are high. However, the number of these programs is rapidly decreasing. As the exposure of general as well as vascular surgical residents to open procedures continues to diminish, many important questions will need to be addressed. The first is whether residents finishing a general surgical training program are qualified to practice vascular surgery in the community. Statistics from the American Board of Surgery show that currently finishing general surgical residents perform on average five vascular cases per year, suggesting that vascular surgery is no longer a dominant part of a general surgeons practice.[5] Impediments that will increasingly mitigate against finishing general surgeons performing vascular surgery include:

1. *Lack of endovascular skills*—The GSR training data were clear in illustrating that general surgical residents will be deficient in this skill set. Even certified vascular surgeons who are not fully endocompetent are finding it difficult to compete with other specialists for patients with vascular disease.
2. *The increasing complexity of open cases*—General surgeons in the past performed "routine" infrarenal AAA repair, fem-pop bypasses, or straightforward carotid endarterectomies. Over time, these open procedures will be replaced with pararenal aneurysm repairs, complex lower extremity revascularizations, and challenging open carotid interventions.
3. *The high cost of malpractice insurance*—In most states the cost of malpractice insurance is substantially greater for vascular surgeons versus general surgeons making it difficult for general surgeons to justify this additional cost unless a substantial portion of their practice is vascular.

Even though it is increasingly unlikely that a large number of finishing GSRs will practice vascular surgery, GSRs can still gain tremendously by being exposed to vascular procedures, both open and endovascular. Arguments in favor of continuing this exposure include: a) gaining technical expertise, b) exposure to complex anatomy, c) experience in control of major arteries and veins, and d) knowledge of remote access to arteries that may translate into valuable skills that can be applied to other areas of general surgery.

Although exposure to vascular procedures will be of substantial benefit to GSRs, it is most important that vascular fellows who will be the future vascular surgeons, leave training with a broad understanding of open vascular surgery. There are, perhaps, a number of mechanisms that can be adopted that will allow excellent training of vascular fellows coupled with exposure of GSRs to vascular cases.

1. Vascular fellows should be given priority to scrub on increasingly scarce open cases.
2. GSRs could be encouraged to double-scrub and participate in these cases with VSFs. In complex open cases, there is usually more than one anastamosis to be

constructed, more than one anatomic site to be dissected, and a great amount to be learned through participation. Thus, sharing of these increasingly rare open cases should be encouraged.

3. There should be an increasing emphasis on teaching open vascular surgical techniques through simulation, which will benefit both vascular and general surgical residents.[11]

4. GSRs should be exposed, even during their early years, to catheter-based interventions. Through this exposure, residents will gain experience with remote access and minimally invasive surgery. This might be accomplished by adding an endovascular case requirement to the curriculum for GSRs. As a side product, this exposure may increase the number of general surgical residents interested in developing a career in vascular surgery.

5. General surgical residents should still be fully exposed to vascular procedures commonly performed by community general surgeons including AV access and amputation.

WHO SHOULD BE PERFORMING COMPLEX OPEN VASCULAR RECONSTRUCTIONS IN THE FUTURE?

It seems inevitable that as open surgery becomes more infrequent and yet the cases become more complex, patients will be directed to centers of excellence (COE). There is no dispute that institutions that perform a specific type of procedure in high volume achieve better results.[12] At present, however, there is no designation of a center of excellence in vascular disease. Probably the most well-known endeavor to identify centers of excellence was started in 1998 by the Leapfrog Group, which is a conglomeration of over 150 large U.S. health care purchasers representing over 40 million people in the United States. The impetus for the creation of the Leapfrog Group was to champion change in the delivery of health care through evidence-based referral and subsequent identification of COE. Hospitals were motivated to meet standards in five invasive surgical procedures that would bring to their institutions public respect and higher reimbursement premiums for both the hospital and the physicians. Elective AAA repair was one of the procedures chosen by the group, and as of 2003, the revised Leapfrog criteria for AAA repair called for a hospital volume requirement of 50 cases per year with the stipulation that 80% of eligible patients receive beta blockers postoperatively.[13] Although the Leapfrog initiative stimulates hospitals to strive for excellence, it has fallen short in terms of changing the paradigm of aneurysm surgery. First, the Leapfrog criteria does not account for surgeon volume as opposed to hospital volume. In the landmark paper by Birkmeyer et. al., the data confirm the inverse relationship between hospital volume and procedure related mortality.[14] However, they also show that this effect can be explained because patients at high volume hospitals are likely to be treated by high volume surgeons. Second, Leapfrog criteria do not make a distinction among the *types* of surgeons performing the procedure. It has been shown that vascular surgeons, in contrast to cardiac and general surgeons, have better outcomes for AAA repairs.[15] Finally, the type of aneurysm repair has not been included in the criteria, and as was stated above, open AAA repairs are not all equal and are gradually becoming more challenging. Therefore, a distinction should be made between uncomplicated infrarenal open AAA repairs and AAA repairs with more complexity when determining a pattern of referral. We believe that the future centers of excellence for AAA or any complex open vascular procedure will employ surgeons with high volume experience and outstanding outcomes for these procedures.

CONCLUSION

It is clear that the field of vascular surgery is currently undergoing a metamorphosis. Having now become endocompetent, vascular surgeons are able to function as complete vascular specialists, providing all levels of care to patients. It is critically important, however, that vascular surgeons maintain a high level of competence with open vascular procedures as it is these skills that continue to define vascular surgery as a distinct specialty compared to other interventionalists that perform just catheter-based intervention. Although it has been estimated that 80–90% of vascular interventions in 10 years will be catheter-based, there will continue to be a need for traditional open vascular surgery. As open cases increase in complexity and also become increasingly rare, it will be necessary that the first priority for training be given to surgeons who specialize in vascular intervention. Even then, it is not clear that there will be a sufficient number of cases to train all vascular surgeons to take on the most complex of open vascular interventions. It may then be incumbent on us to encourage the referral of complex cases to vascular centers of excellence where surgeons maintain expertise in a given complex procedure. The future of general and vascular surgical training is clearly in flux. However, one certainty is that with the evolution of all of surgery, the way we train in the future will not likely resemble the past.

REFERENCES

1. Parodi JC, Palmaz JC, Barone HD. Transfemoral intraluminal graft implantation for abdominal aortic aneurysms. *Ann Vasc Surg*. 1991;5(6):491–9.
2. Zarins CK, White RA, Schwarten D, et al. AneuRx stent graft versus open surgical repair of abdominal aortic aneurysms: multicenter prospective clinical trial. *J Vasc Surg*. 1999;29(2): 292–305; discussion 306–8.
3. Matsumura JS, Brewster DC, Makaroun MS, Naftel DC. A multicenter controlled clinical trial of open versus endovascular treatment of abdominal aortic aneurysm. *J Vasc Surg*. 2003;37(2):262–71.
4. Costin JA, Watson DR, Duff SB, et al. Evaluation of the complexity of open abdominal aneurysm repair in the era of endovascular stent grafting. *J Vasc Surg*. 2006;43(5):915–20; discussion 920.
5. Grabo DJ, Dimuzio PJ, Kairys JC, et al. Have Endovascular Procedures Negatively Impacted General Surgery Training? *Ann Surg*. 2007;246(3).
6. Lin PH, Bush RL, Milas M, et al. Impact of an endovascular program on the operative experience of abdominal aortic aneurysm in vascular fellowship and general surgery residency. *Am J Surg*. 2003;186(2):189–93.
7. Sternbergh WC 3rd, York JW, Conners MS 3rd, Money SR. Trends in aortic aneurysm surgical training for general and vascular surgery residents in the era of endovascular abdominal aortic aneurysm repair. *J Vasc Surg*. 2002;36(4):685–9.
8. Choi ET, Wyble CW, Rubin BG, et al. Evolution of vascular fellowship training in the new era of endovascular techniques. *J Vasc Surg*. 2001;33(2 Suppl):S106–10.
9. Johnson CM, Hodgson KJ. Advanced endovascular training for vascular residents: what more do we need? *Semin Vasc Surg*. 2006;19(4):194–9.

10. Goldstone J, Wong V. New training paradigms and program requirements. *Semin Vasc Surg*. 2006;19(4):168–71.
11. Chaer RA, Derubertis BG, Lin SC, et al. Simulation improves resident performance in catheter-based intervention: results of a randomized, controlled study. *Ann Surg*. 2006; 244(3):343–52.
12. Birkmeyer JD, Siewers AE, Finlayson EV, et al. Hospital volume and surgical mortality in the United States. *N Engl J Med*. 2002;346(15):1128–37.
13. Birkmeyer JD, Dimick JB. Potential benefits of the new Leapfrog standards: effect of process and outcomes measures. *Surgery*. 2004;135(6):569–75.
14. Birkmeyer JD, Stukel TA, Siewers AE, et al. Surgeon volume and operative mortality in the United States. *N Engl J Med*. 2003;349(22):2117–27.
15. Dimick JB, Cowan JA, Jr., Stanley JC, et al. Surgeon specialty and provider volumes are related to outcome of intact abdominal aortic aneurysm repair in the United States. *J Vasc Surg*. 2003;38(4):739–44.

2

How to Train Surgeons in Open Procedures in the Era of Endovascular Surgery

Christopher M. Chambers, M.D., Ph.D.
Gregorio A. Sicard, M.D.

The last 50 years has brought dramatic change to the field of vascular surgery. Prior to the maturity into its own specialty, vascular surgery was performed by general and cardiovascular surgeons. As surgeons began to limit their practice to those patients with arterial and venous disease, the development of vascular surgery specialty training followed, and in 1982, the first vascular surgery certificate was awarded by the American Board of Surgery. Since then, vascular surgery, as a specialty, has evolved to include multiple complex open and endovascular treatment options. As a consequence of the increased complexity and in an attempt to adapt to new educational challenges, vascular surgery training paradigms have recently undergone significant modification, culminating in the approval by the Accreditation Council for Graduate Medical Education (ACGME) in February 2006 of the primary certificate in vascular surgery. Historically, training in vascular surgery was obtained through an additional one or two years after successful completion of a five-year general surgery residency. Because of the increasing educational demand associated with the increase of endovascular and decrease of open procedures, two-year training programs were approved in 2000. And as of July 1, 2007, the Surgery Residency Review Committee (RRC-S) will *only* accredit two-year vascular surgery training programs. Currently, there are four potential options to become board eligible in vascular surgery. Two options that also allow for general surgery board eligibility include the traditional two years of training after five years of general surgery (5+2), or the early specialization program that incorporates two years of vascular surgery training after four years of general surgery (4+2). The early specialization program individual candidates can only be approved by the RRCs if they apply within the same surgery program and are in target to complete the minimum requirements in general surgery within the first four years. The additional options, made possible by the approval of the primary certificate in vascular surgery, include three years of general surgery training followed by three years of vascular surgery training (3+3) and an integrated five-year vascular training program, of which two years must consist of general surgery (0+5). These last two options both require matching into the program from medical school. These multiple options are a result of attempts to maximize the educational component of vascular surgery resident (VSR) training, and minimize both the service component and exposure to an operative experience with little translation to vascular surgery.

The recent changes in training will have a profound impact on the future of the specialty of vascular surgery. Besides shortening the training period to become a vascular surgeon, the new training paradigms provide two new options for medical students to enter vascular surgery training either directly from medical school or after three years of general surgery. Evaluation of the attractiveness and success of the current options will undoubtedly lead to one or two training modalities that will further define the needs of our specialty as an independent area of medicine. These changes will likely require continued modification in order to contend with the many new challenges that lie ahead, including the integration of new training paradigms into existing programs, attracting well-qualified medical school graduates, and ensuring adequate case volume of both open and endovascular procedures. One initial concern during the last several years was weather programs would be able to provide adequate experience for the development and training of endovascular skills. This concern has largely been eliminated as the endovascular surgery volume has increased and as vascular surgeons across the country have developed significant expertise in this field. In fact, one element of training that has now become an area of significant concern, especially during an era of endovascular surgery, is the development of the technical skills needed for open vascular surgery. In order to adequately train tomorrow's VSRs in *open* surgery, current validated methods of examining technical competence should be evaluated and implemented, existing and potential new technology used for simulation in open surgery should be explored and expanded, and the operative experience must be preserved.

TECHNICAL COMPETENCE

Competency of a surgeon in training is complex and difficult to objectively measure. Competency requires a broad spectrum of skills and includes patient care, medical knowledge, practice-based learning, communication skills, and professionalism. While these core competencies are assessed throughout training through written evaluations and annual examinations, technical competency due to the lack of reliable metrics is not formally evaluated. In an era of increasing public demand and the implementation of pay for performance, VSRs will likely be required to demonstrate basic technical skill in order to advance within or move beyond training. Furthermore, in an era of endovascular surgery, operating room time constraints, changing training paradigms, and increasing work hour restrictions, new efficient teaching modalities will become necessary. Currently, eligibility for the vascular surgery Qualifying Exam requires case log submission and minimum requirements in seven categories. Minimum requirements for open procedures include 30 abdominal, 25 cerebrovascular, and 45 peripheral cases. Relying on case log submission and direct observation can be subjective, and assumes that technical competence is achieved by all individuals who meet these minimum requirements.

Clearly, technical competence is variable among trainees, and a significant effort has been put forth in order to develop and validate methods of technical skill evaluation that can be used in the operating room or on various simulation models. Validation of rating scales is necessary for examination purposes, and multiple systems have been created. The Objective Structured Assessment of Technical Skill (OSATS) for surgical residents was developed by the University of Toronto and has been validated as a reliable method for testing operative skill in multiple studies.[1-3]

This method uses a Likert scale for a checklist of surgical maneuvers or surgical behaviors such as economy of motion and appropriate use of assistants. Another validated method of surgical skill assessment is the Imperial College Evaluation of Procedural Skill (ICEPS) that also uses a Likert scale, and is procedure-specific and can be used in conjunction with the OSATS scale.[4] Several studies have been done that demonstrate the improved technical skill attained through the use of simulation in multiple areas of surgery. In particular, the simulation of endovascular surgery, an area well suited for simulation training, was recently demonstrated in a randomized controlled study to improve resident performance.[5] At the same time, several studies have shown the application of simulation models specific to open vascular surgery using commercially available models. Multiple commercially available models have been created. Limbs and Things,[6] a U.K, company specializing in training and demonstration materials for health care professionals, has synthetic simulation devices for several open vascular surgery procedures. These include abdominal aortic aneurysm repair, carotid endarterectomy, femoral popliteal bypass, femorodistal anastomosis, and saphenofemoral ligation. One of the most important considerations when assessing the utility of time spent using simulation as a means of education or assessment of technical skill is whether or not the skills are able to be translated into improved operating room performance. In fact, this has been demonstrated using a synthetic simulation model of the saphenofemoral groin dissection (Limb and Things, U.K.) and compared to performance of a saphenofemoral ligation in the operating room.[7] Rating scores significantly correlated with experience for both simulation and operative procedures. Additionally, a recent study using a commercially available abdominal aortic simulator (Annexart, UK) demonstrated a significant improvement in the performance of a proximal anastomosis of an aortic aneurysm repair after an intensive training course using video assessment scores in an open aneurysm simulator.[8] In summary, various studies have validated the use of simulation for the assessment and development of technical skill of open vascular surgery procedures, and as suggested in a recent review on teaching surgical skill by Reznick et. al. published in *The New England Journal of Medicine*;[9] "Residents would thus be trained in the laboratory until preset criteria had been met and would only then be allowed to participate in the graduated performance of procedures in patients. Competence-based advancement, rather than time served or minimum number of procedures performed would become standard of surgical training."

OPERATIVE EXPERIENCE

Recent developments in vascular surgery training are the result of significant changes in the practice of modern vascular surgery. Endovascular surgery has become a significant portion of the procedures performed, and, therefore, apprehension exists regarding the ability to provide VSRs with enough exposure to complicated open procedures.

In fact, approximately 70% of all abdominal aortic aneurysms (AAA) to which surgical trainees are exposed are repaired endovascularly in the United States.[10] As a consequence, only the most complicated aortic procedures such as pararenal aortic aneurysms are repaired through an open procedure. This significant of a trend has not been seen in all countries however, which raises the possibility for training programs to increase VSRs exposure to open surgery through rotations abroad. Several years ago, we reviewed the experience of our VSRs and found that despite the decrease in infrarenal AAA repairs, total volume of open aortic procedures did not change significantly.[11] This was secondary to the increase in suprarenal aortic repairs and the sustained experience in open repair of aortoiliac occlusive disease. On the other hand, a recent review by Cronenwett examined the experience of AAA repairs performed by VSRs from 1994 to 2005 tracked by the Residency Review Committee (RRC).[10] Since 2001, the RRC has tracked both the open and endovascular AAA repairs, and from 2001 to 2005, VSRs have seen a mean decrease of 27% of open AAA repairs. This decrease, however, has not been as significant as one might predict, given the percentage of AAA repairs done endovascularly (70% in 2005) because of the dramatic increase in endovascular AAA repairs (212% increase from 2001–2005). We have recently reviewed our volume for the treatment of open infrarenal and pararenal AAA, EVAR for the last 10 years (Figure 2–1), and our infrainguinal open and endovascular experience (Figure 2–2). Our experience demonstrates a dramatic increase in EVAR and infrainguinal endovascular repairs and a decrease in open repairs, similar to the experience seen at the national level. We then examined the operative experience of different types of surgical trainees. Figure 2–3 shows the experience of the general surgery chief residents for both open AAA and EVAR, and Figure 2–4 shows the experience of the VSR during the last 10 years. Our experience matches the nationwide trend, and underscores the concern for adequate case volume and the need to develop strategies to preserve ample education in open surgery for the VSRs. One strategy to maintain an experience in open procedures is to sustain an active interest and gain national recognition in procedures that only have an open approach. We have been able to develop a unique volume for the surgical treatment of Thoracic Outlet Syndrome, increasing the exposure to open techniques for our VSRs (Figure 2–5).

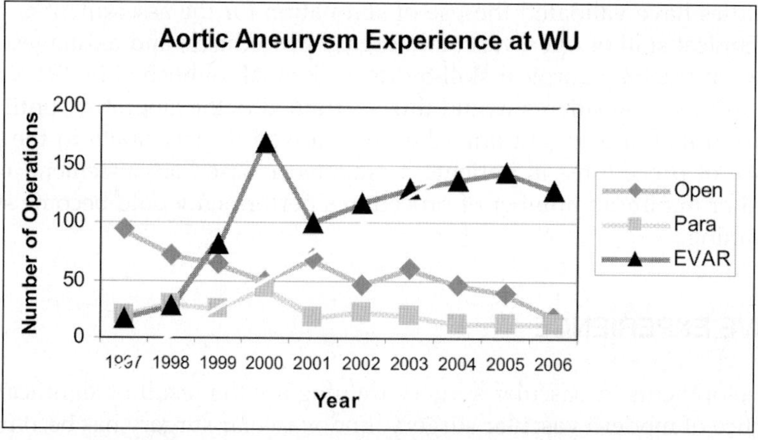

Figure 2-1. Ten-year experience for open (♦), pararenal (■), and EVAR (▲) at Washington University School of Medicine, Barnes-Jewish Hospital.

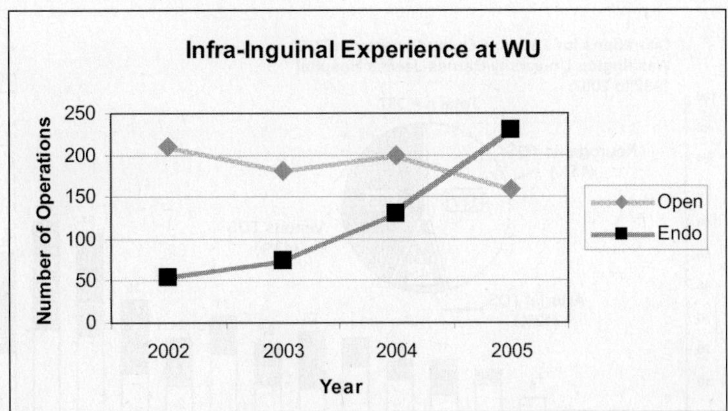

Figure 2-2. Four-year experience for open (◆) and endovascular (■) treatment of infrainguinal occlusive disease at Washington University School of Medicine, Barnes-Jewish Hospital.

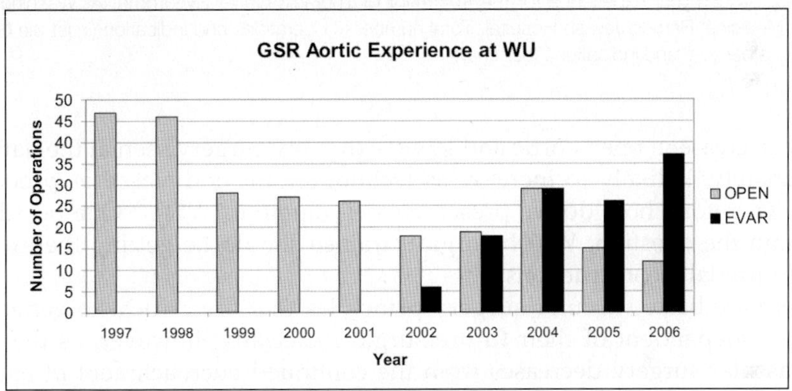

Figure 2-3. Ten-year experience for open infrarenal AAA (gray) and EVAR (black) for general surgery chief residents (GSR) at Washington University School of Medicine, Barnes-Jewish Hospital.

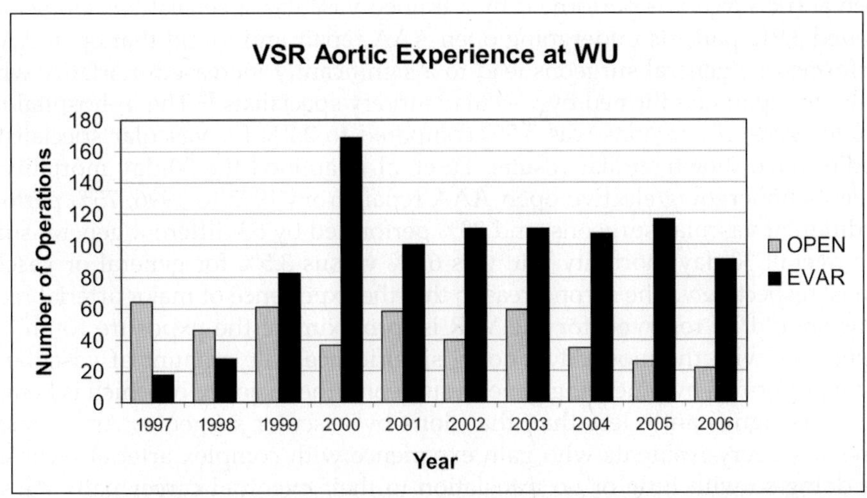

Figure 2-4. Ten-year experience for open infrarenal AAA (grey) and EVAR (black) for vascular surgery residents (VSRs) at Washington University in St. Louis School of Medicine.

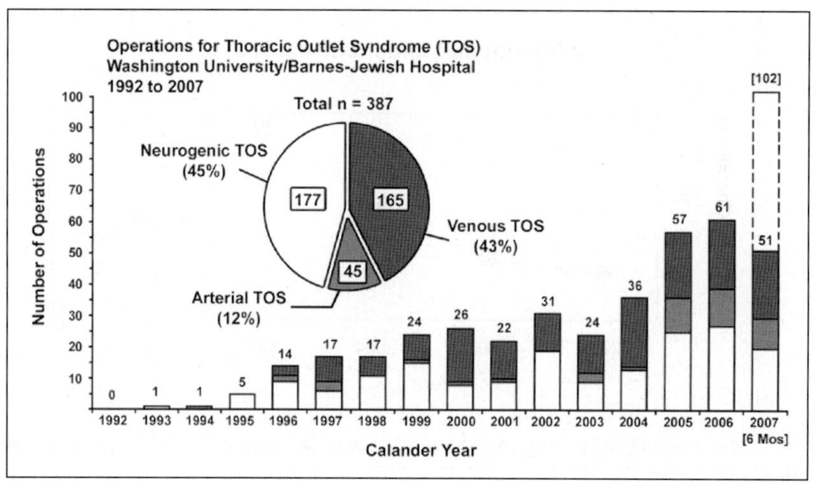

Figure 2-5. Sixteen-year experience for the treatment of Thoracic Outlet Syndrome. At Washington University School of Medicine, Barnes-Jewish Hospital. Total number of operations and indication (inset pie chart). Number of operations per year and indications (bar chart).

The decrease in open aortic and lower extremity surgery seen at the national level, unfortunately, is likely to increase as technology for endovascular procedures advances. Therefore, how do we preserve case volume for VSRs? One possible answer lies within the question, Which surgical trainee should be getting the experience of complex arterial reconstructions?

There are basic vascular surgery principles that are critical to general surgery training, independent of their future surgical specialty; however, as the amount of open vascular surgery decreases from the continued encroachment of endovascular surgery, vascular surgery programs must preserve the experience of complex arterial reconstructions for the VSR. There are two reasons why this should be done. First and foremost, studies have shown that patients' mortality is significantly improved when open aortic surgery is performed by a trained vascular specialist.[12,13] Dimick et. al. reviewed 3,912 patients undergoing open AAA repair and found that open AAA repair performed by general surgeons lead to a significantly increased mortality when compared to repairs performed by vascular surgery specialists.[12] The in-hospital mortality rate for general surgeons was 5.5% compared to 2.2% for vascular specialists. Other studies have shown similar results. Tu et. al. examined the 30-day mortality of 5,878 patients undergoing elective open AAA repair from 1992 to 1996, 75% performed by 63 different vascular surgeons, and 20% performed by 53 different general surgeons.[13] The overall 30-day mortality rate was 6.2% versus 3.5% for general or vascular surgeons, respectively. The second reason that the experience of major arterial reconstructions should be reserved for the VSR is to maximize the exposure to an operative experience with the most educational significance. The amount of vascular surgery being performed by practicing general surgeons, the majority of which is hemodialysis access, is significantly less than that done by vascular surgeons. As a consequence, general surgery residents who gain experience with complex arterial reconstructions are doing so with little or no translation to their eventual career path. As such, decreasing the number of complex arterial reconstructions performed by general surgery trainees does not negatively impact their experience as has been suggested.[14] Taken together, general surgery training should not include an experience with complex aortic reconstruction in the presence of an available VSR in order to maximize the educational experience, especially since this will translate into decreased patient mortality.

CONCLUSIONS

The practice of vascular surgery has undergone dramatic changes over the last several years following the FDA approval of the first endovascular aortic endograft and subsequent widespread application of this technique for the repair of aortic aneurysms. As a result, the training of vascular surgeons has also had to undergo changes in order to maintain an adequate training environment. We have now moved into the endovascular era, and as a result, the numbers of open vascular surgery procedures have decreased. Despite these decreases in open vascular procedures, vascular surgery training programs must find a way to continue to develop surgeons competent in complex open vascular reconstructions. This will be accomplished by reserving the experience of these complex arterial reconstruction cases for the training VSR, fostering potential rotations abroad in locations that use EVAR less commonly, utilizing currently available and validated simulation techniques, and considering the addition of technical skill assessment in addition to current written and oral examinations for career advancement.

REFERENCES

1. Martin JA, Regehr G, Reznick R et al. Objective structured assessment of technical skill (OSATS) for surgical residents. *Br J Surg*. 1997;84:273–278.
2. Reznick RK, Regehr G, MacRae H et al. Testing technical skills outside the operating room: an innovative bench model examination. *Am J Surg*. 1997;173:226–230
3. Anastakis DJ, Regehr G, Reznick RK et al. Assessment of technical skills transfer from the bench training model to the human model. *Am J Surg*. 1999;177:167–170.
4. Pandey V, Wolfe JHN, Moorthy K et al. Technical skills continue to improve beyond surgical training. *J Vasc Surg*. 2006; 43:539–545.
5. Chaer RA, DeRubertis BG, Lin SC et al. Simulation improves resident performance in catheter-based intervention. *Ann Surg*. 2006; 244:343–352.
6. Limbs & Things - Medical Training Models - Medical Simulation Models. Available at www.limbsandthings.com. Accessed August, 2007.
7. Datta V, Simon B, Beard J et al. Comparison of bench test evaluations of surgical skill with live operating performance assessments. *J Am Coll Surg*. 2004;199:603–606.
8. Pandey VA, Black AM, Lazaris JR et al. Do workshops improve the technical skill of vascular surgical trainees? *E J Vasc Endovasc Surg*. 2005;30:441–447.
9. Reznick RK, MacRae H. Teaching surgical skills-changes in the wind. *N Eng J Med*. 2006;355:2664–2669.
10. Cronenwett JL. Vascular surgery training: is there enough case material? *Semin Vasc Surg*. 2006;19:187–190.
11. Choi ET, Wyble CW, Rubin BG et al. Evolution of vascular fellowship training in the new era of endovascular techniques. *J Vasc Surg*. 2001;33:S106–S110.
12. Dimick JB, Cowan JA, Stanley JC et al. Surgeon specialty and provider volumes are related to outcome of intact abdominal aortic aneurysm repair in the United States. *J Vasc Surg*. 2003;38:739–744.

13. Tu JV, Austin PC, Johnston KW. The influence of surgical specialty training on the outcomes of elective abdominal aortic aneurysm surgery. *J Vasc Surg*. 2001;33:447–452
14. Grabo DJ, DiMuzio PJ, Kairys JC et al. Have endovascular procedures negatively impacted general surgery training? Presented at American Surgical Association, 128th Annual Meeting, Colorado Springs, Colorado, April 26–28, 2007.

3

Hospital Volume and Operative Mortality with Abdominal Aortic Aneurysm Repair in the Endovascular Era

Justin B. Dimick, M.D., M.P.H., John A. Cowan, Jr., M.D., and Gilbert R. Upchurch, Jr., M.D.

Elective abdominal aortic aneurysm repair is often the focus of quality assessment and improvement activities.[1] In part, the interest in this operation comes from the simple fact that it is both common and high risk. Thus, ensuring optimal outcomes would avoid many preventable deaths each year in the United States.[2] Much of the enthusiasm also comes from the large body of evidence showing variations in mortality rates between high and low volume hospitals for this operation.

Despite continued emphasis on volume as a proxy for quality with aortic surgery, most of the evidence linking hospital and surgeon volume to outcomes is outdated. In particular, no study has addressed the impact of volume on outcome since the introduction of endovascular approaches to the management of aortic disease. In the present paper, we will first review the extensive body of evidence linking volume to outcome for open abdominal aortic aneurysm (AAA) repair. Finally, new national data showing the relationship of hospital volume on mortality rates after the introduction of endovascular repair will be examined.

REVIEW OF EXISTING LITERATURE

Two recent structured literature reviews provide a comprehensive picture of the large body of evidence linking volume to outcome.[3,4] In the first review, Dudley and colleagues identified all studies published over a 10-year period (1988 and 1998) investigating hospital volume and mortality for numerous surgical and medical conditions.[3] After excluding poor quality studies, 72 articles addressing 40 different procedures and diagnoses were identified. For elective open AAA repair, there were a total of nine studies that all showed a statistically significant difference in mortality between high and low volume hospitals. Based on the highest quality evidence available, the authors estimated that low volume hospitals have a 64% higher mortality compared to higher volume hospitals (Odds Ratio, 1.64; 95% CI, 1.18-2.27).[3]

In the second review, Halm and colleagues identified volume outcome studies published over a 20-year period (1980–2000)[4]. Of 272 studies reviewed, 135 met the inclusion criteria that were based largely on methodological rigor of the studies. In general, the results were similar to the previous review, with most studies showing a strong positive effect of increasing volume on improved mortality. Specifically for open AAA repair, seven of eight studies showed a statistically significant difference in mortality between high and low volume hospitals.[4] The threshold defining high volume varied across the studies from five cases per year to 50 cases per year with a median of 20 cases per year. In addition, this review included the magnitude of the effect (differences in mortality between high and low volume hospitals), which varied depending on the procedure. The median overall mortality rate for open AAA repair in these studies was 7.5% (range 3.8% to 7.6%), and the median absolute difference between the highest and lowest volume hospitals was 3.3% (range 1.1% to 11.6%).

Although these reviews provide a balanced overview of the existing literature, it is worth considering one individual study in more detail. In the largest and most comprehensive volume outcome study, Birkmeyer and colleagues evaluated 14 high-risk operations in the national Medicare population.[5] Consistent with the reviews cited above, they found a significant effect of volume on outcome for elective open AAA repair. The highest volume hospitals (>79 cases per year) had mortality rates of 3.9% compared to 6.5% at the lowest volume hospitals (<17 cases per year). The strength of the relationship between hospital volume and mortality for elective open AAA repair was larger than some operations (e.g., carotid endarterectomy), but much smaller than that for high-risk cancer operations (e.g., pancreatic and esophageal resection).

Largely because hospital volume is more easily determined, many previous studies have not considered the role of individual surgeon volume. In the review by Halm and colleagues, a much shorter list of studies investigated the impact of surgeon volume. For those operations where surgeon volume was considered, most also showed a significant effect on mortality.[4] Few of these studies, however, had sufficient sample size or used appropriate multilevel modeling methods to determine the relative impact of hospital and surgeon volume in contributing to low operative mortality.

In a subsequent study using the national Medicare population from 1998–1999, Birkmeyer and colleagues overcame many of the limitations of previous studies of surgeon volume and outcomes. The authors found that surgeon volume was a strong independent predictor of operative mortality for elective open AAA repair.[6] The authors were also able to estimate the relative importance of surgeon and hospital volume on determining operative mortality. For open abdominal aortic aneurysm repair, hospital volume accounts for almost half of the surgeon volume effect. In contrast, hospital volume accounted for none of the surgeon volume effect for carotid endarterectomy. This finding has strong face validity since carotid endarterectomy requires few resources beyond the skill of the individual surgeon. In contrast, AAA repair requires optimal functioning of a broad range of resources (e.g., anesthesia staff and intensive care units).

In summary, the existing literature shows a consistent inverse relationship between provider experience and operative mortality for elective open AAA repair. Almost every study revealed a statistically significant association between volume and mortality. However, most of these studies were conducted in the 1990s, well before endovascular approaches were widespread.

METHODS FOR THE UPDATED ANALYSIS

We used a nationally representative database—the Nationwide Inpatient Sample—to investigate the relationship of hospital volume to outcome in the contemporary era (2001–2003). This dataset is a stratified, random sample of 20% of the hospitals in the United States. Using analysis techniques designed for complex sampling, national estimates of outcomes and utilization can be obtained. We used the appropriate procedure and diagnostic codes to identify all patients in the dataset who underwent either open or endovascular AAA repair during 2001 to 2003. Patients with an International Classification of Diseases, Ninth Revision, Clinical Modification (ICD-9-CM) primary procedure code for resection of abdominal aorta with replacement (ICD-9-CM 38.44), endovascular implantation of a graft in the abdominal aorta (ICD-9-CM 39.71), or aortoiliac bypass (ICD-9-CM 39.25) were initially selected. We then selected those patients who also had a primary diagnostic code for AAA without mention of rupture (ICD-9-CM 441.4) for inclusion in the data sample. We excluded patients with a diagnostic code for ruptured AAA (ICD-9-CM 441.3).

We first studied the change in marketshare occupied by endovascular repair. We then examined the impact of hospital volume on outcome for overall AAA repair, and then stratified by the type of repair (open and endovascular). Our primary outcome was in-hospital mortality (death prior to hospital discharge). We calculated the annual hospital volume for each hospital during each year of the three-year study period. For the present analyses, we converted the volume variable into a categorical variable by creating five equal size patient groups (quintiles) for each volume measure (total, open, and endovascular volume). Risk-adjusted analysis was performed, accounting for differences in baseline patient characteristics using logistic regression. All statistical analyses were performed using STATA version 8.0 (Stata Corp, College Station, Texas).

TRENDS IN THE USE OF ENDOVASCULAR REPAIR

Using the national dataset, we estimate that 158,800 abdominal aortic aneurysm repairs were performed in the United States during the three year period 2001-2003 (sample size from the NIS = 32,543 patients with an average discharge weight of 4.88). Of the total repairs performed, 44,800 (27%) had the endovascular approach and 114,000 (73%) had the conventional open approach. Patients undergoing endovascular repair were older, more likely to be male, and less likely to be of nonwhite races (Table 3–1). Although most admissions for both types of repair were elective, patients undergoing endovascular repair were less likely to be admitted in an urgent or emergent fashion (Table 3–1).

Over the study period, endovascular repair assumed a larger proportion of the marketshare (from 23% to 33% of total repairs, $P<.001$). The increase in use of the endovascular approach was much greater among older patients compared to younger patients (Figure 3–1). For patients greater than 80 years old, the use of an endovascular repair increased from 37% to 54% from 2001–2003 ($P<.001$). In contrast, for patients younger than 65, the increase was only from 12% to 15% of total repairs ($P<.001$).

TABLE 3-1. CHARACTERISTICS OF PATIENTS UNDERGOING OPEN AND ENDOVASCULAR REPAIR OF ABDOMINAL AORTIC ANEURYSM FROM 2001-2003.

Characteristic	Open (N=23,573)	Endovascular (N=8,962)	P-value
Patient age, mean (SD)	68 (10.5)	73 (8.2)	<.001
Age greater than 80 years	2,109 (9.0%)	1,760 (10.0%)	<.001
Female gender	7,434 (31%)	1,455 (16%)	<.001
Nonwhite race	2,187 (13%)	649 (10%)	<.001
Urgent admission	2,158 (10%)	478 (6%)	<.001
Emergent admission	2,175 (10%)	407 (5%)	<.001

SD = Standard Deviation

Higher volume hospitals (based on total AAA repair volume) were much more likely to use the endovascular approach than lower volume hospitals (Figure 3–2). The highest volume hospitals (>58 per year) employed the endovascular approach 39% of the time compared to only 14% at the lowest volume hospitals (<9 per year). There was a strong correlation between total volume and both open volume (Spearman's rho = 0.88, P<.001) and endovascular volume (Spearman's rho = 0.71, P<.001). Most high and very high volume hospitals for total volume were also high or very high for both endovascular and open volume (Table 3–2).

MORTALITY RATES FOR OPEN AND ENDOVASCULAR REPAIR

Endovascular repair was associated with a much lower in-hospital mortality rate compared to open repair (4.4% vs. 1.2%, P<.001). This finding is particularly striking given the higher average age among patients undergoing endovascular repair. Older

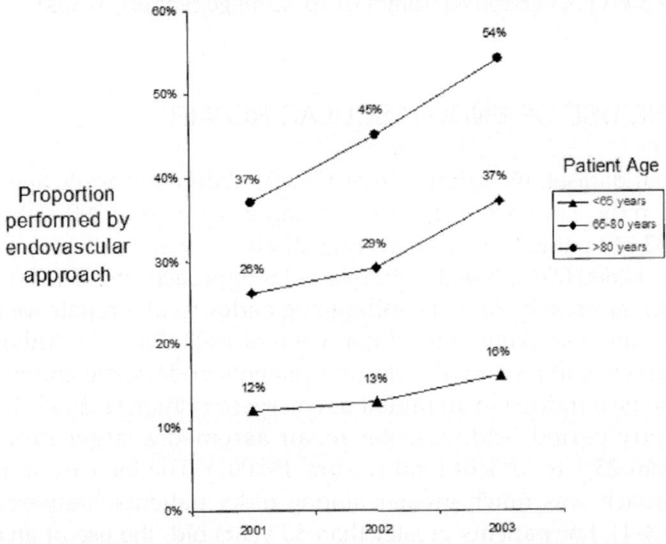

Figure 3-1. Increasing proportion of abdominal aortic aneurysm repairs performed by an endovascular approach (2001–2003).

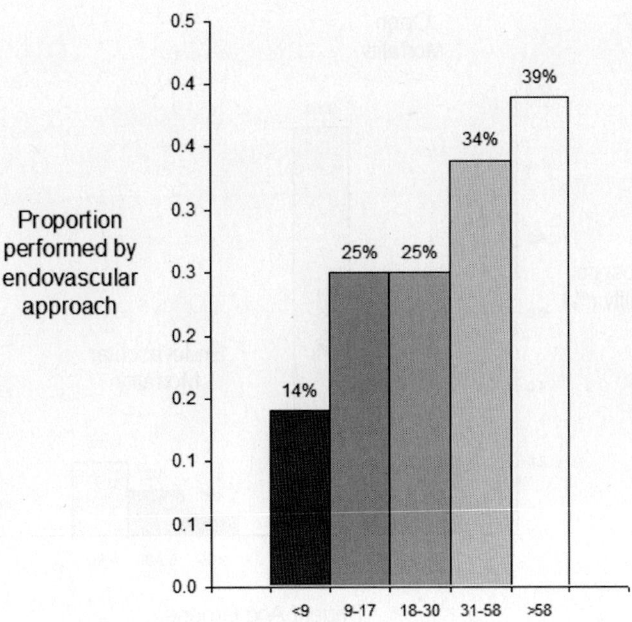

Figure 3-2. Proportion of abdominal aortic aneurysm repairs performed by an endovascular approach across total hospital volume categories (2001–2003).

TABLE 3-2. RELATIONSHIP BETWEEN TOTAL HOSPITAL VOLUME AND BOTH OPEN AND ENDOVASCULAR VOLUME

Total volume (Average annual volume)	Number of hospitals (% total hospitals)	Open Volume Quintiles	Endovascular Volume Quintiles
Very high (>58)	27 (3%)	19 very high 6 high	20 very high 4 high 1 medium
High (31-58)	53 (5%)	8 very high 29 high 12 medium 1 low	8 very high 32 high 5 medium 4 low 1 very low
Medium (18-30)	94 (9%)	18 high 59 medium 17 low 1 very low	15 high 47 medium 24 low 9 very low
Low (9-17)	185 (17%)	23 medium 121 low 34 very low	3 high 60 medium 67 low 48 very low
Very low (<9)	718 (67%)	46 low 683 very low	14 medium 133 low 582 very low

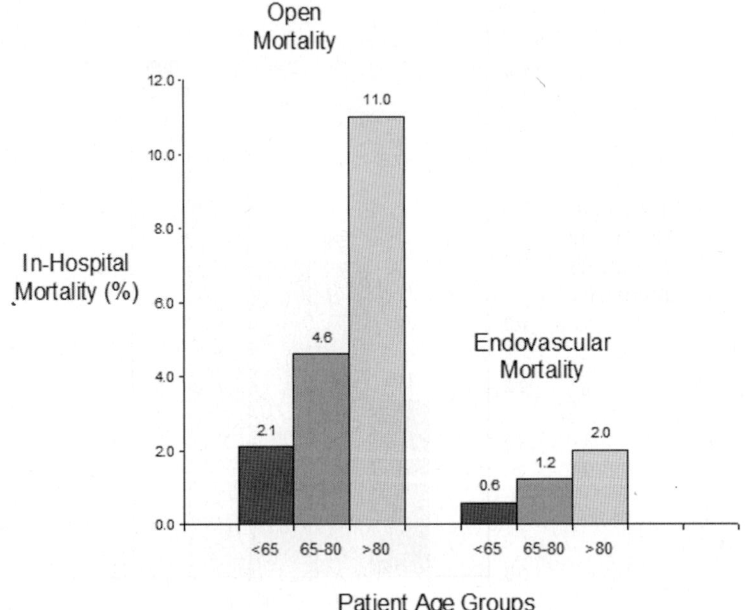

Figure 3-3. Relationship of patient age to in-hospital mortality after open and endovascular aneurysm repair.

patients had much higher in-hospital mortality compared to younger patients for both types of repair (Figure 3–3) (*P*<.001 for all comparisons). However, the difference in mortality rates in the oldest age group is much larger than other age groups (2.0% for endovascular repair vs. 11.0% for open repair, *P*<.001).

HOSPITAL VOLUME AND MORTALITY

Figure 3–4 shows the relationship of hospital volume and in-hospital mortality for three scenarios: 1) overall AAA repair mortality vs. overall AAA volume; 2) open AAA repair mortality vs. open AAA volume; and 3) endovascular AAA repair mortality vs. endovascular AAA repair volume. We found a strong inverse relationship between hospital volume and unadjusted mortality rates in all three comparisons (*P*<.001 for all volume variables). In addition, we also found that overall AAA volume was associated with both open and endovascular repair mortality rates. In other words, overall AAA mortality is a good proxy for quality of care for both types of repair.

In the risk-adjusted analysis, mortality rates were 40% higher at hospitals in the lowest quintile of total volume when considering all types of repair together (OR, 1.40; 95% CI, 1.14-1.73). A similar relationship between total volume and mortality was found when examining each approach separately: open repair (OR, 1.32; 95% CI, 1.06-1.32) and endovascular repair (OR, 2.55; 95% CI, 1.31-4.97). The relationship between operation-specific volume and mortality was similar to that observed for total volume with both approaches.

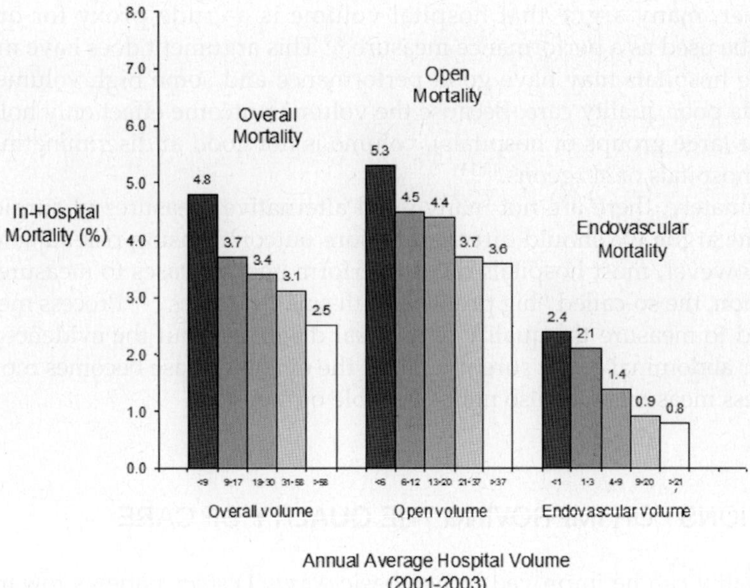

Figure 3-4. Relationship of hospital volume to in-hospital mortality for abdominal aortic aneurysm repair.

COMMENTS

The endovascular approach to AAA repair continues to take up a larger marketshare in the United States. In the present study, we have shown that this change in practice has not meaningfully altered the observed impact of hospital volume on operative mortality. We examined the relationship between three volume variables (total, open, and endovascular) and found each to be related inversely to operative mortality. We also found that a hospital's overall or total abdominal aortic aneurysm repair volume is a good proxy for quality with each individual type of repair; that is, most hospitals with high total volume are also high volume for both open and endovascular repair.

Our updated analysis is important because many existing quality assessment and improvement activities use volume as a proxy for quality for open abdominal aortic surgery. In the remainder of this paper, we will discuss the advantages and disadvantages of this approach, and review existing activities in this area.

ADVANTAGES AND DISADVANTAGES OF USING VOLUME AS A QUALITY MEASURE

Using provider volume as a proxy for quality with abdominal aortic aneurysm repair has several advantages compared to other approaches.[7] First, volume is easily determined from readily available data sources. In contrast, direct outcomes measurement requires detailed clinical data for risk adjustment that is not widely available. Second, provider volume is meaningful to patients. Unlike many complex quality measures used in some hospital report cards, patients can grasp the value of "experience" with a specific procedure.

However, many argue that hospital volume is a crude proxy for quality and should not be used as a performance measure.[8,9] This argument does have merit. Some low volume hospitals may have good performance and some high volume hospitals may provide poor quality care. Because the volume-outcome effect only holds true on average (for large groups of hospitals), volume is not good at discriminating between individual hospitals or surgeons.[10,11]

Unfortunately, there are not many good alternative measures of surgical performance. Some argue we should directly measure outcomes using risk-adjusted mortality rates. However, most hospitals do not perform enough cases to measure mortality with precision, the so-called "big problem with small samples."[12] Process measures are widely used to measure the quality of medical diagnoses, but the evidence base does not exist for abdominal aortic surgery.[7] Until the evidence base becomes more mature, using process measures will also not be a viable option.

IMPLICATIONS FOR IMPROVING THE QUALITY OF CARE

Surgical quality can be improved in two basic ways: 1) steer patients toward the best hospitals, or 2) improve care in all hospitals. The observed relationship between hospital volume and mortality for abdominal aortic aneurysm repair can be used in both contexts.

Selective Referral

Many deaths could be prevented by steering patients to hospitals with low mortality rates.[1,3] Because hospital volume is readily available from administrative data, it is used as a proxy for quality in several public reporting initiatives. Using national administrative databases, a growing number of proprietary Internet sites now provide hospital volume for many operations (e.g., Healthgrades.com). In addition, the Agency for Healthcare Research and Quality (AHRQ) has included the hospital volume of several surgical procedures in their *Inpatient Quality Indicators*.[13] These quality indicators have subsequently been used by payers (e.g., Blue Cross Blue Shield in New York State) and state health organizations (e.g., Texas Inpatient Hospital Association) for public reporting of volume. However, despite the increasing availability of information on hospital volume, the public doesn't seem to be using it to help choose hospitals.[14,15] Future investigations should explore how patients choose hospitals. Specifically, they should address why patients don't use this information. Is it because they don't know about it? Or, even if they have the information, would they prefer to go to a local hospital?

Although public reporting appears to have limited impact on patients choosing hospitals, the landscape may be changing as payers get involved. Some health care payers are working to create financial incentives for patients to choose high volume hospitals. Health care payers selectively contract with providers based on the quality of care they provide (value-based purchasing). As the most visible of these efforts, the Leapfrog Group represents many large employers interested in creating incentives that result in directing more patients to the highest quality hospitals.[16] The Leapfrog Group's initial patient safety practices recommended selective referral to high volume hospitals for five procedures: coronary artery bypass grafting, percutaneous coronary interventions, esophageal resection, AAA repair, and carotid endarterectomy. Significant changes in both the included operations and the quality measures have been made since the initial release of the standards.[1] For abdominal aortic aneurysm repair, the standard includes a minimum volume requirement (more than 50 cases per year) and a new process measure, use of perioperative beta-blockade. Hospitals must demonstrate that at least 80% of patients receive beta-blockers to be fully compliant.

Quality Improvement

The applicability of information on hospital volume to quality improvement is less obvious than selective referral. Yet, we know that hospital volume in and of itself does not produce better outcomes; there are underlying processes of care that differ between high and low volume settings responsible for the differences in outcomes. If we can discover these details, we can disseminate them and improve the quality of care for all patients in need of elective AAA repair. A precedent for this type of quality improvement exists in The Northern New England Cardiovascular Disease Study Group. This group of hospitals collected data in a prospective fashion and described threefold variation in risk-adjusted mortality rates across the five hospitals performing coronary artery bypass graft surgery (range 2% to 6%), and sixfold variation among surgeons (1.6% to 10%).[17] To better understand sources of variation, these investigators conducted site visits and focused on identifying processes of care potentially related to mortality. In this way, the researchers identified numerous processes linked to lower rates of mortality. Examples include continuation of aspirin, beta-blockers, and intravenous heparin until incision in patients with unstable angina is begun; maintaining hematocrits above 24% during cardiopulmonary bypass; minimizing cross-clamp time and specific techniques related to cardioplegia, hypothermia, and intraoperative myocardial protection; and use (or avoidance) of specific inotropic medications during and after surgery. Once identified, these processes were implemented across the entire region and mortality rates dropped dramatically from 5% to under 2% by the end of the 1990s, and continue to be among the lowest in the United States.[18]

However, it is likely that some of the observed differences in mortality rates between high and low volume providers are likely due to differences in the skills of the surgeons and care team (i.e., "practice makes perfect"). Low volume providers may, therefore, never reach the same high quality as high volume providers.

SUMMARY

Our updated analysis reveals that higher hospital volume continues to be related to lower operative mortality for abdominal aortic surgery. In addition, we demonstrated that total hospital volume (the number of open and endovascular repair combined) is a reasonable proxy for mortality for both open and endovascular surgery. Because the relationship appears to persist in the current era of endovascular surgery, volume will likely continue to be an important proxy for quality with abdominal aortic surgery.

Many policy and advocacy efforts include public reporting of volume and selective referral of patients for abdominal aortic aneurysm repair. However, because of the practical limitations of regionalization, this approach has limited benefits. Importantly, we need to learn the processes of care that lead to superior outcomes at high volume centers. Discovering and disseminating these best-practices has the potential to improve care at all hospitals.

REFERENCES

1. Dimick JB, Upchurch GR Jr. The quality of care for patients with abdominal aortic aneurysms. *Cardiovasc Surg*. 2003;11:331–336.
2. Birkmeyer JD, Dimick JB. Potential benefits of the 2003 Leapfrog standards: effect of process and outcomes measures. *Surgery*. 2004;135: 569–575.
3. Dudley RA, Johansen KL, Brand R, et al. Selective referral to high-volume hospitals: estimating potentially avoidable deaths. *JAMA*. 2000;283:1159–1166.
4. Halm EA, Lee C, Chassin MR. Is volume related to outcome in health care? A systematic review and methodologic critique of the literature. *Ann Intern Med*. 2002;137:511–520.
5. Birkmeyer JD, Siewers AE, Finlayson EV, et al. Hospital volume and surgical mortality in the United States. *N Engl J Med*. 2002;346:1128–1137.
6. Birkmeyer JD, Stukel TA, Siewers AE, et al. Surgeon volume and operative mortality in the United States. *N Engl J Med*. 2003;349:2117–2127.
7. Birkmeyer JD, Dimick JB, Birkmeyer NJ. Measuring quality in surgery: structure, process, or outcomes? *J Am Coll Surg*. 2004;198:626–632.
8. Khuri SF. Invited commentary: Surgeons, not General Motors, should set standards for surgical care. *Surgery*. 2001;130:429–431.
9. Christian CK, Gustafson ML, Betensky RA, et al. The volume-outcome relationship: don't believe everything you see. *World J Surg*. 2005;29:1241–1244.
10. Rathore SS, Epstein AJ, Volpp KG, Krumholz HM. Hospital coronary artery bypass graft surgery volume and patient mortality, 1998–2000. *Ann Surg*. 2004;239:110–117.
11. Krumholz HM, Rathore SS, Chen J, et al. Evaluation of a consumer-oriented internet health care report card: the risk of quality ratings based on mortality data. *JAMA*. 2002;287:1277–1287.
12. Dimick JB, Welch HG, Birkmeyer JD. Surgical mortality as an indicator of hospital quality: the problem with small sample size. *JAMA*. 2004;292:847–851.
13. AHRQ Quality Indicators-Guide to Inpatient Quality indicators: Quality of Care in Hospitals-Volume, Mortality, and Utilization, Rockville. MD: Agency for Healthcare Research and Quality, 2002. AHRQ pub. No. 02–R0204.
14. Romano PS, Zhou H. Do well-publicized risk-adjusted outcomes reports affect hospital volume? *Med Care*. 2004;42:367–377.
15. Marshall MN, Shekelle PG, Leatherman S, Brook RH. The public release of performance data: what do we expect to gain? A review of the evidence. *JAMA*. 2000;283:1866–1874.
16. Galvin R, Milstein A. Large employers' new strategies in health care. *N Engl J Med*. 2002; 347:939–942.
17. O'Connor GT, Plume SK, Olmstead EM, et al. A regional intervention to improve the hospital mortality associated with coronary artery bypass graft surgery. The Northern New England Cardiovascular Disease Study Group. *JAMA*. 1996;275:841–846.
18. Malenka DJ, O'Connor GT. The Northern New England Cardiovascular Disease Study Group: a regional collaborative effort for continuous quality improvement in cardiovascular disease. *Jt Comm J Qual Improv*. 1998;24:594–600.

Contemporary Open Techniques For Abdominal Aortic Aneurysms

The Retroperitoneal Approach for Abdominal Aortic Surgery

R. Clement Darling, III, M.D. Philip S. K. Paty, M.D., Stephanie Saltzberg, M.D.

INTRODUCTION

The retroperitoneal approach to the abdominal aorta and its branches can be used for all types of aortic reconstruction. Retrospective and prospective studies have documented technical and physiological advantages of the retroperitoneal approach over the conventional transabdominal exposure.[1-5] When executed properly, the extended left posterolateral retroperitoneal approach can provide excellent exposure of the entire infradiaphramatic aorta. This exposure facilitates infrarenal, juxtarenal, and suprarenal aortic repairs, as well as concomitant reconstruction of the visceral, renal, and iliac arteries.[6,7]

In addition to the technical advantages, physiologic disturbances might be reduced with the retroperitoneal approach. Decreased fluid requirements, blood loss, ileus, and pulmonary complications, resulting in fewer postoperative ICU days and shorter hospital lengths of stay, have all been demonstrated.[1-5]

INDICATIONS AND CONTRAINDICATIONS

The indications for aortic and visceral artery surgical intervention via retroperitoneal approach are the same as those for transabdominal repair. It is the preferred approach in the hostile abdomen that includes patients with prior intraabdominal surgery resulting in adhesions, the presence of stomas, peritoneal dialysis, prior abdominopelvic radiation treatment, and the morbidly obese. This approach can also provide a clean dissection plane in reoperative aortic procedures and facilitate inline replacement of infected aortic grafts.[8] It is advantageous in inflammatory abdominal aortic aneurysms in which visceral organs might be adherent to the anterior aortic wall. In horseshoe kidneys, a retroperitoneal approach can avoid mobilization and division of the kidney.

At our institution, it has become the preferred method for handling symptomatic and ruptured aortic aneurysms, as well as visceral occlusive disease.[7,9]

Relative contraindications to the retroperitoneal approach include limited exposure of the right renal and iliac arterial systems as well as the inability to fully examine the intra-abdominal cavity for additional pathology at the time of surgical intervention. As we have become more experienced with the extended posterolateral left retroperitoneal approach, we have performed right renal and iliac artery reconstructions without increased risk.[7]

SURGICAL TECHNIQUES

Left Posterolateral Retroperitoneal Approach

Positioning.   After the induction of general anesthesia, the patient is placed on a suction bean bag (Olympic Vac Pac) in a modified right lateral decubitus position. The patient is positioned with the table break 5 to 10 centimeters cephalad to the left iliac crest. The patient's torso is shifted toward the left and rotated until the left shoulder is elevated 45 to 60 degrees from the horizontal position, while the pelvis is rotated 15 to 30 degrees to allow access to both groins. The left upper extremity is brought across the chest and supported by blankets, a sling, or a stand. The left thigh is elevated above the horizontal plane to relax the ipsilateral iliopsoas muscle. This maneuver improves access to the distal aorta and left iliac arteries. To open the space between the iliac crest and the costal margin, the table is flexed at the table break (Figure 4–1).

Incision.   The incision is extended from the lateral edge of the rectus muscle between the umbilicus and pubic symphysis in an oblique fashion posteriorly and superiorly through the 10th or 11th interspace to the mid- to posterior axillary line.

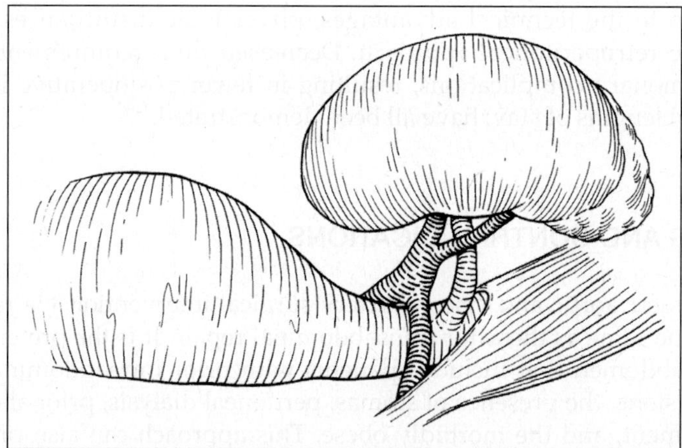

Figure 4-1. Patient in right lateral decubitus position with the table extended in reversed "V" position to open retroperitoneal space. ("With Permission" - Leather RP, Darling RC III, Chang BB, Shah DM. Retroperitoneal approach for elective abdominal aortic aneurysm. In: Ernst CB, Stanley JC, eds. Current *Therapy in Vascular Surgery*. St. Louis: Mosby-Year Book, 1995:238-41.)

The 10th interspace is employed if access to the pararenal or visceral aorta is required. The 11th interspace is adequate for infrarenal aortic reconstruction as it provides access to the infrarenal aorta, proximal right common iliac artery, and left iliac arteries.

Exposure.   The muscle layers of the lateral abdominal wall are divided to the lateral border of the rectus abdominis. This includes the external oblique, internal oblique, transversus abdominis, and transversalis fascia, respectively. The transversus abdominis is initially divided laterally and then medially to separate the peritoneum, which is usually thicker and more discrete laterally, from the underlying muscle. The intercostal muscles are divided on the superior margin of the underlying rib.

The retroperitoneal space is entered posterolaterally to avoid tearing the parietal peritoneum. The posterior peritoneum, posterior layers of Gerota's fascia, and the left kidney are retracted anteriomedially and cephalad to expose the left psoas muscle and periaortic tissue. The fascia remains intact on the psoas, which minimizes dissection-related bleeding from the iliopsoas and cutaneous and genitofemoral nerve injury. Exposure is maintained with a self-retaining retractor (Buchwalter). Care must be taken to avoid vigorous retraction of the anterior and cephalad margin of the incision as this can result in splenic or renal injury.

Distal arterial control is obtained first to prevent embolization. If there is significant involvement of the right iliac arteries, then a small suprainguinal counterincision can be performed on the right to obtain extraperitoneal exposure of these vessels. If necessary, right iliac artery control can also be obtained with a balloon occlusion catheter at the time the aneurysm is entered through the left flank incision. Alternatively, vertical groin incisions can be made to access the femoral arteries. After systemic heparinization, the outflow is occluded and the neck of the aneurysm is approached posterolaterally. The landmarks for the infrarenal neck of the aortic aneurysm are the origin of the left crus of the diaphragm, the lumbar branch of the left renal vein, and the left renal artery (Figure 4–2). The lumbar branch of the left renal vein, which crosses the aorta in a posterior and perpendicular fashion and caudad to the renal artery, is ligated. The lymphareolar tissue is dissected to expose the proximal

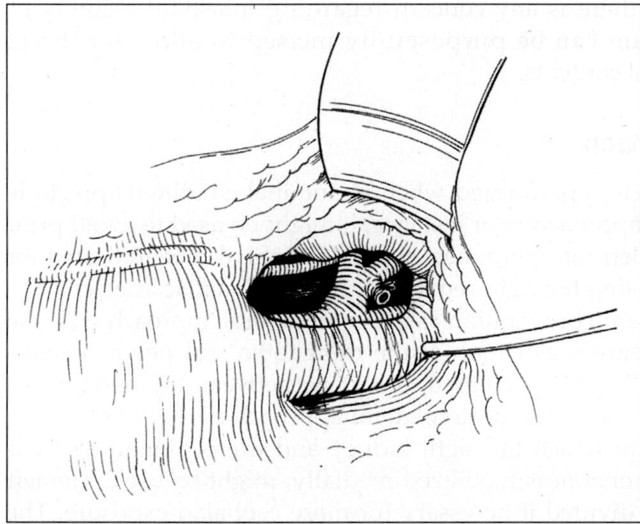

Figure 4-2. The left crus of the diaphragm, the lumbar branch of the left renal vein, and the left renal artery delineate the infrarenal aortic neck. (With Permission – Leather RP, Chang BB, Darling RC III, Shah DM. Retroperitoneal approach to abdominal aortic aneurysms. In: Jamieson CW, Yao JST, eds. *Operative Surgery: Vascular Surgery, 5th* Edition. London: Chapman & Hall Medical, 1994:251-61.)

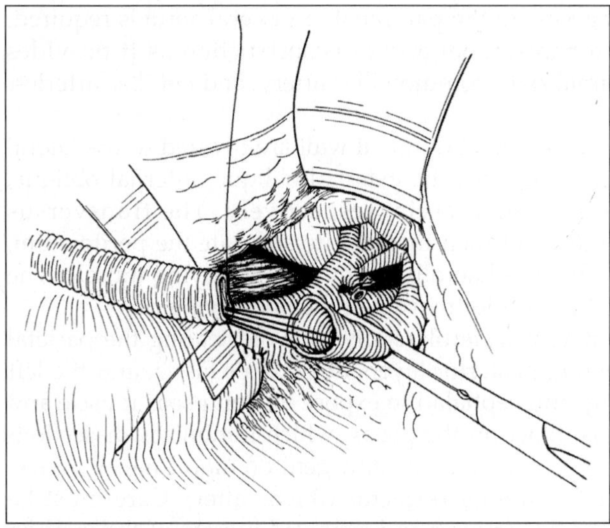

Figure 4-3. Ligation of the lumbar branch of the left renal vein allows access to the pararenal aorta. (With Permission – Leather RP, Chang BB, Darling RC III, Shah DM. Retroperitoneal approach to abdominal aortic aneurysms. In: Jamieson CW, Yao JST, eds. *Operative Surgery: Vascular Surgery, 5th* Edition. London: Chapman & Hall Medical, 1994:251-61.)

infrarenal aorta. The left lateral side of the aorta is dissected, followed by the anterior and then the posterior aspects.

Endoaneurysmorrhaphy.   The superior nonaneurysmal portion of the infrarenal aorta is clamped. The lumbar arteries and the inferior mesenteric artery can be controlled from outside the sac. The sac is then entered and residual backbleeding vessels are ligated with 3-0 polypropylene sutures. The aneurysm neck might be transected completely or partially with the posterior wall remaining intact. Our preference is to completely transect the aorta to allow precise suture placement through the full aortic wall thickness, thus minimizing later development of pseudoaneurysm (Figure 4–3). The proximal graft anastomosis is performed. The aortic clamp is then repositioned from the native aorta to the proximal graft to allow inspection of the proximal anastomosis bleeding. Next, the distal aortic, iliac, or femoral anastomoses are completed. Once the clamps are removed, Doppler interrogation is performed. If there is any concern regarding intestinal viability or traction injury, the peritoneum can be purposefully incised to allow for direct inspection of the intraabdominal contents.

Right Retroperitoneal Approach

A right retroperitoneal approach is performed when abdominal conditions preclude the use of a left retroperitoneal approach.[9] For instance, it might be used to avoid prior surgery or inflammation in the left retroperitoneal space. It might also be indicated for more extensive pathology involving the right renal or right common iliac arteries.

The exposure requires the same preparation as the contralateral approach with the exception of only 30 and 15 degrees elevation of the right torso and pelvis, respectively. When the retroperitoneal space is entered, the plane between the peritoneum and Gerota's fascia is developed. Either a posterolateral approach as described above or an anterolateral dissection, in which the right kidney and ureter remain in their anatomic position and the peritoneum is mobilized medially, might be used. The left renal vein can be mobilized or divided if necessary for more cephalad exposure. The vena cava is gently retracted laterally and small branches are suture ligated. If a posterolateral exposure is used, the gonadal vein should be divided so as to avoid traction injury from more cephalad traction during exposure. This exposes the neck of the aortic aneurysm. The remainder of the operation can be performed as an endoaneurysmorrhaphy. This approach should be avoided in symptomatic or ruptured aneurysm because proximal control is limited to the base of the superior mesenteric artery by fixed structures such as the liver.

Juxtarenal Aortic Exposure

The left posterolateral retroperitoneal approach allows excellent exposure of the suprarenal vessel and supraceliac aorta. Thus, we believe that it is the preferred approach for juxtarenal and suprarenal aneurysms. With the left kidney elevated and division of the lumbar branch of the left renal vein, the left renal artery is easily visualized. With further division of the left crus over the operator's left index finger or a right-angled clamp, the lateral pararenal/visceral aorta is well visualized. Now, an aortic clamp can be placed below the renals, above the left and below the right renal artery, or above the celiac axis for aortic control. This option allows maximal flexibility and reduced visceral ischemic time when performing aortic reconstruction.

Adjunctive Renal and Visceral Artery Reconstruction

The ability to perform simultaneous reconstruction of the renal and visceral arteries is an advantage of the left posterolateral retroperitoneal approach.[7] A 10th interspace incision permits more proximal exposure. The left crus of the diaphragm is divided to expose the visceral portion of the abdominal aorta. Exposure of the celiac, superior mesenteric, and left renal arteries is provided. A right renal artery stenosis can be approached from the left side as long as the lesion is in the proximal half of the artery. Unilateral renal artery stenosis is typically managed with a retroperitoneal approach from the affected side. Renal transaortic endarterectomy or bypass can be performed (Figure 4–4). Isolated visceral artery disease can be treated with endarterectomy or bypass via a retroperitoneal approach. In order to expose the superior mesenteric artery

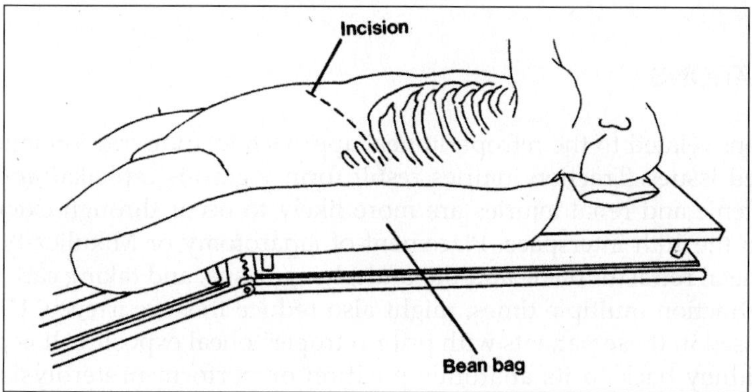

Figure 4-4. The aorta is transected and the proximal aorta anastomosis is performed using a "parachute" technique. (With Permission – Leather RP, Chang BB, Darling RC III, Shah DM. Retroperitoneal approach to abdominal aortic aneurysms. In: Jamieson CW, Yao JST, eds. *Operative Surgery: Vascular Surgery, 5th* Edition. London: Chapman & Hall Medical, 1994:251-61.)

beyond its origin, one must dissect anterior to the kidney and Gerota's fascia with the kidney in its anatomic bed in order to reach the mid-portion of the artery. This will be discussed later in the chapter.

Emergent Repair of Symptomatic and Ruptured Abdominal Aortic Aneurysm

In experienced centers, emergent repair of symptomatic and ruptured abdominal aortic aneurysms can be performed via a left extended posterolateral retroperitoneal approach.[10] In our institution, this is preferred over the traditional transabdominal approach.

As previously described, a left flank incision is made from the ipsilateral rectus to the posterior axillary line along the 10th intercostal space. The retroperitoneum is entered laterally. A hand is inserted to bluntly elevate the peritoneum from the diaphragm while leaving the left kidney in place. Care is taken to not enter the infrarenal retroperitoneal space in order to avoid disturbing the hematoma. The supraceliac aorta is palpated and compressed posteriorly against the spinal column. Thus, manual control of the supraceliac aorta can be obtained within approximately five minutes of intubation. From the right, a handheld deep Dever type retractor is placed to initially retract the peritoneal contents at the level of the supraceliac aorta. The left crus is divided and the aorta is clamped. The retroperitoneal space is opened widely and the peritoneum and left kidney are retracted medially and cephalad. The neck of the aneurysm can then be isolated and clamped in the usual fashion so that the proximal clamp can be removed. The aneurysm is opened and the iliac arteries are controlled, and endoaneurysmorrhaphy is performed as in the elective setting.

Closure

Defects in the peritoneum are closed. If the pleura is violated, this can be closed at the end of the case after suction evacuation over a catheter. The abdominal wall musculature is closed in layers followed by closure of the subcutaneous tissue and skin. Closure is facilitated by taking the flex out of the table and bringing the muscles back into apposition as in the elective setting.

COMPLICATIONS

Complications related to the retroperitoneal approach include traction injuries and incision related issues. Traction injuries result form vigorous cephalad and medial retraction. Splenic and renal injuries are more likely to occur through extension of the incision into the 10th interspace. Placement of laparotomy or Mikulicz-type pads between the metal retractor blade and the underlying tissue, and taking care to minimize changing retraction multiple times, might also reduce this occurrence. Ureteral damage is increased in those patients with prior retroperitoneal exposure. It is preferable to drop the kidney back to its anatomic position or perform ureterolysis to prevent ureteral disruption as the ureter might be tethered to the pelvic brim from adhesions.

In addition to traction injuries, there are several specific wound closure complications related to the retroperitoneal approach. Closure of the retroperitoneal incision can result in incisional hernias, and more commonly, flank bulges. Flank bulge results from division of the 11th or 12th intercostal nerves, which denervates the associated musculature resulting in a diastasis.[11] This complication is best prevented by isolating and protecting this nerve during dissection. If the incision can be extended only to the tip of the rib, this complication might be minimized. Chronic incisional pain from intercostal neuralgia might also occur. The treatment consists of serial nerve injections or operative resection of the intercostal nerve.

Another potential source of injury results from tunneling of the aortic graft to the contralateral limb. Tunneling should be performed manually under direct vision rather than blindly with a blunt instrument.

TECHNICAL CONCERNS

Anatomists have long recognized that the abdominal aorta is a retroperitoneal structure. It is, therefore, no great surprise that early management of aortic and iliac aneurysm pathology by Sir Astley Cooper and Claude Dubost was through a retro- and not transperitoneal approach. As there is no violation of the peritoneal sac and its contents, there is no need to be concerned with any maneuvers to pack or protect the bowel to prevent iatrogenic injury or desiccation during open aortic replacement procedures. In addition, there is no mesenteric traction and thus less physiologic derangements intraoperatively. This, coupled with less fluid requirements as a result of less periprocedure insensible loss, might contribute to a smoother postoperative course.[1-5] Additionally, the facility to avoid contact with large and small bowel results in a reduced chance of enteric contamination of the graft and potential long-term problems of graft enteric interactions and infection.

The ease of exposure of the entire infradiaphramatic aorta and its branches makes the extended left posterolateral approach the procedure of choice in treatment of pararenal and suprarenal/paravisceral aortic aneurysm disease not currently amenable to endovascular aortic repair. Repair of Type IV thoracoabdominal aortic aneurysms is relatively straightforward and is easily performed without the need to divide the diaphragm proper or enter the pleural cavity. In addition, the vascular surgeon can easily address concomitant aneurysmal or occlusive disease in the left renal or iliac arteries.

In certain situations, the posterolateral exposure might not be suitable, and limit proper treatment of the renal or visceral pathology. In these cases, an anterolateral exposure might be used. Examples include the presence of renal venous anomalies such as retroaortic left renal veins or circumaortic renal venous collars. Following the left ureter from its mid-portion cephalad allows the surgeon in these cases to define the plane anterior to Gerota's fascia to complete the anterolateral exposure. If there is any question of the correct lie of a graft limb to the left renal artery, the distal graft to left renal anastamosis can be performed via an anterolateral exposure to avoid the risk of anastamotic kink.

In certain cases, there might be concomitant long segment disease involving the superior mesenteric artery. In this situation, a posterolateral exposure alone will not allow exposure beyond the first few centimeters of this artery. By developing the anterolateral plane as described, one can follow the superior mesenteric artery from its origin, and then anterior to the left renal vein and beyond. In doing so, 10 to 15 centimeters of the superior mesenteric artery beyond its origin might be exposed though a left retroperitoneal approach.

Perceived limitations of the left retroperitoneal approach are involvement of the right renal and iliac arteries. There are several maneuvers that might improve exposure of both these vessels. In procedures where the aorta is exposed from the left side, the usual right-sided counterincision is made either at or one to two centimeters cephalad to the inguinal ligament and centered over the anatomic location of the common femoral artery. This allows adequate exposure of the external iliac artery. A more cephalad and medial incision will allow exposure of the ipsilateral iliac artery bifurcation, hypogastric, and the distal common iliac artery, depending on the patient's girth and the amount the pelvis has been tilted to the right side. The proximal few centimeters of the right common iliac artery are easily exposed through the left retroperitoneum. If further distal exposure is necessary, the left rectus abdominus muscle can be partially divided, and/or the inferior mesenteric artery can be ligated and divided. The depth of the exposure is facilitated with a narrow malleable retractor to elevate the "ceiling" of the field. These maneuvers allow exposure of the entire right common iliac, bifurcation, and hypogastric artery.

The right renal artery might be exposed up to the transverse portion that passes posterior to the inferior vena cava. This exposure is facilitated with placement of a narrow malleable blade to retract the peritoneal contents anteromedially. When it is necessary to divide the right renal artery for bypass, distal control with a curved "C" type Cooley clamp provides stable exposure for anastomosis. Either a right retroperitoneal or transperitoneal exposure should be considered for exposure of the right renal artery distal to the mid-portion of the inferior vena cava.

An additional use of the extended posterolateral left retroperitoneal approach is in the explantation of endovascular grafts in the setting of persistent Type I leak or aneurysm rupture. The operative field in these cases is similar to a reoperative field or that of an inflammatory aortic aneurysm due to the presence of the stent graft. The ability to obtain expeditious control of the suprarenal or supraceliac aorta facilitates the operative repair.

SUMMARY

The retroperitoneal approach has become, for us, the preferred method of exposure of the infradiaphragmatic aorta and its branches. Over the past 25 years, 3,304 abdominal aortic aneurysms have been repaired via this approach; 2,667 for elective AAAs, 281 for symptomatic AAAs, and 356 were repaired in patients presenting with ruptured AAAs. Mortality was 2.6%, 9.5%, and 34.7%, respectively. In addition, 1,426 aortic reconstructions for occlusive disease were performed with 1,379 survivors (97%). Additionally, there were 911 renal artery reconstructions performed using the retroperitoneal approach as well as over 258 visceral aortic reconstructions.

Complications related to the retroperitoneal approach include 17 incisional hernias, (17/4730) (0.4%). The incision might often produce a bulge from the area of operation that is noticeable to the patient. However, these are not true hernias and might be present in approximately 6% to 8% of patients. Incidence of late graft infection was seen in 27 (27/4730) (0.57%) patients, and aortoenteric fistulas were only seen in four patients in this series. More onerous complications include nine splenectomies: four organs ruptured by overzealous retraction and five ureteral injuries, all occurring in reoperative exposures, and nonfatal cardiac complications occurred in 3.6% of patients.

In conclusion, the retroperitoneal approach provides a surgeon with the ability to expose the entire infradiaphragmatic aorta and its branches. Its flexibility, one of the principle advantages of this approach, serves to simplify the operative conduct of these cases. The retroperitoneal exposure of the abdominal aorta is a versatile, safe, and viable exposure for aortic reconstructions. It has significant technical benefit to the surgeon and physiologic benefit to the patient. Therefore, knowledge of the use of this approach can only benefit the surgeon and should prove to be an impetus to familiarize oneself with this valuable technique.

REFERENCES

1. Sicard GA, Freeman, MB, VanderWoule et al. Comparison between the transabdominal and retroperitoneal approach for reconstruction of the infrarenal abdominal aorta. *J Vasc Surg.* 1987;5:19–27.
2. Leather RP, Shah DM, Kaufman JL, et al. Comparative analysis of retroperitoneal and transperitoneal aortic replacement for aneurysm. *Surg Gynecol Obstet.* 1989;268:387–393.
3. Gregory RT, Wheeler JR, Snyder SO, et al. Retroperitoneal approach to aortic surgery. *J Cardiovasc Surg.* 1989;30:185–189.
4. Darling RC III, Shah DM, Chang BB, et al. Current status of the use of retroperitoneal approach for reconstructions of the aorta and its branches. *Ann Surg* 224: 501–508, 1996.
5. Sicard GA, Reilly JM, Rubin BG, et al. Transabdominal retroperitoneal incision for abdominal aortic surgery: report of a prospective randomized trial. *J Vasc Surg.* 1995;21:174–181.
6. Williams GM, Ricotta J, Zinner M, et al. The extended retroperitoneal approach for treatment of extensive atherosclerosis of the aorta and renal vessels. *Surgery.* 1980;88:846–55.
7. Darling RC III, Shah DM, Chang BB, et al. Retroperitoneal approach for bilateral renal and visceral artery revascularization. *Am J Surg.* 11994;68:148–151.
8. Darling RC III, Resnikoff M, Kreienberg PB, Chang BB, Paty PSK, Leather RP, Shah DM. Alternative approach for management of infected aortic grafts. *J Vasc Surg.* 1997;1:106–12.
9. Chang BB, Shah DM, Paty PSK, et al. Can the retroperitoneal approach be used for ruptured abdominal aortic aneurysms? *J Vasc Surg.* 1990;11:326–30.
10. Chang BB, Paty PSK, Shah DM, et al. The right retroperitoneal approach for abdominal aortic surgery. *Am J Surg.* 1989;158: 156–158.
11. Gardner GP, Josephs LG, Rosca M, et al. Flank bulge associated with retroperitoneal incisions: an anatomical and neuruphysiological evaluation. *J Vasc Surg.* 1993;18: 321–322.

5

Modified Retroperitoneal Approach for Aortic Aneurysm Repair: An Improved Approach to Deal With Unfavorable Anatomical Considerations

Frank J. Veith, M.D., Palma M. Shaw, M.D.,
Evan C. Lipsitz, M.D., and
Nicholas J. Gargiulo III, M.D.

The increasing availability of endovascular grafts has substantially altered the management of abdominal aortic aneurysms (AAAs). As more patients with favorable anatomy undergo endovascular graft AAA repair (EVAR), abdominal aortic aneurysm (AAA) repair via an open approach is being performed less often and mostly in patients with complex unfavorable anatomy. Many of these patients are also poor candidates for open repair because of anatomic considerations such as pararenal aortic involvement, extensive iliac disease, abdominal wall deformity, or serious medical comorbidities.

Since Rob[1] reported his early experience with an extraperitoneal approach to the abdominal aorta, the retroperitoneal (RP) approach has been evaluated by various investigators.[2-4] Several distinct advantages have been suggested when compared to the transperitoneal (TP) approach.[5] Over the past 15 years, we have been using EVARs in an increasing percentage of our AAA patients. We have also used increasingly the RP approach in the open treatment of the remaining AAAs, many of which have had complex or difficult anatomy often coupled with serious comorbidities. The aim of the current analysis was to evaluate the role of open AAA repair in the endovascular era as well as the indications for and the advantages and effectiveness of a modified RP approach for these repairs.

MATERIALS AND METHODS

Patients

Four hundred and three elective AAA repairs were performed at our institution from December 1994 thru January 2001. Patients with infrarenal or pararenal AAAs > 5 cm (range 5–10 cm) in diameter who had complex aortic or iliac anatomy precluding EVAR and those who preferred not to have EVAR underwent open repair (n = 175, 43%) via either a TP (n = 118, 67%) or a modified RP approach (n = 57, 33%). There were 81 men (69%) and 37 women (31%) in the TP group and 41 men (72%) and 16 women (28%) in the RP group. The mean age in the TP group was 73 years and in the RP group was 77.5 years. Of the patients who underwent open repair, 32% (38/118) in the TP group and 61% (35/57) in the RP group had one or more major medical or anatomic factors (Tables 5–1 and 5–2), which increased their risk, made open repair more difficult, and/or precluded EVAR. In the RP group, these medical factors included diabetes mellitus (DM) in 8 (14%), previous coronary artery bypass grafting (CABG) in 10 (18%), previous myocardial infarction (MI) in 14 (25%), end-stage renal disease (ESRD) in 1 (2%), an ejection fraction less than 30% (EF < 30%)[6] in eight (14%), and forced expiratory volume at one second of less than 55% (FEV$_1$ <55% [7,8]) in two (4%). The TP group had 14 (12%) diabetics, 29 (25%) patients with previous CABG,

TABLE 5-1. UNFAVORABLE ILIAC ANATOMIC VARIATIONS

Risk Factors	Retroperitoneal (n = 57) Number of patients (%)	Transperitoneal (n = 118) Number of patients (%)	P value
Iliac Occlusive Disease	28 (49%)	10 (19%)	< .0001*
Small Iliac Arteries (<6mm)	1 (2%)	1 (1%)	0.55
Tortuous (>90°) or Heavily Calcified Iliac Arteries	3 (5%)	3 (3%)	0.39
Large Right Iliac Aneurysm (>4.5cm)	3 (5%)	5 (4%)	0.72

*statistically significant

TABLE 5-2. OTHER UNFAVORABLE ANATOMIC VARIATIONS

Risk Factors	Retroperitoneal (n = 57) Number of patients (%)	Transperitoneal (n = 118) Number of patients (%)	P value
Large Ventral Hernia Involving the Left Side of the Abdomen	7 (12%)	1 (1%)	.001*
Failed Attempt at EVAR	3 (5%)	2 (2%)	.17
Failed Attempt at Open Repair	2 (4%)	0 (0%)	.09
Previous Left Colectomy	8 (12%)	3 (3%)	.01*
Prior Major Laparotomy	8 (14%)	10 (9%)	.28
Previous Pelvic Irradiation	4 (7%)	0 (0%)	0.01*
Morbid Obesity*	7 (12%)	3 (3%)	.01*
Average Number of Risk Factors/Patient[a]	1.7	1.1	.01*

* statistically significant;
# a body mass index of >34[REFE09];
[a] risk factors derived and calculated from tables I,II,III,IV

37 (31%) with previous MI, one (1%) with ESRD, six (5%) with EF <30% and two (2%) with FEV_1 <55%. Anatomically, in the RP group, 22 (39%) patients had absent or short aortic neck (<1.0 cm in length) versus 23 (20%) in the TP group, and 17 (30%) had large (< 30mm), angled (>60%), and/or flared aortic neck versus 15 (13%) in the TP group.

Risk Factors and Complications

Patient data, including risk factors, were obtained prospectively. Thirty-day morbidity and mortality rates and length of hospital stay (LOS) were analyzed. Operative parameters including estimated blood loss (EBL), length of stay (LOS), intensive care unit (ICU) stay, transfusion requirement, length of operative time, size of aneurysm, and American Society of Anesthesiologists (ASA) score are shown in Table 5–3. Operative and postoperative complications are detailed in Table 5–4. Iliac occlusive disease was defined as an occluded common and/or external iliac artery unsuitable for percutaneous transluminal angioplasty. Tortuosity of the iliac vessels may make it difficult to obtain clamp control of the hypogastric arteries. Significant scarring was fibrous in nature with obliteration of easy dissection planes.

Operative Approaches

Two different open surgical approaches were utilized: a standard TP exposure via a midline incision and an RP approach via a left posterolateral incision. The RP approach was used in patients with serious comorbidities and those with anatomically unfavorable aortic neck anatomy. The TP approach has been described elsewhere.[9,10] In brief, the patient is placed supine for the TP approach and a midline abdominal incision from the xiphoid process to the pubis is made. The bowel is packed to the right side and the abdominal aortic aneurysm is exposed by opening the retroperitoneum. The aorta is dissected free above and below the aneurysm.[9] The status of the iliac vessels as determined by CT scan preoperatively and intraoperatively by inspection dictates whether a tube or bifurcated graft is used. The classical RP approach is performed with the patient on a "bean-bag" device (Olympic Vac-Pac #68035) with the hips parallel to the table and the trunk and left shoulder elevated to 75 degrees. The incision begins midway between the umbilicus and the symphysis pubis at the lateral border of the rectus muscle anteriorly and extends in a curvilinear fashion, 5 cm medial to the anterior iliac spine, posteriorly to the tip of the eleventh rib.[11]

TABLE 5-3. OPERATIVE VARIABLES DURING OPEN AAA REPAIR BY THE RP AND TP APPROACH

Perioperative Factors	Overall	Retroperitoneal	Transperitoneal	P value
EBL (L)	2.6 (2.0	2.4 (1.8	2.7 (2.1	0.82
LOS (d) mean	12.1(7.3	11.2 (8.3	12.4 (6.9	0.84
median	10	9	10	
ICU Stay (d) mean	5.6 (5.5	5.6 (7.8	5.6 (4.1	0.50
median	4	6	6	
Packed red cell Requirement(units)	2.0.(2.2	1.8 (1.9	2.1 (2.3	0.80
Size of Aneurysm(cm)	6.2 ± 1.2	6.3 ± 1.2	6.1 ± 1.25	0.84
American Society of Anesthesiologists Score	3.0 ± 0.5	3.0 ± 0.6	3.0 ± 0.5	0.50
Age (y)	73.6 ± 9.1	74.5 ± 8.64	73.2 ± 9.34	0.40

TABLE 5-4. MORTALITY, MORBIDITY AND COMPLICATIONS OF OPEN AAA REPAIR

Complication	Retroperitoneal (n/57) Number of patients(%)	Transperitoneal (n/118) Number of patients(%)	P value
30-day Mortality	3.77%	3.39%	1.00
Bleeding	1 (1.7)	3 (2.5)	1.00
Sepsis	0 (0)	5 (4.2)	0.17
C. Difficile Colitis	2 (3.5)	6 (5.1)	1.00
UTI	0 (0)	3 (2.5)	0.55
Pneumonia	5 (8.8)	8 (6.8)	0.76
Respiratory Failure	2 (3.5)	7 (5.9)	0.72
ATN	1 (1.7)	5 (4.2)	0.67
Arrythmia	2 (3.5)	10 (8.5)	0.34
CHF	0 (0)	2 (1.7)	1.00
MI	0 (0)	2 (1.7)	1.00
MOSF	1 (1.7)	2 (1.7)	1.00
Ischemic Colitis	1 (1.7)	3 (2.5)	1.00
Limb Ischemia/ Embolism	1 (1.7)	2 (1.7)	1.00
CVA	1 (1.7)	1 (0.8)	0.53
Incidental Splenectomy	1 (1.7)	1 (0.8)	0.53
Deep Venous Thrombosis	1 (1.7)	2 (1.7)	1.00
Wound Infection	1 (1.7)	0 (0)	0.31

Bleeding- requiring return to OR; Sepsis- documented by clinical findings and positive blood cultures; UTI- urinary tract infection; Respiratory Failure- requiring > 4 days mechanical ventilatory support; ATN- Acute Tubular Necrosis; CHF- congestive heart failure; MI- myocardial infarction; MOSF- Multi-Organ System Failure; Ischemic Colitis- documented by endoscopy; CVA- cerebrovascular accident.

Our modification of the RP approach was particularly useful when there were difficult aortic neck characteristics or when pararenal or suprarenal clamping was required. It was also useful if the abdomen was scarred, a large ventral hernia was present (Figures 5–1 and 5–2) or the patient was morbidly obese. The decision to use the RP instead of the TP approach was influenced by these anatomic factors more so than by surgeon choice. The patient was positioned in the standard fashion with a 30-degree elevation of the left hip and 90 degree elevation of the left shoulder. An S-shaped incision extends just below and halfway along the distal half of the 9th rib more posteriorly and laterally than the classical incision (Figure 5–3). Seven to eight centimeters of the 10th rib may be resected to provide better exposure and increase the space available for clamp application to the pararenal aorta. In the presence of midline abdominal scarring or a large ventral hernia, the inferior portion of this incision is carried more posterolaterally. With this 9th interspace incision, the pleura was often entered but this did not cause increased morbidity in our patients. When the incision was closed, the diaphragm was repaired and a tube was placed to evacuate air as the anesthesiologist hyperinflated the lungs. The tube was removed after closure of the diaphragm and posterior muscle layers.

Statistical Evaluation

Risk factors and operative variables such as length of stay (LOS) and ICU stay were correlated with operative (30-day) mortality using multiple forward stepwise logistic

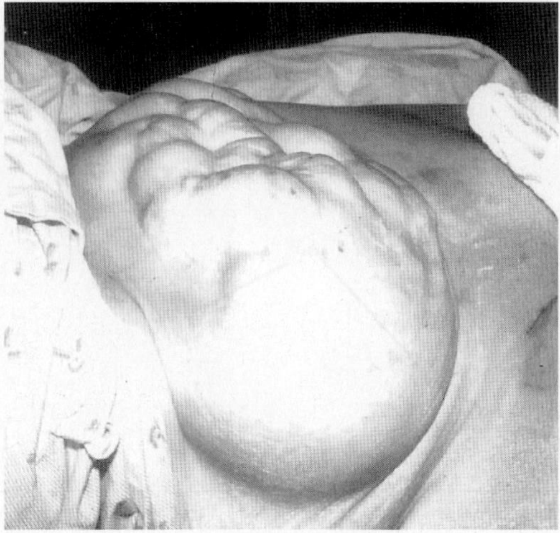

Figure 5-1. A patient with a hostile abdomen and a 6.5 cm AAA, and a 6.0 cm right common iliac aneurysm and a 4.5 cm left common iliac aneurysm. All aneurysms were successfully treated with a modified RP approach.

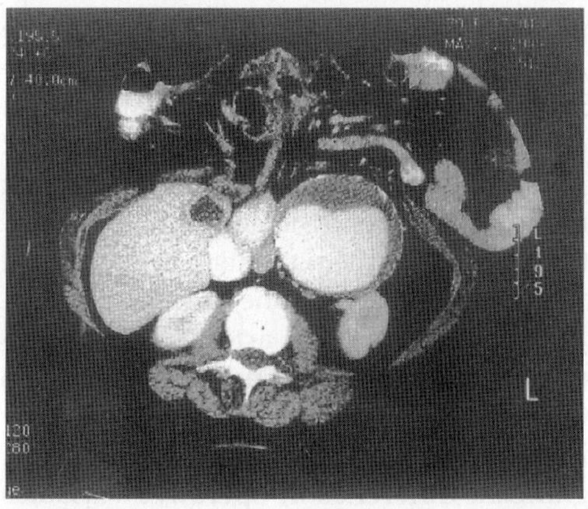

Figure 5-2. Computed Tomographic Scan of the abdomen from a patient with a 7.5 cm pararenal AAA and a large ventral hernia containing most of the abdominal viscera. The AAA was successfully repaired via a modified RP approach.

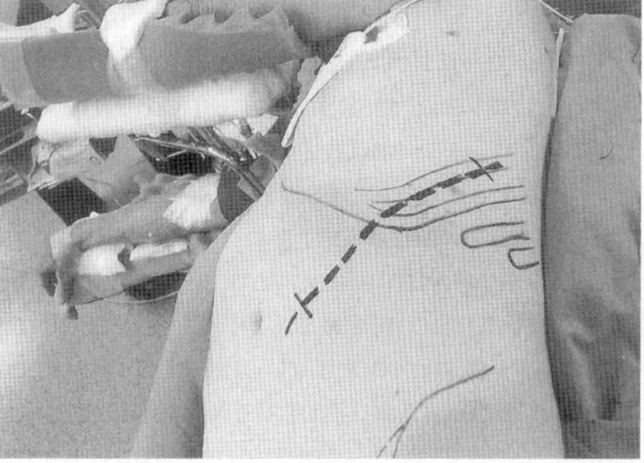

Figure 5-3. Positioning for a modified RP approach in an obese patient. Anatomic landmarks are drawn.

regression. Comparison between the groups with regard to categorical variables was performed using Fisher's Exact or Chi Square tests as appropriate. Comparisons between the groups for continuous variables were performed using t-tests for independent samples.

RESULTS

In our total group of 403 patients undergoing elective AAA repair between December 1994 and January 2001, 228 (57%) had elective EVARs and 175 (43%) had open AAA

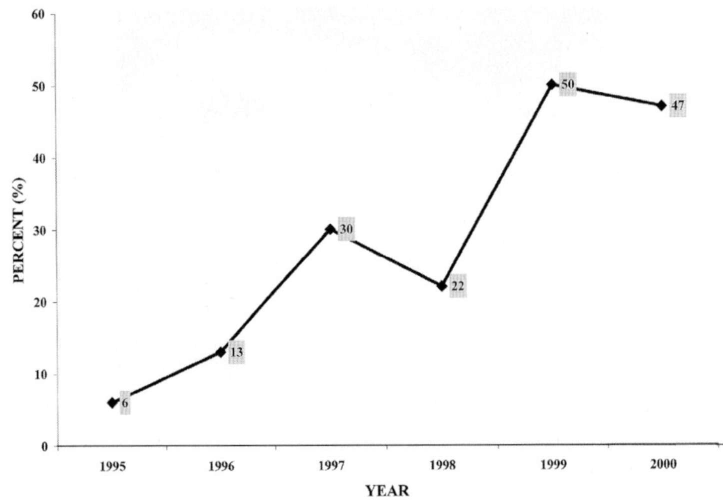

Figure 5-4. Graph showing the increasing use of a RP approach for open AAA repair over a six-year period.

repairs. Of the 175 open repairs, a TP approach was used in 118 (67%) and a RP approach in 57 (33%). There was an increasing trend to use a RP approach over time (Figure 5–4). Between the TP and RP groups, there was a statistically significant difference in several risk factors including a low EF (15–30%) (P = .04), anatomical risk factors such as a short (< 1cm) or absent aortic neck, large angled or flared aortic neck (P = .01), iliac occlusive disease (Table 5–1), a large ventral hernia involving the left side of the abdomen, a previous left colectomy, previous pelvic irradiation, and morbid obesity with a body mass index of >34[12] (Table 5–2). Of the patients with an absent or short aortic neck, 25% (12/45) required aortic clamping above one or both renal arteries (two supraceliac, one above the SMA, nine above the renal arteries). The duration of proximal suprarenal aortic clamping ranged from 24–29 minutes (mean 26 min.). Aortic neck angulation may increase the difficulty of the operation particularly when it deviates to the right and increased dissection is required to gain control.

As shown in Table 5–3, there was no significant difference in operative variables between the RP and TP groups. Despite the fact that the modified RP approach was used predominately in anatomically difficult patients with a large incidence of medical comorbidities and other unfavorable conditions, operative mortality and the incidence of most complications were acceptably low in the RP group and comparable to those in the TP group (Table 5–4).

DISCUSSION

Patients with AAAs and favorable anatomy are increasingly undergoing EVAR. Accordingly, traditional open repair is being used more often for patients with unfavorable aortoiliac or AAA morphology. In addition, many of these patients also have serious medical comorbidities. We found that the RP approach, especially our modification with a higher incision, made more posterolaterally permitted better exposure of the pararenal aorta and was helpful in AAA patients with unfavorable aortic neck anatomy requiring pararenal exposure and suprarenal clamping, especially in muscular or obese individuals. This approach was also useful in the presence of other anatomical conditions such as a hostile abdomen with large ventral hernias involving the left side of the abdomen (Figure 5–1), and/or intraperitoneal scarring due to previous surgery or pelvic irradiation. In all of these situations, the modified RP approach with its more posterior and higher location facilitated safe AAA repair with acceptably low morbidity and mortality. Similar advantages of the classical RP approach in medically high-risk patients have been described by others.[13-16] Other anatomic advantages of the classical and modified RP approach include easier control of the visceral aorta and its vessels when atherosclerotic occlusive disease is present[17] and obviation of the need to retract or divide the left renal vein for high proximal control in the case of juxta or pararenal aneurysmal disease.[11, 14] Moreover, the RP approach allows avoidance of tedious lysis of intraperitoneal adhesions and decreased risk of graft contamination from inadvertantly opened bowel in patients with previous laparotomy.[18] In complex situations with major contraindications to using the TP approach, the RP approach could be utilized with good outcomes in three of our patients who had large right-sided common iliac artery aneurysms (> 4 cm).

We recognize that our study did not include an adequate number of patients to demonstrate statistical superiority or equivalence of our modified RP approach. However, there was no difference in morbidity and mortality rates between the RP and TP groups, even though the RP group contained many more high-risk patients with unfavorable anatomic features.

Two of the patients who would have been candidates for EVAR had chosen to have open surgery. While not including these two patients in the analysis might create a more pure cohort of high-risk patients, eliminating them would not alter our analysis or conclusions.

Several studies by others have claimed physiologic advantages of the RP approach over a TP approach. Patients in the latter group had an increased intraoperative blood loss, fluid requirement, and need for transfusion. Prolonged ileus and nasogastric tube requirement, increased intensive care unit stay, duration of hospitalization, and complication rate were all more common in their patients with the TP approach.[10,18] One group has demonstrated negative physiologic effects such as a decreased systemic vascular resistance that can result in increased myocardial oxygen demand using the TP approach. They attribute this to mesenteric traction and intestinal manipulation.[19] However, one prospective randomized study comparing the TP and RP approach could not confirm these differences. Yet, the latter authors advocated preferential use of the RP approach in cases with a multiple operated abdomen or morbid obesity.[4]

Disadvantages of this RP approach have also been well described. These include inability to inspect the abdominal contents, and limited access to the right renal artery and the distal right common iliac artery (CIA) and its branches. However, with interruption of the inferior mesenteric artery and careful medial mobilization of the ureter and peritoneal contents, the right CIA can often be adequately exposed. When it cannot be, the origin of the right CIA can be oversewn and the right limb of a bifurcated graft can be tunneled along the iliac arteries in a retroperitoneal plane and anastomosed, end-to-side to the right common femoral artery or right external iliac artery accessed via a right lower quadrant incision. In such circumstances, the right external iliac artery must be ligated proximally so that the CIA suture line will not be subjected to systemic arterial pressure. Preservation of the ipsilateral hypogastric circulation is advocated when possible. The internal iliac artery can be revascularized in some cases by various methods such as external-to-internal iliac artery bypass or translocation of the internal iliac artery to the external.[20] In our experience, sacrifice of the internal iliac artery can be tolerated in selected cases with minimal morbidity.[21] If the right hypogastric artery is aneurysmal, the approach described for exclusion of the entire right iliac system may be used. However, more recently, we have used preoperative coil embolization of the hypogastric or its branches to prevent continued pressurization of the hypogastric aneurysm from collateral backflow.[22, 23] One disadvantage of this approach is that right iliac exposure can be difficult. When it is, the incision can be extended inferiorly and medially. This modification of the RP approach may not be necessary in all cases, but it has advantages over the conventional RP approach when patients have difficult aortic neck anatomy, a hostile abdomen, or morbid obesity. We, therefore, believe that this modification of the RP approach will prove useful to others, particularly in the endovascular era when many patients requiring open AAA repair have unfavorable anatomical features.

Those patients in whom this modified RP approach was used had certain anatomic characteristics such as an aortic neck that was absent, short, large, flared or angulated, or other unfavorable anatomic factors such as, a large ventral hernia involving the left side of the abdomen, a previous failed attempt at open repair with periaortic scarring, a previous left colectomy, major laparotomy, pelvic irradiation, or morbid obesity. In these circumstances, we felt that this modification provided an advantage over the TP or standard 10th or 11th interspace RP approaches. Patients in whom these anatomic conditions are absent may be managed with either the standard TP or RP approach. The TP approach was preferred in cases in which inspection of intraperitoneal viscera might be necessary or in the presence of a large right common iliac artery aneurysm, particularly when its bifurcation or the hypogastric artery was involved. The presence of iliac occlusive disease is a relative indication for using the TP approach. Despite this, our comparison of the anatomical risk factors in each group showed that in our patients the RP group had a significantly greater incidence of iliac artery occlusive disease.

High usage of the TP approach occurred because it was initially the favored approach for AAA repair and was generally used on the simpler better-risk patients encountered more frequently in the earlier years of the study. Our increasing experience with high-risk more difficult aneurysms developed as we were referred more patients unsuitable for standard open TP or endovascular repair.

In conclusion, our data shows that the morbidity and mortality of RP AAA repairs in high-risk patients with more unfavorable medical, anatomic and abdominal wall factors were acceptably low and comparable to morbidity and mortality in a better risk group of patients undergoing contemporary TP open repair. We believe that our modification of the RP approach is particularly useful during this period of endovascular enthusiasm when many candidates for open repair will have serious medical comorbidities coupled with difficult and challenging aortoiliac anatomy.

SUMMARY

To evaluate elective open abdominal aortic aneurysm (AAA) repair and the role of a modified retroperitoneal approach in a high volume endovascular center we reviewed prospectively collected data on 175 elective infrarenal open AAA repairs performed during the last six years. A transperitoneal approach was used in 118 cases and a modified retroperitoneal approach in 57. The incisional modification that facilitated repairs in the presence of massive obesity, scarring, and ventral hernias included a higher more posterolateral incision in the 9th intercostal space. Risk factors that added to the difficulty of the repair included aneurysms with a short (< 1cm) or no aortic neck in 45 patients, large angled or flared aortic neck in 32, tortuous and calcified iliac arteries in six, morbid obesity in 10, low ejection fraction (15-30%) in 14, COPD with FEV_1 <55% in four, prior laparotomy in 18, previous left colectomy in 11, a large right iliac aneurysm in eight, large ventral hernias in eight, pelvic irradiation in four, failed endovascular repair in five, and prior failed open repair attempt in two. Many of these factors occurred with significantly greater frequency (P = .04-.001) in the retroperitoneal group. All these factors were correlated with outcome.

Despite these risk factors, overall 30-day mortality was 3.5% (retroperitoneal 3.8%) and mean length of stay (LOS) was nine days (retroperitoneal, eight days). There was no significant correlation between mortality or LOS and any of the above-mentioned risk factors (P> .2).

In the era of endovascular aneurysm exclusion, open AAA repair is generally applied to anatomically complex or difficult aneurysms, many of which are present in high-risk patients. Despite this combination of anatomical and systemic risk factors, the modified retroperitoneal approach facilitates treatment in difficult circumstances and allows open AAA repair to be performed with acceptable mortality and morbidity rates.

REFERENCES

1. Rob C. Extraperitoneal approach to the abdominal aorta. Surgery. 1963;53:87–89.
2. Shepard AD, Tollefson FJ, Reddy DJ, et al. Left flank retroperitoneal exposure: a technical aid to complex aortic reconstruction. *J Vasc Surg*. 1991;14:283–291.
3. Sicard GA, Reilly JM, Rubin BG, et al. Transabdominal versus retroperitoneal incision for abdominal aortic surgery: report of a prospective randomized trial. *J Vasc Surg*. 1995;21: 174–183.
4. Cambria RP, Brewster DC, Abbott WM, et al. Transperitoneal versus retroperitoneal approach for aortic reconstruction: a randomized prospective study. *J Vasc Surg*. 1990;314–325.
5. Sicard GA, Allen BT, Munn JS, Anderson CB. Retroperitoneal versus transperitoneal approach for repair of abdominal aortic aneurysms. *Surg Clin No Am*. 1989;69(4)795–806.
6. Pasternack PF, Imparato AM, Bear G, Riles TS, Baumann FG, Benjamin D, et al. The value of radionuclide angiography as a predictor of perioperative myocardial infarction in patients undergoing abdominal aortic aneurysm. *J Vasc Surg*. 1984;1:320–325.
7. Holden DA, Rice TA, Stelmach K, Meeker DP. Exercise testing, 6-min walk, and stair climb in the evaluation of patients at high risk for pulmonary resection. *Chest*. 1992;102:1774–1779.
8. Kroenke LTC K, Lawrence VA, Theroux JF, Tuley MR. Operative risk in patients with severe obstructive pulmonary disease. *Arch Intern Med*. 1992;152:967–971.
9. Veith FJ. Vascular Surgical Techniques. In: Veith FJ, Hobson RW, Williams RA, Wilson SE, editors. *Vascular Surgery Principles and Practice, 2nd ed*. New York: McGraw-Hill; 1984:166–1173.
10. Sicard GA. Surgical techniques for repair of abdominal aortic aneurysms. In: Gewertz BL, Schwartz LB, editors. *Surgery of the aorta and its branches. 1st ed*. Philadelphia: WB Saunders Company; 2000:124–136.
11. Williams GM , Ricotta J, Zinner M, Burdick J. The extended retroperitoneal approach for the treatment of extensive atherosclerosis of the aorta and renal vessels. *Surgery*. 1980;88(6): 846–855.
12. Kellum JM, DeMaria EJ, Sugerman HJ. The surgical treatment of morbid obesity. *Curr Problems Surg*. 1998;35(9):791–858.
13. Sicard GA, Freeman MB, VanderWoude JC, Anderson CB. Comparison between the transabdominal and retroperitoneal approach for reconstruction of the infrarenal abdominal aorta. *J Vasc Surg*. 1987;5:19–27.
14. Shepard AD, Scott GR, Mackey WC, et al. Retroperitoneal approach to high-risk abdominal aortic aneurysms. *Arch Surg*. 1986;121:444–449.

15. Darling III RC, Shah DM, Chang BB, et al. Current status of the use of retroperitoneal approach for reconstructions of the aorta and its branches. *Ann Surg*. 1996;224(4):501–506.
16. Arko FR, Bohannon WT, Mettauer M, et al. Retroperitoneal approach for aortic surgery: is it worth it? *Cardiovasc Surg*. 2000;9(1):20–26.
17. Ricotta JJ, Williams GM. Endarterectomy of the upper abdominal aorta and visceral arteries through an extraperitoneal approach. *Ann Surg*.1980;192:633–638.
18. Leather RP, Shah DM, Kaufman JL, et al. Comparative analysis of retroperitoneal and transperitoneal aortic replacement for aneurysm. *Surg Gynecol Obstet*. 1989;168:387–393.
19. Hudson JC, Wurm WH, O'Donnell TF, et al. Hemodynamics and prostacyclin release in the early phases of aortic surgery: comparison of transabdominal and retroperitoneal approaches. *J Vasc Surg*. 1988;7:190–198.
20. Faries PL, Morrisey MD, Burks JA, et al. Internal iliac artery revascularization as an adjunct to endovascular repair of aortoiliac aneurysms. *J Vasc Surg*. 2001;34:892–899.
21. Mehta M, Veith FJ, Ohki T, et al. Unilateral and bilateral hypogastric artery interruption during aortoiliac aneurysm repair in 154 patients: a relatively innocuous procedure. *J Vasc Surg*. 2001;33:S27–S32.
22. Cynamon J, Lerer D, Veith FJ, et al. Hypogastric artery coil embolization prior to endoluminal repair of aneurysms and fistulas: buttock claudication, a recognized but possibly preventable complication. *J Vasc Intrev Radiol*. 2000;11(5):543–545.
23. Henretta JP, Karch LA, Hodgson KJ, et al. Special iliac artery considerations during aneurysm endografting. *Am J Surg*. 1999;178(3):212–8.

6

Open Repair of Complex Aortic Aneurysm in the Era of Endovascular Repair

Kenneth J. Cherry, M.D.

Operations on aneurysms of the juxta- and suprarenal aorta (and on the visceral branches of the upper abdominal aorta) are performed much less frequently than reconstructions confined to the infrarenal aorta. There is evidence that more juxtarenal aneurysms are being diagnosed and repaired in absolute numbers.[1] The sophistication of modern imaging modalities, especially computed tomagraphic angiography (CTA), allows more precise assessment of the paravisceral aorta than in years past, making diagnosis of these aneurysms easier.

Endovascular treatment of infrarenal abdominal aortic aneurysms is currently performed for 40–80% of patients undergoing aneurysm repair at referral centers. A larger relative percentage of the aortic aneurysms now repaired conventionally are juxta- or suprarenal. In a recent series from the Cleveland Clinic, the repair of juxtarenal aneurysms accounted for 10.8% of their total repairs in 1995 and 31.7% in 2000.[2] Undoubtedly, these figures are even more pronounced in 2007. This relative increase in juxtarenal reconstructions reflects the active endovascular practice of surgeons for the treatment of infrarenal aortic aneurysms, and the well-recognized and steep decline in open repairs. That relative increase does not make up for the nationwide decline in the absolute number of conventional repairs of infrarenal abdominal aneurysms. Vascular surgery fellows are exposed to much less aortic surgery than in years past. That topic is beyond the scope of this chapter, but there are problems in teaching mastery of aortic surgery to residents and fellows who are exposed to the "simple" cases less and less. Innovative solutions, such as "Aortic Fellowships," may be anticipated.

The endovascular repair of juxtarenal, suprarenal, and paravisceral abdominal aortic aneurysms with fenestrated grafts and branch graft technology in this country is confined to a few centers. For the foreseeable future, fenestrated and branched grafts will continue to be placed for complex pararenal aortic aneurysms in these select referral centers only. The preoperative assessment and planning and construction of these grafts is labor-intensive and time-consuming, and even with FDA approval, endovascular repair of complex aortic aneurysms is not likely to be practiced everywhere. Long-term results are lacking. Therefore, open reconstruction of these complex aneurysms remains a necessary part of vascular surgery.

ANATOMIC HINTS AND OBSERVATIONS

Surface anatomy is important in planning approaches for these patients. Narrow, asthenic patients are best served by vertical or oblique incisions such as are used for lateral retroperitoneal approaches. Transverse incisions in such patients limit the surgeon's options. On the other hand, obese individuals, encountered all too often in practice now, may benefit from transverse incisions, especially if their transverse abdominal width is greater than the distance from xyphoid to symphysis (Figure 6–1).

The two extremes of body habitus, the asthenic and the morbidly obese, are probably both best served by lateral retroperitoneal, thoracoretroperitoneal, or thoracoabdominal incisions for work on the paravisceral aorta. In the thin patient, there is little flaring of the costal margin, and the lower rib cage and iliac crest are very close to one another, leaving little room for maneuver. Midline incisions in these patients, even with medial visceral rotation (MVR), do not allow comfortable handling of the upper abdominal aorta and its branches in this tight and angulated area (Figure 6–2).

The xyphoid is the lynchpin of upper aortic exposure through a midline incision. If a surgeon is to work effectively on the suprarenal aorta through a midline incision, it is imperative that the incision extend alongside the xyphoid process such that the abdominal cavity is opened all the way to the dome of the diaphragm. The incision along the xyphoid transects the transverses thoracis muscle, diaphragmatic fibers, the ventral costoxyphoid ligament, the dorsal costoxyphoid ligament, the rectus abdominis muscle, and the aponeuroses of the abdominal muscles. Attention to this detail of the incision allows for much more craniad, and hence more comfortable and effective exposure of the paravisceral aorta, as well as easier and wider retraction (Figure 6–3).

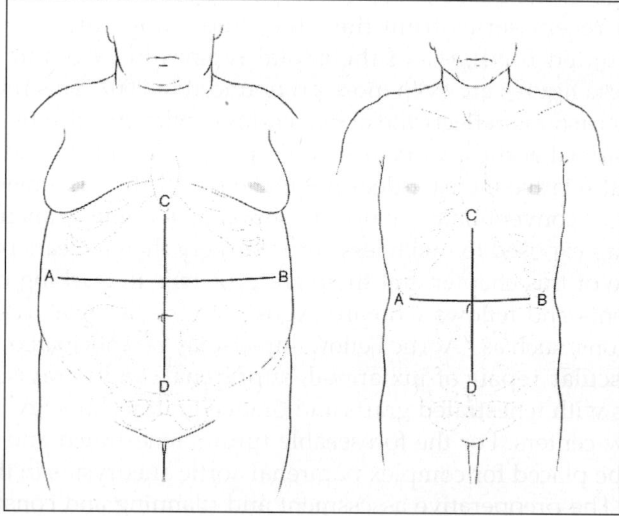

Figure 6-1. Vertical and horizontal axes.

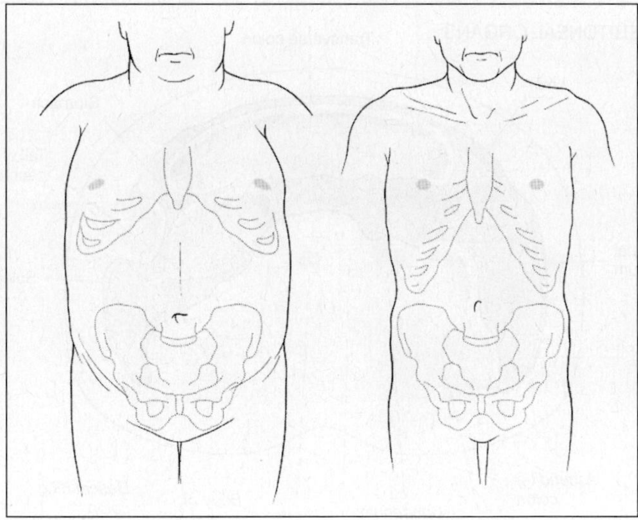

Figure 6-2. Costal flaring.

The upper abdominal aorta is intimate with the diaphragm, esophagus, stomach, vagus nerves, portal circulation, bile ducts, liver, spleen, pancreas, duodenum, colon, adrenals, and kidneys. It is these associations and the risk of injury to these structures that contribute in large part to the difficulty of performing operations on the paravisceral aorta.

A recitation of the retroperitoneal contents may sound simplistic but bears repeating as a reminder of the basics. Those structures and organs in the retroperitoneum of

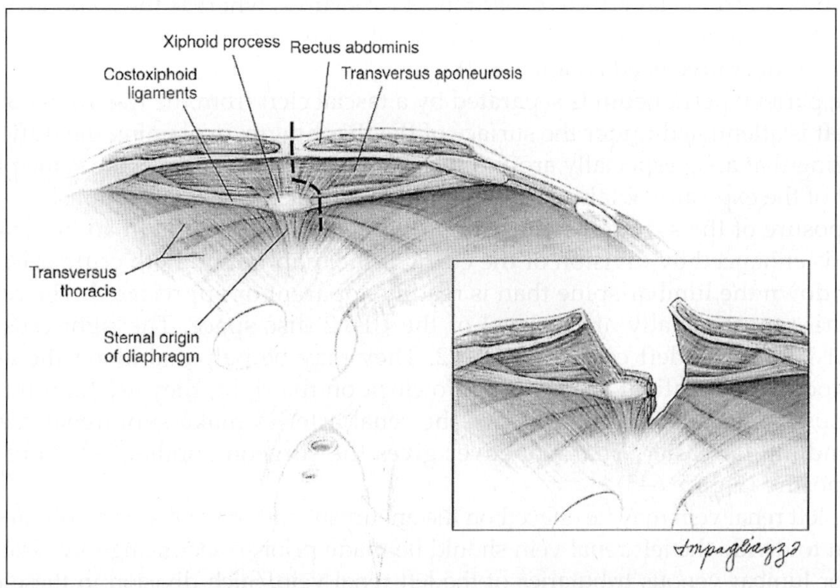

Figure 6-3. Incision along xyphoid.

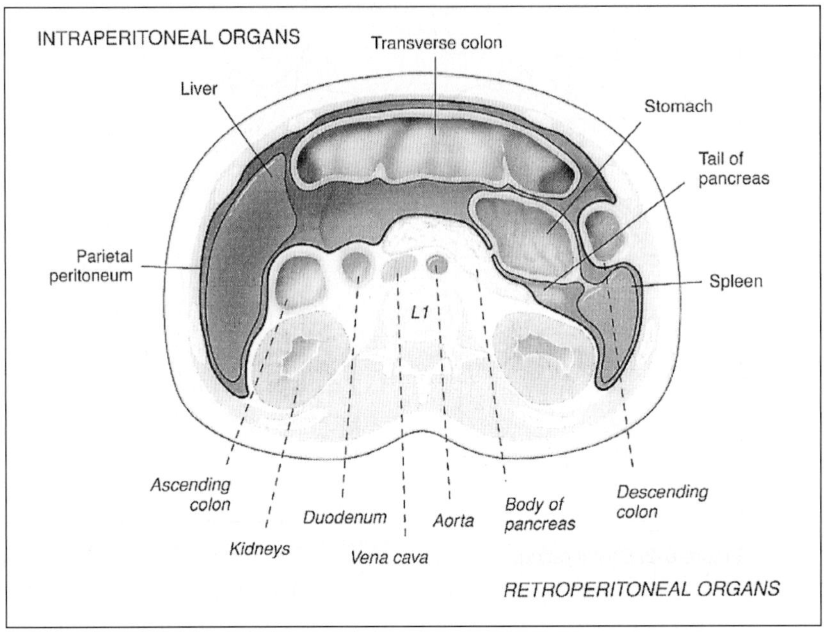

Figure 6-4. Retro/intraperitoneal organs.

interest to the performance of complex aortic surgery are the ascending and descending colon, the inferior vena cava (IVC), the aorta, the kidneys and ureters, the adrenal glands, the horizontal portion of the duodenum, and the pancreas, excepting the tail which is intraperitoneal. Of note, the transverse colon, the spleen, and the tail of the pancreas are within the peritoneal cavity. Thus, there are subtle differences between lateral retroperitoneal approaches and MVR. The descending colon and the left kidney are not mobilized in classical retroperitoneal exposures, whereas the colon is in MVR, and the left kidney may be. The kidney may be left in situ or mobilized because of anatomy or operative needs (Figure 6–4).

The parietal peritoneum is separated by a fascial cleft from the transversalis fascia. This cleft is attenuated under the surface of the diaphragm, explaining the difficulty in mobilizing that area, especially around the spleen, and remaining in the same plane as the rest of the exposure obtained with MVR and retroperitoneal dissections.

Exposure of the suprarenal aorta and the renal arteries through an infracolic approach is enhanced by division of the crura of the diaphragm. Both crura arise much further down the lumbar spine than is readily apparent or appreciated. The renal arteries arise most usually at the level of the L1-L2 disc space. The right crus arises from L1-L3 and the left crus from L1-L2. They may be palpated along the aorta at 4–5 o'clock on the patient's left and 7–8 o'clock on the right; they are tight musculotendinous bands. Cutting them above the renal arteries make suprarenal clamping and handling far easier. That maneuver gives the surgeon another 1-2 cm of proximal exposure (Figure 6–5).

The left renal vein may be effaced on the aneurysm and may need to be divided. That decision to divide the left renal vein should be made prior to sacrificing the adrenal, gonadal, or lumbar venous tributaries of the left renal vein. Such division in these elderly patients is associated with increased pulmonary complications and postoperative renal

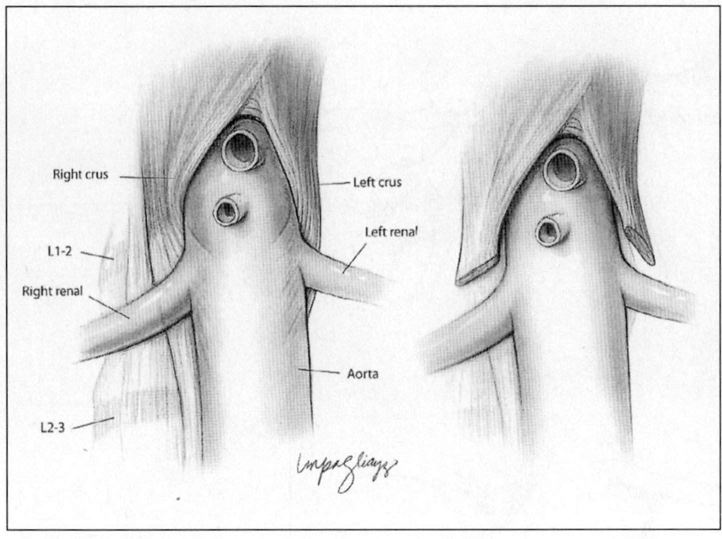

Figure 6-5. Division of Crura.

insufficiency, and should be utilized only if absolutely necessary. The vein may be re-anastomosed to avoid those increases in morbidity (Figures 6–6, 6–7, and 6–8).

Lateral retoperitoneal and thoracoretroperitoneal approaches may extend as high as T8-T12. Some authors have defined thoracoabdominal incisions as those involving T10 or higher.[3] Classically, thoracoretroperitoneal (Pillsbury) incisions are performed with the hips as flat as possible, that is, with the patient torqued. Thoracoabdominal incisions utilize a full decubitus approach with the hips as well as the trunk turned (Figure 6–9).

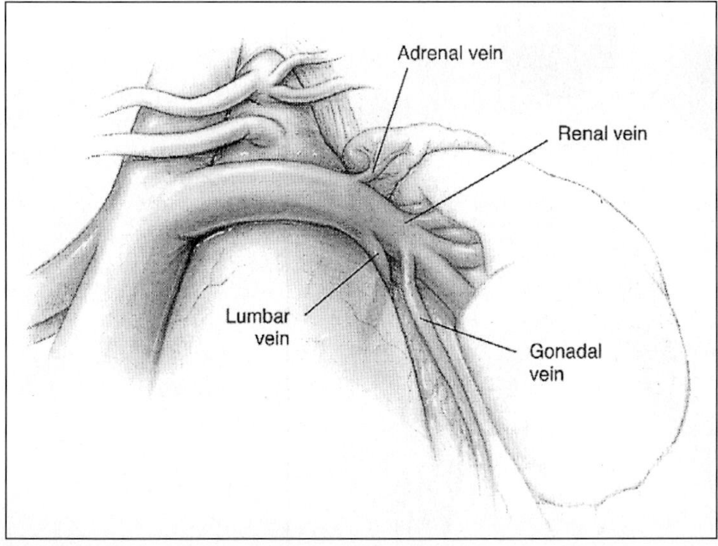

Figure 6-6. Left renal vein tributaries.

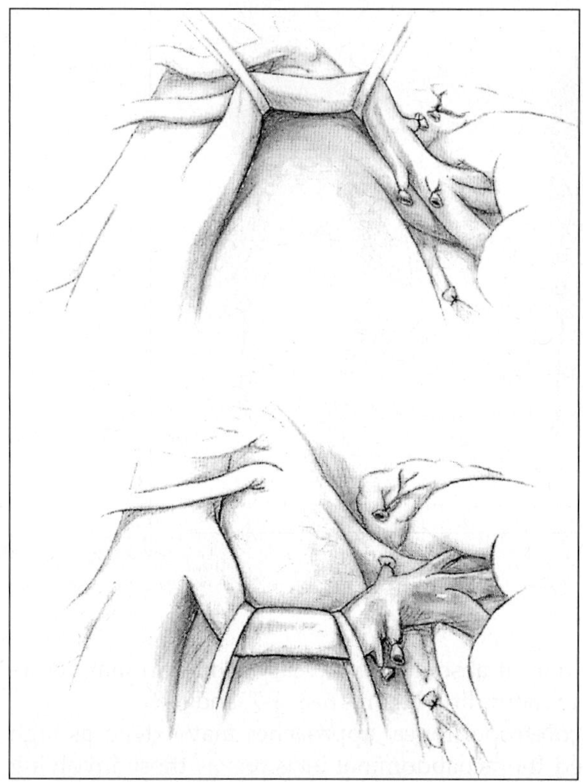

Figure 6-7. Left renal vein retraction

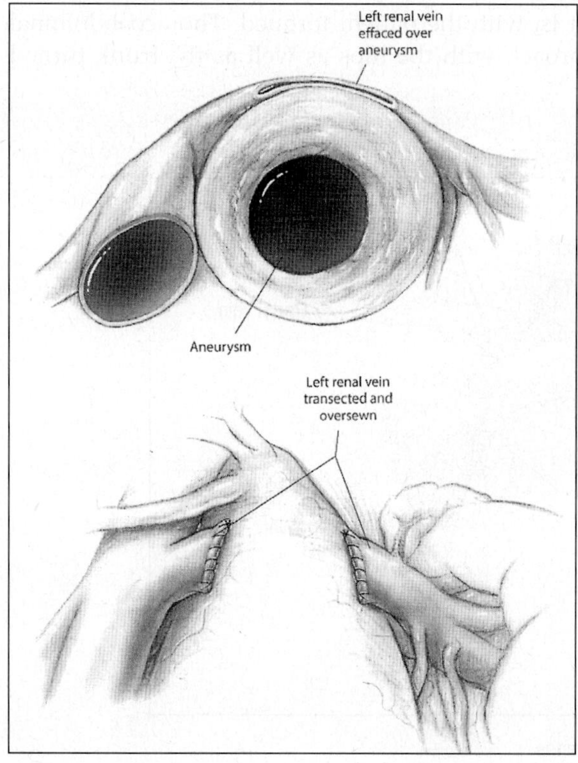

Figure 6-8. Left renal vein division.

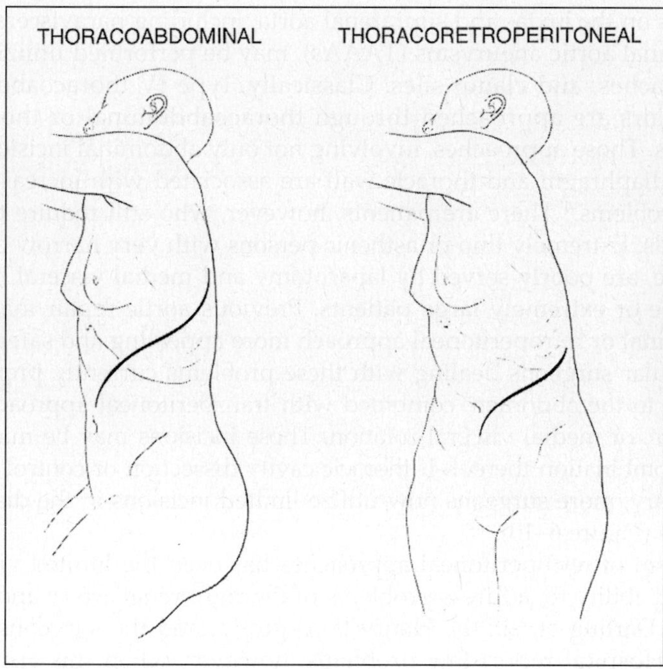

Figure 6-9. Thoracoabdominal and Thoracoretroperitoneal positioning

Dependent on the operation planned, the left kidney may be mobilized anteriorly or left in situ with either retroperitoneal or visceral rotation exposures. With an anterior left renal vein, anterior mobilization is helpful. The lumbar tributary must be divided and ligated. In the presence of a posterior left renal vein, a better exposure is obtained leaving the kidney in its bed. If adjunctive reconstruction of the superior mesenteric artery is necessary to the aneurysm repair, the kidney should be left in situ to allow the surgeon full lateral access to that artery.

TECHNIQUES

The crux of complex aortic surgery is the paravisceral aorta. The vascular surgeon must be able, with the least anatomic and physiologic trauma to the patient, to expose the celiac artery, the superior mesenteric artery, the renal arteries, and the corresponding proximal aortic segments to the extent that allows safe and complete performance of the planned operation.

The ability to access these areas, not so they are barely seen but are available to repair, is what allows safe upper abdominal aortic surgery. Furthermore, the choice of aortic clamp level, made preoperatively, is the single biggest determinant of success or failure. Moving the proximal clamp caudad during the course of the operation at planned stages is helpful, restoring arterial flow to the viscera and reducing cardiac afterload. Very much in contrast to that, moving the proximal clamp craniad during the operation is usually an indicator of an incorrectly chosen clamp site, and raises the likelihood of serious complications, usually atheroembolic, to the viscera.

Operations on the juxta- and suprarenal aorta, including paravisceral and Type IV thoracoabdominal aortic aneurysms (TAAAs), may be performed utilizing various incisions, approaches, and clamp sites. Classically, type IV thoracoabdominal aortic aneurysm repairs are approached through thoracoabdominal or thoracoretroperitoneal incisions. Those approaches, involving not only abdominal incisions but also incisions of the diaphragm and thoracic wall are associated with increased pulmonary and wound problems.[4] There are patients, however, who still require these more extensive methods. Extremely thin or asthenic persons with very narrow costal margins, as stated above, are poorly served by laparotomy and medial visceral rotation, as are morbidly obese or extremely large patients. Previous aortic repair may also make a thoracoabdominal or retroperitoneal approach more appealing and safer.

Most vascular surgeons dealing with these problems currently prefer to use incisions confined to the abdomen, combined with transperitoneal approaches, retroperitoneal exposure, or medial visceral rotation. Those incisions may be midline, traverse, oblique, or a combination thereof. If thoracic cavity dissection or control of the thoracic aorta is necessary, more surgeons now utilize limited incisions in the diaphragm to reduce morbidity (Figure 6–10).

The criticism of retroperitoneal approaches has been the limited visualization of, and the limited ability to, address problems of the right renal artery and the right iliac artery system. Darling et. al., the Henry Ford group, and the surgeons at Massachusetts General Hospital report few problems, however, when this approach is used preferentially and frequently.[3,5-7]

The operative results for pararenal aneurysm repair at large referral centeres are good to excellent, with mortality averaging approximately 5%. Qvarfordt et. al.

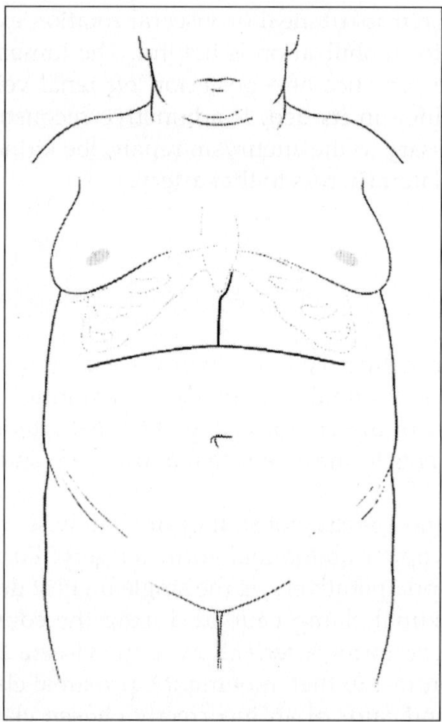

Figure 6-10. Subcostal incision with "T."

from the University of California–San Francisco (UC–SF) reported a 1.3% mortality for 77 patients, an even more salutary figure when one considers that 70% of those patients had concomitant renal artery reconstructions.[8] Allen and colleagues from Washington University–Barnes Hospital had a mortality of 1.5% in their patients and likewise reconstructed the renal arteries.[9] Jean-Claude et. al., continuing the work from UC–SF, reported a mortality of 5.8% in 257 patients.[10] Sarac and colleagues at the Cleveland Clinic reported a very similar mortality of 5.1% for 138 patients with juxtarenal aneurysms, contrasting with a mortality of 2.8% for their open infrarenal repairs.[2]

West et. al. from the Mayo Clinic, in their 2005 report on 247 pararenal aneurysm repairs, detailed a 30-day mortality of 2.8%, contrasting with their open infrarenal mortality of 1.1%.[11]

Shepard et. al., at the New England Medical Center, used an extended left lateral retroperitoneal exposure in 23 high-risk patients with abdominal aortic aneurysms, 14 of whom had pararenal occlusive and aneurysmal problems. There was only one death (4%).[6] Shepard and coworkers, continuing their work at Henry Ford Hospital, reported the same approach for 85 patients with complex occlusive and aneurysmal aortic problems. The elective mortality in their series was 2.4%.[7]

The series from UC–SF, Barnes, and Mayo are remarkable not only for the low mortality reported but also for their use of the supramesenteric clamp level, in addition to the suprarenal and supraceliac levels. None of these authors found any increase in morbidity or mortality with that clamp site.[8,9,11]

The incisions used are primarily surgeons' preference. All are used to good effect by their proponents and none has been shown to be superior or inferior to the others. The incision, approach, and clamp site are determined by the multiplicity of reasons mentioned in this chapter. Body habitus, previous operation, comorbidities (e.g., pulmonary disease), and the segment of aorta needing repair all impact on those decisions. The coexistence of aortic or branch vessel calcific and/or thrombotic occlusive disease is a huge factor in deciding the best operative plan.

Paravisceral aortic aneurysms may be exposed via MVR, laterlal retroperitoneal approach, or thoracoabdominal incisions. Body habitus is probably the key determinant here. These aneurysms are subtly different from Type IV TAAAs. The latter usually require separate proximal aortic and visceral anastomoses, whereas the former may be repaired utilizing one anastomosis involving the visceral origins and the aorta. Debranching for Type IV TAAAs has been described, but this author fails to see the benefit of that approach for a process confined entirely to the abdomen.

Supramesenteric aneurysms may be approached similarly, with MVR or lateral retroperitoneal exposure. Some, in thin patients, may be approached via an infracolic route. Clamp placement may be suprmesenteric or supraceliac. If an infracolic route is chosen, suprceliac clamping through the lesser omentum may be the best approach.

Suprarenal aneurysms may be approached by any of the above methods. Clamping may be at an interrenal, suprarenal, supramesenteric, or supraceliac level. For more proximal repairs, medial visceral rotation allows exposure of the entire abdominal aorta; this is our preferred approach for upper abdominal operations. West et. al. from Mayo, reporting on their 247 pararenal aneurysms (not including paravisceral aneurysms), used a midline transabdominal approach in 200 (81%), a midline approach with MVR in 30 (13%), a lateral retroperitoneal incision in 14 (6%), and a thoracoabdominal incision in 2 (0.8%).Clamp sites in that series were supraceliac in 34 (14%), supramesenteric in 49 (20%), and suprarenal in 164 (67%).[11]

COMPLICATIONS

All three methods of exposure—transperitoneal, retroperitoneal, and MVR—offer excellent choices for the correct patient populations. All are subject to complication. Thoracoabdominal incisions and oblique lateral oblique incisions are subject to flank herniation or laxity of the flank muscles because of division of the nerves. There is also the potential problem of costochondral pain or instability.[4,7] Splenic and renal injury is more likely to occur with either MVR or a lateral retroperitoneal exposure than with a transperitoneal approach.

Of most importance is the choice of the proximal aortic clamp site. It is on this issue that success or failure hinges. Crawford preferred supraceliac clamping and used it almost exclusively.[12] As stated previously, the surgeons at UC–SF, Washington University–Barnes, and Mayo applied clamps at suprarenal, supramesenteric, and supraceliac sites. West and colleagues reported an association of supraceliac clamping with renal insufficiency and visceral ischemia, but like the other two studies, found no increase in mortality.[8,9,11] In contrast to those findings, Green et. al. from the University of Rochester reported a 10-fold higher mortality with suprarenal clamps, 32%, in comparison to a 3% mortality for supraceliac clamping, and a sevenfold increase in frank renal failure with suprarenal clamping. Eleven patients included in that suprarenal group were initially clamped at the infrarenal level, and the clamp level changed during the course of the operations.[13] That fact underscores the absolute necessity for precise judgment in choosing the proximal aortic clamp site preoperatively. That judgment is much easier in 2007 with CTA than it was at the time of that report.

Renal artery atheroembolization is the most feared sequela of improper clamp placement; it was felt by Green et. al. to account for their poor results with suprarenal clamping.[13] The group from Mayo felt they had more problems with the supraceliac clamp, with three of their six deaths thought to be secondary to mesenteric embolization or thrombosis.[11] Jean-Claude et. al. from UC–SF, attributed six of their 15 deaths (40%) to visceral ischemia or infarction; atheroembolization was thought to be responsible in five of those six patients.[10] Like the authors from Mayo, they found that atheroembolization was more likely with supraceliac clamping or supramesenteric clamping than with suprarenal clamping (9.1, 6.3, and 0.6% respectively). Similarly, Sarac and colleagues from the Cleveland Clinic found supraceliac clamping more problematic than suprarenal clamping.[2]

Cardiac disease, of course, remains a primary cause of perioperative morbidity and mortality. However, in that large group of patients from the Mayo Clinic, the most common complication was renal insuffiency in 54 patients (22%), followed by pulmonary complications in 38 (16%), and myocardial infarction in 32 (13%).[11]

In most series, renal insufficiency is indeed the leading complication of juxtarenal aortic operations; it is certainly the most analyzed and the most feared. It was the leading complication in the majority of the series cited with transient rises of serum creatinine in 12.3–30.4% of patients, and led to the need for new dialysis in 0–28.3% of patients.[2,4-11] In the Mayo Clinic series, no patients required new onset permanent dialysis, however. Preoperative renal dysfunction is felt by most to be the best predictor of postoperative renal dysfunction, but others have not been able to demonstrate that association. Concomitant renal artery operations are felt by several groups to be a major cause of renal insufficiency, whereas others feel that attention to renal artery disease improves results(16) (15) Mayo. Jean-Claude and colleagues also found statistical correlation with crossclamp time. Seventy-five percent of their patients improved; they felt acute tubular necrosis and not atheroembolization was the disease mechanism.[10] On the other hand, the group from Barnes found no correlation between crossclamp time and renal insufficiency.[9]

Shepard et. al. use hypothermic renal perfusion, as does the group at Barnes.[7,9] We also prefer its use. Some surgeons at our institution use a continuous drip, while others perfuse the kidneys with boluses of ice-cold heparinized saline on a periodic basis such as every 15 minutes.

Renal dysfunction may, therefore, safely be said to result from any one or combination of the following: prolonged ischemia, embolization, renal artery occlusive disease, artery or graft thrombosis, hypovolemia, hypoperfusion and shock, reperfusion, or multisystem organ failure with its cytokine response. Renal failure is more likely with proximal aortic repair, known renal insufficiency, intraoperative complications, especially hemorrhage, and comorbidities including cardiac disease and diabetes.

All things considered, renal ischemic issues relate most probably to the patient's preoperative renal and cardiac status; renovascular disease; the site, sequence, and time of crossclamping; and the patient's hemodynamic status intraoperatively. Hydration, preoperatively as well as intraoperatively, with determination and maintenance of the patient's best hemodynamic parameters and appropriate fluid and blood replacement during the operation, are essential to lessening the incidence of renal insufficiency. Pulmonary artery catheters should be used in all patients undergoing complex aortic reconstructions. Transesophageal echocardiography may be added to those patients with known cardiac disease, though we used few in our series from Mayo. Lasix and mannitol are used to induce diuresis prior to clamping. Mannitol is also given to decrease renovascular resistance and provide free radical scavenging. It also increases the glomerular filtration rate during periods of hypoperfusion. Vasodilators are given prior to clamping. Many surgeons, ourselves included, favor the use of intraoperative dopamine in low doses for its dopaminergic type 1 effects, despite the lack of level 1 evidence. Heparin is, of course, used for these repairs.

In regard to intraoperative cardiac function, there may be real benefit in applying a supramesenteric rather than a supraceliac clamp if the anatomy will allow. Jean-Claude et. al. have pointed out that they had only one death from myocardial infarction in their series of 257 patients.[10] The increased stress on the heart seen with supraceliac clamping is mitigated in part by supramessenteric clamping, allowing afterload reduction through the mesenteric circulation.

Pulmonary dysfunction is another frequent and serious complication of complex pararenal aortic reconstructions. In the UC–SF review of their 108 operations with MVR, 31% of patients had pulmonary complications.[4] Postoperative pulmonary failure is the most commonly seen complication at UC–SF, Barnes, and the Henry Ford hospital, and the second leading complication in the Mayo Clinic series.[7,9-11] Renal failure, of course, compounds the issue, often leading to prolonged intubation.

Pulmonary insufficiency is much more likely with a thoracoabdominal incision than it is with a purely abdominal approach.[4] Patients known preoperatively to have chronic obstructive pulmonary disease (COPD) may be pretreated with mechanical pulmonary toilet and/or steroids if the latter have been shown to be helpful on preoperative pulmonary function testing. Transverse abdominal incisions, postoperative epidural analgesia, and retroperitoneal exposures are all thought to benefit patients with COPD, and are used preferentially for patients with known pulmonary compromise.

Gastrointestinal complications after pararenal abdominal aortic surgery occur less frequently than either renal or pulmonary complications. Two notable exceptions are the reports from UC–SF in which visceral ischemia was the cause of death in 40% of their mortality, and the report from the Mayo Clinic, in which three of their six deaths were attributed to mesenteric ischemia.[10,11] Careful attention preoperatively to all of the mesenteric circulation, including the inferior mesenteric artery and the hypogastric arteries, is important.

The group at Parkland Hospital looked at pancreatitis following aortic reconstructions.[14] They found that 1.8% of their patients undergoing aortic reconstructions of all types experienced pancreatitis. None died. These patients were approached from a transperitoneal infracolic route. Reilly et. al. reported pancreatitis in six (6.8%) of their 88 patients undergoing MVR and suprarenal clamping, and two of those six died of pancreatitis.[4] It is probable that the combination of ischemia and local trauma attendant to MVR (from dissection, mobilization, and retraction) is responsible for that difference.

Splenic injury with its usual sequela, splenectomy, is reported for both retroperitoneal exposure and MVR.[4,7] Anecdotally, it occurs occasionally with a transperitoneal infracolic approach.

End-organ failure, and especially hepatic failure, is seen with supraceliac clamping, and is related directly to ischemia time. Patients with hepatic dysfunction, cirrhosis, or hepatitis are particularly susceptible to ischemic liver failure. Selective mesenteric shunting is appropriate for patients with types I to III TAAAs but is not entirely applicable for patients with pararenal aneurysms (33). Ballard has developed a trifurcated graft technique, with separate grafts to branch vessels in addition to the aortic replacement graft, to reduce ischemic time (34). His principle may be useful for patients with known liver or renal dysfunction if prolonged supraceliac clamping is anticipated.[15] This author has found it a useful technique.

Pseudoaneurysm, or anastomotic aneurysm, is the most common long-term problem with aortic grafts, occurring in approximately 4–10% of patients (35). When an aggressive follow-up protocol utilizing new imaging modalities is utilized, the prevalence of anastomotic aneurysms may be higher than has been suspected.

The repair of recurrent juxtarenal aneurysms is attended by higher morbidity and mortality than is primary reconstruction.

CONCLUSIONS

Successful operation on complex aneurysms of the pararenal and paravisceral aorta requires thoughtful preoperative assessment, planning, and execution. Accurate preoperative assessment of the upper abdominal aorta and the branch vessel anatomy, including the extent and type of of associated aortic and visceral artery atherosclerosis, by CTA is the single most important aspect of preoperative care.

Studies cited above from centers with real and sustained expertise in aortic surgery reveal that these aneurysms may be repaired conventionally with a mortality of 3–5%.

The site, sequence, and timing of aortic and branch vessel clamping is the prime determinant of success or failure. The different incisions and approaches discussed above may all be utilized to achieve excellent results. Surgeon preference, the extent of aneurysmal and occlusive disease, the patient's body habitus, and comorbidities are all factors in that decision process.

Renal, pulmonary, mesenteric, and cardiac problems are the most serious and feared of the complications of complex aortic surgery, but the incidence of each may be minimized by attention to pre-, intra-, and postoperative care.

The number of open repairs for infrarenal aortic aneurysms is in decline. Training the next generation of vascular surgeons to operate on these complex aortic aneurysms, certainly a more challenging task than infrarenal repair, not just to maintain the excellent results currently obtained but to improve on them, is problematic, and deserves the attention of vascular surgery leaders.

REFERENCES

1. Taylor SM, Mills JL, Fujitani RM. The juxtarenal abdominal aortic aneurysm. *Arch Surg* 1994; 129:734737.
2. Sarac TP, Clair DG, Hertzer NR, et al. Contemporary results of juxtarenal aneurysm repair. *J Vasc Surg* 2002; 36: 1 1041 11 1.
3. Clouse WD and Cambria RP. Complex aortic aneurysm: pararenal, suprarenal, and thoracoabdominal. In: Hallett JW, Mills JL, Earnshaw JJ, Reekers JA, eds, *Comprehensive Vascular and Endovascular Surgery*. New York, New York: Mosby, 2004: 445–478.
4. Reilly LM, Ramos TK, Murray SP, et al. Optimal exposure of the proximal abdominal aorta: A critical appraisal of transabdominal medial visceral rotation. *J Vasc Surg* 1994; 19:375–390.
5. Darling RC III, Shah DM, Chang BB, et al. Retroperitoneal approach for bilateral renal and visceral artery revascularization. *Am J of Surg* 1994; 168 (2): 148–151.
6. Shepard AD, Scott GR, Mackey WC, et al. Retroperitoneal approach to high-risk abdominal aortic aneurysms. *Arch Surg* 1986; 121: 444–448.
7. Shepard AD, Tollefson DF, Reddey DJ, et al. Left flank retroperitoneal exposure: a technical aid to complex aortic reconstruction. *J Vasc Surg* 1991; 14: 283–291
8. Qvarfordt PC, Stoney RJ, Reilly LM, et al. Management of pararenal aneurysm of the abdominal aorta. *J Vasc Surg* 1986; 3: 84–93
9. Allen BT, Anderson CB, Rubin BG, et al. Preservation of renal function in juxtarenal and suprarenal abdominal aortic aneurysm repair. *J Vasc Surg* 1993; 17: 944–959.
10. Jean-Claude JM, Reilly LM, Stoney RJ, Messina LM. Pararenal aortic aneurysms: the future of open aortic aneurysm repair. *J Vasc Surg* 1999; 29: 902–912.
11. West CA, Noel AA, Bower TC, et al. Factors affecting outcome of open surgical repair of pararenal aortic aneurysms: a 10-year experience. *J Vasc Surg* 2006; 43: 921–927
12. Crawford ES, Beckett WC, Greer MS. Juxtarenal infrarenal abdominal aortic aneurysm. Special diagnostic and therapeutic considerations. *Ann Surg* 1986; 203:661–670.
13. Green RM, Ricotta JJ, Ouriel K, DeWeese JA. Results of supraceliac aortic clamping in the difficult elective resection of infrarenal abdominal aortic aneurysm. *J Vasc Surg* 1989; 9: 124–134.
14. Burkey SH, Valentine RJ, Jackson MR, et al. Acute pancreatitis after abdominal vascular surgery. *J Am Coll Surg* 2000; 191:373–380.
15. Ballard JL. Thoracoabdominal aortic aneurysm repair with sequential visceral perfusion: A technical note. *Ann Vasc Surg* 1999; 13:21&221.

7

Minimal Incision Aortic Surgery (MIAS)

William D. Turnipseed, MD

Until the introduction of catheter based alternatives for treatment of aortic aneurysms and iliac occlusive disease, most efforts to improve the safety and efficiency of aortic surgery were directed towards improving perioperative care and the development of postoperative clinical pathways. The rapid growth and development of endovascular stent graft technology and improvements in vascular imaging techniques used for the selection and surveillance of patients treated with endografts have generated great enthusiasm for less invasive means of treating aortic disease. This enthusiasm had been fueled by Phase II clinical trials in our country demonstrating morbidity and mortality statistics that rival those well accepted for standard open aortic repair.[1-2] However, recently published information regarding the mid-term performance of endovascular devices suggests that there are predictable patterns of failure, which may not become apparent for up to twenty-four months after implantation. These observations have caused even the most enthusiastic proponents of endovascular therapy to: reemphasize the need for life long CAT scan surveillance of patients currently treated with stent endografts, and to call for judicious selection of patients to be treated.[3-7]

Uncertainty, regarding the durability of currently available endoaortic devices in this country has stimulated a small number of vascular surgeons to address the question whether alternative technologies or procedural modifications might be possible so as to: improve patient satisfaction; shorten hospital stay; reduce health care cost; yet maintain quality outcomes. The purpose of this article is to evaluate the clinical and economic impact of using alternative less invasive techniques for aortic repair.

Until Parodiís introduction of endoaortic stent grafts, the only significant procedural change directed towards improving recovery from aortic surgery was the retroperitoneal aortic exposure.[8] This technique modification effectively reduced postoperative ileus and seemed to enhance recovery of patients with chronic respiratory problems. Despite apparent benefits, few surgeons routinely employ the retroperitoneal approach for treatment of aortic aneurysms and iliac occlusive disease because of the extensive dissection and retraction requirements and because of limited access to the visceral arteries and or contralateral pelvic vessels in patients with complex iliac and aortic disease. One of the more innovative concepts to be introduced since the development of the retroperitoneal exposure has been laparoscopically assisted aortic surgery. Video assisted techniques in general surgery have rapidly developed because of electrocautery and auto suture devices which have enabled effective hemostasis and the ability to easily perform gastrointestinal anastomoses. Unfortunately, application of laparoscopic techniques to abdominal vascular surgery has been less effective. Although, current instrumentation can be useful for dissection and exposure of the aorta, auto suture devices for performing vascular anastomoses have not been perfected. As a result, intraperitoneal hand sewn anastomoses performed through a laparoscope are extremely tedious and require high technical skill levels. This critical shortcoming has in part been overcome by the use of a small midline periumbilical abdominal incision, which allows direct access to the dissected aorta and direct suture techniques to be used for arterial anastomoses. One of the first published reports of laparoscopically assisted open aortic aneurysm repair was made by Klein & Cohen et al. in 1998.[9] Aortic dissection was performed through multi port laparoscopy and a traditional open graft repair was performed through a small laparotomy incision. Successful repair was accomplished in eighteen of twenty consecutive patients. The majority of patients were fed clear liquids on the second postoperative day, and hospital length of stay reduced from 10 to 5.8 days. There were no perioperative deaths and the major complication rate was 28%. This clinical study demonstrated that laparoscopically assisted aortic surgery was technically feasible and that a reproducible, less invasive approach for treatment of elective aneurysms could be developed. The authors concluded that minimal small bowel manipulation and the smaller abdominal incision accounted for most of the observed improvements in patient recovery. Since this report, there has been increasing interest in the use of video assisted techniques in aortic surgery. Castronuovo and Edoga have developed a retroperitoneal gas insufflation technique, for aortic exposure.[10-11] Video assisted aortic cross-clamping, autosuture occlusion of the common iliac arteries, opening of the aortic sac, control of back-bleeding lumbar vessels, and proximal aortic anastomosis are performed in the gas environment. Retroperitoneal or femoral incisions are used for open exposure of the common iliac or femoral arteries depending on the preferred site for distal graft anastomoses. Although, total procedural times are quite long (460 minutes), significant reductions in ICU stay, hospital length of stay, and return to oral feeding have been achieved. Perioperative mortality was 10%, and associated major morbidity 25%. More recent clinical outcome data from these authors suggest that further improvement may be possible as experience with this technique increases. Dion has confirmed biological stress reduction using a closed laparoscopic technique for repair of aortoiliac occlusive disease.[12] More recently, Alimi has documented reduced hospital stay and resource utilization for patients treated with transperitoneal laparoscopically assisted open aneurysm repair.[13] Despite the fact that laparoscopically assisted aortic repair techniques may reduce hospital stay and facilitate patient recovery; until dependable auto suture devices which are capable of securely bonding prosthetic graft material to host aortic wall become available, this approach will remain a treatment option used by only the most skilled laparoscopic surgeons for the elective treatment of low to moderate risk patients who can tolerate long periods of anesthesia.

Shortly after the publication of the Kline/Cohen article,[9] I became intrigued with the possibility of performing aortic repairs through a mini laparotomy incision without the use of laparoscopic aortic dissection. The major problem with a small abdominal incision is maintaining an uncluttered surgical field within which to work. Trial and error has resulted in the use of a very simple collection of surgical tools that makes the minimal incision aortic approach possible. These include: the Bookwalter retractor, Cosgrove vascular clamps, the Fish abdominal closure pad, and long surgical instrumentation. The use of the small midline periumbilical incision offers the surgeon flexibility to easily expand the incision should more exposure or open conversion be necessary. The Bookwalter retractor and Cosgrove vascular clamps are useful because vertical instrument clutter in the surgical field can be eliminated. After making a small midline incision, the left hand is inserted into the abdomen and the small bowel finger manipulated to the right of abdominal aorta. The Fish abdominal closure pad is then scrolled and inserted into the abdomen, to the right of the aorta, then allowed to expand vertically, acting as a semi-rigid retaining wall that keeps the small bowel out of the surgical field. The long instrumentation allows the surgeon to work at or above the level of the abdominal wall. Exposure of the aorta is achieved with the use of electrocautery and sharp dissection. When the patient is adequately relaxed, the abdominal wall and its incision can be moved caudad and cephalad to facilitate exposure of the aortic neck, and the bifurcation distally. Once the patient has been anti-coagulated and the aorta cross-clamped, the aneurysm is opened and its clotted contents removed. Decompression of the aneurysm affords plenty of workroom to complete the arterial reconstruction. A small butterfly retractor can be inserted into the aneurysm sac which facilitates exposure of back bleeding lumbar vessels and provides clear visualization of the proximal and distal anastomotic sites. Aortic anastomoses are performed using 2-0 Prolene. Anastomoses distal to the aortic bifurcation can be easily performed to level of the mid-common iliac artery. However, when complex pelvic disease is present, it is easier to ligate the iliac arteries and to tunnel a bifurcation graft into the groin and perform distal anastomoses at the common femoral artery level. Wound closure is performed with absorbable sutures. Epidural anesthesia is not routinely used for postoperative pain control because it restricts early patient mobility and the removal of Foley catheters. At the termination of the procedure 0.5% Marcaine is injected into the abdominal incision and intravenous PCA anesthesia is used for 24-48 hours postoperatively. The patients are extubated in operating room, nasogastric tubes removed in recovery or on rounds the first postoperative day and patients are usually started on p.o. fluids the first day after surgery. Regular diets are started on the second or third day. The average hospital length of stay from uncomplicated patients treated with the MIAS procedure is 3.1 days.

Over the past three years, minimal incision aortic surgery (MIAS) has been used at the University of Wisconsin for the elective treatment of patients with infrarenal aortic aneurysms and aortoiliac occlusive disease.[14] There has been no effort to select MIAS candidates based on risk category, body weight, or aneurysm size. Exclusion criteria have included ruptured aneurysms, suprarenal and pararenal aneurysms, and patients with aneurysm aortoiliac occlusive disease that might require concomitant renal mesenteric, or infrainguinal vascular reconstruction. Individuals that were candidates for endoaortic grafting or MIAS had both procedures explained and patients were allowed to select one over the other. Clinical outcome for patients treated with MIAS were compared with the results of standard open aortic surgery performed by surgeons in our clinical group that had not adopted the MIAS technique and to endoaortic repair as well. The open surgical repair included both retroperitoneal incisions and use of long midline abdominal incisions and extra cavitary small bowel retraction. Postoperative management was standardized by care pathways. Demographics for the MIAS, standard, and endovascular repairs were compared. Outcome analysis included: OR time, intraoperative fluid resuscitation, transfusion requirements, ICU stay, time to general dietary feeding, hospital length of stay, as well as morbidity, mortality, and total hospital cost. Patient demographics were compared with a Fisher's Exact Test. Operative parameters were compared with a two-tailed student T-test, performed on NSTAT software. Average time interval to regular diet, ICU stay and length of hospital stay were compared using the Wilcoxan Rank/Sum Test. Other analysis were performed using SAS statistical software (SAS Institute Inc.). The data analyzed by students T-test considered p-valves less than 0.05 to be significant.

Medical hospital reimbursement recorded as Total Standard Cost per patient for the principle diagnosis of unruptured abdominal aortic aneurysm (ICD-9 #444.1) was calculated based on metric mean length of stay, which is a statistically adjusted value for all cases of a given DRG (110, 111 = AAA with or without complications). Cost data was provided by the University Health System Consortium, which is the national agency that provides cost-related data for all major university health care providers in the United States. Cost determination (Total Direct and Indirect Cost) for patient populations, is built from costs of individual encouters; cost of an individual patient encounter is estimated from the sum of costs assigned to each billable item or service that the patient received during the stay. Our total actual cost is an approximate measure of fully allocated costs of providing services to patients including all direct costs of care (patient care staff, disposable medical supplies, drugs, medical equipment) plus an allocation of indirect or support costs (administration, medical records, information systems, facility cost such as building depreciation and utilities, etc.) Actual direct cost plus actual indirect cost equals actual total cost. Net hospital revenue is a product of the total hospital reimbursement minus the total actual cost per patient.

There was no significant difference between MIAS, standard repair, and endoaortic repair with regards to age, gender distribution, aneurysms size or body weight. Comorbid risk factors were similar between comparison groups (Table 7–1). Tube graft repairs were more prevalent in the MIAS and standard repair groups where as, bifurcated stent grafts were used in all endoaortic repairs. Surgical exposure of the common femoral arteries was required more commonly in the MIAS and endoaortic groups than in standard open repair. Although, procedural times tended to be longer for the

TABLE 7-1. PROSPECTIVE NON-RANDOMIZED STUDY DEMOGRAPHICS

	MIAS	Std. Open Repair	Endo Repair
#PTS. Age (yrs.)	65±10	67±12	71 (+/−) 9.8)
SEX Male	57	61	30
Female	23	19	2
AAA SIZE (cm)	4.0-8.2	4.2-9.0	(4.5-8.4)
Median	5.7	6.2	6.2
BODY WT (kg)	52-110	60-105	(70-150)
Median	87.5	85.0	91.9
COMORBID RISKS			
CAD	52%	33%	72%
HBP	70%	67%	38%
AODM	9%	10%	28%
COPD	26%	24%	44%
PREV. ABD. SURG	20%	24%	12%

TABLE 7-2. PROSPECTIVE NON-RANDOMIZED STUDY RESULTS

	MIAS	Std. Open Repair	Endo Repair
INTRAOPERATIVE			
OR TIME (min)	157±37	200±44	257 ± 44
IV FLUID (cc)	4375±1583	5304±2433	3483 ± 1562
TRANSFUSION (units)	1.1±1.3	1.7±2.0	1.0 ± 0.7
POSTOPERATIVE			
*ICU STAY (days)	1.0±1.2	3.0±3.5	1.1 ±0.7
*POSTOP GEN. DIET (days)	3.4±1.2	5.4±4.7	2.0 ± 0.5
*TOTAL LOS (days)	4.1±1.4	7.2±3.4	4.3 ± 3.7
	[3.1]	[5.8]	[3.0]
MORBIDITY	15%	26%	19%
MAJOR COMPLICATIONS			
ILEUS	(2)	(6)	(2)
↑VENT. ASSIST.	(1)	(5)	(1)
WOUND COMP,	(1)	(1)	(2)
LEG EMBOLUS	(1)	(-)	(3)
Mortality	1.3%†	2.5%*	3%*

* = p≤0.001
[ ] = uncomplicated recovery
† = myocardial infarct

endograft repair, there was no significant difference in operating room time between the three groups (157 +/− 37 Min = MIAS, 257 +/− 93 = endograft, 190 +/− Min = 64 standard repair). Furthermore, there was no significant difference in intraoperative fluid use or transfusion requirements between treatment groups. Blood transfusion was based on calculated loss. Auto transfusion was used in the MIAS and standard repair group. ICU stay, return full general dietary feeding, and hospital length of stay for the MIAS and endoaortic techniques were significantly lower than those in the standard open repair group. Morbidity and mortality rates; however, were not significantly different in the three groups (Table 7–2). Total standard cost was lowest for the MIAS procedure and highest for the endoaortic repair technique, despite the fact that, ICU utilization and hospital length of stay were comparable for both methods of aortic repair. This discrepancy is explained by increased direct costs incurred in the operating room because of stent graft delivery systems and imaging requirements. Our hospital recognized a greater net profit for the MIAS procedure than for standard open repair because of reduced resource utilization and reduced hospital length of stay (Table 7–3).

Although, there is little question that endovascular stents will prevail as an option for the repair of aortic aneurysms, mid-term performance standards have not matched expectations, and give rise to concern about the durability of currently available device technology. Until long term efficiency and durability of endoaortic repair techniques can be clearly established it seems logical that an array of alternative, less invasive procedures for treatment of abdominal aneurysm and aortic occlusive disease would be in the patient's best interest. Currently, the major advantages MIAS has over video assisted techniques are that: laparoscopic surgical skills and equipment are not

TABLE 7-3. PROSPECTIVE NON-RANDOMIZED STUDY FISCAL ANALYSIS (UW HOSPITAL)

	MIAS	Std. Open Repair
HOSPITAL REIMBURSEMENT	$20,879	$22,621
TOTAL STANDARD COST	$13,731	$17,751
OR COST	$3,036	$3,431
NET HOSPITAL REVENUE	$7,148	$4,870
		p=0.0326

	MIAS	Endoaortic Repair
HOSPITAL REIMBURSEMENT	$20,879	$24,777
TOTAL STANDARD COST	$13,731	$32,040
OR COST	$3,036	$24,562
NET HOSPITAL REVENUE	+$7,148	−$,7,263
		p=0,0001

required; anastomoses are easier to perform; and surgical times are significantly shorter. The major advantages of the MIAS procedure over endovascular stent graft repair are that; that fewer patients are rejected because of vessel morphology, or limited device availability; that advanced catheter management skills as well as expensive imaging and device delivery accessories are not required; and that less economic stress is exerted on hospital resources. When compared to the standard open aortic repair group, all of the less invasive alternatives have reduced postoperative morbidity, and shortened hospital stay, but not significantly changed mortality statistics.

REFERENCES

1. Zarins CK, White RA, Schwarten D. AnwuRx stent graft versus open surgical repair of abdominal aortic aneurysms: Multicenter prospective clinical trial. *J Vase Surg.* 1999;29(2): 292–305.
2. Moore WS, Rutherford RB. Transfemoral endovascular repari of abdominalaorti aneurysm: results of the North American EVT phase 1 trial. *J Vase Surg.* 1996;23:543–553.
3. Bush RL, Lumsden AB, Dodson TF. Midterm results after endovascular repair of the abdominal aortic aneurysm. *J Vase Surg.* 2001;33(2):S70–S76.
4. Holzenbein TJ, Kretschmer G, Thurnher S. Midterm durability of abdominal aortic aneurysm endograft repair: A word of caution. *J Vasc Surg.* 2001;33(2):S46–S54.
5. Beebe HG, Cronenwett JL, Katzen BT. Results of an aortic endograft trial: Impact of device failure beyond 12 months. *J Vase Surg.* 2001;33(2):S55–S63.
6. Moore WS, Brewster DC, Bernhard VM. Aorto-uni-iliac endograft for complex aortoilia aneurysms compared with tube/bifurcation endografts: Results of the EVT/Guidant trials, *J Vase Surg.* 2001;33(2)S11–S20.
7. Makaroun MS. The Ancure endografting system: An update. *J Vasc Surg.* 2001;33(2): S129–S134.
8. Parodi JC. Endovascular repair of abdominal aortic aneurysm and other arterial lesions. *J Vase Surg.* 1995;21(4)549–555.
9. Kline RG, D, Angelo AJ, Chen MHM. Laparoscopically assisted abdominal aortic aneurysm repair: First 20 cases. *J Vase Surg.* 1998;27(l):81–88.

10. Castronuove Jr JJ, James KV, Resnikoff M. Laparoscopic- assisted abdominal aortic aneurys-mectomy. *J Vase Surg.* 2000;32(2):224–233.
11. Edoga J K, Asgarian K, Singh D et al. Laparoscopic surgery for abdominal aortic aneurysms. *Surg Endosc.* 1998;12:1064–1072.
12. Dion YM, Gracia CR. A new technique for laparoscopic aortobifemoral grafting in occlusive aortoiliac disease. *J Vasc Surg.* 1997;26:685–692.
13. Alimi YS, Hartung O, Valerio N. Laparoscopic aortoiliac surgery for aneurysm and occlusive disease: When should a minilaparotomy be performed? *J Vase Surg.* 2001;33(3):469–480.
14. Tunipseed WD. A less invasive minilaparotomy techniques for repair of aortic aneurysm and occlusive disease. *J Vase Surg.* 2001;33(2):431–434.

Open Surgical Treatment of Thoracoabdominal Aortic Aneurysms

8

Open Surgical Treatment of Thoracoabdominal Aortic Aneurysms

Anthony L. Estrera M.D., M.D., Tam T. T. Huynh, M.D., Charles C. Miller, III, Ph.D., and Hazim J. Safi, M.D.

Repair of thoracic aortic aneurysm is a major challenge for the aortic surgeon. Since its inception, the repair of thoracic aortic aneurysm has been plagued with a major complications; one of the most catastrophic events is paralysis or paraparesis from the waist down. Because of these fearsome complications, many methods have been implemented in attempts to protect the spinal cord. In the beginning, a shunt was employed from the subclavian artery or ascending aorta into the infrarenal aorta while the repair of the descending thoracic aorta or the thoracoabdominal aorta was being performed.[1] A Dacron graft was used in the descending to infrarenal and sequentially bypassing the celiac axis, superior mesenteric, and both renal arteries, as described in the early 1950s, to lessen the ischemic time to end-organs, the bowels, the liver, stomach, and kidneys.[2] Regional hypothermia to the spinal cord, as well as systemic profound hypothermia, have been applied to thoracoabdominal aneurysm repairs but have been associated with complications of bleeding, prolonged operative time, stroke, and temporary neurological deficits. Cerebrospinal drainage alone was used in the early period as was left heart bypass with variable success.[3-4]

In the last decade and a half, we settled on the adjunct consisting of three elements: distal aortic perfusion, in which oxygenated blood is taken from the left atrium directly to the femoral artery via the left lower pulmonary vein using the centrifugal pump; cerebrospinal fluid drainage; and moderate passive hypothermia in which core temperature is allowed to drift to 33–34°C. We have employed this method to protect the spinal cord and the descending thoracic aortic aneurysm as well as the thoracoabdominal aorta since 1992. We chose this avenue based on a study that showed a great impact of protecting the spinal cord by using these three modalities.[5]

In this chapter, the adjunct refers to the combination of distal aortic perfusion as described above, cerebrospinal drainage, and moderate hypothermia. We refer to them as a single adjunct because the emergent protective effect of these three elements, when used together, is greater than their individual efficacies. We also will report on our experience with repairs of the descending thoracic and the thoracoabdominal aorta. We will mention briefly our experience with repairs of extensive aneurysms of the aorta that includes the ascending, transverse arch, and thoracoabdominal aorta or descending thoracic aorta with special emphasis on second-stage repair. The ascending aorta and transverse arch will not be included in this chapter because it is beyond the scope of this report.

Currently, there is a vascular revolution happening with regard to the vascular management of aortic aneurysm, the infrarenal abdominal aorta, the descending thoracic aorta, the abdominal aorta with involvement of the celiac axis, and superior mesenteric artery using endovascular techniques. It is an evolving technology that has not reached maturity as it is fraught with some complications, but has the promise of simplifying the procedure beyond the scope of open reduction as well as potentially lessening dreaded complications such as neurological injury and mortality rate. We are going to emphasize our techniques and results with open repair, the current methods of protecting the spinal cord using the adjunct, and other approaches to multiorgan protection (i.e., hepatic, visceral, and renal protection).

CLASSIFICATION

In the decades following the inception of descending thoracic and thoracoabdominal aortic aneurysm repair (1960s, 1970s, and early 1980s), the results varied tremendously from center to center. This was probably due to the lack of coherent methods of reporting and an agreed-upon classification of the aneurysms. As such, we are going to describe our rationale for classifications of the descending thoracic and thoracoabdominal aortic aneurysm. In the last decade, we began classifying descending thoracic aneurysms based on whether they affect the upper half, lower half, or entire thoracic aorta known as types A, B, and C, respectively (Figure 8–1). Type A involves the upper half, type B involves the sixth intercostal space to T12, and type C comprises the entire thoracic aorta. In the past, during the era of clamp-and-sew technique, some reported cases showed that the maximum incidence of neurological deficit involved types B and C. We will readdress that issue in the results section when we compare our results with regard to the clamp-and-go technique and the modern results of the descending thoracic aorta. Thoracoabdominal aortic aneurysm is an extensive aneurysm involving the thoracic aorta and varying degrees of the abdominal aorta. We categorize these using the modified "Crawford classification" (Figure 8–2). Extent I is from the left subclavian to above the renal arteries. Extent II is from the left subclavian artery below the renal arteries, and Extent III is from the sixth intercostal space to below the renal arteries. Extent IV involves the total abdominal aorta from T12 to below the renal arteries. Extent V, which has been described in the last half decade, is from the upper extent of the sixth intercostal space to the lower extent above the renal arteries. In the past, we found that the extent of the aneurysm correlates with a high incidence of neurological deficit, the highest being in Extent II and then Extent I, III, and IV. In the era of the clamp-and-sew technique, the clamp time and the extent of the aneurysm correlated to neurologic deficit. In Extent II, the overall incidence of neurological deficit was 31%.[6]

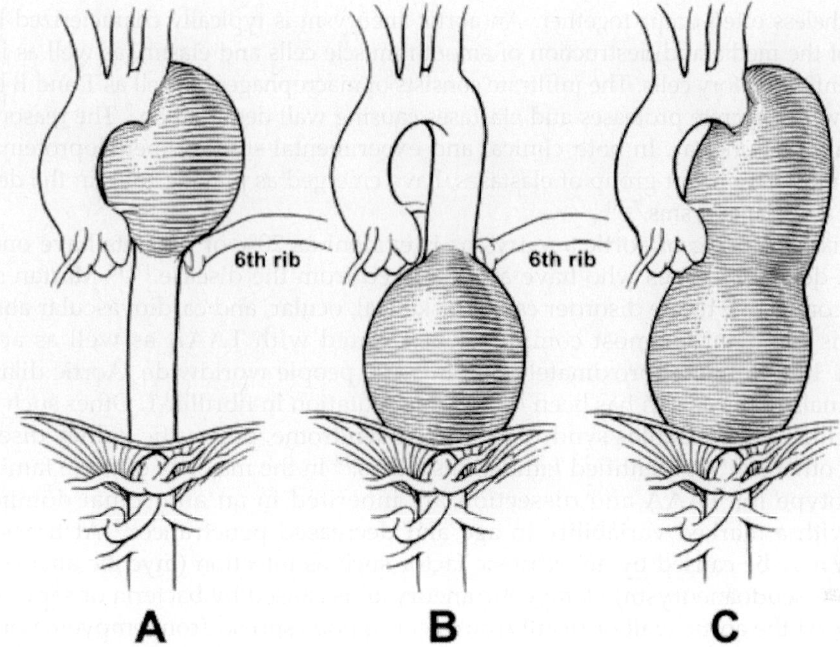

Figure 8-1. Classification of descending thoracic aortic aneurysm.

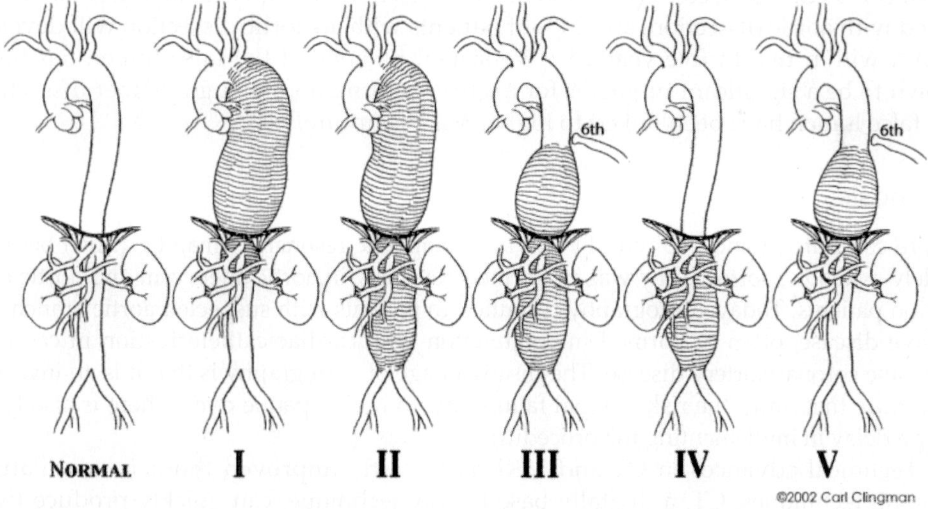

Figure 8-2. Modified Crawford Classification of thoracoabdominal aortic aneurysms.

Etiology

Arteriosclerosis has long been implicated with the aortic aneurysm, but each affects different layers of the aortic wall; arteriosclerosis affects the intima causing occlusive disease while aortic aneurysm is a disease of the media and adventitia. They are distinct conditions that nonetheless often occur together. An aortic aneurysm is typically characterized by a thinning of the media and destruction of smooth muscle cells and elastin, as well as infiltration of inflammatory cells. The infiltrate consists of macrophages as well as T and B lymphocytes, which excrete proteases and elastases causing wall degradation.[7] The reason for this migration is unclear. In both clinical and experimental studies, metalloproteinases (MMP), a most prominent group of elastases, have emerged as playing roles in the development of aortic aneurysms.[7-10]

Familial clustering of aortic aneurysms is evident as 20% of patients have one or more first-degree relatives who have also suffered from the disease.[11-13] Marfan syndrome, a connective tissue disorder causing skeletal, ocular, and cardiovascular abnormalities, is the disorder most commonly associated with TAAA as well as aortic dissection. It occurs in approximately one in 5,000 people worldwide. Aortic dilation in individuals with Marfan has been linked to a mutation in fibrillin-1. Other such disorders include Ehlers-Danlos syndrome, Turner syndrome, polycystic kidney disease, as well as other not yet identified familial disorders.[14] In the majority of these families, the phenotype for TAAA and dissection are inherited in an autosomal dominant manner with a marked variability in age and decreased penetrance.[14] At times, an aneurysm may be caused by an extrinsic factor such as infection (mycotic aneurysm) or trauma (pseudoaneurysm). A mycotic aneurysm is caused by bacteria or septic emboli that seed the aortic wall or result from a contiguous spread from empyema or adjacent infected lymph node. Though any organism can be the cause of a mycotic aneurysm, the most commonly described are salmonella, hemophilus influenza, staphylococcus, tuberculus, and treponema pallidum spirochetes species.[15-16] There is also a connection between TAAA and aortic dissection. One quarter of TAAA are associated with aortic dissection, and 24% of patients with an aortic dissection will develop TAAA within two to five years.[11-13] Persistent patency of the false lumen has been shown to be a significant predictor for aneurysm formation, though neither dissection nor false lumen have been linked to higher risk of rupture.[17-19]

Diagnosis

Before computed tomography (CT) and later magnetic resonance imaging (MRI) became widely available, aortography was performed routinely in aortic aneurysm and aortic dissection patients. Today, aortography is limited to patients with suspected aortic branch occlusive disease, often performed in conjunction with cardiac catheterization in cases of occlusive coronary artery disease. The disadvantage of aortography is that it is an invasive procedure that raises the risk of renal failure due to radio-opaque dyes. There is also typically a delay in implementing the procedure.

Technical advances in CT and MRI have vastly improved thoracic vasculature imaging techniques. CT, a digitally based X-ray technique, can quickly produce two- and three-dimensional digital images of multiple slices of the body's soft tissue organs. It is less invasive, faster, safer, and cheaper than aortography. CT evaluates systemic vasculature (defining aortic anomalies, dissection aneurysm, clots, and calcification) and pulmonary vasculature (depicting lung disease and thoracic venous anomalies such as pulmonary arteriovenous malformation). The more rapid CT angiography (CTA) has virtually supplanted conventional CT. It acquires axial images during the arterial phase following a bolus of intravenous contrast.[20-22] The scan determines aneurysm extent by recording aortic diameter serially, from the ascending aorta to the arch and thoracoabdominal aorta. CTA can distinguish the difference between the false and true lumen in aortic dissection, and can also reveal associated thrombus and inflammatory changes in the aortic wall. In cases of acute and chronic aortic dissection, CTA can accurately detect the proximal location of the intimal tear and thereby the dissection classification (DeBakey I, II, or III; Stanford A or B). For patient follow-up, the CT scan is indispensable in tracking aortic aneurysm growth rate. CT scan is contraindicated in patients with renal insufficiency or who have allergies to contrast agents, but otherwise is our preferred technique for imaging the thoracic aorta.

Unlike the CT scan, MRI can be performed safely in patients with impaired renal function because it does not require intravenous radio-opaque contrast. An image is detected by radio frequency signals when the body's hydrogen atoms react to the MRI's strong magnetic field. MRI, particularly three-dimensional gadolinium-enhanced MRI angiography (MRA), can clearly identify the morphology of the aortic and pulmonary vascular supply. Although yet unable to match the definition clarity of more invasive imaging techniques such as intravascular ultrasound (IVUS), MRA can image plaques smaller than 1 mm and assess the level of atherosclerosis throughout the body. This helps to gauge the risk of heart attack and stroke that can result from plaque rupture in the carotid arteries and aorta. MRA can reliably assess the site and extent of nonvalvar obstructive lesions of the aorta (i.e., coarctation, interruption of the aortic arch, and supravalvar stenosis). Compared with CT, limitations of MR imaging and MRA include longer examination times. Patients with internal metallic hardware (such as pacemakers, orthopedic rods, and the like) cannot undergo MRI or MRA, and higher cost compared with other imaging techniques is also a limiting factor.

Other imaging modalities for the thoracoabdominal aorta include transesophageal echocardiography (TEE), IVUS, and intraoperative epiaortic ultrasound (IEUS). Whereas aortography can provide an outline of diseased vascular tissue, IVUS can provide an image of the anatomy within the vessel walls. A miniature catheter tip inserted percutaneously, incorporated with an ultrasound device, can identify intimal defects, atheromatous plaques, calcification, and laminated thrombi. TEE uses a miniature high-frequency ultrasound transducer placed on a probe that is inserted into the lower esophagus. Because the lower esophagus is located close to the posterior of the heart, there is no image interruption by lung tissue. TEE has the advantage of portability and quick execution. TEE is highly sensitive in aortic pathology diagnosis, and is an excellent intraoperative tool, able to report cardiac structure and function. It can assess ventricular function and can reliably survey aortic valve disease, aortic dilatation, ascending aortic aneurysm, dissection, thrombi, atherosclerotic disease, and mitral valve disease. Of particular value during cardiac operations that employ cardiopulmonary bypass, TEE—and also IEUS—can detect atheromas of the thoracic aorta. Aortic aneurysms below the diaphragm and in the transverse aortic arch cannot be identified by TEE because of the interposition of the air-filled trachea and primary bronchi. Although TEE can be done at the bedside or intraoperatively, the technique requires a skilled cardiologist to interpret study data. Contraindications are esophageal obstruction, diverticulum or varices, active upper gastrointestinal bleed, and cervical spine disease.

Extensive Aortic Aneurysms

The management of extensive aortic aneurysms poses a challenge to all persons involved, demanding multiorgan protection and maximum technical support. Graft replacement of the ascending aorta, arch, and descending thoracic aorta performed in a single operation

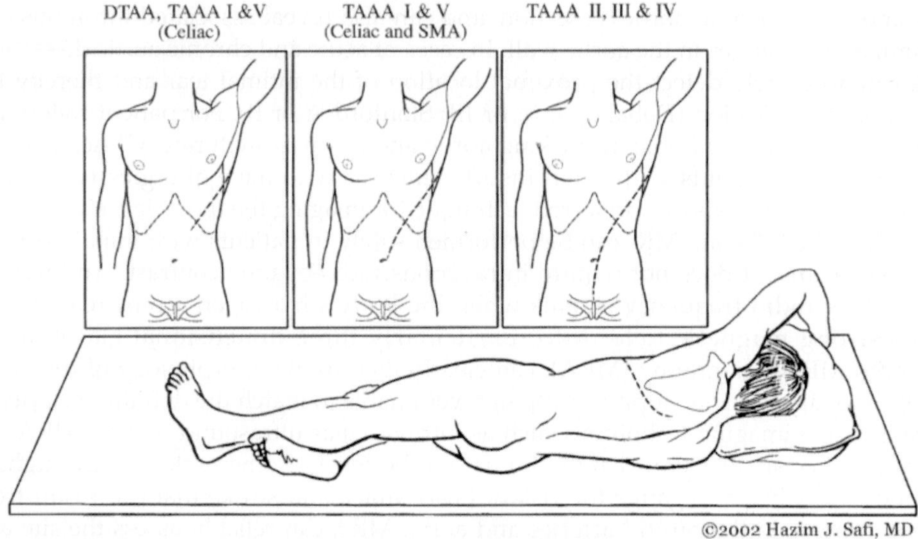

Figure 8-3. Patient positioning and incision selection for thoracoabdominal aortic aneurysm repair.

can exaggerate potential hazards. The patient is submitted to a lengthy procedure, requiring multiple incisions, an increased number of protective surgical adjuncts, longer clamp times, and greater blood loss. Prior to the introduction of the elephant trunk technique in 1983[23], staged repair was also fraught with complications, particularly in the second stage when aortic dissection to gain proximal control caused excessive bleeding. Frequently, the pulmonary artery or the aorta would be entered, causing catastrophic bleeding. The elephant trunk technique permitted the surgeon to avoid cross-clamping of the highly vulnerable proximal descending aorta in the second stage and obviated the bleeding problem. We have routinely used the elephant trunk technique since 1991 (Figure 8–3).[24–27] In the first stage, cardiopulmonary bypass, profound hypothermia, circulatory arrest, and retrograde cerebral perfusion provide protection to the brain and guard against stroke. In the second stage, distal aortic perfusion and perioperative cerebrospinal fluid (CSF) drainage provide protection to the spinal cord and defense against paraplegia or paraparesis. In the second stage, we also use passive core cooling as well as active visceral cooling with excellent results in renal protection.

TREATMENT

The treatment of thoracoabdominal aortic aneurysm and descending thoracic aortic aneurysms is graft replacement. The technique is as follows. The patient is brought to the operating room and placed in the supine position. A thermodilution catheter (Swan-Ganz catheter) with a large bore needle is placed in the jugular vein. A bifurcated intubation tube is inserted into the trachea to collapse the left lung. The patient is placed in the right lateral decubitus fashion and the anesthesiologist inserts a catheter in lumbar space 3–4 or 4–5, advancing it 5–10 centimeters (Figure 8–4). The cerebrospinal fluid is drained intraoperatively and for three days postoperative. For distal aortic perfusion, once the patient is open, we prefer to cannulate either the left atrium or the left lower pulmonary vein connected to a centrifugal Biomedicus pump, and then an in-line heart exchanger and cannulate the

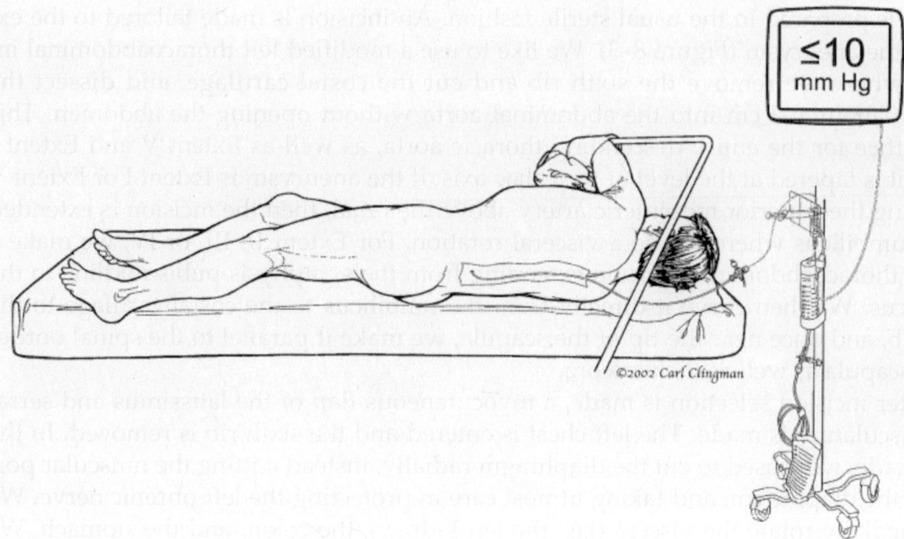

Figure 8-4. Insertion of the cerebrospinal fluid drain.

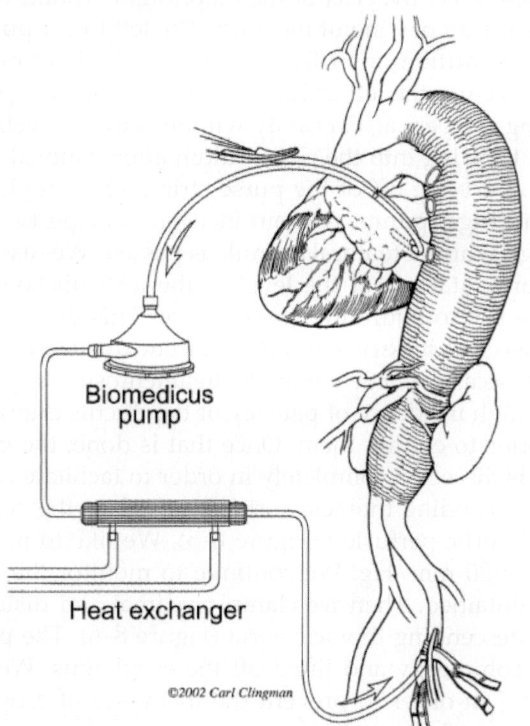

Figure 8-5. Distal aortic perfusion with placement of cannulas in the left atrium and left common femoral artery.

femoral artery (Figure 8–5). If the femoral artery is occluded or cannot be used, the distal thoracic aorta or abdominal aorta will be used for the arterial inflow.

Once in the thoracoabdominal position, with shoulders at right angles to the bed and the hip rotated 60° in order to get access to both right and left femoral arteries, the patient is prepared in the usual sterile fashion. An incision is made tailored to the extent of the aneurysm (Figure 8–3). We like to use a modified left thoracoabdominal incision where we remove the sixth rib and cut the costal cartilage, and dissect the incision about 1–2 cm into the abdominal aorta without opening the abdomen. This will suffice for the entire descending thoracic aorta, as well as Extent V and Extent I where it is tapered at the level of the celiac axis. If the aneurysm is Extent I or Extent V involving the superior mesenteric artery above the renal, then the incision is extended to the umbilicus where we do a visceral rotation. For Extent II, III, or IV, we make a formal thoracoabdominal incision extending from the symphysis pubis midline to the umbilicus. We then curve it directly from the umbilicus to the costal cartilage to the sixth rib, and once near the tip of the scapula, we make it parallel to the spinal border of the scapula as well as the vertebra.

After incision selection is made, a myocutaneous flap of the latissimus and serratus musculature is made. The left chest is entered and the sixth rib is removed. In the last decade, we ceased to cut the diaphragm radially, instead cutting the muscular portion of the diaphragm, and taking utmost care in protecting the left phrenic nerve. We then medially rotate the viscera (i.e., the left kidney), the colon, and the stomach. We put the self-retaining retractor in place. This is one of the major advances in dealing with the patients because it keeps the exposure steady and the chest and abdomen are accessible at once. We dissect the crux of the diaphragm around the aorta and expose the aortic hiatus for a future passing of the graft. The left lower pulmonary vein is dissected, opening the pericardium in order to cannulate the left lower pulmonary vein. If that is not suitable, we use the left atrium. We like to open the pericardium in order to prevent cannulating the pericardial cavity without flow, as well as cardiac tamponade caused by blood trickling into the pericardium after removal of the catheter from the pulmonary vein and tying off of the purse string. On completion, the catheter is connected to the centrifugal pump. A groin incision is made to expose the common femoral artery through which a femoral cannula is passed. We dissect the proximal descending thoracic aorta, starting at the level of the left subclavian artery to the diaphragm, taking care not to injure the vagus nerve. This dissection leads to the left recurrent laryngeal nerve as it skirts around the atretic ductus. We ligate the bronchial arteries and on most occasions, cut the atritic ligamentosus. In patients with Marfan syndrome, there is a high incidence of patency of the ductus arteriosus, and care must be taken to secure prior to cutting them. Once that is done, the proximal or distal to left subclavian aorta is dissected completely in order to facilitate clamping. We choose the site on the mid-descending thoracic aorta site to place the clamps. The patient is then placed on distal aortic perfusion (Figure 8–5). We like to maintain the proximal pressure greater than 100 mm/Hg. We continue to monitor the flow until adequate blood pressure is maintained. Then we clamp proximal and distal to the left subclavian artery and mid-descending thoracic aorta (Figure 8–6). The proximal descending thoracic aorta is cut completely and lifted off the esophagus. We have proceeded in this fashion since 1987 in order to prevent the incidence of esophageal graft fistula with fatal outcome (Figure 8–7).

The graft is sutured into the descending thoracic aorta distal to the subclavian using a #3-0 polypropylene suture and we reinforce the anastomosis with a pledgeted suture in order to prevent bleeding. Once this is checked and found to be hemostatic, the mid descending thoracic aortic clamp is moved down either above or below the celiac axis or infrarenal abdominal aorta. Once it is above the renals, the remainder of the aorta is opened longitudinally. An arrow retractor is used to retract the aortic hia-

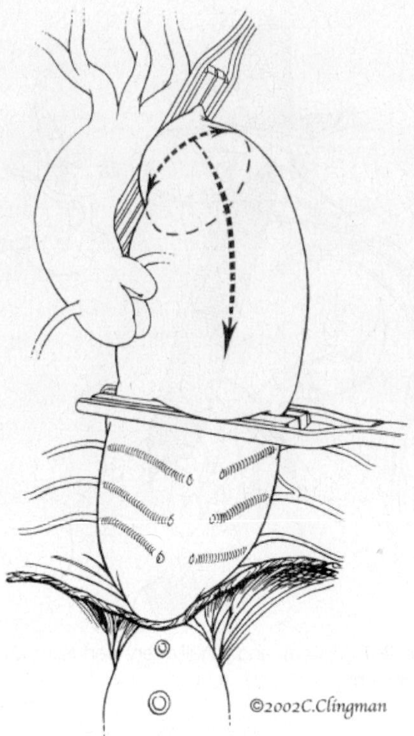

Figure 8-6. Proximal clamping and aortotomy.

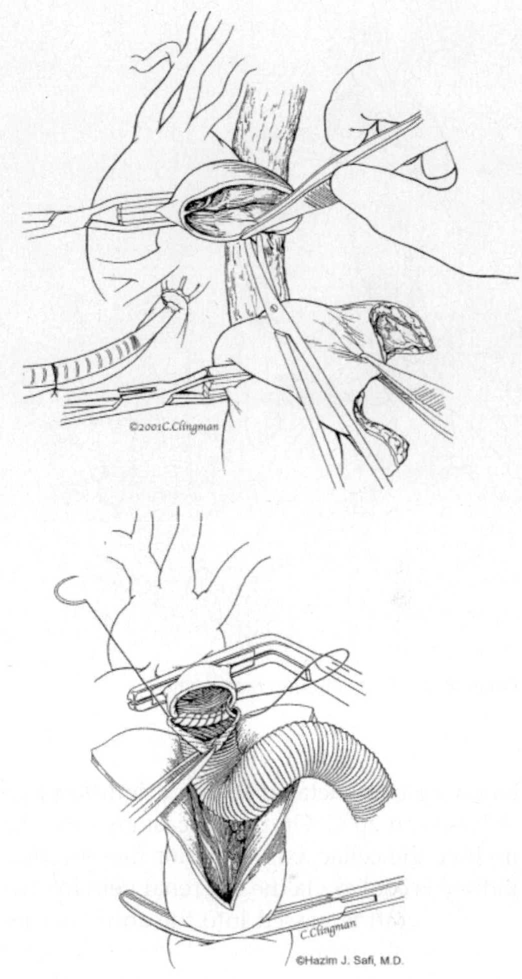

Figure 8-7. Complete dissection of the proximal descending thoracic aorta for the performance of the proximal anastomosis.

tus to expose the entire descending thoracic aorta to the level of the celiac axis. The walls of the aorta are retracted using #2 self-retracting sutures. The intercostal arteries are identified. Any intercostal artery between 8 to 12 that appear patent are secured for future reattachment. The upper intercostal arteries are ligated using 2-0 silk. If the lower intercostal arteries are occluded by clot or atheromatous plaque, then the upper intercostal arteries are reimplanted. We like to stretch the graft and then cut a sidehole opposite the 8th, 9th, 10th, 11th, and 12th intercostal arteries, and we use a #3-0 polypropylene suture (Figure 8–8). We examine the anastomosis and if it is hemostatic, we proceed to put the clamp in the infrarenal abdominal aorta.

We open the remainder of the abdominal aortic aneurysm. The walls are retracted with a #2 self-retracting suture. We mobilize the celiac axis, superior mesenteric, and both renal arteries. These are perfused with a perfusing catheter in the celiac axis, superior mesenteric, and both renal arteries (Figure 8–9). We infuse tepid blood, cold

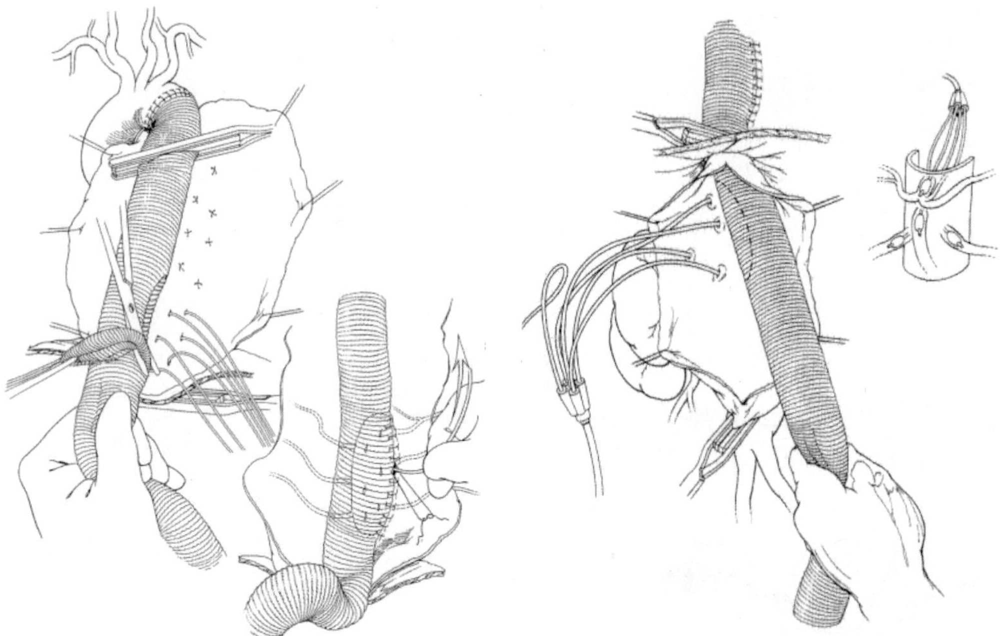

Figure 8-8. Intercostal artery reattachment.

Figure 8-9. Visceral and renal artery perfusion and reattachment.

blood, or cold lactated Ringer's solution to the renal arteries, keeping them protected at less than 20°C. On rare occasions (less than 5% of the time), atheromatous plaques involve the celiac axis, superior mesenteric, and both renal arteries. At this point, the kidney is cooled via the left renal vein in retrograde fashion.

The graft is passed into the aortic hiatus to the abdominal field. An elliptical incision is made opposite the celiac axis, superior mesenteric, and both renal arteries, and #3-0 polypropylene suture is used to reattach the viscera. In case the renal artery, especially the left, is displaced distally, we use a 10–12 mm Dacron graft and reattach it independently. Once the visceral patch is sewn, the descending thoracic aortic clamp is re-applied onto the aortic graft beyond the visceral and renal anastomosis after flushing the graft. The patient is placed in the head-down position and air is evacuated, restoring pulsatile flow to the viscera. The patient is rewarmed. In patients with Ehler-Danlos or Marfan's syndrome, we use a specially constructed branched graft in order to bypass the celiac axis, superior mesenteric, and both renal arteries separately because of higher incidence of patch aneurysm in these patients with connective tissue disorders.

Once that is done, attention is paid to the infrarenal abdominal aorta. On occasion, we cannot clamp the aorta above the iliac bifurcation, so the left iliac is clamped separately. Either #3-0 polypropylene or #2-0 polypropylene suture is used to anastomose the graft into the abdominal aorta above the iliac bifurcation (Figure 8–10). Once this is achieved, the distal clamp is removed, the patient is placed in the head-down position, and pulsatile flow is restored to the viscera. We also use indigo carmine to check the amount of time it takes for urine to appear. The patient is then closed. We use #1 polypropylene suture to close the diaphragm and the abdominal fascial layers. The intercostal space is closed with heavy absorbable braided suture and the chest wall is closed using heavy absorbable monofilament suture. Figure 8–11 illustrates the repair of an extent II thoracoabdominal aortic aneurysm.

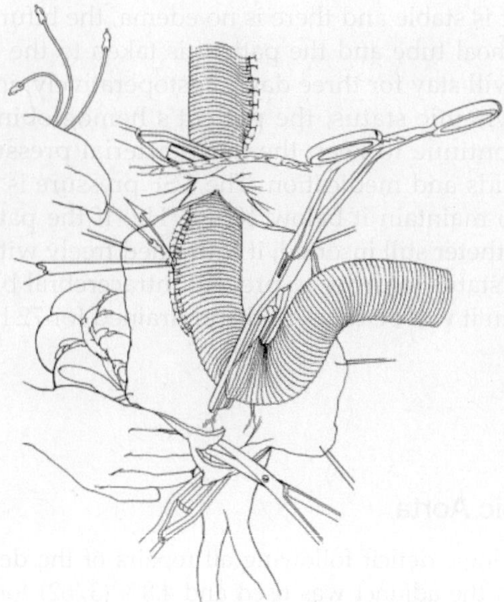

Figure 8-10. Distal abdominal anastomosis.

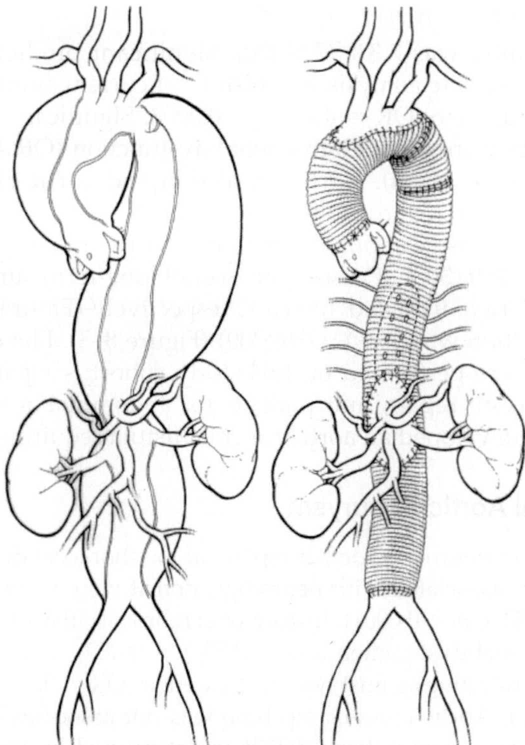

Figure 8-11. Illustration of a patient with extensive aortic aneurysm with chronic dissection before (left) and after (right) treatment. First stage of the procedure was performed on ascending aorta and arch in standard fashion. After a four week recovery period, thoracoabdominal aortic aneurysm (Extent II) graft replacement was performed.

Then if the patient is stable and there is no edema, the bifurcation tube is changed into a single endotracheal tube and the patient is taken to the surgical intensive care unit where he or she will stay for three days. Postoperatively, in addition to maintaining adequate hemodynamic status, the patient's hemoglobin is maintained above 10 mg/dL, and we continue to keep the mean arterial pressure above 80 mm/Hg through the use of fluids and medication. The CSF pressure is measured hourly, and drained 15 cc/hour to maintain it below 10mm/Hg. If the patient develops delayed paraplegia with the catheter still inserted, it is drained freely with close attention to the patient's neurological status in order to prevent intracerebral bleeding. If the catheter has been removed, then it will be reinserted and drained for 72 hours.

RESULTS

Descending Thoracic Aorta

The incidence of neurologic deficit following all repairs of the descending thoracic aorta was 0.8% (2/238) when the adjunct was used and 4.8% (3/62) for the nonadjunct group, $p < 0.02$.[28] All neurologic deficits in the series of descending thoracic aortic repairs occurred in patients with aneurysmal involvement of the entire descending thoracic aorta (extent C). Predictors significantly associated with neurologic deficit by univariate analysis were the use of the adjunct, OR = 0.19, $p < 0.02$, previous repaired abdominal aortic aneurysm, OR = 7.0, $p < 0.005$, extent C aneurysm, OR = 13.73, 0.02, and cerebrovascular disease history, OR = 4.7, $p < 0.03$.

Thirty-day mortality was 7.3% (22/300). Significant predictors associated with early mortality by univariate analysis was history of current smoking, OR = 4.27, $p < 0.001$, and renal dysfunction, OR = 4.71, $p < 0.0008$. Significant independent predictors of early mortality were preoperative renal dysfunction (OR 4.6, $p < 0.01$) and female gender (OR 2.9, $p < 0.03$). Aortic dissection and aortic clamp time were not significant risk factors with regards to patient outcome.

Median follow-up was 97 months; range one to 165 months. Survival follow-up was obtained in 96% (289/300) of cases. The overall long-term survival was 79%, 76%, 64%, and 35% at one, two, five, and 10-years, respectively (Figure 8–2). Freedom from aortic related reoperation was 96.3% (289/300) (Figure 8–3). Eleven subsequent aortic related procedures were performed on this study cohort: six patients for thoracoabdominal aortic aneurysm repair, four patients for abdominal aortic aneurysm repair, and one patient who developed an aortobronchial fistula requiring a pneumonectomy.

Thoracoabdominal Aortic Aneurysm

The overall incidence of neurologic deficit repairs of the thoracoabdominal aorta was 3.3% (36/1106). Risk factors associated with neurologic deficit were age (OR = 1.03, $p = 0.02$), TAAA extent II (OR 8.09, $p < 0.0001$), history of cerebrovascular disease (OR = 2.49, $p = 0.03$), and history of renal dysfunction (OR = 2.55, $p = 0.007$). The use of the adjunct and female gender were protective against neurologic deficit (OR = 0.42, $p = 0.008$, OR = 0.40, $p = 0.04$, respectively). Aortic cross-clamp time was not associated with ND ($p = 0.11$). Independent risk factors for neurologic deficit as determined by multiple logistic regression were extent II TAAA and renal dysfunction.

Aortic cross-clamp times have increased significantly (34 seconds/year, $p < 0.0001$) since 1991 during the study period. Despite this increase in aortic cross-clamp time, neurologic deficit rates have declined for the period of surgery, $p = 0.02$ (Figure 8–3). Of note, the incidence of neurological deficit has declined to 1.1% during the last quartile with the use of the adjunct. This decrease in neurologic deficit is most pronounced with the Extent II thoracoabdominal aortic aneurysms (21.1% to 3.3%). The use of the adjunct has increased the aortic cross-clamp time by a mean of 12 minutes ($p = 0.0001$), but is associated with a significant protective effect against neurologic deficit (OR = 0.4, $p = 0.0002$). Although other previously established risk factors have remained significantly associated with neurologic deficit, aortic cross-clamp time is no longer significant.[29]

Extensive Aortic Aneurysms

Thirty-day mortality was 19/218 (8.7%) in first-stage repair and 10/103 (9.7%) in second stage repair. During the interval, or 31 days to six weeks following stage 1, mortality was 10/124 (8%). Seven of the 10 interval deaths were due to rupture of the untreated aortic segment. Over the entire course of follow-up, the mortality rate was 18.4% (18/98) in the group of the patients who did not return for the second-stage repair. Three of 218 (2.7%) first-stage patients who were evaluable suffered postoperative stroke. No spinal cord dysfunction occurred in second-stage patients (0/103).

Update on Outcome Predictors

In the past, we used serum creatinine as a measure for preoperative renal function. We have found that about 9% of patients undergoing TAAA have preexisting renal disease, which in turn is a risk factor for postoperative paraplegia and mortality.[30] We recently reviewed the incidence of preexisting renal disease in our cumulative experience with 1,106 TAAA and descending thoracic aortic aneurysm patients. We found that the glomerular filtration rate (GFR) as estimated from the Cockroft-Gault equation, which takes into account the patient's age, weight, and gender, is superior to the serum creatinine both in detecting subclinical renal disease and predicting mortality. Based on GFR, approximately two-thirds of our patients had stages 2 and 3 preexisting renal disease according to the National Kidney Foundation. More importantly, the study showed that 30-day mortality ranges from 5% in the best GFR quartile to 27% in the worst.[31]

CONCLUSION

Remarkable progress in the treatment of thoracoabdominal aortic aneurysms has been achieved in the last decade. Morbidity and mortality have declined, which we attribute to the adoption of the adjuncts distal aortic perfusion and CSF drainage, as well as the evolution of surgical techniques to include sequential aortic cross-clamp, intercostal artery reattachment, and moderate hypothermia. Currently, the overall incidence of neurological deficit in descending thoracic aortic aneurysm is 0.8% and mortality rate in patients with normal renal function is 5%. It is these results against which the stent repair of descending thoracic aortic aneurysm should be compared rather than old historical data showing high incidence of neurological deficits/death. We know the adjunct of CSF drainage, distal aortic perfusion, and moderate hypothermia has had a tremendous impact in lowering the incidence of neurologic deficit for the repair of descending thoracic and thoracoabdominal aortic aneurysms. Our continuing goals are to further decrease the incidence of neurologic deficits and to improve renal protection, with particular focus on the Extent II thoracoabdominal aortic aneurysm.

ACKNOWLEDGEMENT

We are grateful to Kirk Soodhalter for his editorial assistance.

REFERENCES

1. Etheredge, S, Yee, J, Smith, et al. Successful resection of a large aneurysm of the upper abdominal aorta and replacement with homograft. *Surgery*. 1955;138:1071–1081.
2. DeBakey ME, CD, Crawford ES, Morris Jr GC. Clinical application of a new flexible knitted Dacron arterial substitute. *Arch Surg*. 1957;74:713–724.
3. Hollier LH, Money SR, Naslund TC et al. Risk of spinal cord dysfunction in patients undergoing thoracoabdominal aortic replacement. *Am J Surg*. 1992;164(3):210–213; discussion 213–214.
4. Connolly, JE, Wakabayashi, A, German, JC, Stemmer, EA and Serres, EJ. Clinical experience with pulsatile left heart bypass without anticoagulation for thoracic aneurysms. *J Thorac Cardiovasc Surg* 1971;62(4):568–576.
5. Safi HJ, Hess KR, Randel M, et al. Cerebrospinal fluid drainage and distal aortic perfusion: reducing neurologic complications in repair of thoracoabdominal aortic aneurysm types I and II. *J Vasc Surg*. 1996;23(2):223–228; discussion 229.
6. Svensson LG, Crawford ES, Hess KR, et al. Experience with 1509 patients undergoing thoracoabdominal aortic operations. *J Vasc Surg*. 1993;17(2):357–368; discussion 368–370.
7. Ailawadi G, Eliason JL, Upchurch Jr GR. Current concepts in the pathogenesis of abdominal aortic aneurysm. *J Vasc Surg*. 2003;38(3):584–588.
8. Longo GM, Xiong W, Greiner TC, et al. Matrix metalloproteinases 2 and 9 work in concert to produce aortic aneurysms. *J Clin Invest*. 2002;110(5):625–632.
9. Annabi B, Shedid D, Ghosn P, et al. Differential regulation of matrix metalloproteinase activities in abdominal aortic aneurysms. *J Vasc Surg*. 2002;35(3):539–546.
10. McMillan WD, Pearce WH. Increased plasma levels of metalloproteinase-9 are associated with abdominal aortic aneurysms. *J Vasc Surg*. 1999;29(1):122–127; discussion 127–129.
11. Biddinger A, Rocklin M, Coselli J Milewicz DM. Familial thoracic aortic dilatations and dissections: a case control study. *J Vasc Surg*. 1997;25(3):506–511.
12. Coady MA, Davies RR, Roberts M, et al. Familial patterns of thoracic aortic aneurysms. *Arch Surg*. 1999;134(4):361–367.
13. Hasham SN, Willing MC, Guo DC, et al. Mapping a locus for familial thoracic aortic aneurysms and dissections (TAAD2) to 3p24-25. *Circulation*. 2003;107(25):3184–3190.
14. Milewicz, DM, Chen, H, Park, ES, et al. Reduced penetrance and variable expressivity of familial thoracic aortic aneurysms/dissections. *Am J Cardiol*. 1998;82(4):474–479.
15. Jarrett F, Darling RC, Mundth ED, Austen WG. Experience with infected aneurysms of the abdominal aorta. *Arch Surg*. 1975;110(11):1281–1286.
16. Bakker-de Wekker P, Alfieri O, Vermeulen F, et al. Surgical treatment of infected pseudoaneurysms after replacement of the ascending aorta. *J Thorac Cardiovasc Surg*. 1984;88(3): 447–451.

17. Bernard Y, Zimmermann H, Chocron S, et al. False lumen patency as a predictor of late outcome in aortic dissection. *Am J Cardiol*. 2001;87(12):1378–1382.

18. Marui A, Mochizuki T, Mitsui N, et al. Toward the best treatment for uncomplicated patients with type B acute aortic dissection: A consideration for sound surgical indication. *Circulation*. 1999;100(19 Suppl):II275–280.

19. Juvonen T, Ergin MA, Galla JD, et al. Risk factors for rupture of chronic type B dissections [In Process Citation]. *J Thorac Cardiovasc Surg*. 1999;117(4):776–786.

20. Kieffer E, Richard T, Chiras J, et al. Preoperative spinal cord arteriography in aneurysmal disease of the descending thoracic and thoracoabdominal aorta: preliminary results in 45 patients. *Ann Vasc Surg*. 1989;3(1):34–46.

21. Williams GM, Perler BA, Burdick JF, et al. Angiographic localization of spinal cord blood supply and its relationship to postoperative paraplegia. *J Vasc Surg* 1991;13(1):23–33; discussion 33–35.

22. Fillinger, MF. Imaging of the thoracic and thoracoabdominal aorta. *Semin Vasc Surg* 2000; 13(4):247–263.

23. Borst HG, Walterbusch G, Schaps D. Extensive aortic replacement using "elephant trunk" prosthesis. *Thorac Cardiovasc Surg*. 1983;31(1):37–40.

24. Svensson, LG. Rationale and technique for replacement of the ascending aorta, arch, and distal aorta using a modified elephant trunk procedure. *J Card Surg*. 1992;7(4):301–312.

25. Safi HJ, Miller 3rd CC, Iliopoulos DC, et al. Staged repair of extensive aortic aneurysm: improved neurologic outcome. *Ann Surg*. 1997;226(5):599–605.

26. Safi HJ, Miller 3rd CC, Estrera, AL, et al. Staged repair of extensive aortic aneurysms: morbidity and mortality in the elephant trunk technique. *Circulation*. 2001;104(24):2938–2942.

27. Safi HJ, Miller 3rd CC, 3rd, Estrera AL, et al. Staged repair of extensive aortic aneurysms: long-term experience with the elephant trunk technique. *Ann Surg* 2004;240(4):677–684; discussion 684–685.

28. Estrera AL, Miller 3rd CC, Chen EP, et al. Descending Thoracic Aortic Aneurysm Repair: 12-year Experience Using Distal Aortic Perfusion and Cerebrospinal Fluid Drainage. *Ann Thorac Surg*. In Press.

29. Safi HJ, Estrera AL, Miller 3rd CC, et al. Evolution of Risk for Neurologic Deficit following Descending and Thoracoabdominal Aortic Repair. *Ann Thorac Surg*. In Press.

30. Safi HJ, Miller 3rd CC, Huynh TT, et al. Distal aortic perfusion and cerebrospinal fluid drainage for thoracoabdominal and descending thoracic aortic repair: ten years of organ protection. *Ann Surg*. 2003;238(3):372–380; discussion 380–381.

31. Huynh TT, VanEps R, Miller CC, et al. Glomerular Filtration Rate is Superior to Serum Creatinine for Prediction of Mortality Following Thoracoabdominal Aortic Surgery. *J Vasc Surg*. In Press.

9

Open Repair of Thoracoabdominal Aortic Aneurysms (TAAAs): When and How

*Gilbert R. Upchurch, Jr., M.D., Himanshu J. Patel, M.D.,
John E. Rectenwald, M.D., Loay Kabbani, M.D.,
Ramon Berguer, M.D., Ph.D., Enrique Criado, M.D.,
Susan A. Blackburn, R.N., M.B.A., G. Michael Deeb, M.D.*

Thoracoabdominal aortic aneurysms (TAAAs) represent a potentially lethal disease. Patients with untreated large TAAAs have a reported two-year mortality rate of 76%, with nearly one-half dying from rupture.[1] While the data are clear that untreated TAAAs have a very high mortality, even in the elective setting, the surgical repair of these aneurysms represents a most challenging technical procedure. While published early mortality data following repair of intact TAAAs from large, single center institutions of excellence range from 4% to 18%,[2-5] national data suggest a mortality rate greater than 20%.[6] Furthermore, postoperative complications, including acute renal failure, paraplegia, stroke, myocardial ischemia, and prolonged ventilation are common and often severe.

Unlike patients with infrarenal abdominal aortic aneurysms (AAA) and isolated thoracic aortic aneurysms (Crawford type I) where there are a number of FDA-approved endovascular options, there are no endografts in the United States (U.S.) currently available to treat TAAAs. Reports from Europe, Australia, and a few specialized centers in the U.S. have suggested the feasibility of endovascular approaches, but these devices are not widely available. Long-term follow-up of these fenestrated and multibranch endografts is also lacking. In addition, the recent increased use of "hybrid" approaches, in which sequential extra-anatomic bypasses are performed to the mesenteric and renal vessels followed serially by endovascular exclusion of these aneurysms, has gained favor. Unfortunately, the initial "open" stage of this procedure is associated with a mortality rate of 5% to 15% and the long-term patency of these extra-anatomic bypasses to the mesenteric and renal vessels and is also unknown.

Therefore, while gradual and steady progress is being made in this area, surgical repair of TAAAs should still be considered the "gold standard" therapy.

The general consensus is that TAAAs are repaired when the aneurysm reaches a diameter of approximately 6 cm by CT scan. Unlike with infrarenal AAAs in which there is level 1 evidence to support a diameter of 5.5 cm to proceed with aneurysm repair, similar data to guide our clinical decision-making for TAAAs will probably not be produced, mainly because there are so few TAAAs compared to AAAs. In addition to aortic diameter, the determination of when to repair a TAAA is also influenced by a number of clinical risk factors including the patients' history of coronary artery disease, pulmonary disease, renal insufficiency, and a host of other comorbidities. TAAA repair is often performed in patients with atherosclerotic disease in the renal and mesenteric vessels, as well as in patients with connective tissue disorders. The complexity of the decision as to when to operate on these patients is further increased by the observation that a number of these patients also have aortic dissections, making surgical repair of their aneurysm more difficult.

The present review describes our surgical technique for repair of TAAAs with the understanding that a number of endovascular options are being developed. With the addition of hybrid or combined endovascular and open approaches, as well as widespread application of fenestrated and multibranch aortic grafts, one would predict that the number of open TAAA repairs over time will decrease. Finally, in addition to describing the technical aspects of this operation, the University of Michigan and U.S. mortality and morbidity following TAAA will be described.

PREOPERATIVE WORKUP

All patients being considered for TAAA repair should undergo a dedicated CT scan of the chest, abdomen, and pelvis using IV contrast with thin cuts. The use of three-dimensional CT has obviated the need for angiography, even in the setting of occlusive disease of the renal and mesenteric arteries. The preoperative workup of these patients should also include coronary angiography and transesophageal echocardiography to exclude coronary disease and valvular insufficiency or stenosis, respectively. Liberal use of pulmonary function testing and the noninvasive laboratory for carotid artery disease and popliteal aneurysms is appropriate. Patients are routinely placed on a β-blocker and a HMG-CoA reductase inhibitor (statin).

ANESTHESIA

Patients undergoing TAAA repair are typically admitted to the hospital the night before their operations where they undergo a bowel prep, while also receiving adequate intravenous hydration. The morning of surgery, a radial arterial line and pulmonary artery catheter are placed. The patients undergo general endotracheal intubation with a double lumen tube followed by placement of a transesophageal echocardiogram probe. A spinal fluid drain is placed in all patients undergoing open TAAA repair (Figure 9–1). The use of a spinal fluid drain has been studied prospectively following TAAA repair, and appears to decrease the high incidence of paraplegia.[7] Spinal pressures are maintained at 10 mm Hg throughout the case (Figure 9–1). A rapid trans-

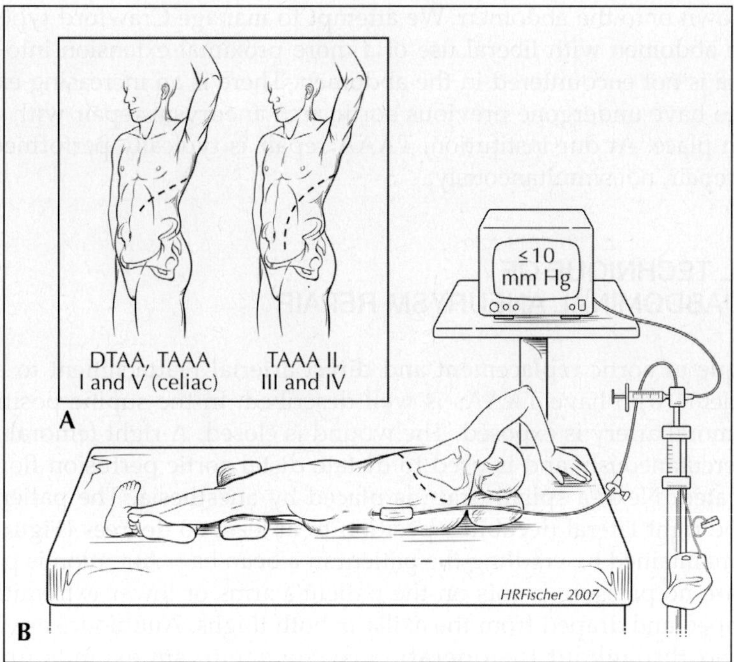

Figure 9-1. (A) TAAA incision based on aneurysm extent. Crawford type I (and Safi V) are typically repaired through an isolated thoracotomy. In contrast, Crawford Type II, III, and IV require a thoracotomy with extension down onto the abdomen. **(B)** Patient placed in right lateral decubitus position with spinal drain in place.

fuser is set up at the start of the case for blood products (packed red blood cells and fresh frozen plasma). Platelets are not given until bypass is completed.

The senior author (GMD) of this experience has preferentially used hypothermic arrest for patients undergoing Crawford type I TAAA repairs to avoid clamping of the proximal aorta near the arch with its attendant increased risk of stroke. Our recent experience has also been to more liberally perform endovascular stent grafting of type I TAAAs if anatomically feasible. Over the last six years, for type II, III, IV, and V TAAA repairs, we have used an atrial-femoral artery bypass system with Carmeda coated tubing, including an oxygenator. This has allowed us to decrease the amount of systemic heparin given prior to the initiation of distal aortic perfusion. Distal aortic perfusion is routinely maintained by an arterial cannula placed in the left common femoral artery and a venous cannula placed in the inferior pulmonary or superior pulmonary vein, the left common femoral vein, or the right internal juglar vein, depending on the extent of the operation.

CLASSIFICATION OF PATIENTS ACCORDING TO EXTENT

The technical performance of TAAA repair is closely aligned with the Crawford Classification, which has been modified by Safi to include a type V aneurysm.[8,9] We repair Crawford type I and Safi type V TAAAs through an isolated thoracotomy (Figure 9–1A). In contrast, Type II, III, and IV TAAAs require a thoracotomy with extension down onto the abdomen. We attempt to manage Crawford type IV TAAAs through the abdomen with liberal use of a more proximal extension into the chest if normal aorta is not encountered in the abdomen. There is an increasing experience in patients who have undergone previous aortic arch aneurysm repair with an elephant trunk left in place. At our institution, TAAA repair is typically performed following aortic arch repair, not simultaneously.

SURGICAL TECHNIQUE OF THORACOABDOMINAL ANEURYSM REPAIR

The technique of aortic replacement and direct arterial reattachment to a prosthetic graft in patients who have TAAAs is well described. In the supine position, the left common femoral artery is exposed. The wound is closed. A right femoral arterial line is placed percutaneously and is used to dictate distal aortic perfusion flows once bypass is initiated. Next, a spinal drain is placed by anesthesia. The patients are then placed in the right lateral decubitus position to at least 60 degrees (Figure 9–1). This position is maintained by cradling the patient in a bean bag. Attention is paid to make sure there are no pressure points on the patient's arms or lower extremities. The patient is prepped and draped from the axilla to both thighs. Antibiotics are used preoperatively and throughout the operation. If the aneurysm extends up to the left subclavian artery, a fourth intercostal space thorocotomy is preferred. If the aneurysm extends into the abdomen, a second thorocotomy in the eighth intercostal space will be performed through the same skin incision. Shingling of ribs is performed to facilitate exposure. We have evolved toward making the abdominal incision in a paramedian fashion in order to avoid a perceived high incidence of ventral hernias with a midline incision. The presence of a LIMA graft for coronary bypass grafting should be noted to allow for preservation of the inferior and superior epigastic arteries, and the subsequent risk of chest wall ischemia.

The remainder of this review will focus on repair of Type II, III, & IV TAAAs, as most of these repairs recently at our institution have been performed using the "pick off" technique using distal aortic perfusion and not hypothermic arrest. Following the thoracotomy, the thoracic aorta is isolated, including all intercostals from the left subclavian artery down to the diaphragm. This allows us to decrease the amount of blood lost on opening the thoracic aortic aneurysm as either permanent or temporary clips can be placed directly on the intercostals. It also facilitates reimplantation of multiple pairs of intercostals between T8 and T12. The transesophageal echo probe helps to isolate the esophagus and allows us to separate it from the aorta. Special attention is paid to the thoracic duct at the level of the diaphragm where we intentionally ligate it. We have moved to sparing the diaphragm rather than dividing it circumferentially or radially to avoid the pulmonary morbidity associated with division of the diaphragm.

The approach to the abdominal portion of the procedure can be accomplished by remaining in the retroperitoneum either behind the left kidney or anterior to it (Figure 9–2). We tend to bring the kidney forward if the left renal artery does not need to be bypassed. On the other hand, we leave the kidney back if a bypass to the left kidney is required or if a retroaortic renal vein is present. In the abdomen, circumferential control of the aorta at the diaphragm and at the distal aortic anastamotic site is obtained. Standardly, the celiac artery, SMA, and left renal artery are all encircled with vessel loops, while the right renal artery is controlled once inside the aneurysm.

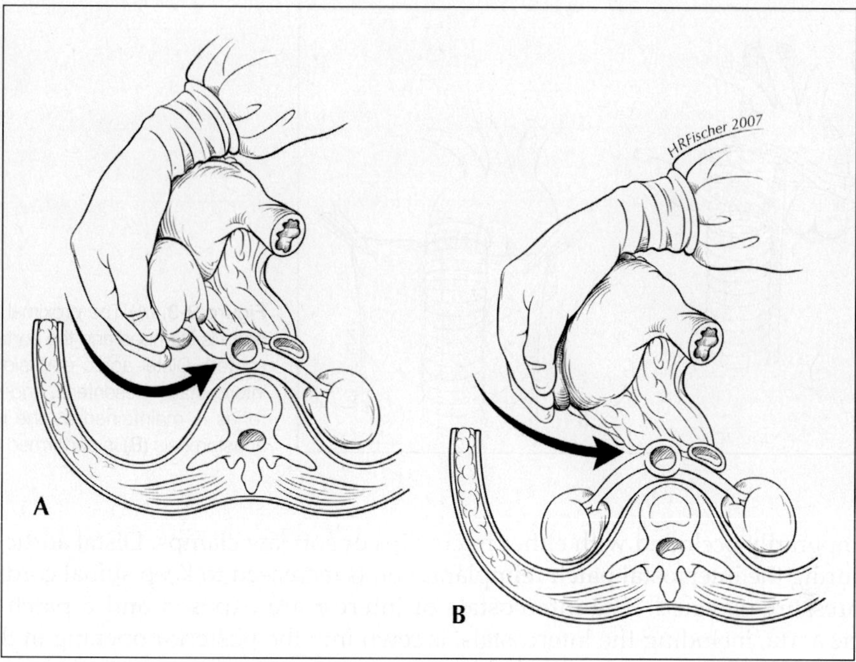

Figure 9-2. The left kidney can be managed from the retroperitoneum and brought forward **(A)**, or a plane can be developed in front of the kidney **(B)**.

Once control of the proximal and distal aorta, intercostals, and mesenteric and renal vessels are obtained, the patient is heparinized to maintain an ACT of greater than 250. Cannulation of the left common femoral artery (CFA) is done via a "stove pipe" graft sewn to the left CFA in order to avoid prolonged left lower extremity ischemia. Typically, the left inferior or superior pulmonary vein is also cannulated. A mean pressure of approximately 60 mm is maintained in the right femoral arterial line using distal aortic perfusion. The oxygenator allows us to maintain normothermia. The proximal anastomosis is performed first clamping either proximal or distal (Figure 9–3) to the left subclavian artery with a soft jaw clamp. The recurrent laryngeal nerve is identified and protected. In addition, the mid-thoracic aorta is clamped with a hinged curved soft jaw clamp. The intercostals are permanently clipped at this level from outside the aorta after the proximal anastamosis is performed. This is especially critical if the proximal clamp is proximal to the left subclavian artery in order to maintain spinal perfusion. The isolated aorta between clamps at this level is subsequently opened. The proximal aortic anastomosis is fashioned to a prefabricated 24 or 28 mm multibranch graft. The graft is cut and sewn in with a running nonabsorbable suture with external felt reinforcement in a direct end-to-end fashion.

The next anastomosis to be performed is the intercostal patch. This is technically challenging and requires the most time of all the anastomoses performed. We have been very aggressive about implanting intercostals in all Crawford type II and III TAAAs. Our preference is to implant at least three pairs of intercostals. The distal aortic clamp is moved to below the diaphragm. The graft is subsequently pulled to length and a posterior portion of the graft is excised with an handheld incandescent cautery to prevent unraveling of the graft. Variably, the intercostals between T8 and T12 level

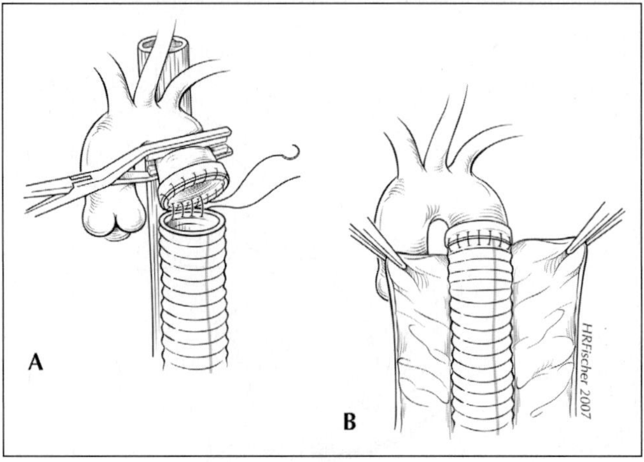

Figure 9-3. (A) The proximal thoracic aorta is clamped and the aorta is transected. Distal aortic perfusion to the intercostals, mesenteric, and renal arteries is maintained as the proximal anastamosis **(B)** is performed.

are temporarily occluded with either microclips or soft jaw clamps. Distal aortic perfusion during the intercostal patch reimplantation is increased to keep spinal cord perfusion pressure elevated. The intercostals of interest are exposed and a patch of the thoracic aorta, including the intercostals, is sewn into the posterior opening in the aortic graft using a running nonabsorbable suture with external felt reinforcement. Once hemostasis is adequate, flow to the intercostals is reestablished by clamping the graft distal to our intercostals patch. The graft is subsequently passed through the diaphragmatic hiatus (Figure 9–4).

While we initially performed the standard Crawford visceral patch including the celiac artery, SMA, and right renal artery, it became apparent that the "pick off" technique was better tolerated by the patients despite taking a longer time to perform indi-

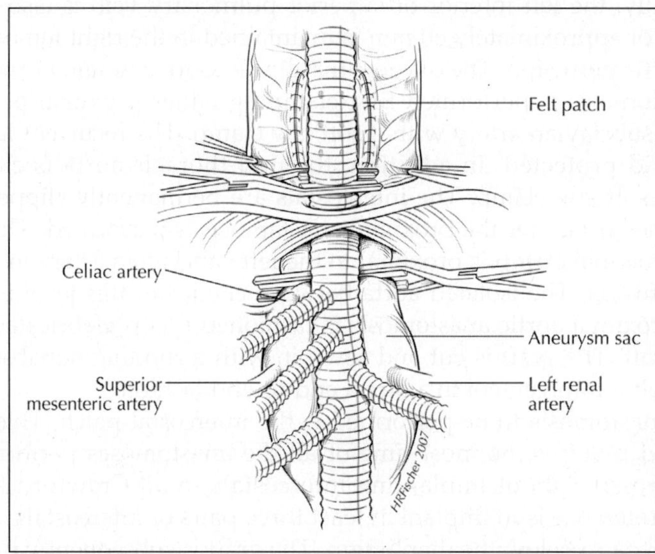

Figure 9-4. Following completion of the intercostal artery patch into the back of the aortic graft, flow is reestablished to the spinal arteries once the distal aortic clamp is moved to the supraceliac aortic position.

vidual anastamoses. In addition, as many of our patients also have aortic dissections or connective tissue disorders in which a visceral patch is contraindicated, we routinely perform individual bypasses to each visceral and renal vessel. We maintain the aortic clamp at the supraceliac aortic position, maintaining perfusion of the celiac artery, the SMA, and both renal arteries through distal aortic perfusion (Figure 9–4). The celiac artery is controlled distally and suture ligated proximally at its orifice on the aorta. An 8 or 10 mm side branch graft is sewn in an end-to-end fashion to the celiac artery using external felt reinforcement (Figure 9–5A). With antegrade flow reestablished to the celiac artery, the SMA is replaced in the same fashion (Figure 9–5B). We next turn our attention to grafting the left renal artery. We give a 100 to 250 ml cold renal preservation solution that includes mannitol and heparin directly into the left renal artery rather than using continuous perfusion. Following cold perfusion of the left kidney, a 6 or 8 mm bypass is performed to the left renal artery (Figure 9–5C). With antegrade flow established in the celiac artery, the SMA, and the left renal artery, the infrarenal aorta is subsequently clamped. Prior to clamping the aorta or the iliacs, distal aortic flow is decreased. All lumbar arteries and the IMA are oversewn at this level. The right renal artery is typically isolated from inside the aneurysm, and this bypass is performed last. Either cold kidney preservation solution is infused directly into the right renal artery as a bolus or a perfusion cannulae from the left heart circuit is inserted to maintain flow to the kidney. This anastamosis is also performed to an end-to-end 6 or 8 mm graft (Figure 9–5D). Finally, the aortic clamp is moved to the terminal aorta or the iliac arteries are clamped individually. After antegrade flow is established to the celiac artery, SMA, and both renals, the distal anastomosis is performed with a running nonabsorbable suture with external felt reinforcement (Figure 9–5E).

Once the repair is completed, flow is confirmed in all bypasses by handheld Doppler interrogation (Figure 9–6). The patient can be rewarmed using distal aortic perfusion. If there is no surgical bleeding, the pulmonary vein and femoral artery cannulae are removed, and the venotomy and arteriotomy closed. At this point, the patient is fully reversed with protamine to allow the ACT to drop below 150. If the patient is thrombocytopenic or coagulopathic, platelets, as well as FFP or cryoprecipitate, are administered. Copious warm irrigation is performed. A significant amount of time is typically required to attain hemostasis given the large surface areas in these incisions. The thoracic aorta is covered with a large bovine pericardial patch, while the graft in the abdomen is closed with the aortic aneurysm to prevent aortoenteric fistulae.

Closure of these large incisions can be daunting, especially as the surgical team is typically fatigued at this time during the operation. Meticulous attention to detail is required. The thoracotomies are closed first with interrupted absorbable suture. A straight and angled chest tube are placed and secured. The retoperitoneal incision is closed with a running suture. The remaining portions of the thoracotomy and abdominal incision are closed in the standard fashion. A sterile dressing is applied and the patient is placed in the supine position. The endotracheal tube is converted to a single lumen tube and the patient is taken to the intensive care unit (ICU).

Protocol driven care of these critically ill patients is important. Once patients are in the ICU, they remain intubated until they are warm. It is important that they are adequately volume resuscitated. It is also critical to avoid hypotension in order to prevent the sequelae of paralysis and renal failure. These patients behave much more like abdominal aortic aneurysm repairs, as opposed to isolated thoracic aneurysm repairs, as they tend to have significant third spacing. These patients are extubated the next morning. The CSF drain is maintained anywhere from 24 to 72 hours.

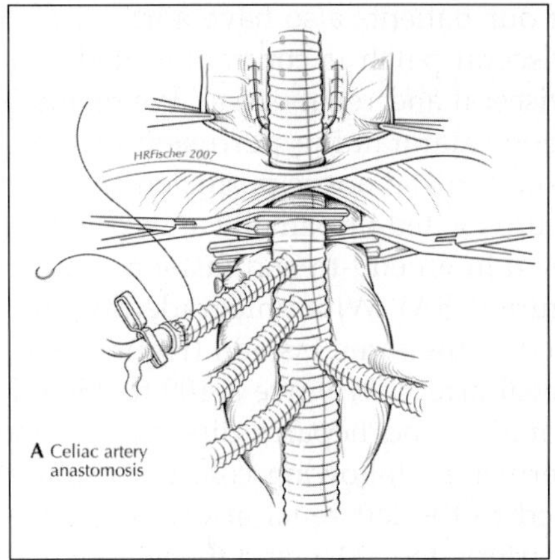

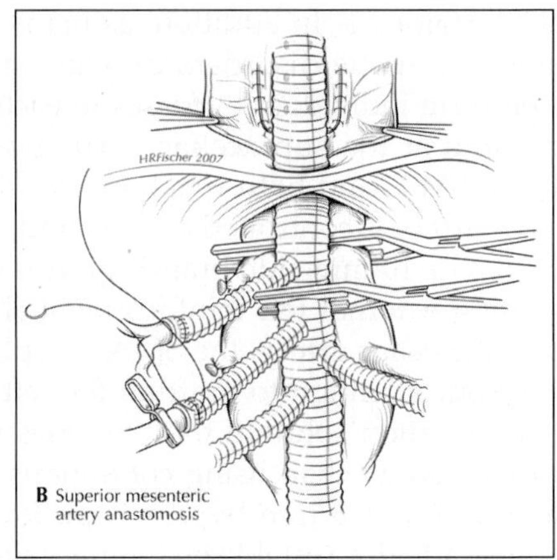

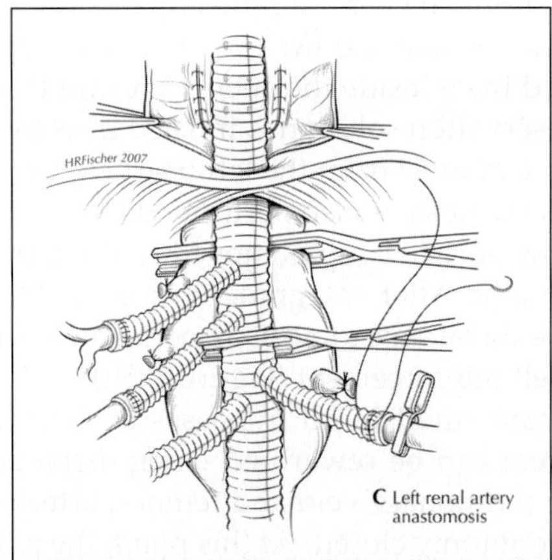

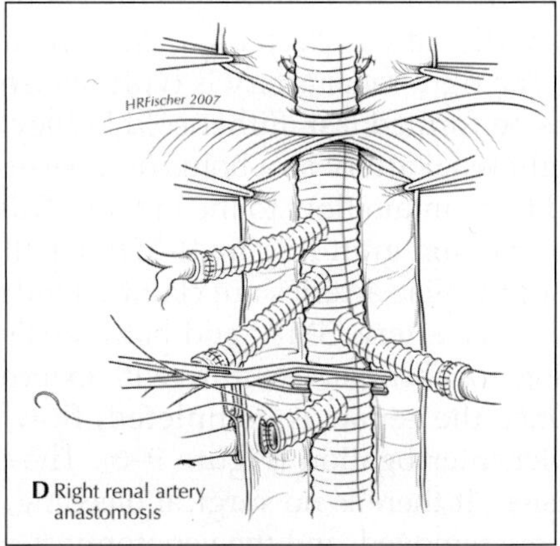

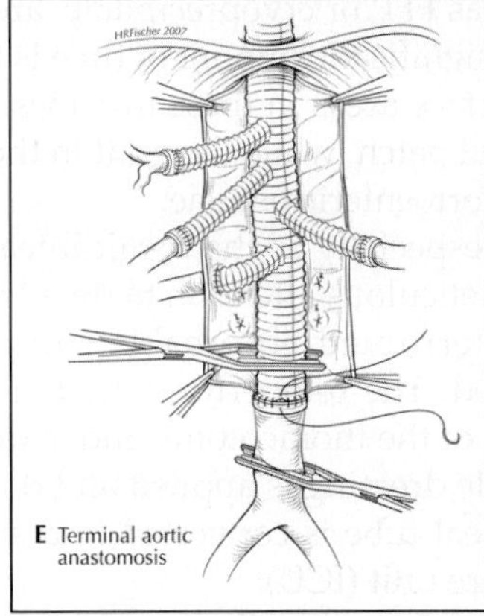

Figure 9-5. Series of diagrams illustrating sequential grafting of the celiac artery **(A)**, SMA **(B)**, left renal artery **(C)**, right renal artery **(D)**, and terminal aorta **(E)**.

UNIVERSITY OF MICHIGAN TAAA EXPERIENCE (2000–2006)

Using the above described approach, we have performed 67 elective, primarily type II-IV TAAA repairs over the last six years (excluding most type I and all endovascular TAAA and pararenal/ suprarenal AAA repairs) (Table 9–1). During this period, the

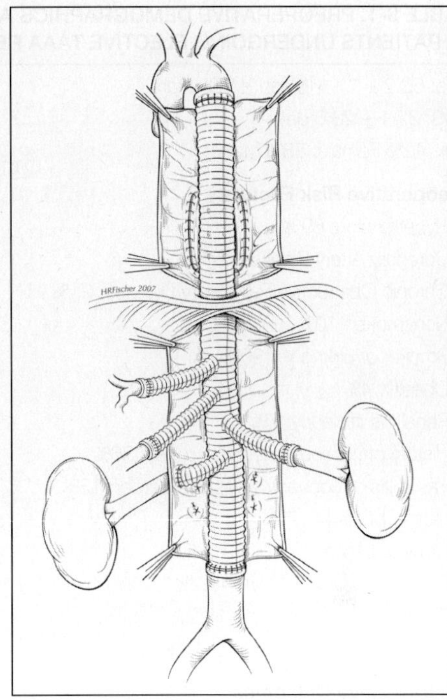

Figure 9-6. Illustration of completed type II TAAA repair.

mortality associated with repair was *only* 3%. However, the incidence of renal failure, requiring either temporary or permanent dialysis, and paraplegia or paraparesis, remain about 10%. This suggests that despite significant advances in the care of these patients, new adjuncts are still needed in order to prevent the devastating complication of renal failure and paralysis following open TAAA repair.

THE DISPARITY BETWEEN TAAA REPAIR NATIONALLY VERSUS CENTERS OF EXCELLENCE

It is suspected that there are few operations performed in the U.S. where the disparity between outcomes in high-volume hospitals (HVHs) by high-volume surgeons (HVSs) and those of low-volume hospitals (LVHs) and surgeons (LVSs) are so dramatically different. For example, a large single institution series reported a low 4.8% mortality rate following TAAA repair.[3] Increasing age, renal insufficiency, and symptomatic enlargement predicted a worse outcome in this experience.

While large, single center experiences dominate the literature, a recent study from our institution used a national database to examine the surgical treatment of TAAAs. This study was performed in order to gain a more realistic evaluation of how surgeons and hospitals across the U.S. were performing. Cowan et. al. examined outcomes following TAAA repair across the U.S. using the National Inpatient Sample.[10] In this study, men outnumbered women 59% to 41%, the majority of whom were Caucasian. Overall in-hospital mortality after TAAA repair was 22.3% in these 1,542 patients. A small, but significant (P = .01), improvement in mortality was observed from 1988 to 1998 (Figure 9–7). Over one-half of all patients suffered at least one postoperative complication after repair of an intact TAAA.

TABLE 9-1. PREOPERATIVE DEMOGRAPHICS AND POSTOPERATIVE COMPLICATIONS ON 67 PATIENTS UNDERGOING ELECTIVE TAAA REPAIR AT THE UNIVERSITY OF MICHIGAN (2000–2006)

Age: 62.2 ± 11.1 (Mean ± SD) years

LOS: 22.1 ± 23.6 days

Sex: 42% Female: 58% Male

Preoperative Risk Factors

Hypertension: 69%

Coronary Artery Disease: 24%

Chronic Obstructive Pulmonary Disease: 21%

Nonsmoker: 10%

Smoker or unknown: 90%

Obesity: 4%

Renal insufficiency: 7%

History of previous aneurysm repair: 36%

Vasculitis or connective tissue disorder: 13%

History of stroke: 7%

Crawford Type   I: 9.2%

                     II: 46.2%

                     III: 16.9%

                     IV: 27.7%

Postoperative Outcomes

Death: 3% (2 patients)

Cardiac complications: all 16%, Atrial Fibrillation 13%, Myocardial Infarction 1.4%

Paralysis or paraparesis: 12%

Dialysis (both temporary and permanent): 10%

Stroke: 4%

Pulmonary Embolus/ Deep Venous Thrombosis: 4%

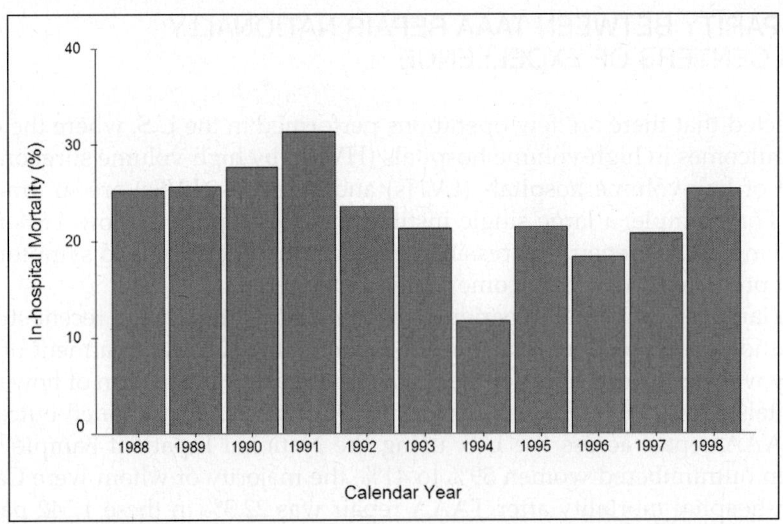

Figure 9-7. In-hospital mortality following TAAA surgical repair from 1988 to 1998 in the United States. Comparing 1988-1993 to 1994-1998, mortality rates improved 25.7% to 19.3% (P = .002). (Reprinted with permission from *J Vasc Surg* 2002; 37: 1169-74.)

Mortality varied significantly for patients undergoing TAAA repair based on hospital caseload volume. LVH experienced a 27.3% mortality rate compared to 15.0% at HVH (P<.001), and a 23.8% mortality rate at medium-volume hospitals (MVH) (P = .001). Significant differences in mortality were also observed by surgeon volume. LVS experienced a 25.6% mortality rate and HVS an 11.0% mortality rate (P<.001). Regression models identified predictors of postoperative mortality, which included postoperative hemorrhage (odds ratio [OR] = 4.4; 95% confidence interval [CI] 3.1-6.2, P<.001), acute renal failure (OR = 3.5; 95%CI 2.4-5.0, P<.001), postoperative cardiac complications (OR = 3.0; 95%CI 2.1-4.2, P<.001), LVS (OR = 2.6; 95%CI 1.7-4.1, P<.001), LVH (OR = 2.2; 95%CI 1.6-3.1, P<.001), MVH (OR = 1.7; 95%CI 1.2-2.4, P = .004), age 65 years and older (OR = 1.6; 95%CI 1.2-2.2, P = .003), non-Caucasian race (OR = 1.5; 95%CI 1.1-1.9, P = .009), and emergent admission (OR = 1.4; 95%CI 1.1-1.9, P = .006).

SUMMARY

Despite improvement in outcomes following intact TAAA repair from 1988 to 1998, the overall morbidity and mortality in the United States continues to be high. In addition, there appear to be large variations in outcomes following elective TAAA repair. As the outcomes following this operation are dependent on a complex balance of outstanding technical detail and skill, and a hospital system that can support these complex procedures, it may be in the patient's best interest to regionalize these operations. At present, while endovascular approaches have significantly impacted isolated thoracic and abdominal aortic aneurysms mortality and morbidity, the technology to repair TAAAs endovascularly is in its early stages. The use of combined open and endovascular approaches in combination, the "hybrid approach," has great appeal because a thoracotomy is not required. However, the open section of this procedure with complex bypasses to the mesenteric and renal arteries is associated with significant mortality and morbidity, and the patient is still left to deal with the pitfalls associated with endografting.

REFERENCES

1. Crawford ES, DeNatale RW. Thoracoabdominal aortic aneurysm: observations regarding the natural course of the disease. *J Vasc Surg*. 1986;3:578–82.
2. Svensson LG, Hess KR, Coselli JS, Safi HJ. Influence of segmental arteries, extent, and atriofemoral bypass on postoperative paraplegia after thoracoabdominal aortic operations. *J Vasc Surg*. 1994;20:255–62.
3. Coselli JS, LeMaire SA, Miller CC 3rd, et al. Mortality and paraplegia after thoracoabdominal aortic aneurysm repair: a risk factor analysis. *Ann Thorac Surg*. 2000;69:409–14.
4. Coselli JS, LeMaire SA, Conklin LD, et al. Morbidity and mortality after extent II thoracoabdominal aortic aneurysm repair. *Ann Thorac Surg*. 2002;73:1107–15.
5. Rectenwald JE, Huber TS, Martin TD, et al. Functional outcome after thoracoabdominal aortic aneurysm repair. *J Vasc Surg*. 2002;35:640–7.
6. Derrow AE, Seeger JM, Dame DA, et al. The outcome in the United States after thoracoabdominal aortic aneurysm repair, renal artery bypass, and mesenteric revascularization. *J Vasc Surg*. 2001;34:54–61.
7. Svensson LG, Crawford ES, Hess KR, et al. Experience with 1509 patients undergoing thoracoabdominal aortic operations. *J Vasc Surg*. Jj1993;17:357–70.

8. Safi HJ, Miller CC 3rd, Huynh TT, et al. Distal aortic perfusion and cerebrospinal fluid drainage for thoracoabdominal and descending thoracic aortic repair: ten years of organ protection. *Ann Surg*. 2003; 238:372–381.

9. Coselli JS, Lemaire SA, Koksoy C, et al. Cerebrospinal fluid drainage reduces paraplegia after thoracoabdominal aortic aneurysm repair: results of a randomized clinical trial. *J Vasc Surg*. 2002;35:631–9.

10. Cowan JA Jr, Dimick JB, Henke PK, et al. Surgical treatment of intact thoracoabdominal aortic aneurysms in the United States: hospital and surgeon volume-related outcomes. *J Vasc Surg*. 2003;37:1169–74.

Reoperative Aortic Surgery

10

Reoperative Techniques in the Management of Aortic Problems

Layne Sandridge, M.D.
and Kenneth J. Cherry, Jr., M.D.

One of the goals of vascular surgery is to provide the patient with a long-lasting surgical revascularization free of complications and the need for reoperations. Unfortunately, the need for repeat aortic operation does occur, and whether or not it results from technical problems, patient risk factors, or the inherent progressive nature of vascular disease, it poses a tremendous challenge for the vascular surgeon. Graft-related and operation-related complications include infection, thrombosis, hemorrhage, fistula, aneurysmal degeneration, intestinal ischemia, and sexual dysfunction. Postoperative complications requiring reoperation ultimately affect long-term morbidity and mortality, whether related to the primary disease process itself or to associated cardiovascular disease. Reoperation in a previous surgical site can be tedious, especially when complicated by intense scarring, inflammation, radiation changes, or infection in the area. Determining the proper care of these patients is often difficult and each case must be approached on an individual basis. Fortunately, refinements in perioperative care, postoperative surveillance, graft materials, and the maturation of surgical technique and approaches have resulted in improved outcomes in these patients. This discussion will address the management of reoperative aortic surgery.

REOPERATION FOR OCCLUDED GRAFTS

Aortoiliac reconstruction and aortofemoral bypasses performed for either occlusive or aneurysmal disease are very durable vascular operations.[1] However, even under ideal circumstances, postoperative complications occur. Hallett et al. reported on 307 patients undergoing AAA repair and found a 9.4% rate of graft-related complications. Anastomotic pseudoaneurysm was the most common complication and occurred in 3% of patients.

Graft thrombosis was the second most common complication and occurred in 2% over a mean follow-up of 5.8 years.[2] Other series have found graft limb thrombosis rates as high as 10%–20% [3]. The majority of these occlusions (72%–82%) occur as late complications, whereas only 18%–28% of these occur perioperatively.[3–5] Graft thrombosis is considered early (perioperative and less than 30 days) or late (occurring months to years after reconstruction), and is caused by very different pathophysiologic mechanisms. Most early thrombotic complications of aortic reconstruction are due to technical problems whereas the causes of late thrombosis tend to be multi-factorial.[6] Late occurrences can result from degeneration of the aortic wall at the proximal anastomosis. Both aneurysmal and occlusive aortic disease involve the whole of the infrarenal aorta; thus, performing the proximal anastomosis as close to the renal arteries as possible is optimal.[1] Recurrent or progressive atherosclerosis can contribute to late graft failure as well. Because reoperative surgery for aortic problems is generally a technically demanding procedure that may put patients at risk for significant morbidity and mortality, high-risk patients without signs and symptoms of limb-threatening ischemia may be treated conservatively.[7]

Although performed less frequently than in years past, an insufficiently performed endarterectomy can also predispose to late reconstructive failure if the disease process is inadequately removed at either the proximal or—more commonly—distal extent of the endarterectomy. Bypass grafting is performed much more frequently. The proximal anastomosis of an aortic graft done in an end-to-end fashion offers favorable hemodynamic flow and is the most often used approach. Sizing of the graft can contribute to reconstructive failure when too large a graft is used as these predispose to low flow. Smaller grafts are preferred and may dilate slightly over time.[1] Grafts should be sized according to the outflow vessels. Rarely, late dilation of these smaller grafts causes sluggish blood flow and results in accumulation of mural thrombus leading to graft occlusion.[7] Layered thrombus can lead to intimal hyperplasia and eventual thrombosis and/or embolization. Late graft failure can also result from improper tunneling or twisting of the graft, inappropriate tension on the graft, or kinking of a limb or the body of the graft itself.[1] Lastly is the importance of the presence of outflow disease. Late graft occlusions can occur secondary to poor distal runoff, and are seen particularly in patients with ongoing risk factors for atherosclerosis including smoking and hypertension.[7]

Management

The treatment of postoperative graft thrombosis is influenced by the timing of occurrence as well as patient symptomatology. Any thrombosis occurring in the early operative period is likely due to a technical error or inadequate outflow, and should be addressed emergently with reoperation. Most of these grafts can be repaired with simple thrombectomy or anastomotic revision. Failure of the technical repair to restore patency of the graft should prompt a work-up for thrombophilic states or for hemodynamic or metabolic factors that may lead to thrombosis.[1] Iatrogenic injuries from interventional radiographic procedures or angiography should not be overlooked as a contributing factor to graft failure.[7] Of course, any patient who presents with an acutely ischemic extremity should be evaluated and treated urgently to prevent progression to limb loss.

Patients with complaints of chronic ischemia can be evaluated on a less urgent basis with a thorough evaluation including angiography in order to better define the inflow and ouflow tracts and guide reoperative decisions.[1] It is essential at the time of first operation to assess the quality of the outflow vessels, in particular the deep and superficial arteries since outflow can be easily improved with endarterectomy or profundaplasty.[6] A majority of patients undergoing aortic reconstruction for occlusive disease will have associated superficial femoral artery stenosis or occlusion; thus, the importance of ensuring adequate profunda femoris arterial flow during the time of initial operation in order to promote long-term patency of the bypass.[8] If preoperative angiography reveals a distal outflow obstruction, then consideration should be given to include a distal bypass procedure in conjunction with the proximal aortic reconstruction if the patient's ischemic symptoms are of a magnitude as to warrant such an extensive operation.[6]

Early thrombosis of an aortic graft usually involves a single limb. Reoperation can often be accomplished through a groin incision only, and involves obtaining control of the common femoral artery, graft limb, and outflow vessels. The graft is opened and a distal thrombectomy is performed prior to restoration of proximal flow. The deep femoral orifice should be visualized to ensure patency. Systemic heparinization should be used with caution in the immediate postoperative period to avoid bleeding complications. Once outflow has been restored, attention should turn to proximal thrombectomy. The graft should be flushed free of any clot before restoration of blood flow and closure of the graft defect.[1]

Patients with late limb thrombosis often present with ischemia of the lower extremity with or without associated sensory or motor paralysis. Dissection may be difficult due to intense scarring. An alternative approach to avoid a scarred field is to enter the anterior surface of the thrombosed graft through a longitudinal incision. Proximal and distal control can be achieved through embolectomy catheters or vessel loops. Adequate inflow may be established by proximal balloon catheter thrombectomy. Once adequate inflow is restored, a patch angioplasty or distal bypass can be performed. This is usually sufficient; however, with some chronic occlusions, limited or localized thrombectomy may not succeed. In this case, graft limb replacement must be undertaken. Another approach with single limb thrombosis is to perform a femoral-femoral artery bypass. Regardless of the technique used, the goal is to ensure excellent inflow and runoff, and to minimize trauma to important collaterals.[1]

Complete aortic graft occlusion is an infrequent event. With complete thrombosis of an end-to-end graft and a juxtarenal aortic occlusion, renal ischemia may be a possibility. Reoperation demands well-planned and executed suprarenal, supramesenteric, or supraceliac exposures with appropriate clamp placement and sequence. Reoperative techniques include direct graft revision and axillo-femorofemoral bypass. Patients considered poor risk for direct aortic reconstruction can be considered for axillo-femorofemoral bypass. However, in addition to poor long-term patency, axillofemoral bypasses for failed aortic reconstruction may allow propagation of the aortic thrombus proximally and compromise renal or visceral circulation.[7] Alternatively, the ascending or descending thoracic aorta may be used as a proximal landing zone with bypass distally.[1,7] All of these techniques may be used. The authors prefer a direct in-line approach if at all possible.

POSTOPERATIVE ANEURYSM FORMATION

Despite improved operative techniques and advances in the development of new prosthetic graft materials, aneurysm formation still occurs after aortic reconstruction and poses a challenge for vascular surgeons. There are three types of recurrent aneurysms following the initial repair of an aortic aneurysm: a true aneurysm developing proximal or distal to the graft, an anastomotic aneurysm, and aneurysmal graft degeneration.[9] The latter is quite rare. Factors implicated in the development of anastomotic aneurysms include perioperative complications, infection, material defects, graft dilation, and improper surgical techniques.[10] A review from the Mayo Clinic found recurrent aneurysms to be the third leading cause of death after coronary artery disease and cancer in patients undergoing abdominal aortic aneurysm repair. Plate et al. reported the results of a series of 1,112 patients who underwent abdominal aortic aneurysm repair and found 55 (5.4%) of these patients developed recurrent aneurysms. Interestingly, a threefold risk of developing aneurysms was noted in patients with associated hypertension.[11] Edwards et al. reported a series of 111 patients with aortic reconstruction who were followed with abdominal ultrasound. Ten percent of patients had recurrent paraanastomotic aneurysms a mean of 144 months postoperatively. Seven aneurysms were at the anastomosis and four were true aneurysms. Three of the total were diagnosed within three years, and the remaining eight occurred between seven and 28 years postoperatively.[12] In contrast to patients with infection or occlusion who are symptomatic, patients who develop recurrent, usually asymptomatic, aneurysms may be lost to follow-up or the imaging studies used for surveillance may not be appropriate for the detection of new pathology.[13] On occasion, patients with recurrent aneurysms will present with ischemic symptoms due to thrombosis and/or embolization of the aneurysm.[9] Newer diagnostic methods, especially computed tomography (CT) and computed tomographic angiography (CTA), have allowed for improved follow-up.[13]

Management

The importance of serial follow-up and early diagnosis of recurrent true and anastomotic aneurysm is underscored by the results seen in several series including that by Plate et al. Twenty-five of 26 patients in this report with recurrent aortic aneurysms presented with rupture and died.[11] Gloviczki et al. reported a 47% mortality rate in patients undergoing emergent repair of recurrent aneurysms.[14] The high rates seen in these series support the early detection and elective repair of these aneurysms. Once recurrent aortic aneurysms have been detected, the next step is thoughtful planning and preparation for repair. Important points to take into account include approach, incision, and extent of exposure, and site and sequence of clamp placement. Any interval development of occlusive disease is important to note and if present, may alter the method of repair. The patient's overall state of health also influences the surgical approach. Consideration should be given to ureteral stenting in reoperations, especially when reconstructions are performed for secondary occlusions or aneurysmal disease distal to a previously placed abdominal aortic graft.[13] Last, any evidence of perigraft infection preoperatively or intraoperatively must be addressed and may alter the course of treatment.[10]

Incision Placement

There are multiple approaches and incisions and all have benefits and disadvantages. Again, thoughtful planning as to incision placement will provide the best exposure to facilitate repair for a particular patient's problem, anatomy, and comorbid conditions. A left flank retroperitoneal approach can be used for suprarenal or supraceliac clamping. The patient should be placed in a modified left thoracotomy position with the shoulders at a 70° to 80° angle to the table, and the hips flat in order to gain access to the groins. The left flank is centered over the break in the table and the table is extended to open the flank space. An oblique incision is then made from the lateral edge of the rectus muscle between the pubis and the umbilicus, and extended to the ninth, 10th, 11th, or 12th intercostal space, depending on the reconstruction necessary.

A midline, extraperitoneal approach with medial visceral rotation provides excellent exposure of the subdiaphragmatic aorta as well as the visceral vessels. The left kidney and adrenal can be left in their bed if exposure of the superior mesenteric artery is required.[13] Medial visceral rotation can be combined with a standard infracolic transperitoneal approach to allow exposure of the entire abdominal aorta and the iliac arteries. This combination of approaches allows adequate visualization and handling of the right iliac vessels and of the right renal artery. The thoracoabdominal approach by Crawford can be used for recurrent aneurysms involving the renal or mesenteric vessels. It is with this approach that the distal portion of the graft is sutured to the previous aortic graft.[9] Each approach provides wide exposure and facilitates repair. Patients with severe lung disease may tolerate an abdominal or flank approach much better than a thoracoabdominal approach. The type of approach should take into account surgeon preference, patient body habitus, and cardiac and pulmonary function, as well as coexisting abdominal pathology.[13]

Reconstruction

Recurrent aneurysms require direct in-line aortic reconstruction. The approaches are similar to those used in primary repair. Infrarenal abdominal aortic aneurysms appearing after repair of thoracic or thoracoabdominal aneurysms can be repaired as an initial aneurysm in a standard approach.[13] Alternatively, patients with previous abdominal aortic aneurysm repair may have a new thoracic or thoracoabdominal aneurysm needing repair.[9,13] This can be treated with the usual repair through a thoracic or thoracoabdominal incision.[13] Segments of healthy aorta should be dissected free of scar tissue to provide an accepatable landing zone for the new graft. Anastomoses should be end to end and tension-free with generous bites of healthy aortic wall. Endarterectomy of the aorta should be avoided to prevent future occurrence of anastomotic aneurysms.[10] When recurrent aneurysms are contiguous with the old graft, the anastomosis can be made to the old graft. If there is normal sized patent aorta between the old graft and the new aneurysm, an attempt should be made to preserve the native aorta and its associated lumbar or intercostal branches.[13]

Recurrent juxtarenal aneurysms may be especially challenging for vascular surgeons whether they are anastomotic or true aneurysms. The approach may be through an abdominal incision. If the aneurysm does not extend suprarenally, it may be approached through a midline, transperitoneal infracolic approach. Supramesenteric clamping can usually be achieved through this incision. Division of the diaphragmatic crura cephalad to the renal arteries allows for easier dissection and clamping of the supramesenteric aorta. If this exposure appears difficult, subdiaphragmatic clamping of the supraceliac aorta may be used. Some advocate a routine retroperitoneal exposure through a flank or thoracoabdominal incision for repair of juxtarenal abdominal aortic aneurysms.[13]

Suprarenal aneurysms require planning for adequate and safe exposure needed for the repair. Aneurysms extending proximally to the celiac level are difficult to approach through a midline transperitoneal infracolic exposure. However, a midline incision with medial visceral rotation can provide excellent exposure of the supraceliac aorta. The disadvantage of this exposure lies in that mobilizing the left kidney makes exposure of the superior mesenteric artery difficult if mesenteric reconstruction is necessary. If the aneurysm extends to the level of the diaphragm as a Crawford type IV thoracoabdominal aortic aneurysm, medial visceral rotation may be employed.[13] A low thoracoabdominal or thoracoretroperitoneal (Pillsbury) incision may be used also if body habitus dictates.

Proper clamp positioning and sequencing is vital to adequate repair of recurrent aneurysms. Proper site placement depends on location and proximal extent of the aneurysm, and of any associated intraluminal thrombus as well as the presence of aortic atherosclerosis. Supramesenteric clamping predisposes to fewer cardiac effects compared to supraceliac clamping. Maintenance of gastric, splenic, hepatic, and mesenteric blood flow helps reduce afterload on the heart, and helps prevent prolonged liver and gut ischemia. The proper clamp placement, sequence of clamp placement, and declamping sequence should be individualized to the patient's pathology, and if well planned and executed, will yield excellent exposure and results.[13] These decisions need to be made preoperatively and the operation performed to meet those planned ends. Changing clamp sites after the aorta is clamped because of poorly anticipated findings or poorly planned clamp level may prove disastrous.[15] Gloviczki et al. reported their results of multiple operations for recurrent aneurysms and found an 8% mortality for elective repairs of thoracic and abdominal aortic aneurysms. With additional procedures, the mortality rate increased from 4.7% for the first operation to 10.4% for the second operation.[14] Since morbidity and mortality increases with each subsequent procedure for recurrent aneurysms, careful preoperative planning regarding proper incision, clamping, and repair should minimize associated morbidity and mortality.

AORTIC GRAFT INFECTIONS

Aortic graft infection occurs in 1% to 2% of prosthetic abdominal aortic reconstructions.[16–17] Several important known risk factors predispose to graft infections. These include skin and subcutaneous wound infection, hematoma, and lymphatic leak, and relate to the time of initial surgery. Contamination can occur when the graft comes in contact with the skin. Breaks in sterile technique also contribute to this problem. Procedures performed emergently increase the risk for postoperative graft infection due to the physical condition of the patient and perhaps hurried attention to sterile prepping and draping. Prolonged operative times contribute to wound and subsequent graft infections.[18] Grafts may become secondarily infected after placement by hematogenous spread from distal sites or by lymphatic or contiguous spread.[19] Edwards et al., in their review assessing risk factors for primary graft infection, found that postoperative wound infection was the predisposing risk factor in 33% of graft infections.[20] Early redo operations are associated with a higher infection rate due to reexposure of the graft to potential contamination and repeated dissection through already once devitalized tissue.[18] Careful attention to wound hemostasis and avoidance of hematomas and seromas should be important surgical techniques, especially with implantation of graft material.[19]

Management

The traditional approach to aortic graft infection is complete excision of the infected graft, debridement, and axillofemoral reconstruction through a noninfected field. However, this reconstruction carries a risk of amputation in 20%–29% of patients, aortic stump blowout in 10%–20%, and graft reinfection in 10%–40%. These results have prompted the search for alternative surgical options for patients with infected aortic grafts. Autogenous reconstruction and in situ prosthetic replacement are alternatives used today. A review by Oderich et al. compared patients undergoing axillofemoral reconstruction with those treated with graft excision and in situ prosthetic reconstruction. Patients with in situ reconstruction had a significantly improved outcome.[21] Young et al. reviewed the data of 25 patients undergoing in situ graft replacement with either standard polyester grafts, or rifampin-soaked collagen or gelatin-impregnated polyester grafts, and found a lower rate of reinfection with rifampin-impregnated grafts.[22] The mortality rate for these patients was 8% with a limb salvage rate of 100%. Clagett et al. reported on their series of patients undergoing autogenous reconstruction with superficial femoral vein for aortic graft infection and found a mortality rate of 10%.[23] The mortality rates for these in-line reconstructions are similar.[22] Extraanatomic reconstruction for an infected aortic graft is associated with a mortality rate as high as 24%.[24]

Graft Excision and Extraanatomic Bypass

The gold standard of treatment for an infected aortic graft involving more than one limb entails complete excision with extraanatomic bypass through clean tissue planes. Data suggest that the postoperative mortality rate is less in patients undergoing revascularization prior to graft excision.[25] When bypass precedes graft excision by a period of 45 days there is less of a physiologic insult to the patient since this approach minimizes extremity ischemia time.[19] Reilly et al. reported a 26% mortality rate in patients receiving bypass prior to excision versus a 43% mortality rate in patients undergoing the "traditional" approach of graft excision initially.[26] The extraanatomic bypass constructed is dictated by the initial operation. An axillobifemoral bypass can be constructed to uninvolved groins in a patient with a previous aortoaortic or aortobi-iliac graft. In the case of initial aortobifemoral bypasses, reconstruction should be redirected around the infected groins. One option is axillary bypass with lateral groin tunneling to the superficial femoral, profunda, or popliteal arteries. Alternatively, native conduits such as the superficial femoral or greater saphenous vein can be used as a cross-femoral bypass after debridement of infected tissue. Use of the saphenous vein should only be used as a temporary conduit as it lacks durability. Extraanatomic bypass for a single infected limb can be accomplished without complete excision of the graft. The infected limb of the graft is approached through the retroperitoneum and divided. The proximal stump is then oversewn and covered with peritoneum. The affected limb is removed through the groin. An axillary bypass or cross femoral bypass can then be performed through clean tissue. Close surveillance of the remaining graft is of the utmost importance since the remaining graft may subsequently exhibit infection.[25]

Graft Excision with In Situ Bypass

Excision of an infected prosthetic graft and immediate replacement of an in situ graft reduces limb ischemia, provides long term patency with improved hemodynamic flow, and eliminates the need for stump closure. However, many surgeons avoid this method because of the subsequent risk of reinfection. In situ graft placement, when performed, should be in a nongrossly contaminated bed and the choice of graft material is important. PTFE may be more resistant to infection than Dacron; however, antibiotic impregnated gelatin-coated Dacron grafts provide an alternative.[25] Rifampin bonded Dacron grafts are easily prepared by soaking the gelatin sealed graft in a rifampin/saline mixture for 15 minutes.[27] Alternative but less widely used grafts include cadaver aortic and venous homografts. These grafts offer resistance to recurrent infection; however, their limited availability prevents widespread use. Clagett described the use of a neoaortoiliac system (NAIS) using autogenous femoropopliteal veins from the lower extremities. NAIS has been placed in infected aortic beds without evidence of graft or anastomotic breakdown. The limitation of this alternative is the potential for intractable lower extremity swelling. To prevent this, the deep and superficial systems should not be harvested from the same lower extremity.[19,25]

When a patient is not a candidate for graft excision because of poor risk or involvement of a visceral segment graft, infections can be treated with antibiotic irrigation through surgically placed catheters.[25] In a study published by Morris et al., eight out of 10 patients were successfully treated for their graft infection by antibiotic irrigation. Two out of the 10 patients died of complications related to their graft infection.[28] Alternatively, coverage of exposed prosthetic material with muscle flaps can be undertaken.[19] These may provide alternatives when surgical graft excision is not an option.

An important adjunct to the surgical management of aortic graft infections includes appropriate antibiotic therapy. The regimen should be tailored to match bacterial susceptibility and a minimum of a two-week course is indicated with negative graft wall cultures. A six-week minimum course is recommended for positive wall cultures or an in situ replacement or treatment using nonexcisional therapy. If biologic material was used or an extraanatomic bypass was placed through clean tissue, then only a few weeks of appropriate antibiotic coverage is necessary.[25]

CONCLUSION

The first step in managing postoperative graft complications begins with prevention during the time of initial operation. Aseptic and flawless surgical technique as well as attention to careful clamp placement will forestall many postoperative complications. The recognition of factors predisposing to surgical failure such as distal outflow disease allows surgeons to act preemptively in maintaining integrity of the reconstruction. The importance of close postoperative follow-up and graft surveillance cannot be overemphasized. Once a graft complication is recognized, it is the responsibility of the vascular surgeon to take prompt but thoughtful measures. The appropriate action depends on the patient's symptoms, overall health, and morbidity and/or mortality associated with reoperation. When these aspects are taken into consideration, patients can be offered the procedure that will be of greatest benefit to them individually.

REFERENCES

1. DePalma RG. Reoperations for Occluded Aortic Grafts. In: Trout HH ed. *Reoperative Vascular Surgery*. New York: Marcel Dekker, Inc; 1987:95–112.
2. Hallett JW, Marshall DM, Petterson TM, et al. Graft-related complications after abdominal aortic aneurysm repair: Reassurance from a 36-year population based experience. *J Vasc Surg.* 1997;25(2):277–286.
3. Brewster DC, Meier GH, Darling RC, et al. Reoperations for aortofemoral graft limb occlusion: Optimal methods and long term results. *J Vasc Surg.* 1987;5(2):363–374.

4. Ernst CB. Aortic graft limb occlusion. In: Ernst CB, Stanley JC eds. *Current Therapy in Vascular Surgery*. Philadelphia: BC Decker; 1991:449–454.

5. LeGrand DR, Vermillion BD, Hayes JP, et al. Management of occluded aortofemoral graft limb. *Surgery*. 1983;93:818–821.

6. Colburn MD, Moore WS. Reoperative Approach for Failed Aortofemoral, Axillofemoral, and Femorofemoral Bypasses. *Semin Vasc Surg*. 1994;7(3):139–151.

7. Brewster DC. Surgery of late aortic graft occlusion. In: Bergan JJ, Yao JST eds. *Aortic Surgery*. Philadelphia: W.B. Saunders, 1989:519–538.

8. Brewster DC, Perler BA, Robison JG, et al. Aortofemoral graft for multilevel occlusive disease: Predictors of success and need for distal bypass. *Arch Surg*. 1982;117:1593–1599.

9. Yao JST, Flinn WR, Rizzo RJ. Recurrent aortic and anastomotic aneurysms. In: Bergan JJ, Yao JST eds. *Aortic Surgery*. Philadelphia: W.B. Saunders; 1989:305–316.

10. Shepard AD, Jacobson GM. Anastomotic aneurysms. In: Towne JB, Hollier LH eds. *Complications in Vascular Surgery*. New York: Marcel Dekker, Inc, 2004:139–153.

11. Plate G, Hollier LA, O'Brien P, et al. Recurrent aneurysms and late vascular complications following repair of abdominal aortic aneurysms. *Arch Surg*. 1985;120:590–594.

12. Edwards JM, Teefey SA, Zierler E, et al. Intraabdominal paraanastomotic aneurysms after aortic bypass grafting. *J Vasc Surg*. 1992;15:344–350.

13. Cherry KJ. Techniques in the management of recurrent aortic aneurysms. In: Yao JST, Pearce WH eds. *Aneurysms new findings and treatments*. Norwalk, CT: Appleton & Lange, 1994:249–256.

14. Gloviczki P, Pairolero PC, Welch T. Multiple aortic aneurysms: The results of surgical Management. *J Vasc Surg*. 1990;11:19–28.

15. Green RM, Ricotta JJ, Ouriel K, et al. Results of supraceliac aortic clamping in the difficult elective resection of infrarenal abdominal aortic aneurysm. *J Vasc Surg*. 1989;9(1):124–134.

16. Bunt TJ. Synthetic vascular graft infections: I. Graft infections. *Surgery*. 1983;93:733–746.

17. Goldstone J, Moore WS. Infection in vascular prosthesis: clinical manifestations and surgical management. *Am J Surg*. 1974;128:225–233.

18. Towne JB. Inguinal wound complications and graft infections. In: Pearce WH, Matsumura JS eds. *Trends in Vascular Surgery*. Evanston, IL: Greenwood Academic; 2005:197–203.

19. Clagett GP. Aortic graft infections. In: Towne JB, Hollier LH eds. *Complications in Vascular Surgery*. New York: Marcel Dekker, Inc, 2004:317–336.

20. Edwards WH Jr, Martin RS III, Jenkins JM et al. Primary graft infections. *J Vasc Surg*. 1987; 6:235–239.

21. Oderich GS, Bower TC, Panneton JM. Comparison of in situ versus axillofemoral reconstruction in the treatment of aortic graft infection. Presented at the 2005 Vascular Annual Meeting of the Society for Vascular Surgery. June 16-19, 2005. Chicago, Illinois.

22. Young RM, Cherry KJ, Davis PM. The results of in situ prosthetic replacement for infected aortic grafts. *Am J Surg*. 1999;178(2):136–140

23. Clagett GP, Valentine RJ, Hagino RT. Autogenous aortoiliac/femoral reconstruction from superficial femoral-popliteal veins: feasibility and durability. *J Vasc Surg*. 1997;25:255–266.

24. Quinones-Baldrich WJ, Hernandez JJ, Moore WS. Long-term results following surgical management of aortic graft infection. *Arch Surg*. 1991;126:507–511.

25. Galt SW, Kraiss LW. Treatment of aortic graft infection. In: Gewertz BL, Schwartz LB eds. *Surgery of the aorta and its branches*. Philadelphia: W.B. Saunders, 2000:397–404.

26. Reilly LM, Stoney RJ, Goldstone J, et al. Improved management of aortic graft infection: The influence of operation sequence and staging. *J Vasc Surg*. 1987;5:421.

27. Gahtan V, Esses GE, Bandyk DF, et al. Antistaphylococcal activity of rifampin bonded gelatin-impregnated Dacron grafts. *J Surg Res*. 1995;58:105.

28. Morris GE, Friend PJ, Vassallo DJ, et al. Antibiotic irrigation and conservative surgery for major aortic graft infection. *J Vasc Surg*. 1994;20: 88.

11

Management of Infected Aortic Grafts by In-situ Grafting

Paul A. Armstrong, D.O. and Dennis F. Bandyk, M.D.

Infection involving an aortic graft placed by an open or endovascular route continues to occur despite advancements in biomaterials, improved grafting techniques, and routine antibiotic prophylaxis. The incidence of infection following aortic prosthetic grafting is low: aortic interposition graft—0.2%–1.3%; aortofemoral bypass—0.7%–3%; aortic stent-graft—0.4%–0.8%; and secondary graft-enteric fistula—0.3%–1.2%.[1-2] When infection involves the intracavitary graft segment, its management is more complex than if localized to an extracavitary segment (i.e., groin, or a single graft limb). The morbidity of aortic graft infection has steadily decreased with time due to the development of effective operative strategies including the application of in situ graft replacement. For example, mortality associated with graft excision and lower limb revascularization has decreased by approximately 20% to the 10%–15% range.[3-8] When confronted with an aortic graft infection, the treatment goals are straightforward: save the patient's life and limbs. The extent of graft involvement needs to be determined since the entire graft may not be infected. All infected graft material must be excised in conjunction with an appropriate arterial reconstruction that maintains circulation to the lower limbs and other vital structures (kidneys, gut, pelvis). Surgical management should be associated with low morbidity/mortality, be durable, and have a low incidence of persistent and recurrent infection.

Aortic graft infections can be classified by extent of graft involvement and the virulence of the infecting organism (Table 11-1). In situ replacement is an appropriate treatment option in the majority of patients with the preferred approach to use lower extremity deep veins (femoropopliteal venous segment) to replace the excised, infected graft segments. Use of an antibiotic (rifampin) impregnated graft for in situ replacement is also an effective option in selected patients presenting with graft biofilm infections caused by *S. epidermidis*.[9-10] In general, in situ replacement is not recommended as treatment option for an aortic graft infected by a contiguous infectious process (diverticulits, abdominal abscess). This type of intracavitary graft infection requires drainage of the intraabdominal abscess, correction of the underlying cause of intraabdominal sepsis followed by aortic graft excision, and when possible, extraanatomic bypass.

TABLE 11-1. CLASSIFICATION OF AORTIC GRAFT INFECTION AND RECOMMENDATION REGARDING IN SITU RECONSTRUCTION

Intracavitary Graft Involvement	In Situ Revascularization Option
Graft-enteric fistula—associated mycotic aneurysm	Not Recommended
GEE (graft erosion into gut)	FPV* grafting
Total graft involvement with infection	
biofilm infection (*S. epidermidis*)	FPV or Rifampin-impregnated graft
virulent bacterial sp.	FPV grafting
Aortofemoral Graft Limb Infection (localized to groin segment)	
Invasive infection	FPV grafting
Biofilm infection (*S. epidermidis*)	Rifampin-impregnated graft
Aortofemoral Graft Limb Infected due to contiguous infection	Not Recommended
Diverticulitis	
Appendicitis	

*FPV, femoropopliteal venous segment

Extraanatomic bypass, usually performed as an axillobifemoral bypass, is an appropriate option for aortic graft infections confined to the abdomen, particularly when associated with a graft-enteric fistula. When performed as staged procedures (i.e., extraanatomic bypass followed by aortic graft excision), lower limb ischemia time is minimized, the patient is better able to tolerate both procedures, and the aortic graft excision procedure can be performed unhurried with careful attention to aortic stump closure, perigraft tissue debridement, and reconstruction of the bowel when graft erosion is present.[4–6] Unfortunately, the majority of aortic graft infections occur following aortofemoral bypass grafting with infection presenting in the groin or involving the entire graft. Extraanatomic bypass with excision of the infected aortobifemoral graft is a more complex procedure than in situ grafting, and is associated with inferior long-term patency and higher reinfection rates.[9–11] Bilateral axillopopliteal bypass to avoid the groin regions involved by infection has been shown not to be a durable treatment option, and this procedure is currently not recommended.[6]

In situ replacement of the infected aortic graft has emerged as preferred treatment at many tertiary vascular centers. Reconstructive options include in situ replacement with lower limb (FPV) deep veins, an arterial allograft, or antibiotic-impregnated prosthetic graft.[7–13] Partial or total excision of the infected aortic graft with immediate in situ grafting avoids several complications associated with ex situ therapy including infrarenal aortic closure with its potential for aortic stump blow-out or renal artery thrombosis, the requirement for multiple or staged procedures, and the need for antithrombotic therapy to maintain extraanatomic graft patency. Importantly, the application of in situ grafting allows the surgeon to develop an "individualized" treatment strategy for each patient based on the anatomic and microbiologic features of the infectious process. Compared to axillofemoral reconstruction with aortic graft excision, in situ replacement has been associated with less graft-related deaths, decreased hospitalization, and improved primary graft patency.[13]

The clinical spectrum of aortic graft infection ranges from biomaterial contamination as a result of a postoperative wound infection to the late appearance of gramnegative infection caused by graft-enteric erosion. Most patients who develop an aortic graft infection are not critically ill on clinical presentation, thus allowing time to formulate and institute a treatment plan than may incorporate in situ graft replacement. The majority of the aortic graft infections are caused by *Staphylococcus epidermidis*, a bacterial strain that is part of normal skin flora but has sufficient virulence to infect a vascular prosthesis. The prosthetic graft is colonized as a "bacterial biofilm" as microcolonies on graft surfaces are protected from host defenses and antibacteria by a mucopolysacharride glycocalyx film produced by the bacteria. The infectious process is indolent in presentation, often involves only a segment of the aortic graft, and is associated with low-numbers of bacteria harbored on the external graft surfaces. This type of graft infection is resistant to antibiotic therapy, but when combined with in situ grafting, it can be successfully eradicated.[9,12] Which in situ replacement procedure (i.e., autogenous versus prosthetic/allograft grafting) is "best" for the patient depends on a number of factors: accurate recovery of infecting organism(s), the nature and extent of graft involvement, and patient-specific conditions such as medical comorbidities, arterial anatomy, and availability of lower limb deep veins for reconstruction of the aortoiliac segment.

PREOPERATIVE ASSESSMENT FOR IN SITU GRAFT REPLACEMENT

Most aortic graft infections present beyond three months of the primary procedure. These late-appearing infections are manifest clinically in several ways: gastrointestinal hemorrhage caused by graft-enteric erosion, unexplained sepsis, or as an infectious process (sinus tract, perigraft abscess, anastomotic pseudoaneurysm) in the inguinal region following aortofemoral bypass. The aortic graft is typically patent, and septic embolization is a rare presenting sign. When an aortic graft infection is manifest early (< three mo.), it is typically associated with a wound infection or a postoperative bowel complication (ischemic colitis, diverticulitis). If groin infection develops following aortofemoral bypass grafting, the surgical site should be promptly explored in the operating room. All ischemic and infected tissue should be debrided, and cultures of deep tissue performed including tissue adjacent to the graft if exposed and involved in the wound infection. Implantation of antibiotic (vancomycin, daptomycin, gentamicin) beads into the surgical site can often sterilize the wound and may avert the need for graft excision.[14] Use of serial wound debridements coupled with coverage of the distal aortofemoral graft limb by a sartorius muscle flap has been shown to be an effective strategy for graft preservation for these early extracavitary graft infections.

Establishing an accurate diagnosis of graft infection and the extent of involvement is paramount for clinical success. Imaging of graft and adjacent vascular structures is performed both for diagnosis as well as for preoperative planning for in situ replacement of an assumed or known aortic graft infection. Contrast-enhanced, thin slice, computed tomography (CT) of the abdomen and extremities provides soft tissue detail and 3-D visualization of the pararenal aorta, visceral/renal arteries, the aortic graft, and lower limb arteries and veins. Graft involvement with an inflammatory process with perigraft air or fluid is highly diagnostic of an infectious process (Figures 11-1 and 11-2). Likewise, the absence of perigraft inflammation with normal retroperitoneal tissues suggests no graft involvement (Figure 11-3). Other important CT signs of aortic graft infection include psoas abscess, pseudoaneurysms, hydronephrosis, hydroureter, graft thrombus, and perigaft fluid.[15] CT angiography provides sufficient anatomic detail of the aorta, iliac arteries, and infrainguinal arterial system to identify significant

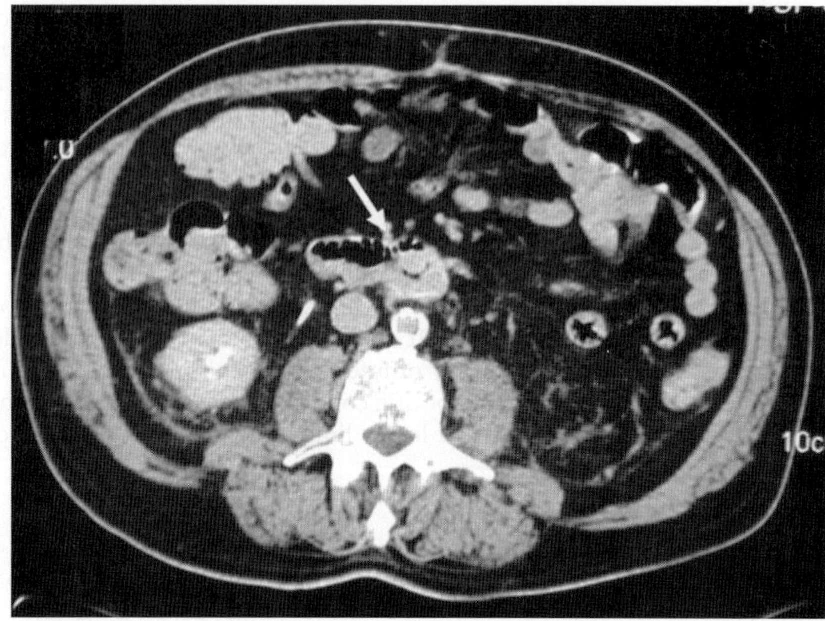

Figure 11-1. Computed tomography (CT) scan of the abdomen demonstrating air (arrow) adjacent to an aortic graft in a patient with a graft-enteric erosion.

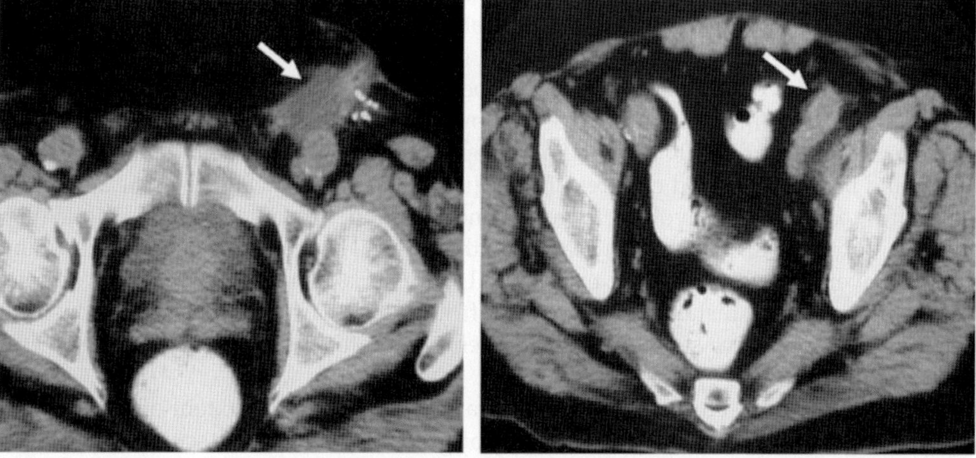

Figure 11-2. Computed tomography (CT) of the groin (left image) and pelvis (right image) demonstrating peri-graft fluid/inflammation (arrows) in a patient with a *S. epidermidis* biofilm infection of the left aortofemoral graft limb. Note absence of graft infection in the right groin.

concomitant occlusive disease and plan arterial reconstruction. In addition, caliber of the lower limb superficial (great saphenous) and deep (common femoral, femoral, popliteal) veins can be assessed. Catheter-based diagnostic arteriography is required in only select cases such as to evaluate the aortic arch and its branches for occlusive disease, and in patients with concomitant aortic and infrainguinal bypass grafts. While magnetic resonance imaging (MRI) provides excellent soft tissue detail and is capable of defining the arterial anatomy, we prefer CT imaging for preoperative planning and

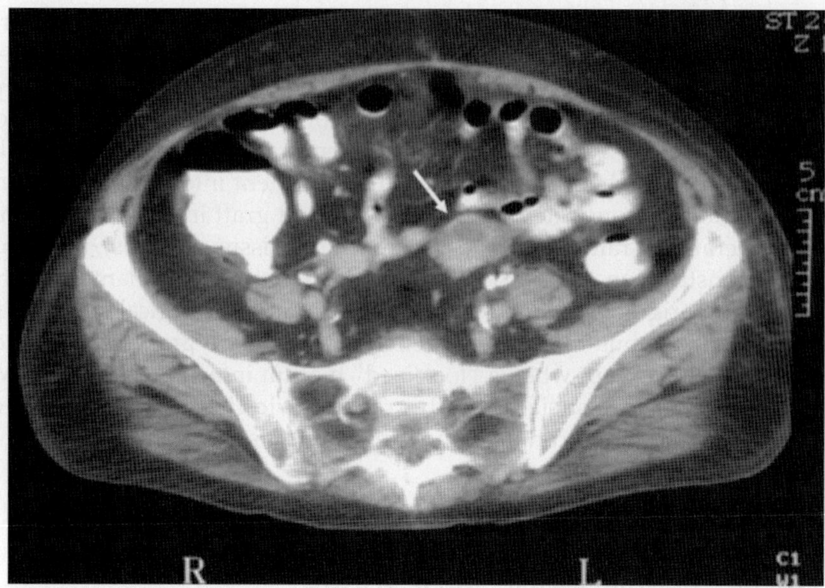

Figure 11-3. Computed tomography (CT) scan of the pelvis demonstrating signs of intracavitry infection of the left aortofemoral graft limb (arrow) with perigraft fluid. No CT abnormality of the right aortofemoral graft limb indicates partial graft involvement.

graft surveillance for recurrent infection. MRI is a useful adjunct in patients with renal insufficiency.

Noninvasive vascular testing is recommended to provide baseline values of ankle-brachial systolic pressure index (ABI), and for imaging of the lower limb deep (femoral, popliteal) and superficial (great saphenous) veins for patency and caliber. If duplex ultrasound demonstrates a recanalized femoropopliteal venous segment, autogenous in situ replacement of the aortoiliac segment is not an option. Finding a large 5–6 mm diameter graft saphenous vein indicates a satisfactory autogenous conduit for femorofemoral bypass, but the great saphenous vein is not suitable as an aortoiliac replacement conduit.

Broad-spectrum, bactericidal, parenteral antibiotic therapy should be started on clinical suspicion of an aortic graft infection. The most common infecting organisms (in decreasing order of prevalence) are staphylococcal strains (*S. aureus, S. epidermidis*), streptococcus, E. coli, Kliebseilla, Pseudomonas strains, and Candida albicans. Methicillin-resistant *S. aureus* (MRSA) now accounts for one-half of early and one-quarter of late aortofemoral graft infections. If *S. aureus* or *S. epidermidis* is most likely a pathogen, parenteral antibiotic therapy with a first- or second-generation cephalosporin and vancomycin is appropriate, although the use of daptomycin or line-zolid is a better, bactericidal therapy for a MRSA graft infection. In patients allergic to penicillin, administration of aminoglycoside or a fluoroquinolone is recommended for extended gram-negative bacteria coverage. Once the infecting organism has been isolated (e.g., by needle aspiration of perigraft fluid or surgical exploration), antibiotic coverage should be modified based on antibiotic susceptibility testing of the recovered strains. Antibiotic therapy is an adjunct to surgical management that includes drainage of perigraft abscesses, debridement of infected tissues, and excision of the infected graft. Both are essential for a successful treatment strategy.

Patient selection for in situ replacement therapy depends on the clinical presentation, extent of graft infection, and its microbiology as determined by operative exploration of the involved graft segment (Figure 11-4). The intent of the evaluation process is to accurately establish whether the infection involves the entire aortic graft or is localized to a graft segment, followed by a determination whether a graft biofilm (amenable to in situ prosthetic grafting) or a more virulent infectious process exists. If surgical exploration demonstrates an invasive, virulent graft infection (organisms present on intraoperative Gram's stain, positive perigraft tissue cultures), an autogenous vein in situ reconstruction should be considered. Preliminary implantation of antibiotic beads in the perigraft space is recommended to aid in surgical site sterilization. When possible, autogenous vein reconstruction of the excised graft segment should be performed in all cases except when a "localized" biofilm infection is present. When an aortic graft infection is associated with graft-enteric fistula, extraanatomic (axillofemoral) reconstruction in conjunction with graft excision and aortic stump closure should be considered.

IN SITU GRAFT REPLACEMENT PROCEDURE

Removal of an infected aortic graft and in situ reconstruction is associated with prolonged exposure of abdomen and lower limbs. To avoid reduction in core body temperature below 35°C, air warming blankets should be placed on the upper body, intravenous fluids warmed, and the room temperature kept above 22°C. In order to minimize lower limb ischemia time, the sequence for aortic graft excision and in situ autogenous recon-

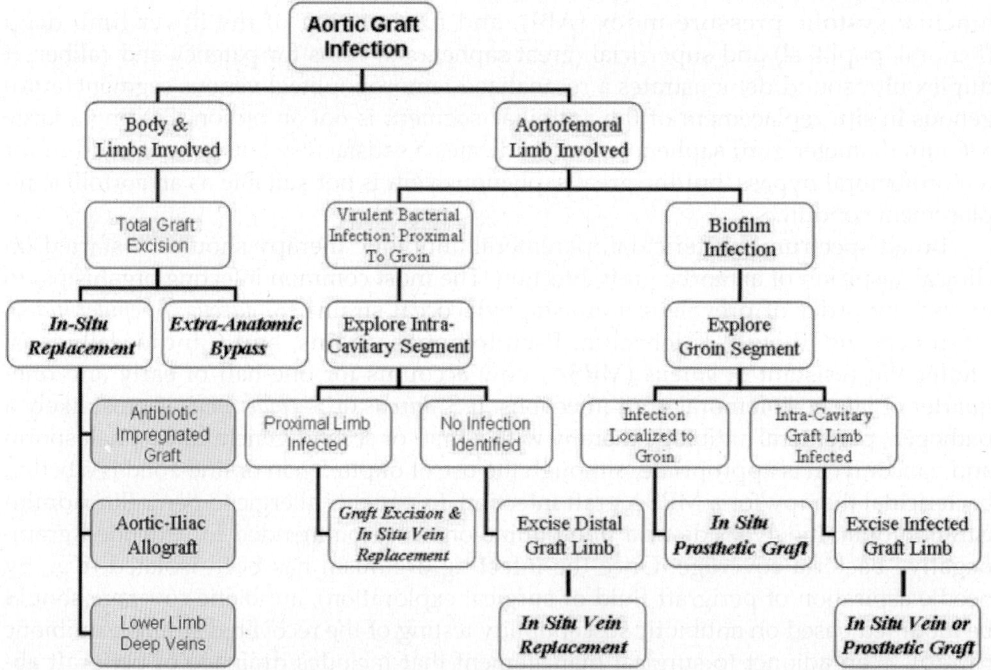

Figure 11-4. Algorithm for deciding on the type (vein versus rifampin-soaked prosthetic graft) of in situ grafting procedure based on extent (entire versus partial) graft involvement and type (biofilm versus virulent) of infection.

struction is dissection of lower limb deep veins, dissection and control of femoral vessels, abdominal exposure of the infrarenal aorta and graft, and graft excision followed by in situ reconstruction.

Surgical exposure for excision of the infected aortic graft depends on the type of previous aortic reconstruction and the availability of the infrarenal aorta for cross-clamping. Retroperitoneal approach is necessary for exposure of the pararenal, supraceliac, or thoracic aorta, and is recommended when extensive exposure of the right iliac vessels is not necessary. Proximal aorta control must be at a level to permit graft excision, debridement of the aorta to noninfected wall, and a redo graft-aorta anastomosis. Prior to cross-clamping, the femoral-popliteal veins are harvested from the profunda vein to the popliteal vein, and valves excised under direct vision. Vein grafts are then distended using a solution containing Dextran-40 (500 ml), heparin (5,000 IU), and papaverine HCl (60 mg). All side branches should be suture ligated using 5-0 or 6-0 polypropylene suture.

The proximal aorta and graft limbs are clamped after the patient has been heparinzed (activated clotting time > 200 sec). The intracavitary aortic graft (interposition, aortoiliac) is then excised including all suture material at the anastomosis. Graft specimens should be submitted for culture in a tryptic soy broth media. If a graft-enteric erosion is present, the bowel should be repaired, and the graft bed debrided and irrigated with a solution of one-half strength hydrogen peroxide containing 10 ml of Betadine per 500 ml. This solution, termed the "brown volcano," is used to cleanse retroperitoneal tissue and the exposed aorta. In the case of an infected aortofemoral graft, the limbs are left in place while the proximal aortic anastomosis is performed by either end-to-end or end-to-side techniques. Multiple graft configurations can be used to reconstruct the neoaortoiliac or aortofemoral segment using the lower extremity FPV segments, including aortobiiliac, aortobifemoral, or aortofemoral with femoro-femoral bypass (Figure 11-5). The proximal aorta-FPV anastomosis is performed with

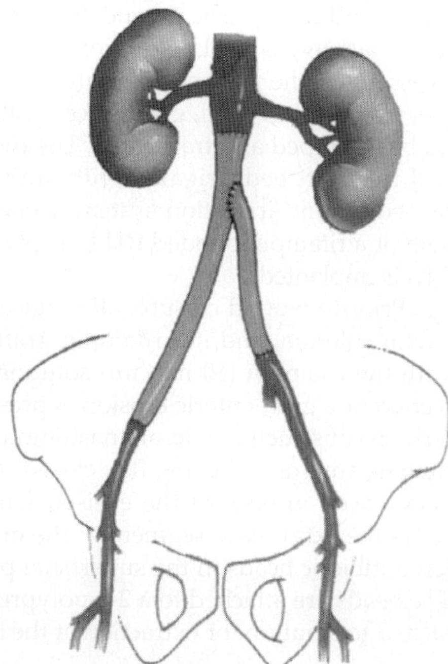

Figure 11-5. Most common grafting configuration used for lower extremity femoropopliteal vein reconstruction following excision of an infected aortofemoral graft.

continuous 4-0 or 5-0 polypropylene suture. Caliber mismatch between the femoral vein and aorta is handled by spatulation of the vein, placation of the aorta, or use of a triangular vein-patch angioplasty at the proximal aspect of the vein graft.[16]

If an antibiotic-impregnated graft is selected for in situ replacement, we recommend use of a gelatin-impregnated polyester graft (Gelsoft, Vascutek Ltd, Glasgow, UK), which has been soaked in 60 mg/ml solution of rifampin for 15 min. Use of this graft is associated with at least two days of bactericidal activity toward gram-positive (staphylococcus, streptococcus) and some gram-negative (E. coli, Proteus sp.) bacteria. The greater omentum should be mobilized, passed through the transverse mesocolon, and wrapped around in situ aortic reconstruction to cover the graft and prevent bowel adherence.

The aortofemoral graft limbs are removed by excising them from the distal anastomotic sites, and then via the groin, twisting the graft into a chord and pulling them from the retroperitoneum. Graft tunnels are debrided by repeated passage of betadine-soaked 4x4 gauze pads. Vein grafts may be tunneled through the existing tunnels as it may be difficult to create new tunnels through the scarred retroperitoneum. If the existing tunnels are too small, a lateral tunnel should be created. New, lateral tunnels are recommended for in situ rifampin-impregnated aortofemoral reconstruction. Bypass to femoral arteries is performed using standard anastomotic techniques once all prosthetic graft and inflamed perigraft tissue has been excised, and the wound cleansed with clorpactin (3 gm/L) irrigation. When possible, end-to-side femoral anastomoses should be performed to preserve retrograde pelvic perfusion.

When the infectious process is isolated to an aortofemoral graft limb, a combined inguinal and lower abdominal oblique ("transplant") retroperitoneal incision can be used for surgical exposure. In the presence of extensive inguinal inflammation or abscess, a staged operative approach is recommended. At the initial operation, the perigraft abscess is drained, necrotic tissue excised, and the cavity irrigated with the "brown volcano" solution. Antibiotic beads (vancomycin [3 gms] mixed with polymethylmethacrylate in a bead mold) are then placed adjacent to the infected graft and the wound closed. The second stage is performed three to five days later after culture results are available. Exploration of the proximal aortofemoral graft limb is performed to assess for the presence of graft incorporation. If found to uninvolved with infection (i.e., no perigraft fluid, graft incorporated with surrounding tissue), the proximal graft limb is clamped and transected. The distal graft is then excised to femoral anastomosis and the graft bed irrigated with antibacterial solution (clorpactin, 3 gm/L) using a pulsed wound irrigation system. Depending on the prior culture results, either deep vein or a rifampin-bonded PTFE (6 or 7 mm diameter, Gel-Seal, Vascular Ltd, Galsgow, UK) is implanted.

Prior to wound closure, all surgical fields are pulse lavaged again with the chlorpactin solution, and if a rifampin graft is used, the external graft surface is resoaked with the rifampin (60 mg/ml) solution. If Gram's stain indicates a gram-negative infection or a graft-enteric erosion is present, tobramycin powder is spread along the arterial reconstruction and at anastomotic sites. Perigraft fluid cavities and empty grafts tunnels are drained using flat, closed-suction drain systems. Closed suction drains are also placed in beds of the excised femoral vein and the sartorius muscle if used to cover the extracavity segment of the in situ graft reconstruction. On occasion, we have left antibiotic beads in the superficial portion of the groin wound for seven to 10 days. The beads are attached to a 2-0 polypropylene suture brought through the skin and attached to a button for extraction at the bedside.

POSTOPERATIVE CARE

Parenteral antibiotic therapy administration is modified based on the explanted graft cultures with the intent to maintain bactericidal levels for four to six weeks after the in situ grafting procedure. Prior to discharge from the hospital, a baseline CT scan of the abdomen and femoral regions is obtained. This scan is repeated at three months and then every six to 12 months depending on the type of in situ reconstruction. In general, prolonged oral antibiotic therapy is not prescribed following FPV reconstruction, but used for at least three months after in situ prosthetic reconstruction. The oral antibiotic prescribed is selected based on graft culture results and antibiotic susceptibility testing.

UNIVERSITY OF SOUTH FLORIDA EXPERIENCE

Over a 12-year period (1992–2004), our vascular surgery division has treated 145 aortic graft infections, including 30 patients presenting with secondary aortoenteric erosion or fistula. In situ grafting was selected for treatment in 96 (66%) of the 145 patients. Infection involving an aortofemoral prosthetic graft was present in 90 (94%) cases; the remaining infections involved a thoracofemoral (n = 2), aortoiliac (n = 2), or aortic interposition (n = 2) graft. Patient evaluation using contrast-enhanced CT graft imaging, in conjunction with "selected" graft surgical exploration, demonstrated either intra- or both intra- and extracavitary aortic graft involvement in 26 (28%) patients, with the remainder having infection limited to one or both aortofemoral graft limbs. Four patients treated by in situ grafting had a graft-enteric erosion.

The pathogens isolated relative to the type (total or partial graft replacement; FPV versus rifampin-bonded grafting) of in situ reconstruction are shown in Table 11-2.

TABLE 11-2. PATHOGENS ISOLATED RELATIVE TO TYPE OF IN SITU REPLACEMENT PROCEDURE

Total Graft Replacement (n = 26)

FPV* replacement (n = 11)	
FPV—Rifampin graft (n = 3)	
Biofilm infection (n = 6):	
MRSA	3
S. epidemidis	2
S. aureus	1
Virulent infection (n = 8)+	
E. coli	3
Klebsiella sp.	1
Multiple sp.	4
Rifampin graft replacement (n = 12)	
Biofilm infection:	
S. epidemidis	5
MRSA	3
S. epidermidis/S. aureus	1
Clostridium sp.	1
No Growth	2

(Continued)

TABLE 11-2. PATHOGENS ISOLATED RELATIVE TO TYPE OF IN SITU REPLACEMENT PROCEDURE (CONTINUED)

Partial Graft - Limb Excision (n = 70)	
FPV replacement (n = 12)	
Biofilm infection (n = 2):	
S. epidermidis/MRSA	2
Virulent infection:	
E. coli	4
Pseudomonas sp	3
Klebsiella sp	1
Multiple sp	2
PTFE replacement	10
Rifampin graft replacement	48
Biofilm infection:	
S. epidemidis	27
S. aureus	6
MRSA	12
Multiple staphylococcal sp.	3
Candida sp.	2
No growth	6
Virulent infection:	
E. coli	1
Klebsiella	1

* FPV, femoropopliteal venous segment
+ Four graft infections associated with graft-enteric erosion.
MRSA, methicillin-resistant S. aureus

Although the clinical presentation suggested a graft biofilm infection (i.e., caused by *S. epidermidis* or candida sp., in 78 [81%] patients), surgical exploration of CT abnormal graft segments identified infection caused by more virulent bacteria (MSSA, MRSA) in 25 cases. MRSA bacteria were isolated from 20 (21%) of 96 explanted graft segments. Lower extremity FPV reconstruction was performed in 14 (54%) of 26 total graft and 12 (24%) of 70 partial graft in situ replacement procedures based on findings of total graft involvement, or cultures isolating more virulent bacteria than *S. epidermidis*. A rifampin-impregnated (n = 60) or plain PTFE (n = 10) graft was used in the remainder of the procedures. Five patients treated by total graft excision and in situ rifampin graft replacement were not candidates for FPV reconstruction because of inadequate lower extremity deep veins.

Five patients died within 30 days of the procedure, including two (8%) following total graft replacement and three (4%) following partial graft replacement (Table 11-3). No deaths or limb amputations occurred in the rifampin graft group within 30 days. Overall, limb loss was 4% (two patients). No replacement demonstrated signs of infection at 30 days, but procedures to treat a graft or in situ replaced graft infection were required following 7% of the repairs; higher following partial graft excision and rifampin graft placement. Secondary procedures were performed in six patients for reinfection of the in situ rifampin graft caused by a rifampin resistant *S. epidermidis* in four patients, and in two patients, persistent MRSA infection in the retained, nonexcised polyester graft was treated. When possible, recurrent infection was treated by autoge-

TABLE 11-3. 30-DAY MORTALITY AND GRAFT RE-INFECTION RATES RELATIVE TO IN SITU GRAFT
REPLACEMENT PROCEDURES FOR 96 AORTIC GRAFT INFECTIONS

Procedure Type	30-day Mortality	Limb Loss	Reinfection*	Mirobiology
Total graft S.epidermidis[+] replacement (n = 26)	2 (8%)	2 (8%)		1 (4%)
Partial graft-limb (n = 70) Replacement	3 (4%)	0	5 (7%)	S. epidermidis-3+ MRSA—2 Candida sp—1
Total	5 (5%)	2 (2%)	6 (7%)	

*all re-infections associated with in situ grafting with a rifampin-impregnated (n = 4) or PTFE (n = 2) replacement conduit
[+] rifampin-resistant S. epidermidis strain isolated

nous deep vein reconstruction and total graft excision. During a mean follow-up
period of 40 months, six patients died of nongraft related causes and four patients required revision of the in situ reconstruction for graft stenosis.

In a prior report on the expanded application of in situ replacement for prosthetic
graft infection, our group reported the use of in situ grafting to treat one-half (35 of 68)
of aortoiliofemoral graft infections.[11] Outcomes included a 30-day mortality of 4% and
amputation rate of 2%. Since that report, we have increased our application FPV in
situ reconstruction and implanted antibiotic beads into infected vascular surgical sites
of patients presenting with virulent graft infection prior to the in situ grafting procedure. In situ replacement with a rifampin-bonded graft continues to be effective treatment for low-grade graft infections caused by *S. epidermidis* with a late reinfection rate
< 10% (follow-up extending beyond four to five years).

OUTCOMES FOLLOWING IN SITU GRAFTING FOR AORTIC GRAFT INFECTION

In situ grafting incorporates several recent advances in the treatment of aortic graft infections, including the use of antibiotic-bonded grafts and autogenous reconstruction with
lower limb FPV as described by Clagett and Nevelsteen.[7-8] Clinical experience with in situ
rifampin-bonded grafting remains anecdotal, but the reports originating from multiple vascular centers indicate clinical success in > 80% of cases with a mortality and morbidity
comparable or lower than axillofemoral reconstruction. Our group has limited in situ prosthetic grafting to treatment of "biofilm" graft infections and thus the operative mortality in
this "selected" patient group has been < 2%. A recent report from the Mayo Clinic indicated significantly improved clinical outcomes following in situ replacement compared to
axillofemoral reconstruction. Treatment of 52 of 101 patients with aortic graft infection with
in situ grafting (rifampin grafts, n = 43; allograft, n = 6; FPV, n = 3) resulted in less graft-
related deaths ($p < 0.001$), decreased hospitalization, and improved primary graft patency
($p < 0.001$) and limb salvage ($p < 0.03$) rates.

Outcomes following conventional management of aortic infection have also
improved, especially with the use of staged reconstruction. Procedural and graft-
related mortality rates were in the range of 10%–15% with the majority of deaths in
patients presenting with secondary aortic enteric fistula (AEF). Our group continues
to use staged axillofemoral grafting, followed by aortic graft excision in patients
presenting with AEF or a virulent intracavity infection of an endovascular stent-graft,

aortic interposition graft, or aortoiliac graft. Our outcome associated with the axillofemoral reconstruction of 26 secondary AEF infections included a 23% (six deaths) 30-day or in-hospital mortality, and one case of aortic stump blow-out during follow-up. Overall, procedural mortality in the treatment of aortic graft infection has occurred more frequently in the secondary AEF group (20%, six of 30) than in patients without this graft complication (4%, five of 119).

Our group advocates in situ grafting in the patient presenting with an aortofemoral graft infection because it provides the surgeon with more options regarding reconstruction. Neoaortoiliac reconstruction has an excellent track record. Vascular surgeons have learned to harvest and use the FPV to bypass from the infrarenal aorta to common femoral artery bifurcation. The FPV conduits are resistant to infection, durable (primary patency >80%), and their harvest are not associated with significantly lower limb morbidity. Use of in situ prosthetic grafting is more controversial, but in appropriately selected patients, use of the rifampin-soaked gelatin-impregnated polyester or PTFE grafts has also been successful in treating aortic graft infection. Because of patient selection criteria, it use has been associated with the lowest procedural mortality and morbidity rates. The most frequent failure mode of rifampin grafting is emergence of a rifampin-resistant staphylococcal strain than reinfects the in situ graft.

Our group has no experience using arterial allograft in the treatment of aortic graft infection. Outcomes from the United States cryoperserved aortic allograft registry (51 patients treated at 31 institutions) indicated use of this conduit was associated with a 13% mortality rate, but most deaths were not the result of allograft failure. Late-graft complications (infection, thrombosis, aneurysmal degeneration) occurred in 20% of patients. These early results led the authors to conclude that preferential use of cryoperserved arterial allograft was not justified in the treatment of aortic graft infection.

SUMMARY

In devising an operative strategy for the treatment of infected aortic graft infection, the surgeon should consider all surgical options, then select one that optimizes patient survival and limb salvage, and is associated with the least procedural morbidity. In our experience, in situ grafting has been the best treatment option in the majority of patients. Our treatment algorithm has evolved over the past decade, and when possible, in situ grafting with FPV is the preferred treatment. Unfortunately, this type of reconstruction is not possible in many patients either for anatomic reasons or patient factors. For "selected" patients, in situ rifampin grafting, performed in conjunction with excision of all clinically infected graft, has proven to be safe and associated with low (< 10%) reinfection rate when treating a biofilm graft infection. In situ grafting avoids multiple or staged procedures, imparts less physiologic stress on the patient, and avoids the complications of aortic stump disruption and extraanatomic graft failure due to thrombosis or infection.

REFERENCES

1. Bandyk DF, Back MR. Infection in prosthetic vascular grafts. In: Rutherford (ed) : *Vascular Surgery (Sixth Edition)*, Philadelphia, Elsevier Saunders, 2005:875–894.
2. Ducasse E, Calisti A, Speziale F, et al. Aortoiliac stent graft infection: current problems and management. *Ann Vasc Surg.* 2004 Sep;18(5):521–526.

3. O'Hara PJ, Hertzer NR, Beven EG, et al. Surgical management of infected abdominal aortic grafts: Review of a 25-year experience. *J Vasc Surg.* 1986;3:725.
4. Reilly LM, Stoney RJ, Goldstone J et al. Improved management of aortic graft infection: The influence of operative sequence and staging. *J Vasc Surg.* 1987;5:421–431.
5. Yeager RA, Moneta GL, Taylor LM et al. Improving survival and limb salvage in patients with aortic graft infection. *Am J Surg.* 1990;159:466–469.
6. Seeger JM, Pretus HA, Welborn MB, et al. Long-term outcome after treatment of aortic graft infection with staged extra-anatomic bypass grafting and aortic graft removal. *J Vasc Surg.* 2000;32:451–461.
7. Nevelsteen A, Lacroix H, Suy R. Autogenous reconstruction with the lower extremity deep veins: An alternate treatment of prosthetic infection after reconstructive surgery for aortoiliac disease. *J Vasc Surg.* 1995;22:129–134.
8. Clagett GP, Valentine RJ, Hagino RT. Autogenous aortoiliac/femoral reconstruction from superficia femoral-popliteal veins: Feasibility and durability. *J Vasc Surg.* 1997;25:255–70.
9. Bandyk DF, Novotney ML, Johnson BL et al. Use of rifampin-soaked gelatin-sealed polyester grafts for in situ treatment of primary aortic and vascular prosthetic infections. *J Surg Res.* 2001;95(1):44–49.
10. Hayes PD, Nasim A, London NJM et al. In situ replacement of infected aortic grafts with ri-fampicin-bonded prostheses: the Leicester experience (1992 to 1998). *J Vasc Surg.* 1999;30:92–98.
11. Bandyk DF, Novotney ML, Back MR,. Expanded application of in situ replacement for prosthetic graft infection. *J Vasc Surg.* 2000;32:451–461.
12. Leseche G, Castier Y, Petit MD et al. Long-term results of cryopreserved arterial allograft reconstruction in infected prosthetic grafts and mycotic aneurysms of the abdominal aorta. *J Vasc Surg.* 2001;34(4):616–622.
13. Noel AA, Gloviczki P, Cherry Jr., KJ et al. Abdominal aortic reconstruction in infected fields: Early results of the United States cryopreserved aortic allograft registry.*J Vasc Surg.* 2002;35:847–852.
14. Benaerts PJ, Ridler BMF, Vercaeren P et al. Gentamicin beads in vascular surgery: long-term results of implantation. *Cardiovasc Surg.* 1999;7(4):447–450.
15. Egun A, O'Neill H, Ward AS. Intragraft thrombus: an early CT finding in aortic graft infection. *Eur J Vasc Endovasc Surg.* 2000;20:482–483.
16. Clagett GP. Treatment of aortic graft infection. In: Ernst CB, Staey JC, eds. *Current therapy in vascular surgery, 4th ed.* Philadelphia: Mosby. 2001;pp.422–428.

In Situ Prosthetic Repair of an Aortic Graft

12

Thomas C. Bower, M.D.

In situ replacement of an aortic graft is used to repair proximal aortic anastomotic pseudoaneurysms, aneurysms that extend to involve the pararenal or paravisceral aorta, and is an option to treat selected patients with prosthetic aortic graft infection involving the thoracic, thoracoabdominal, suprarenal, or infrarenal aorta. The discussion of repair of complex aneurysms of the abdomen and the thoracoabdominal aorta is discussed in other chapters. This chapter will focus on in situ prosthetic replacement of infected aortic grafts. Fortunately, the incidence of these problems is rare. A 10-year, population-based study by Hallett et. al. at the Mayo Clinic estimated the long-term incidence of abdominal aortic graft infection to approach 5%, or less than a 1% risk per year.[1] The incidence of thoracic or thoracoabdominal graft infections is less than 2%.[2,3] Currently, aortic graft infections are best treated by open techniques, though endovascular repair has been reported and might serve as a "bridge" until definitive therapy can be provided.

The goals of surgical treatment are to eradicate aortic infection by removing the infected prosthesis; to revascularize the aorta and its branches, ensuring that pelvic, visceral, and renal perfusion is maintained; and to minimize the risk of perioperative complications and late recurrent graft infection.[2-4] Successful treatment requires assessment of patient comorbidities preoperatively if time allows, definition of the location and extent of infection based on imaging studies, and careful planning of operation to ensure that the operation will achieve the aforementioned goals.

The time-honored method of treatment is extra-anatomic bypass with resection of the involved prosthesis.[2,4-8] In situ reconstruction with autogenous or prosthetic materials are alternatives in selected patients.[2-19] The use of prosthetic in situ grafts to replace infected aortic grafts was first introduced by the University of Texas-Houston group in the late 1980s.[20] We prefer the use of a Rifampin-bonded prosthesis, in which the polyester graft is soaked in a solution of Rifampin (Rifandin IV; Merrill Dow Pharmaceutical, Kansas City, MO) at a concentration of 2.5 mg/ml for a minimum of 30 minutes prior to implantation.[4] These grafts have been shown experimentally to resist infection.[4] Silver-impregnated grafts might be another option in the future, though these are currently unavailable for routine use in the United States.[19]

PREOPERATIVE ASSESSMENT

It is important to thoroughly evaluate a patient's cardiac, pulmonary, and renal function preoperatively, but only if time allows it. We rarely obtain functional cardiac stress tests but will obtain a resting transthoracic echocardiogram to gauge left ventricular function. Pulmonary reserve is assessed with the use of pulmonary function studies and a resting arterial blood gas. Patients with a forced expiratory volume less than 1 liter, or those on home oxygen, face a higher risk of postoperative pulmonary complications. Renal insufficiency (creatinine ≥ 1.5 mg/dL), small renal size (< 8 cm) or thin parenchyma, or elevated renal resistive indices increases the patient risk of postoperative renal failure. Most of these evaluations can be done quickly, will help assess perioperative risk, and any improvement in organ function that can be gained preoperatively might help lessen major morbidity with operation. Blood cultures are drawn and broad-spectrum intravenous (IV) antibiotics are initiated if the causative organism is undefined.

IMAGING

Either CT or MR imaging can be used to determine the extent of infection, and to provide detail of the aortic branches, pelvic circulation, and the runoff arteries in the extremities. CT imaging has a sensitivity of 80–100% and specificity of 50–90% for confirming the presence of infection.[2] Signs include periaortic and perigraft soft tissue stranding, edema, fluid, enhancing soft tissue rind, or air. The latter is a sine qua non of infection. Lack of a fat plane between the aortic graft, its limbs, and the adjacent intestine is worrisome for graft enteric erosion (AGEE) or fistula (AGEF) in patients with fever of unknown origin or repetitive episodes of gastrointestinal blood loss. Indium 111-labeled neutrophil-specific white blood cell scans may be beneficial in these circumstances.[4,17] These scans have a positive predictive value of 80–90%.[2] However, we have treated patients with negative indium scans who later proved to have a graft infection. Extended upper gastrointestinal (GI) endoscopy is an important adjunct for individuals suspected of having AGEE or AGEF. Endoscopy is done in hemodynamically stable patients and helps exclude other sources of blood loss. Upper endoscopy should be done in the operating room if patients are thought to have an AGEF, and have recent blood loss requiring transfusion or have active rapid hemorrhage.[2] Bronchoscopy is done for patients with hemoptysis and suspected thoracic aortic graft infection, using the same management principles as for GI endoscopy.[3] Duplex ultrasonography is rarely used to confirm aortic graft infection, other than to image the limbs of an aortoiliac or aortofemoral graft, and to assess patency of the deep veins should autogenous in situ reconstruction be necessary.

THORACIC AND THORACOABDOMINAL AORTIC GRAFT INFECTIONS

Prosthetic graft infections in these locations are some of the most formidable procedures to undertake.[3,18] Patients may present with acute gastrointestinal hemorrhage from aorto-esophageal or aortoduodenal fistulas, hemoptysis from aortobronchial or aortopulmonary fistula, septic emboli, or nonspecific symptoms with perigraft fluid.[3] Multirow (64-row) computed tomographic angiography (CTA) has been the most useful diagnostic imaging modality in our experience.

Treatment options are limited, and in most cases require prosthetic replacement of the infected graft and autogenous tissue coverage of the new prosthesis. Whenever possible, the new graft should be routed away from the infected field. An antibiotic-bonded prosthesis from the ascending aorta to the upper abdominal aorta may be used for patients with isolated infections of a descending thoracic aortic graft.[2,3] This operation is accomplished via median sternotomy and midline abdominal incision. That option, as well as extra-anatomic bypass from the axillary artery, is inadequate for patients with thoracoabdominal graft infections because of the need to maintain renal, visceral, and spinal cord perfusion. In addition, the small size of an axillofemoral graft does not provide enough retrograde blood flow to ensure good perfusion to these end organs.[3]

The way the new in situ graft is configured depends on the extent of the original operation, the extent of infection, and the hemodynamic stability of the patient. In stable patients with prior type III or IV thoracoabdominal repairs, the visceral and renal arteries can be reconstructed with a trifurcated graft taken from the uninvolved mid- or upper descending thoracic aorta (Ballard technique), or retrograde from the native iliac arteries, prior to resection of the infected prosthesis. The new aortic graft is routed more lateral than normal. The critical intercostal arteries require separate interposition grafts. Graft coverage with muscle (latissimus dorsi, rectus abdominis), perinephric or pericardial fat, parietal pleura, bovine pericardium, or omentum is an important adjunct to protect the graft from contamination. In some cases, irrigation-suction drains are left in the infected bed through which a dilute povidone-iodine or antibiotic solution is infused.[2,3]

Kieffer and associates, in a report of arterial allografts used in 11 patients to treat infected grafts in these positions, highlight the primary problems in treatment.[3] Proximal aortic control can be difficult in those with upper thoracic aortic anastomoses and in patients who have rupture or active hemorrhage from aortobronchial or aortoesophageal fistulas. Secondly, reperfusion of the visceral, renal, and spinal cord beds is important but often difficult to achieve in an expeditious manner. Kieffer has used cardiopulmonary bypass and deep hypothermic circulatory arrest, accepting the higher risk of hemorrhagic complications in order to protect the spinal cord and other aortic branch territories. This technique may be the only option in those with grafts involving the entire thoracic and thoracoabdominal aorta, and those in whom proximal aortic control is difficult.

There are anecdotal reports of graft salvage using perigraft debridement and drainage, irrigation of the graft with antibiotics or dilute povidone-iodine solutions, and coverage of the prosthesis with muscle or omentum.[2,3] Broad-spectrum IV antibiotics are changed to organism-specific antibiotics once culture results are available. We continue IV antibiotics for six to eight weeks via a central or peripherally inserted central line.

INFRARENAL AORTIC GRAFT INFECTION

These infections usually occur at a mean of 40 months postoperatively and have a bimodal distribution.[2] Some patients present within months of surgery, which is usually related to a break in sterile technique or inadequate coverage of the proximal aortic anastomosis. Most other patients present four to seven years after surgery, and the cause of infection is either bacterial seeding from a remote site of infection, secondary involvement from a contiguous infection such as diverticular abscess, or mechanical erosion of the graft into the adjacent intestine when inadequate soft tissue coverage of the graft anastomosis was done at the original operation, or if an indolent infection develops in the area.[2,4] Malnutrition, chronic immunosuppression from corticosteroids, chemotherapy, diabetes mellitus, renal failure, or autoimmune or lymphoproliferative disorders are systemic factors that predispose patients to either early or late graft infection.[2] Infections may be polymicrobial or monomicrobial with the former occurring most frequently in a recent report from the Mayo Clinic.[4] Monomicrobial infections in that series were due to coagulase-negative staphylococcus species in 33%, *Streptococcus viridans* in 20%, enterococcus in 15%, and methicillin-resistant *Staphylococcus aureus* in 9%. *Escherichia coli*, *Klebsiella*, and enterobacter species were the most common Gram-negative infections. The presence of anaerobic or fungal organisms was noted in approximately one-fourth of the patients. The bacteriology is dependent on the location of the infection with Gram-positive species most prevalent in localized infection, and polymicrobial and Gram-negative species more common in patients with AGEF or AGEE. Gram-negative species, especially *pseudomonas*, are particular virulent.[2,3]

The type, location, and extent of infection determine whether partial or total graft excision is needed. By definition, primary graft infection refers to individuals who have no enteric involvement. An aortic graft-enteric fistula is communication between the aortic suture line and adjacent bowel. Many individuals with AGEF have a proximal anastomotic pseudoaneurysm. Aortic graft-enteric erosion implies enteric contamination away from an anastomosis. Partial graft infection indicates isolation to one limb or an anastomosis, in contrast to total graft infection.

Ideal candidates for in situ prosthetic replacement of an abdominal aortic graft are those with localized biofilms due to low-grade virulent organisms such as *Staphylococcus epidermidis*. These patients usually present years after initial implantation and have no active systemic signs of bacteremia or sepsis.[2] In situ reconstructions also have been used to treat AGEE or AGEF, and have been applied to patients with total graft infection and frank perigraft purulence.[2,4,7,8,16,17,19]

PARTIAL GRAFT EXCISION

If the infection is localized to a portion of one graft limb, which is often the distal segment or femoral anastomosis, that segment of graft can be resected and replaced, provided the intraoperative findings confirm good soft tissue incorporation around the uninvolved graft[4,9] (Figure 12–1). Typically, these patients will only have small amounts of perigraft fluid on imaging or a pseudoaneurysm at the distal anastomosis (often the femoral).

In these cases, the distal limb of the graft can be approached through a lower quadrant retroperitoneal incision. The incorporated limb of the graft is isolated, the patient is given intravenous heparin, and the graft is divided. The distal end of the graft is oversewn and pushed into the tunnel. If a biofilm is encountered, the resection must extend proximally. If the area is clean, the Rifampin-soaked graft is sewn end to end to the old graft limb. If the reconstruction is carried to the distal external iliac

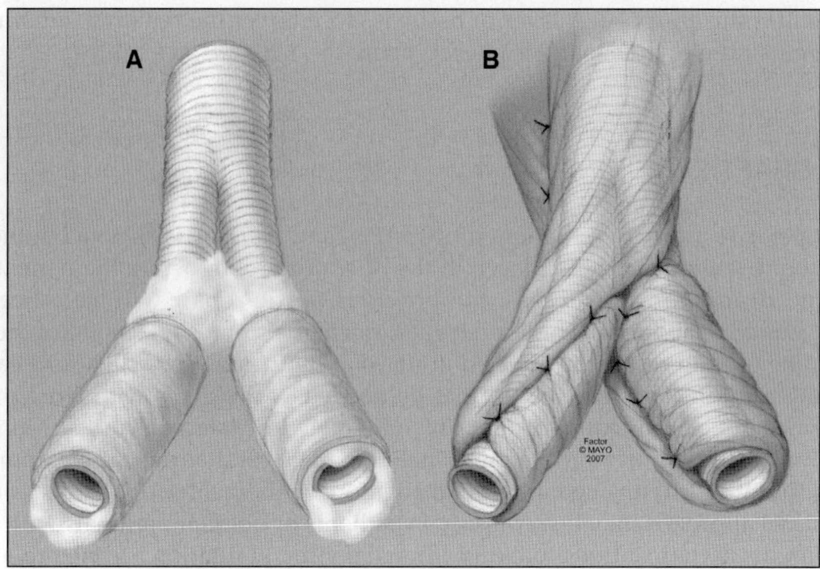

Figure 12-1. Schematic representation of primary graft infection of the distal limbs replaced with a Rifampin-bonded prosthesis, wrapped circumferentially with omentum.

artery, it is done end to side to maintain pelvic perfusion. The infected graft is resected after the new graft has been covered by autogenous tissue, if that is available. If the infection extends to the groin, the graft is wrapped in antibiotic-soaked salts and the wound is covered with an iodine-impregnated Steri-Drape. The groin incision is opened, and the deep and superficial femoral arteries are dissected free through a clean tissue plane. These vessels are crossclamped, and the infected portion of the femoral graft limb or the pseudoaneurysm is resected. If there is no purulent material in the groin, the wound is debrided and copiously irrigated with antibiotic solution. The old tunnel tract is debrided using a rongeur. Gowns, gloves, and instruments are changed before the new graft is passed into the groin. The new graft is passed through a clean tunnel whenever possible and sewn either end to end or end to side to the femoral artery, whichever is required to maintain pelvic perfusion. A portion of the femoral artery is sent to pathology to be certain there are no micro abscesses within the vessel wall. This helps ensure that the distal anastomosis is sewn to healthy tissue. We have a low threshold to rotate a rectus femoris muscle flap to cover the femoral anastomosis,[4] and prefer this muscle to sartorius. This is certainly necessary in patients who have scarred, nonpliable adjacent soft tissues or those who require resection of a large femoral anastomotic pseudoaneurysm where there is concern about dead space in the wound if it were closed primarily. Cultures of the graft and biofilm are taken so that organism-specific intravenous and oral antibiotics can be administered.

In patients with purulent infections in the groin, the new graft should be tunneled either through the obturator foramen or laterally along the psoas muscle so it can be sewn to an uncontaminated deep or superficial femoral artery. In these cases, the tissues are closed over the new graft before the groin incision is reopened and the infected graft is resected. An autogenous patch is used to close the common femoral artery so that perfusion can be maintained into both femoral branches. Bovine pericardium, saphenous vein, or a piece of endarterectomized superficial femoral artery work well for this purpose. A layer of tissue is closed over the repaired femoral artery and the remainder of the wound is packed open.

TOTAL GRAFT EXCISION

The preoperative patient evaluation, preparation, and imaging is as noted in the previous section. Ureteral stents are placed in the operating room before the patient is prepared and draped. In most cases, the previous aortic repair will have been done through a midline abdominal or left retroperitoneal incision. While either of these incisions can be used to resect the infected graft, a midline approach will afford easier access to the right iliac system should that be needed. Individuals with large proximal aortic anastomotic pseudoaneurysms, which involve the juxtarenal aorta or those with aneurysmal change involving the pararenal or paravisceral aorta, can be approached transperitoneally or with medial visceral rotation. A thoracoretroperitoneal or thoracoabdominal approach may be necessary in asthenic or obese individuals with narrow costal margins in these latter situations. If medial visceral rotation is contemplated and the patient has a wide costal margin, a "bump" (30°) placed under the left side prior to draping might aid in this exposure. With the knees strapped to the operating table, the table can be rotated so that the surgeon can work from a left semilateral position or directly via the midline.

The key to exposure of the juxtarenal or suprarenal aorta is the ability to obtain upward and lateral retraction of the abdominal wall and costal margin. Retraction can be accomplished with the use of a variety of self-retaining retractors.

Location for proximal aortic control is dictated by the proximity of the old graft anastomosis to the renal arteries, the presence of a proximal anastomotic pseudoaneurysm or suprarenal aneurysm, and the presence of any intraluminal atheromatous debris or thrombus on the preoperative imaging study. Our preference is to gain control of the supraceliac aorta in most patients before any attempt is made to dissect free the juxtarenal or suprarenal aorta. This can be done by opening the lesser sac and splitting the fibers of the crura of the diaphragm longitudinally, taking care to protect the esophagus (nasogastric tube in place). Thereafter, the suprarenal aorta can usually be dissected free via an infracolic approach. If the inferior mesenteric vein has not been ligated or divided previously, this needs to be done to allow incision of an avascular plane of tissue at the base of the left transverse mesocolon, which allows upward and somewhat lateral retraction of the colon and pancreas, thereby widening the field of view.

The left renal vein must be mobilized for adequate exposure, which requires ligation and division of the adrenal, gonadal, and lumbar branches (Figure 12–2). If there is intense scar between the aorta and renal vein, the vein can be divided as long as its branches are preserved. We reconstruct the renal vein after the proximal anastomosis is completed in patients with preoperative renal insufficiency. Often, the renal arteries require control but the visceral arteries are dissected free only if there is aneurysmal involvement at that level. In the latter case, medial visceral rotation aids this exposure. Similar exposure of the pararenal or paravisceral aorta can be achieved through retroperitoneal or thoracoretroperitoneal incisions, as discussed elsewhere. The crura of the diaphragm should be divided on either side of the renal arteries to provide a secure place for the proximal aortic crossclamp at the suprarenal level (Figure 12–3). We

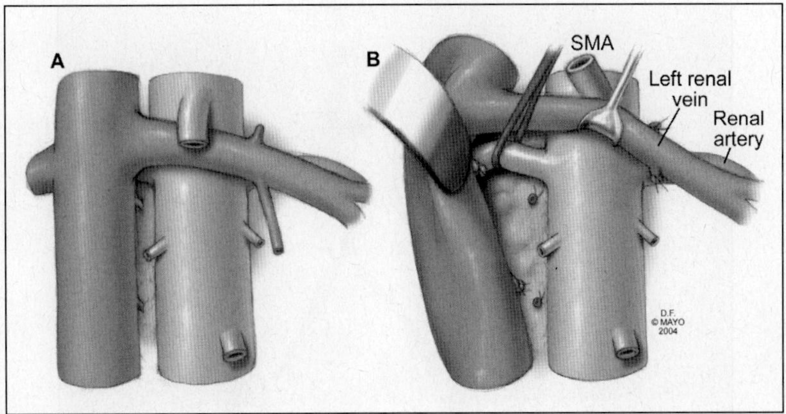

Figure 12-2. The left renal vein requires mobilization for exposure of the juxtarenal or suprarenal aorta. The branches of the vein require ligation and division.

have little experience isolating this portion of the aorta via a right retroperitoneal or infraduodenal approach.

The next step is to isolate the uninfected iliac or femoral arteries, taking care to protect the ureters. Intravenous heparin and mannitol are administered. The sequence of clamping involves the distal iliac or femoral arteries, the renal arteries if suprarenal clamping is necessary, followed by the proximal aortic clamp. The capsule of the graft is opened, and the entire graft is resected. Graft material, periaortic tissue, and any perigraft fluid or purulence are sent for Gram stain and culture. The aorta is resected to healthy tissue as are the periaortic soft tissues. No effort is made to resect the entire aortic wall if it is densely adhered to the major veins. A piece of the proximal aorta is sent for microscopic analysis to determine if there are microabscesses or bacterial colonies within the aortic wall. After the periaortic tissues have been debrided and the tunnel tracts curetted, the wound is irrigated copiously with liters of antibiotic and povidone-iodine solutions. Gowns, gloves, and instruments are changed. The Rifampin-soaked

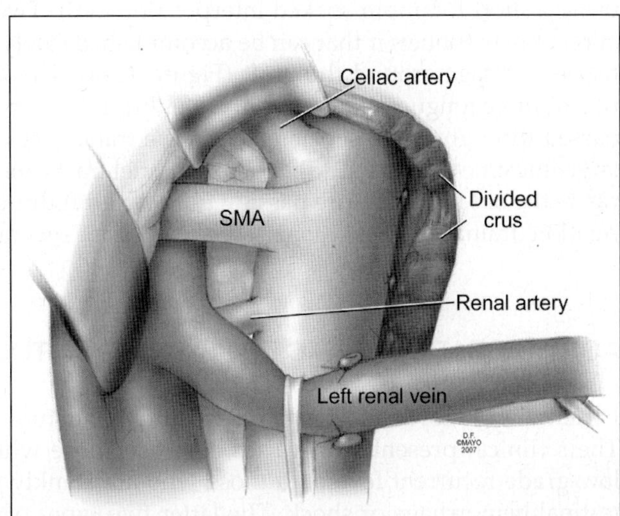

Figure 12-3. In many cases, the suprarenal aorta must be crossclamped. Mobilization of the left renal vein and division of the crura of the diaphragm on either side of the aorta are necessary steps, as illustrated here.

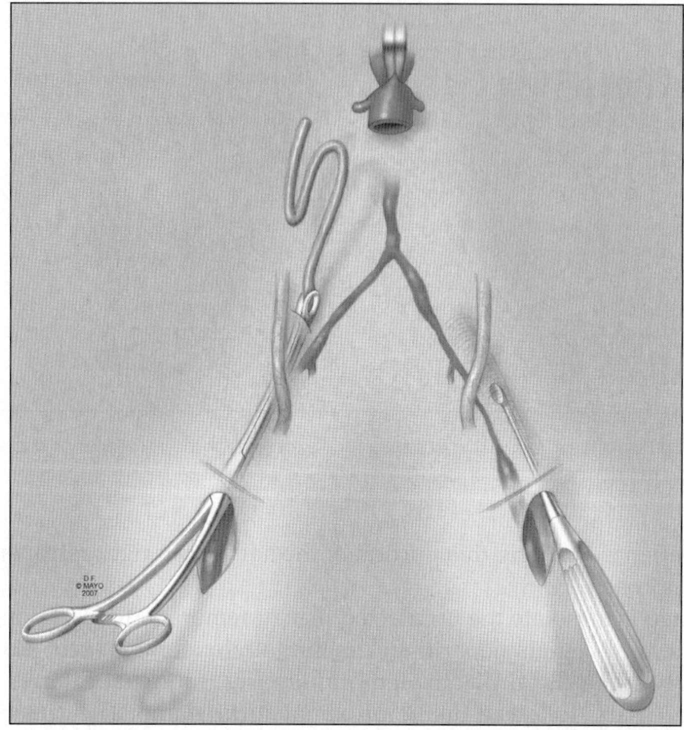

Figure 12-4. Schematic representation showing debridement of a tunnel tract on the left and creation of a new tunnel on the right. Rubber tubing is placed through the new tunnel to facilitate passage of the new graft.

prosthesis is sewn end to end to the aorta and then appropriately to the distal target arteries. It is important to maintain pelvic perfusion, which often necessitates an end-to-side anastomosis to the distal external iliac or femoral arteries if there has been a previous bifurcated graft, or directly to the common iliac arteries if a straight graft had been placed. In some circumstances, the internal iliac artery requires reconstruction using a short Rifampin-soaked interposition graft. Two important adjuncts include creation of new tunnels if that can be accomplished safely, and circumferential autogenous tissue coverage around the graft (Figure 12–4). The latter is best accomplished using two or three tongues of omentum, either brought over the top of the colon or preferably passed through an avascular plane in the transverse colon to avoid constriction of the large intestine[4] (Figure 12–5). If a new tunnel tract cannot be created, we debride and irrigate the old tunnel before passing the new graft through it, and will leave a suction irrigation drainage system along side the graft for several days.

AORTIC GRAFT-ENTERIC EROSION OR FISTULA

Patients with aortic graft-enteric erosions or fistulas have polymicrobial infections. Their clinical presentation varies between those who have indolent infections with low-grade recurrent fevers, to those who are frankly septic or have massive gastrointestinal hemorrhage or shock. The latter two types of patients are difficult to manage,

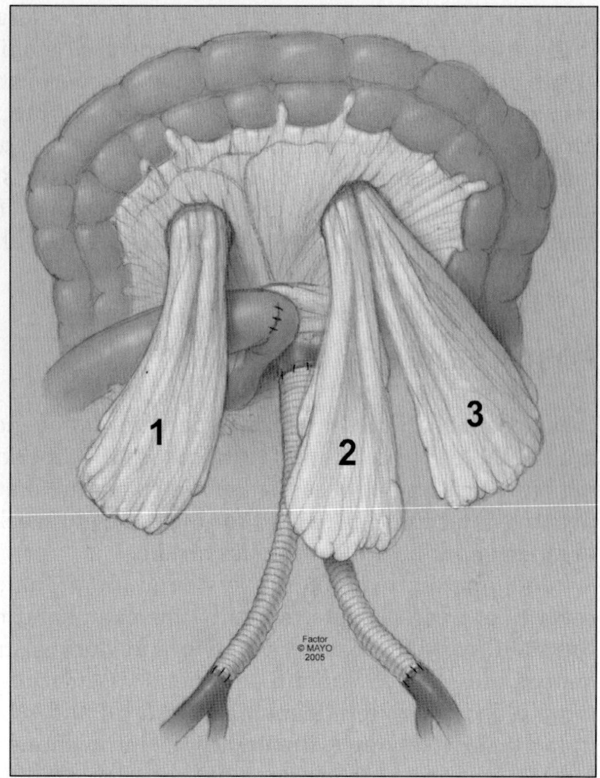

Figure 12-5. Two or three tongues of omentum are passed through a vascular plane in the transverse mesocolon in preparation to wrap the new graft.

and have the highest risk of perioperative mortality and morbidity, regardless of the type of aortic reconstruction used.

If patients are hemodynamically stable when the diagnosis is made and there is no evidence on CT imaging of a large aortic pseudoaneurysm or signs of contained rupture, the patient's risk for operation is assessed, and efforts are made to optimize cardiac, pulmonary, and renal function preoperatively. For patients who have large perigraft abscesses but none of the aforementioned findings on imaging studies, percutaneous drainage is used when possible to gain better control of the infection and reduce the bacterial burden. In this latter case, staged axillofemoral reconstructions followed by resection of the graft is preferable, in our opinion, to the use of prosthetic in situ reconstruction.

Proximal aortic control in a hemodynamically stable patient with AGEF or AGEE is approached as it is in a patient who requires total excision of the aortic graft, either at the suprarenal or supraceliac level, depending on the conditions encountered once the abdomen is opened. Either supraceliac or intraluminal balloon occlusion are necessary for unstable patients. In many cases, the infection is localized to the site of erosion or to the body of the graft and the proximal anastomosis. In these cases, the incorporated uninfected old graft limbs are dissected free. The area of the erosion or fistula should not be disturbed. Sequence of crossclamping is as noted previously, after heparin and mannitol have been administered. The graft is transected distal to the point of intestinal involvement, and the native aorta is transected above the old anastomosis in the case of a fistula. No effort is made to mobilize the intestine at this point, but rather povidone-iodine soaked salts are placed against the bowel, and it is retracted out of the field. Rarely, the intestinal opening is large and will contaminate the field if it is not controlled. In this case, the bowel is mobilized so that an atraumatic bowel clamp can be placed across the opening. The reconstruction proceeds as outlined in the previous section, including the 360° omental wrap. Antibiotic-soaked salts are placed on top of the omental wrap, and the intestine is repaired in two layers. In some cases, intestinal resection with end-to-end anastomosis is necessary. An additional piece of omentum can be placed over the intestinal repair. The abdomen is closed in standard fashion, preferably with monofilament sutures for the fascia and skin.

POSTOPERATIVE MANAGEMENT

Patients are continued on broad spectrum intravenous antibiotics until culture results are available. We continue IV antibiotics for a period of four to eight weeks, depending on which type of organism grows in culture. Patients with polymicrobial or Gram-negative infections are treated for the full eight weeks. Patients are then maintained on organism-specific oral antibiotics for life.

Most patients develop a systemic inflammatory response after operation, the severity of which is determined by the extent and type of preoperative infection, and the stability of the patient prior to and during surgery. Many patients need intravenous pressors to maintain peripheral vascular resistance, and to provide a mean arterial blood pressure adequate for visceral and renal perfusion. The more severe the inflammatory response, the higher the intravenous volume requirements will be early after operation. A widening $A\text{-}aO_2$ gradient, falling platelet counts, high-volume requirements extending beyond three to four days, or a leukopenic response are ominous signs, and indicate ongoing sepsis or intestinal ischemia. In general, patients should begin to spontaneously diurese within two to four days of operation. We have found the use of a Lasix drip to provide more even diuresis than intermittent boluses once the patient is ready to give up fluid. For patients with renal failure who need diuresis, continuous veno-venous hemodialysis works well and causes less hemodynamic insult than standard hemodialysis.

Follow-up with CT imaging is important and is done within the first three postoperative months, sooner for those who had more extensive or virulent infections. Thereafter, follow-up is dictated by the clinical status of the patient and the initial postoperative CT scan.

OUTCOMES

Table 12–1 lists the contemporary outcomes for patients with aortic graft infections treated by a variety of techniques, including axillofemoral, autogenous, and prosthetic in situ reconstructions.[4-6,10-16] We recently reported the results of 52 patients treated with in situ techniques, of which 30 (56%) had graft enteric erosions or fistulas.[4] The overall mortality rate was 8%. All four deaths occurred in those with AGEF or AGEE, and the cause of death was multisystem organ failure in two and intraoperative coagulopathy and myocardial infarction in one each. The operative mortality rate was 22% for those with AGEF or AGEE who required emergency operation, but only 9.5% for

TABLE 12-1. CONTEMPORARY RESULTS OF AXILLOFEMORAL AND IN SITU RECONSTRUCTIONS FOR AORTIC GRAFT INFECTION.

Author (Year)	n	Mean FU (months)	Operative mortality n (%)	Procedure-related death n (%)	Graft disruption/ stump blowout n (%)	Graft reinfection n (%)	Primary patency	Limb salvage
Axillofemoral reconstruction								
Yeager et al (1999)[5]	60	41	8 (13)	11 (18)	1 (1.5)	6 (10)	73% at 5 years	82% at 5 years
Seeger et al (2000)[6]	36	32	4 (11)	7 (19)	1 (3)	1 (3)	64% at 5 years	80% at 5 years
Oderich, et al (2006)[4]	34	41	5 (12)	9 (26)	4 (12)	5 (15)	48% at 5 years	88% at 5 years
In situ reconstruction								
Femoral-popliteal vein graft								
Clagett et al (1993)[10]	41	32	3 (7)	3 (7)	0	0	83% at 5 years	86% at 5 years
Nevelsteen et al (1995)[11]	15	17	1 (7)	1 (7)	0	0	94%*	94%*
Arterial allograft								
Verhelst et al (2000)[12]	90	36	16 (18)	20 (22)	8 (9)	2 (2)	98%*	100%*
Noel et al (2002)[13]	56	5	7 (13)	14 (25)	5 (9)	5 (9)	91%*	91%*
Vogt et al (2002)[14]	14	22	2 (14)	3 (21)	1 (7)	1 (7)	NR	NR
Kieffer et al (2004)[15]	179	46	36 (20)	39 (22)	9 (5)	4 (2)	NR	99%*
Prosthetic rifampin-soaked graft								
Bandyk et al (2001)[16]	27	17	2 (8)	2 (8)	0	2 (7)	100% at 17 months	100% at 17 months
Oderich, et al (2006)[4]	52	41	4 (8)	4 (8)	0	6 (11.5)	89% at 5 years	100% at 5 years

NR, not reported

**Kaplan-Meier analysis not reported

patients with those problems operated on electively. The elective mortality rate for the entire cohort was 5.1%. Recurrent graft infection occurred in approximately 11% of patients and was highest in those (18.5%) who had gross perigraft purulence. This subset of patients may be best treated with femoropopliteal vein reconstruction or axillofemoral reconstructions staged by graft excision. While some surgeons might argue with in situ reconstruction for patients with AGEF or AGEE, only one of our surviving 26 patients with this problem developed recurrent graft infection. The risk of major cardiac, pulmonary, renal, or vascular morbidity ranged between 10-14%, which highlights the importance of appropriate preoperative patient preparation whenever possible.

The great advantage of prosthetic in situ reconstruction for aortic graft infection is that it is quicker than the other techniques, and it has excellent primary patency (89%) and limb salvage (100%) at five years. These rates are as good as those reported for other in situ techniques and superior to those reported for axillofemoral grafts.

In summary, successful in situ prosthetic replacement of an infected aortic graft requires appropriate patient selection, thorough preoperative evaluation if possible, and careful planning and execution of the operation.

REFERENCES

1. Hallet JW, Marshal DM, Peterson TM, et al. Graft-related complications of the abdominal aortic aneurysm repair: Population-based experience. *J Vasc Surg.* 1977;25:277
2. Bandyk DF, Buckner . Infection in prosthetic vascular graft. In: Rutherford *Vascular Surgery Sixth Ed.* Philadelphia. Elsevier Sander; 2005:875–894.
3. Kieffer E, Sabatier J, Plissonnier D, Knosalla C. Prosthetic graft infection after descending thoracic/thoracoabdominal aortic aneurysmectomy: Management with in situ arterial allografts. *J Vasc Surg.* 2001;33:671–678.
4. Oderich GS, Bower TC, Cherry KJ, et al. Evolution from axillofemoral to in situ prosthetic reconstruction for the treatment of aortic graft infections at a single center. *J Vasc Surg.* 2006;43:1166–1174.
5. Yeager RA, Taylor LM, Moneta GL, et al. Improved results with conventional management of infrarenal aortic infection. *J Vasc Surg.* 1999;30:76–83.
6. Seeger JM, Pretus HA, Welborn MB, et al. Long-term outcome after treatment of aortic graft ifnections with staged extra-anatomic bypass grafting and aortic graft removal. *J Vasc Surg.* 2000;32:451–459.
7. Armstrong PA, Martin RB, Wilson JS, et al. Improved outcomes in the recent management of secondary aortoenteric fistula. *J Vasc Surg* 2005;42:660–666.
8. Seeger JM, Back MR, Albright JL, et al. Influence of patient characteristics and treatment options on outcome of patients with prosthetic aortic graft infection. *Ann Vasc Surg.* 1999;4:411–420.
9. Calligaro KD, Veith FJ, Yuan JG, et al. Intra-abdominal aortic graft infection: complete or partial graft preservation in patients at very high risk. *J Vasc Surg.* 2003;38:1199–1204.
10. Clagett GP, Bowers BL, Lopez-Viego MA, et al. Creation of a neo-aortoiliac system from lower extremity deep and superficial veins. *Ann Surg.* 1993;218:239–248; discussion 248–9.
11. Nevelsteen A, Lacroix H, Suy R. Autogenous reconstruction with the lower extremity deep veins: an alternative treatment of prosthetic infection after reconstructive surgery for aortoiliac disease. *J Vasc Surg.* 1995;22:129–34.
12. Verhelst R, Laxroix V, Vraux H, et al. Use of cryopreserved arterial homografts for management of infected prosthetic grafts: a multicentric study. *Ann Vasc Surg.* 2000;14(6):602–607.

13. Noel AA, Gloviczki P, Cherry KJ Jr., et al. United Stated Cryopreserved Aortic Allograft Registry. Abdominal aortic reconstruction in infected fields: early results of the United States cryopreserved aortic allograft registry. *J Vasc Surg*. 2002;35(5):847–852.

14. Vogt PR, Brunner-LaRocca HP, Lachat M, et al. Technical details with the use of cryopreserved arterial allografts for aortic infection: influence on early and midterm mortality. *J Vasc Surg*. 2002;35(1):80–86.

15. Kieffer E, Gomes D, Chiche L, et al. Allograft replacement for infrarenal aortic graft infection: early and late·results in 179 patients. *J Vasc Surg*. 2004;39(5):1009–1117.

16. Bandyk DF, Novotney ML, Johnson BL, et al. Use of Rifampin-soaked gelatin-sealed polyester grafts for in situ treatment of primary aortic and vascular prosthetic infections. *J Surg Res*. 2001;95(1):44–49.

17. Young RM, Cherry KJ Jr, Davis PM, et al. The results of in situ prosthetic replacement for infected aortic grafts. *Am J Surg*. 1999 Aug;178(2):136–140.

18. Oderich GS, Panneton JM, Bower TC, et al. Infected aortic aneurysms: aggressive presentation, complicated early outcome, but durable results. *J Vasc Surg*. 2001;34:900–908.

19. Batt M, Magne JL, Pierre A, Muzj A, et al. In situ revascularization with silver-coated polyester grafts to treat aortic infection: Early and midterm results. *J Vasc Surg*. 2003;Nov;35(5);983–989.

20. Walker EW, Cooley DA, Duncan JM, et. al. The management of aortoduodenal fistula by in-situ replacement of the infrarenal abdominal aortic graft. *Ann Surg*. 1987;205:727–732.

13

Aortic Reconstruction with Cryopreserved Human Allografts in the Setting of Infection

Mark D. Morasch, M.D

Aortic reconstruction following arterial or prosthetic graft excision in the setting of infection remains one of the most challenging problems encountered by surgeons. While primary arterial infections are uncommon, infection associated with bioprosthetic material can occur in up to 3% of implanted materials.[1-2] Accepted methods of vascular reconstruction in the setting of sepsis have been associated with high rates of major complications including graft failure, graft reinfection, amputation, hemorrhage, and death. Promising results with the use of cryopreserved human allografts for in-situ arterial reconstruction have been reported by some centers. On the other hand, there have also been reports of human allograft arterial degeneration, hemorrhage and thrombosis which have prevented widespread use

The ideal solution to revascularization in the setting of arterial infection would be an operation in which elimination of arterial sepsis and restoration of in-line flow could be performed in an expedient manner using a readily available conduit that is resistant to reinfection, thrombosis and is free from late aneurysmal degeneration. Biological tissue in the form of cryopreserved human allografts may be a conduit with these desired properties and thus can be used in this high risk population of patients with arterial infection in an expedient manner with acceptable peri-operative morbidity and mortality and long term durability when compared to the traditional ex-situ bypass grafting.

Cryopreserved human allografts have gone through a number of modifications since transition from the use of fresh human allografts for aortic reconstruction. Fresh allograft rupture, disintegration and, aneurysmal degeneration resulted in post-operative catastrophic events that caused their use to be abandoned after early cases of arterial reconstruction for infection.[3] The use of cryopreserved cadaveric allografts by cardiovascular surgeons for arch and valve reconstruction in the setting of endocarditis[4-5] have stimulated new interest for use in other anatomical locations. Cryopreservation techniques have permitted the preparation, storage and sterilization of human arterial and venous segments from brain dead donors for future use in live patients without risk of a host immune response or donor to recipient infection. Fresh human allografts are no longer used for arterial reconstruction thus eliminating many of the previous complications such as immune-mediated degeneration and aneurysmal degeneration with subsequent rupture.[6]

The most widely accepted procedure for arterial reconstruction in the setting of vascular sepsis is extra-anatomic bypass grafting in a sterile field with either immediate or staged complete excision of infected prosthetic material or arterial tissue. This method of reconstruction requires prolonged operative time and the long term patency of these grafts is less than optimal. In addition, aortic excision carries the risk of fatal aortic stump blow-out with reported rates as high as 20%.[2, 7] Five year patency rates of 73% have been reported, while other groups have reported patency as low as 43% at 3 years.[8-10] We also have noted an extra-anatomic graft thrombosis rate of 5% in the immediate post-operative period with additional 5% thrombosis rate after 30 days. On the other hand, we have noted no graft thromboses or amputation in early and late follow-up in a cohort treated with cryopreserved allograft. Some reports have suggested that allografts are prone to thrombosis because of a host response to the substance of the graft but most report allograft failure is very rare and usually occlusive failure is not secondary to the conduit but rather to the patient condition.

Autogenous deep femoral veins for the creation of a neoaortoiliac system (NAIS) have been used because of the obvious benefits of use of non-prosthetic or biological tissue for arterial in-situ reconstruction. Clagett et al.[11-12] described this procedure and reported acceptable patency rates in the short term without evidence of graft reinfection and a recent study by Beck et al.[13] reviewed long term data for over 240 NAIS reconstructions and reported a 5 year primary patency rate of 82%. In exchange for the benefits of in-situ reconstruction with biological tissue, this procedure requires more operative time and can be complicated by venous insufficiency and lower extremity compartment syndrome.[14] Cryopreserved allografts, provided they can be readily accessed for implantation, allow for markedly shorter operative times as the two staged approaches used for extra-anatomic reconstruction with aortic exclusion and for the NAIS procedure can be avoided.

Antibiotic soaked polyester prosthetic graft is an alternate conduit which can be used for in-situ aortic reconstruction. Despite the benefits of expedient restoration of in-line flow to the lower extremities, reinfection rates exceed 10%[15-17] and thus have not been widely implanted for arterial sepsis. While reinfection of cryopreserved allografts can occur, it is much less common than is seen with in-situ prosthetic reconstruction. One consideration, however, is that with the use of in-situ prosthetic, reinfection is rarely associated with acute hemorrhage. When allograft becomes infected, especially with fungal species, graft degeneration with acute bleeding episodes is not unheard of.

Anastamotic disruption has been described with the use of cryopreserved human allografts. Vogt et al.[18] reported complications of allograft degeneration in inadequately drained operative fields specifically with intra-abdominal infection and suggested additional post-operative drainage to control sepsis. Allograft aortic anastomotic disruption has been reported in the setting of allograft reconstruction for aortoenteric fistulae[19-23] and it has been hypothesized that in addition to virulent organisms, contamination from enteric contents may accelerate allograft degeneration.

Anastomotic disruption secondary to allograft anastomosis to non-autogenous tissue was has been noted in our institutional series and been described in one other report.[24] It remains to be seen if allograft can be anastomosed successfully to any tissue other than non-infected native arterial tissue. Vogt et al.[18] have also proposed gentamycin bonded fibrin glue and allograft strip reinforcement of a tension-free anastomosis and allograft to recipient appropriate sizing to prevent anastomotic disruption. Our center's practice now is to perform only native arterial to allograft anastomoses because of our experience with failed prosthetic-allograft anastomoses.

In our institutional series, we have seen no cases of true aneurysmal degeneration during allograft follow-up. The durability of allografts has been excellent since the advent of cryopreservation.[6, 22, 25-27] Since the diameters of an arterial allograft conduit are large, allograft stenoses appear rare. In our experience, such lesions can be treated endoluminally with angioplasty and stents.

We recently reviewed our patients with aortic infection and were able to compare a group treated with allografts to a similar cohort treated over the same time period with the more traditional approaches (mostly extra-anatomic reconstruction with aortic exclusion) and found an statistically significant improvement in mortality, amputation and wound complication rates.[28] This would suggest that there may be a benefit to CHA reconstruction as it pertains to reoperative procedures and the fate of the graft in the short term.

While our comparison was small, retrospective and non-randomized, our early data revealed an acceptable peri-operative risk of major complications and death in patients treated for aortic infection with allografts when compared to other accepted methods of revascularization.

In conclusion, cryopreserved human allograft reconstruction in the aortic position offers the benefit of in-situ reconstruction with biological tissue and is associated with low risk of reinfection, thrombosis and aneurysmal degeneration in mid-term follow-up. Arterial reconstruction with allografts in the setting of persistent arterial sepsis or direct anastomosis of allograft to non-arterialized tissue may result in a higher risk of anastomotic disruption and thus should not be performed. However, the use of allograft material seems as an acceptable method or arterial reconstruction when compared to the standard treatment methods. Long term follow-up and larger patient groups are required for improved outcome data.

REFERENCES

1. Ducasse E, Calisti A, Speziale F, et al. Aortoiliac stent graft infection: current problems and management. Ann Vasc Surg 2004; 18(5):521–6.
2. O'Hara PJ, Hertzer NR, Beven EG, Krajewski LP. Surgical management of infected abdominal aortic grafts: review of a 25-year experience. J Vasc Surg 1986; 3(5):725–31.
3. Szilagyi DE, Rodriguez FJ, Smith RF, Elliott JP. Late fate of arterial allografts. Observations 6 to 15 years after implantation. Arch Surg 1970; 101(6):721–33.
4. O'Brien MF, Harrocks S, Stafford EG, et al. The homograft aortic valve: a 29-year, 99.3% follow up of 1,022 valve replacements. J Heart Valve Dis 2001; 10(3):334–44; discussion 335.
5. Sabik JF, Lytle BW, Blackstone EH, et al. Aortic root replacement with cryopreserved allograft for prosthetic valve endocarditis. Ann Thorac Surg 2002; 74(3):650–9; discussion 659.
6. Kieffer E, Gomes D, Chiche L, et al. Allograft replacement for infrarenal aortic graft infection: early and late results in 179 patients. J Vasc Surg 2004; 39(5):1009–17.
7. Reilly LM, Altman H, Lusby RJ, et al. Late results following surgical management of vascular graft infection. J Vasc Surg 1984; 1(1):36–44.
8. Quinones-Baldrich WJ, Hernandez JJ, Moore WS. Long-term results following surgical management of aortic graft infection. Arch Surg 1991; 126(4):507–11.

9. Seeger JM, Pretus HA, Welborn MB, et al. Long-term outcome after treatment of aortic graft infection with staged extra-anatomic bypass grafting and aortic graft removal. J Vasc Surg 2000; 32(3):451-9; discussion 460–1.

10. Yeager RA, Taylor LM, Jr., Moneta GL, et al. Improved results with conventional management of infrarenal aortic infection. J Vasc Surg 1999; 30(1):76–83.

11. Clagett GP, Bowers BL, Lopez-Viego MA, et al. Creation of a neo-aortoiliac system from lower extremity deep and superficial veins. Ann Surg 1993; 218(3):239-48; discussion 248–9.

12. Clagett GP, Valentine RJ, Hagino RT. Autogenous aortoiliac/femoral reconstruction from superficial femoral-popliteal veins: feasibility and durability. J Vasc Surg 1997; 25(2):255-66; discussion 267–70.

13. Beck AW, Murphy EH, Hocking JA, et al. Aortic reconstruction with femoral-popliteal vein: graft stenosis incidence, risk and reintervention. J Vasc Surg 2008; 47(1):36–43; discussion 44.

14. Modrall JG, Sadjadi J, Ali AT, et al. Deep vein harvest: predicting need for fasciotomy. J Vasc Surg 2004; 39(2):387–94.

15. Bandyk DF, Novotney ML, Back MR, et al. Expanded application of in situ replacement for prosthetic graft infection. J Vasc Surg 2001; 34(3):411-9; discussion 419–20.

16. Oderich GS, Bower TC, Cherry KJ, Jr., et al. Evolution from axillofemoral to in situ prosthetic reconstruction for the treatment of aortic graft infections at a single center. J Vasc Surg 2006; 43(6):1166–74.

17. Young RM, Cherry KJ, Jr., Davis PM, et al. The results of in situ prosthetic replacement for infected aortic grafts. Am J Surg 1999; 178(2):136–40.

18. Vogt PR, Brunner-LaRocca HP, Lachat M, et al. Technical details with the use of cryopreserved arterial allografts for aortic infection: influence on early and midterm mortality. J Vasc Surg 2002; 35(1):80–6.

19. Gabriel M, Pukacki F, Dzieciuchowicz L, et al. Cryopreserved arterial allografts in the treatment of prosthetic graft infections. Eur J Vasc Endovasc Surg 2004; 27(6):590–6.

20. Pirrelli S, Arici V, Bozzani A, Odero A. Aortic graft infections: treatment with arterial allograft. Transplant Proc 2005; 37(6):2694–6.

21. Teebken OE, Pichlmaier MA, Brand S, Haverich A. Cryopreserved arterial allografts for in situ reconstruction of infected arterial vessels. Eur J Vasc Endovasc Surg 2004; 27(6): 597–602.

22. Verhelst R, Lacroix V, Vraux H, et al. Use of cryopreserved arterial homografts for management of infected prosthetic grafts: a multicentric study. Ann Vasc Surg 2000; 14(6):602–7.

23. Vogt PR, Brunner-La Rocca HP, Carrel T, et al. Cryopreserved arterial allografts in the treatment of major vascular infection: a comparison with conventional surgical techniques. J Thorac Cardiovasc Surg 1998; 116(6):965–72.

24. Noel AA, Gloviczki P, Cherry KJ, Jr., et al. Abdominal aortic reconstruction in infected fields: early results of the United States cryopreserved aortic allograft registry. J Vasc Surg 2002; 35(5):847–52.

25. Chiesa R, Astore D, Piccolo G, et al. Fresh and cryopreserved arterial homografts in the treatment of prosthetic graft infections: experience of the Italian Collaborative Vascular Homograft Group. Ann Vasc Surg 1998; 12(5):457–62.

26. Leseche G, Castier Y, Petit MD, et al. Long-term results of cryopreserved arterial allograft reconstruction in infected prosthetic grafts and mycotic aneurysms of the abdominal aorta. J Vasc Surg 2001; 34(4):616–22.

27. Zhou W, Lin PH, Bush RL, et al. In situ reconstruction with cryopreserved arterial allografts for management of mycotic aneurysms or aortic prosthetic graft infections: a multi-institutional experience. Tex Heart Inst J 2006; 33(1):14–8.

28. Brown KE, Heyer K, Rodriguez H, et al. Arterial reconstruction with cryopreserved human allografts in the setting of infection: A single-center experience with midterm follow-up. J Vasc Surg 2009; 49(3):660–6.

Clinical Trials on Open Versus Endovascular Repair in AAA

14

The VA Open versus Endovascular Repair (OVER) Trial for AAA

Frank A. Lederle M.D.

Four randomized clinical trials have been undertaken to compare standard open repair of abdominal aortic aneurysm (AAA) with endovascular repair (EVR).[1] The Dutch DREAM trial and the British EVAR[1] trial have recently reported their results.[2-3] The French ACE trial is still recruiting patients. The purpose of this chapter is to describe the VA Open Versus Endovascular Repair (OVER) Trial for AAA, the only U.S. trial of EVR. The trial is solely funded by the Department of Veterans Affairs Cooperative Studies Program.

Patients

Inclusion Criteria

Patients will be eligible for randomization if they meet the following criteria:

1. Patient meets the following conditions:
    a) AAA with a maximum external diameter in any plane of ≥ 5.0 cm
or
    b) an iliac aneurysm (associated with an AAA) with a maximum external diameter in any plane of ≥ 3.0 cm
or
    c) AAA ≥ 4.5 cm, if the AAA has increased by 0.7 cm in diameter in six months or 1.0 cm in 12 months, is saccular, or is associated with distal embolism
and
2. Patients must:
    a) have completed all preoperative evaluation such that no further testing is required prior to undertaking either procedure
    b) be a candidate for both procedures in the opinion of the Participating Investigator
    c) meet the manufacturers' indications for the endovascular system that would be used if the patient were randomized to EVR

Exclusion Criteria
   Patients with any of the following will be excluded from entry:

1. Previous abdominal aortic surgery
2. Evidence of AAA rupture or other reason for urgent repair
3. Inability or unwillingness to give informed consent or follow study protocol

Interventions

Enrolled patients will be randomized to open AAA repair or EVR. Open AAA repair is the conventional elective treatment of AAA and will be performed as usual at each VA clinical site. We define open repair as a procedure with sutured anastomoses of a standard anatomically placed vascular graft and ligation of branch vessels of the infrarenal AAA sac through an abdominal incision (which may be small) and may include minimal incision aortic surgery, left and right retroperitoneal approach, laparoscopically assisted arterial exposure and endoaneurysmorraphy, internal iliac artery embolization, ligation or bypass, inferior mesenteric artery reimplantation, clipped or sutured anastomosis, inferior pole renal artery revascularization or ligation, infrarenal aorta, iliac, or femoral artery endarterectomy for preparation for anastomosis, femoral-femoral bypass, balloon occlusion of iliac vessels for vascular control, application of fibrin glues/sealants, and profundaplasty/endarterectomy.

For the purposes of this study, open repair does *not* include celiac, superior mesenteric artery, or primary renal artery endarterectomy/bypass, aortic ligation/ exclusion and bypass, stapled anastomosis, axillofemoral bypass, popliteal or distal by-pass/thrombectomy/angioplasty/stenting, completely laparoscopic AAA repair, partial or complete cardiopulmonary bypass, or thoracotomy.

EVR generally involves the transluminal introduction of an expandable graft system through the femoral or iliac arteries into the aneurysmal region of the aorta and iliac arteries without an aortic clamp. The AAA is excluded from the arterial pressure with the intention that further AAA growth and rupture will be avoided. For the purposes of this study, EVR may include hypogastric artery embolization, reimplantation or sleeve extender coverage, branch artery embolization, aortic and iliac extenders or bell bottoms, iliac cutdown or conduits, iliac angioplasty, endarterectomy or stenting, pull-down maneuver, percutaneous closure, femoral artery patch closure, femoral-femoral bypass, endovascular clips/suture devices, laparoscopic branch vessel ligation, and profundaplasty/endarterectomy. For the purposes of this study, EVR does *not* include laparoscopic banding or suturing of the aorta, celiac, superior mesenteric artery or primary renal artery endarterectomy/bypass, renal artery stenting, axillofemoral bypass, popliteal or distal bypass/thrombectomy/angioplasty/stenting, aortic clamping, or aortic cut-down.

Only FDA-approved EVR systems will be used in the study. Newly approved EVR systems will be incorporated on an ongoing basis throughout the enrollment period. As new techniques become available, the definitions above may be revised by the executive committee. The choice of the EVR system to be used for a particular patient will be made prior to randomization by the individual investigator based on that physician's judgment of what system would be optimal for that patient. Because a particular EVR system may be selected based on patient characteristics that might affect outcome, identification of the intended EVR system prior to randomization permits identification of corresponding patients assigned to open repair for subgroup comparisons based on an EVR system.

A vascular surgeon (or interventional radiologist) approved by the Executive Committee must be scrubbed in on all study procedures. Criteria used for approval included vascular surgery fellowship, certificate, or equivalent (including equivalent training for interventional radiologists). In addition, to be approved to perform EVR, the proceduralist should have performed at least 12 EVR procedures with adequate supervision.

Outcomes

The primary outcome of the OVER trial is long-term all cause mortality.

Secondary outcome measures include:

1. Procedure failure; defined as failure to complete the initial procedure, any additional aortic procedures at any time during the study, any unplanned surgical procedures within 30 days of the initial procedure, or any secondary procedures resulting directly or indirectly from the initial procedure
2. Short-term (first 12 months after initial AAA repair defined as the day the patient enters the procedure suite for the initial procedure regardless of outcome) major morbidity; defined as clinical diagnosis of myocardial infarction, clinical diagnosis of stroke, amputation, or renal failure requiring dialysis. Myocardial infarction is defined as at least two of the following three criteria: (1) angina or anginal equivalent, (2) troponin or CK MB elevation, and (3) EKG changes consistent with ischemia. Stroke is defined as the rapid onset of a persistent neurological deficit attributed to obstruction or hemorrhage that is not due to brain trauma, tumor, infection, or other cause.[4] The deficit must last more than 24 hours unless death intervenes, and must be confirmed by imaging (head CT, MRI) and/or neurologist's written opinion.
3. Untreated aortoiliac abnormalities detected by close-out imaging studies.
4. Numbers of hospital and ICU days associated with the initial procedure or any additional procedures as listed under "Procedure failure" above.
5. Costs.
6. Health-related quality of life.
7. Erectile dysfunction.
8. Other procedure-related morbidities (e.g., incisional hernia, new claudication).

The advantages of using all-cause mortality as the primary outcome are (1) it is usually the patient's chief concern, (2) reducing mortality is the reason for performing AAA repair, so that any other outcome would be surrogate (though if there is no difference in mortality, the other outcomes may become decisive), (3) it can be assessed with a high degree of accuracy, and (4) it includes outcomes indirectly (but not obviously) caused by the interventions (e.g., late death due to undetected perioperative cardiac damage). Disadvantages include a relative insensitivity to detect differences due to the diluting effect of deaths unrelated to the intervention, and failure to count procedure failures not resulting in death such as conversion of EVR to open repair. Additional procedures will be recorded as secondary outcomes, and conversion of EVR to open repair in particular is associated with a high mortality rate, and so is likely to be reflected in the primary outcome.

Outcomes are adjudicated by an Outcomes Committee. Clinical and technical success rate for EVR will also be reported, as defined by the Ad Hoc Committee for Standardized Reporting Practices in Vascular Surgery of the Society for Vascular

Surgery/International Society for Cardiovascular Surgery.[5] Clinical success is defined as an excluded aneurysm and a patent graft without significant kinks, twists, or obstruction without death or secondary procedure at 30 days. Technical success is defined as a clinical success that is also without endoleak (leakage of blood into the space between the graft and the aortic wall, usually through the graft attachment areas or through back-bleeding by tributary arteries). While these rates will be reported, they are not listed as outcomes since they pertain only to the EVR group of the trial.

One-year outcomes will be published when available on all patients who had the initial procedure within the time period allowed by the protocol, and prior to the availability of long-term outcomes.

Methods

Patients provide informed consent for preoperative evaluation and for randomization. Entry evaluation includes demographics, comorbidities, medications, surgical risk using criteria developed by the RAND Corporation (Table 14-1), and results of preoperative evaluation (including anatomical compatibility with the EVR system to be used).

All preoperative evaluation must be completed and the information sent to the study central office prior to randomization, including requisite imaging studies to determine AAA diameter and suitability for both procedures. Records are kept as to why each pre-operative study was obtained (i.e., needed for EVR, open repair, or both) for future cost accounting. AAA repair must be done as soon as possible and not more than six weeks after randomization. Randomization is by telephone to the coordinating center, using computer-generated random numbers. After review of eligibility, the coordinating center randomly assigns the patient to open surgery or EVR, with an equal probability of receiving either assignment. Once assignment is made, it is final

TABLE 14-1. RAND CRITERIA FOR SURGICAL RISK

A. High risk (any one of the following):

    i. Renal: Renal dialysis or serum creatinine > 3.0 mg/dl

    ii. Hepatic: Child's Class C

    iii. Cardiac: New York Heart Association Class IV or myocardial infarction within three months

    iv. Respiratory (one of the following):

        a). Ventilator dependency

        b). $P_aO_2 < 50$ torr (room air at sea level)

        c). Dyspnea at rest

    v. ASA physical status: Category IV or higher

B. Low risk (all of the following):

    i. Renal: serum creatinine < 2.0 mg/dl

    ii. Hepatic: Child's Class A

    iii. Cardiac: no cardiac disease or New York Heart Association Class I

    iv. Respiratory (all of the following):

        a). $P_aO_2 > 70$ torr (room air at sea level)

        b). $FEV_1 > 2.0$

    v. ASA physical status: Category I or II

C. Intermediate risk (all other patients)

Ballard DJ, et al. Abdominal Aortic Aneurysm Surgery: A Literature Review and Ratings of Appropriateness and Necessity. Santa Monica; California: RAND. JRA-04;1992.

and the patient will be analyzed in that group regardless of future events or information, in accordance with the intent-to-treat principle.

Details of procedures and operative and postoperative complications and transfusions will be recorded. Troponin (or cardiac enzymes) and electrocardiograms must be obtained daily for at least two days (unless the patient is discharged sooner than this) and when clinically indicated.

Health-related quality of life is assessed using two brief questionnaires, the SF-36 and EuroQoL (EQ-5D), which are completed at baseline and at follow-up visits. The SF-36 covers eight areas: physical functioning, role limitations due to physical problems, social functioning, bodily pain, general mental health, role limitations due to emotional problems, vitality, and general health perceptions. It has been extensively tested and used in numerous studies, resulting in more than 1500 publications.[7] The SF-36 has been used to measure change in health-related quality of life after AAA repair in several studies, including the ADAM study,[8] and appears to be sensitive for this purpose though uncertainty remains due to lack of a gold standard. The EuroQoL (EQ-5D) questionnaire[9] will also be used to facilitate derivation of a utility score to assist the cost-effectiveness analysis. Erectile function will be assessed using the previously validated five-item International Index of Erectile Dysfunction (IIEF-5).[10]

Patients with AAA (5 cm (or who are planning AAA repair) who refuse randomization are invited to participate in a registry/observational study to assess long-term outcomes.

Follow-up

Follow-up will consist of visits at the following intervals: within 1 month after AAA repair, six and 12 months after enrollment, then yearly until the end of the study. All follow-up visits will include history, serum creatinine, and (except at the one month visit), the SF-36, EQ-5D, and IIEF-5. Patients randomized to endovascular repair have CT scans and plain radiography (four views of the abdomen) at all follow-up visits and any other tests recommended by the device manufacturer. Patients randomized to open repair have follow-up CT scans at one year and at the end of the study. The unequal use of CT scans in the two groups reflects clinical practice (many vascular surgeons obtain no follow-up CT scans after open repair), so any secondary procedures prompted by results of these CT scans also reflect what would occur in practice. Patients will be called monthly during the first 14 months after AAA repair and at 18, 30, 42, and 54 months to identify outcomes and costs, and will be asked to log all health care visits to facilitate these monthly reports. The follow-up described above will be conducted by study coordinators under the direction of the Participating Investigators.

Additional follow-up information will be obtained by the coordinating center from the following national datasets: the VA Beneficiary Identification and Records Locator Subsystem (BIRLS), the VA Patient Treatment File (PTF), the VA Outpatient file, the National Death Index (NDI), and MEDICARE inpatient files (it is expected that nearly all patients will be over 65 years old). At present, AAA treatment is done on an in-patient basis only.

BIRLS has a 94.5% sensitivity for identification of death in veterans who have ever been admitted to a VA hospital.[11] PTF contains dates of admission and discharge for each VA medical center, survival status at discharge, and ICD-9 classification of discharge diagnoses and procedures performed. PTF and BIRLS combined have a 97.4% sensitivity for identification of death in veterans.[11] In addition, by reporting patient contacts, PTF can be used to establish that a patient was alive at a given time. NDI has a 96.7% sensitivity for identifying deaths when the Social Security number is known,[11] and can also provide underlying and multiple causes of death. By using BIRLS and PTF (combined sensitivity 97.4%) and NDI (sensitivity 96.7%) together, the combined sensitivity should be greater than 99.9% if false negatives are independent by the two methods. Even if the sensitivity of NDI is as low as 60% for BIRLS/PTF false negatives (i.e., if false negatives are not independent between the two databases), the combined sensitivity will still be 99%. Cost data will be collected prospectively using methods based on previous experience in the Cooperative Studies Program.[12]

Statistics and Recruitment

Five-year survival rates after open repair of unruptured AAA reported in studies available when the trial was designed are shown in Table 14-2.[13–19] Five-year mortality varies from 28% to 37%.

The primary hypothesis to be tested in the study is whether EVR and open repair vary in the primary outcome of all-cause mortality. Using a cumulative five-year event rate of 28% for open repair, we are interested in detecting a 25% reduction in five-year survival with EVR; these estimates result in eight-year event rates of 30.4% and 23.1%, an absolute difference of 7.3% and a relative difference of 24.0%. Assuming a 4.5 year enrollment period, a minimum follow-up of 3.5 years, 5% lost to follow-up, and using a two-sided test of significance at the 0.05 level, these rates indicate that a sample size of 1,260 will provide 85% power. With this sample size, we expect a total of 337 events.

The average participating VA repaired 18 AAA per year before the study and we estimated that about a third of these would be anatomically unsuitable for EVR, and that based on ADAM study experience, about a third of the remainder (the eligible patients) would refuse, resulting in about eight patients enrolled per year. Thirty-four VA medical centers were needed, each enrolling at least 37 patients during 4.5 years of intake.

Prespecified subgroup analyses are planned for age (tertiles), AAA diameter (tertiles), EVR graft system (specified before randomization, so patients randomized to open repair also have EVR system assigned), VA medical center, and calendar year.

Figure 14-1 shows enrollment progress, which has been slower than planned. Reasons for this include high patient refusal rates at some sites, often due to preference for EVR, and competition with community practitioners, particularly for EVR.

TABLE 14-2. SURVIVAL FOLLOWING OPEN ELECTIVE AAA REPAIR

Study) (Author	Years of Study Entry	Patient Population	Number of Patients	Five-year Survival
Roger[13]	1971–1987	Olmsted County	131	63%
Johnston[14]	1986	Canadian Vascular Society	680	68%
Feinglass[15]	1985–1987	Academic VA Medical Centers	280	64%
Koskas[16]	1989	French Vascular Society	834	64%
Cappeller[17]	1978–1987	University Hospital in Munich	545	65%
UKSAT[18]	1991–1995	Trial Participants	563	72%
Moore[19]	1992–1998	UCLA	100	72%

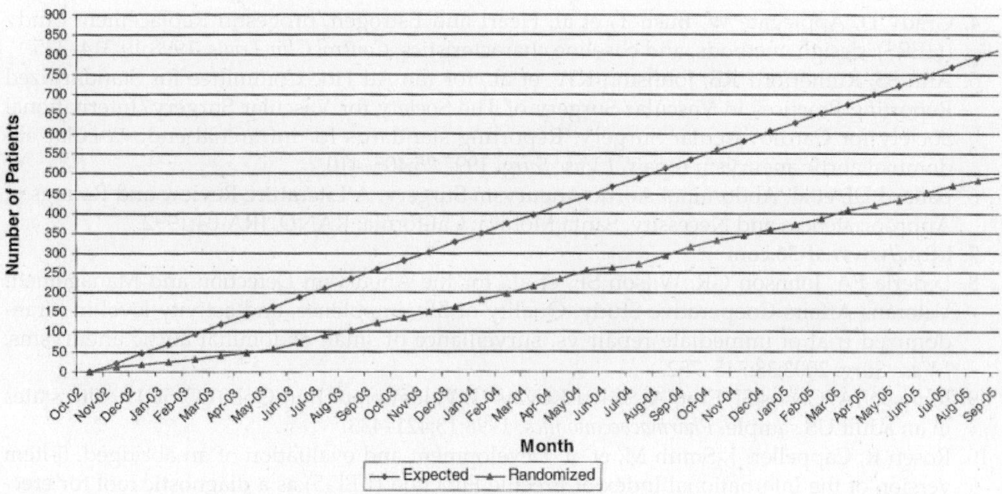

Figure 14-1. Shows enrollment progress, which has been slower than planned. Reasons for this include high patient refusal rates at some sites, often due to preference for EVR, and competition with community practitioners, particularly for EVR.

DISCUSSION

EVAR and DREAM each reported mid-term results in June 2005.[2-3] Both trials reported that the substantial reduction in all-cause mortality seen with EVR at 30 days had disappeared after two years of follow-up. This occurred because there were more late deaths in the EVR group. It remains to be seen if this was just the EVR group catching up on delayed deaths, or if late mortality is increased due to complications or failure to prevent rupture. On the positive side, both studies continue to show some advantage for EVR in AAA-related deaths. While this may be because all early postoperative deaths were classified as AAA-related and late true AAA-related deaths are easily misclassified as something else, it may also reflect a real benefit from EVR.

The answers to both questions, whether EVR increases late mortality or reduces AAA-related mortality, will require data from more randomized patients and longer follow-up. OVER will serve both of these needs, and the importance of OVER appears to have increased, rather than decreased, with the publication of the other two studies. At the end of June 2005, 450 patients had been randomized into OVER.

REFERENCES

1. Lederle FA. Abdominal aortic aneurysm - open versus endovascular repair. *N Engl J Med*. 2004;351:1677–1679.
2. Blankensteijn JD, de Jong SECA, Prinssen M, et al. Two-year results of a randomized trial comparing conventional and endovascular repair of abdominal aortic aneurysms. *N Engl J Med*. 2005;352:2398–2405.
3. EVAR trial participants. Endovascular aneurysm repair versus open repair in patients with abdominal aortic aneurysm (EVAR trial 1): randomised controlled trial. *Lancet*. 2005;365: 2179–2186.

4. Grady D, Applegate W, Bush T, et al. Heart and Estrogen/progestin Replacement Study (HERS): design, methods, and baseline characteristics. *Control Clin Trials*. 1998;19:314–335.

5. Ahn SS, Rutherford RB, Johnston KW, et al., for the Ad Hoc Committee for Standardized Reporting Practices in Vascular Surgery of The Society for Vascular Surgery/International Society for Cardiovascular Surgery. Reporting standards for infrarenal endovascular abdominal aortic aneurysm repair. *J Vasc Surg*. 1997;25:405–410.

6. Ballard DJ, et al. Abdominal Aortic Aneurysm Surgery: A Literature Review and Ratings of Appropriateness and Necessity. Santa Monica; California: RAND. JRA-04;1992.

7. **http://www.sf-36.com**

8. Lederle FA, Johnson GR, Wilson SE, et al., for the Aneurysm Detection and Management Veterans Affairs Cooperative Study. Quality of life, impotence, and activity level in a randomized trial of immediate repair vs. surveillance of small abdominal aortic aneurysms. *J Vasc Surg*. 2003;38:745–752.

9. Johnson JA, Coons SJ, Ergo A, Szava-Kovats G. Valuation of EuroQoL (EQ-5D) health states in an adult US sample. *Pharmacoeconomics*. 1998;13:421–433.

10. Rosen R, Cappelleri J, Smith M, et al. Development and evaluation of an abridged, 5-item version of the International Index of Erectile Function (IIEF-5) as a diagnostic tool for erectile dysfunction. *Int J Impotence Res*. 1999;11:319–326.

11. Fisher SG, Weber L, Goldberg J, Davis F. Mortality ascertainment in the veteran population: alternatives to the National Death Index. *Am J Epidemiol*. 1995;141:242–250.

12. Hynes D, Reda D, Giobbie-Hurder A, et al. Measuring costs in multisite randomized controlled trials: lessons from the VA Cooperative Studies Program. *Med Care*. 1999;37: AS27–36.

13. Roger VL, Ballard DJ, Hallett JW, et al. Influence of coronary artery disease on morbidity and mortality after abdominal aortic aneurysmectomy: a population-based study, 1981-1987. *J Am Coll Cardiol*. 1989;14: 1245–1252.

14. Johnston KW, and the Canadian Society for Vascular Surgery Aneurysm Study Group. Nonruptured abdominal aortic aneurysm: six-year follow-up results from the multicenter prospective Canadian aneurysm study. *J Vasc Surg*. 1994;20:163–170.

15. Feinglass J, Cowper D, Dunlop D, et al. Late survival risk factors for abdominal aortic aneurysm repair: experience from fourteen Department of Veterans Affairs hospitals. *Surgery*. 1995;118:16–24.

16. Koskas F, Kieffer E. Long-term survival after elective repair of infrarenal abdominal aortic aneurysm: results of a prospective multicentre study. *Ann Vasc Surg*. 1997;11:473–481.

17. Cappeller WA, Holzel D, Hinz MH, Lauterjung L. Ten-year results following elective surgery for abdominal aortic aneurysm. *Internat Angiol*. 1998;17:234–240.

18. UK Small Aneurysm Trial Participants. Mortality results for randomised controlled trial of early elective surgery or ultrasonographic surveillance for small abdominal aortic aneurysms. *Lancet*. 1998;352:1649–1655.

19. Moore WS, Kashyap VS, Vescera CL, Quinones-Baldrich WJ. Abdominal aortic aneurysm: a 6-year comparison of endovascular versus transabdominal repair. *Ann Surg*. 1999;230: 298–308.

15

Population-based Comparison of Open Repair and EVAR

Marc L. Schermerhorn, M.D.
Kristina A. Giles, M.D.

The first endovascular aortic aneurysm repair (EVAR) was reported by Juan Parodi in 1991.[1] FDA approval was then attained in September of 1999 and a specific ICD-9-CM was assigned in October of 2000 (International Classification of Diseases, 9th Revision, Clinical Modification). In 2004, two studies analyzing databases from the earliest years of EVAR were published showing a lower perioperative mortality after EVAR versus conventional open repair. Anderson et al. used the 2000–2002 New York State discharge dataset while Lee et al. used the 2001 Nationwide Inpatient Sample (NIS).[2,3] In the same year, European randomized controlled trials (RCT) demonstrated a similar mortality benefit with EVAR (1.6–1.7% vs. 4.6%).[4,5] Within five years of FDA approval, EVAR became the dominant repair technique spread to both academic and community hospitals in the United States.[2,6-8] This rapid growth emphasizes the importance of population database analysis as single or multi-institutional series from academic medical centers as well as RCTs may not be representative of expected national outcomes. Population-based studies allow us to see if these results are generalizable to the U.S. population.

POPULATION-BASED DATABASES

Many population-based databases exist and all have differences whether in collection, organization, or patient distribution (Table 15–1). There are advantages and disadvantages of each. Medicare, managed by the Centers for Medicare and Medicaid Services, includes both Part A and Part B files based on Medicare claims data and denominator files (www.cms.hhs.gov). Parts A and B refer to hospital inpatient claims and physician inpatient and outpatient claims, respectively. Of the hospital files, a 100% dataset or a random 5% sample can be used for analysis. The dataset's defining asset is its ability to link the hospital records via a unique patient identifier to Part B files in order to ensure accuracy of comorbidities and complications. Longitudinal follow-up is also

TABLE 15-1. POPULATION-BASED DATABASES

	Medicare Part A	Medicare Part B	Nationwide Inpatient Sample (NIS)	National Surgical Quality Improvement Program (NSQIP)	Statewide
Population representation	(100% or random 5% sample)	100%	20% stratified sample of all-payer community hospitalizations (non-federal)	All veterans hospitals and select "Private Sector" Approximately 20% of selected surgical cases	Variable
Codes utilized	ICD-9	CPT	ICD-9	ICD-9; CPT	ICD-9
Etiology	Inpatient claims	Inpatient and outpatient claims	Inpatient	Inpatient chart review	Inpatient, Ambulatory surgery, Emergency
Age	> 65, < 65 if ESRD or disability	> 65, < 65 if ESRD or disability	All	All	All
Identifiers	Patient, physician, hospital identifier	Patient, physician, hospital identifier	Physician, hospital identifier	Hospital identifier	Physician, hospital identifier
Longitudinal follow-up	Indefinite via patient identifier (100% only)	Indefinite via patient identifier	None	30-days	None

Resources Medicare: "http://www.cms.hhs.gov/home/medicare.asp"
NIS: "http://www.hcup-us.ahrq.gov/databases.jsp"
NSQIP: "http://www.acsnsqip.org"
Statewide: variable
ICD-9 International Classification of Diseases, 9th Revision
CPT Current Procedural Terminology

possible with parts A and B as well as the denominator file, giving this database the added ability to assess long-term outcomes, whereas the remaining databases are limited to hospital stays only or to a 30-day postoperative period. The Medicare population is predominately ages above 65 years; therefore, use of this resource to generalize to younger populations is limited.

The National Surgical Quality Improvement Program (NSQIP) was developed specifically for quality assessment for surgical outcomes originally within the Department of Veterans Affairs (VA). It was extended to the private sector (NSQIP-PS) hospitals by the American College of Surgeons in a pilot study of three medical centers beginning in 1999, and now includes 193 participating hospitals with a more comprehensive population representation. It is a prospectively collected and validated database with 30-day follow-up available. Data are entered from chart review by trained data-entry nurses rather than taken from administrative discharge data. Specific operative and perioperative information are available, along with other variables that do not exist in administrative datasets.[9]

The Nationwide Inpatient Sample (NIS) is a 20% stratified sample of all-payer nationwide hospitalizations collected and managed by the Healthcare Cost and Utilization Project (HCUP) of the Agency for Healthcare Research and Quality. Researchers have used the NIS database extensively to assess both elective and ruptured AAA outcomes as well as epidemiological trends across the United States. The NIS currently includes 37 states (1,054 hospitals) containing discharge data from approximately eight million hospitalizations. This is created from discharge data and audited for accuracy. Sampling weights are included to allow extrapolation to representative population numbers. It has been available since 1988 and thus allows time trend analysis to be done.[10] Some statewide datasets from HCUP and other agencies, as well as other national survey results, are available as well.[11]

Most population-based datasets use ICD-9-CM (International Classification of Diseases 9th Revision, Clinical Modification) and DRG (Disease Related Group) coding for diagnoses and procedures. Comparison studies between open and EVAR using these databases are possible for the time period after October 2000 as that was when a procedure code from the ICD-9-CM was assigned specifically for EVAR (39.71). Medicare has the added ability to include CPT coding from physician inpatient and outpatient claims to allow for even greater sensitivity and accuracy of procedures, and diagnoses including pre-existing comorbidities and follow-up complications. The NSQIP also uses CPT codes to identify inpatient procedures.

Table 15–2 outlines some of the major population-based studies that have been performed using the databases outlined above. The first population-based study was published in 2004 from the New York State hospital discharge database (Statewide Planning and Research Cooperative System [SPARCS]), which contains information on all nonfederal hospitalizations in New York. This looked at open repair and EVAR for elective aneurysms in the years 2000 to 2002, examining the adoption of EVAR in the state as well as the associated mortality rates for each year.[2] Following this, Lee et al. published a broader, national outcomes study using the NIS from 2001, comparing over 7,000 elective aneurysm repairs performed via EVAR or open repair.[3] Many subsequent studies using the NIS in addition to other database resources have followed these in an attempt to show real-world outcomes in the United States.

We previously identified patients in the Medicare population undergoing open repair or EVAR from 2001–2004. The dataset was further limited to only those patients for whom two years of preoperative data and at least one year of postoperative follow-up were available in order to have reliable preoperative comorbidity and postoperative complication variables. In order to control for the differing patient characteristics of the two procedures, the cohorts were matched via propensity score matching, resulting in a comparative study population of 45,660. This allowed for a more direct and valid comparison of outcomes. Perioperative and long-term outcomes out to four years were analyzed, including survival and AAA or laparotomy related complications requiring re-operation or rehospitalization.[6] Dillavou et al. employed the 5% Medicare beneficiary sample from 2000–2003, and analyzed preoperative differences and perioperative outcomes of open repair and EVAR, and looked at trends in repair utilization. Ruptured AAA was also included in this analysis.[12,13]

Hua et al. and Bush et al. both used the NSQIP database to assess comparisons between open repair and EVAR.[14,15] Hua et al. used private sector data from 2000–2003 when up to 14 academic medical centers were participating and identified 1,042 elective AAA repairs.[14] Bush et al. used the VA hospital data (123 hospitals) from 2001 through 2004. This study was limited to high-risk patients and included 2,368 elective

TABLE 15-2. EXAMPLES OF POPULATION-BASED STUDIES EXAMINING ELECTIVE ANEURYSM REPAIR UTILIZING DATABASE RESOURCES.[2,3,6-8,13,14]

	Anderson et al. (2004)	Lee et al. (2004)	Hua et al. (2005)	Dillavou et al. (2006)	McPhee et al. 2007)	Schermerhorn et al. (2008)	Giles et al. (In submission)
Years of study	2000–2002	2001	2000–2003	2000–2003	2001–2004	2001–2004	2001–2005
Database	New York State	NIS	NSQIP	5% Medicare	NIS	Medicare A & B	NIS
N	4,770	7,172	1,042	113,020	183,387	45,660 (matched) 61,598 (unmatched)	194,507
EVAR mortality	3.1% (2000) 1.1% (2001) 0.8% (2002)	1.3%	2.8%	1.9%	1.0%	1.2% (matched) 1.7% (unmatched)	1.1%
Open repair mortality	4.1% (2000) 3.6% (2001) 4.2% (2002)	3.8%	4.0%	5.2%	4.5%	4.8% (matched) 4.6% (unmatched)	4.6%
Other outcomes	Complications LOS	Complications LOS Discharage destination Hospital charges	Complications LOS	LOS Discharge destination Hospital charges and reimbursement		Complications LOS Disscharge destination Long-term mortality Reinterventions	LOS Discharge destination Hospital charges

NSQIP National Surgical Quality Improvement Program
NIS Nationwide Inpatient Sample
LOS Length of stay

repairs.[15] Any AAA repair comparisons representing the more extensive current private sector database are as yet unpublished.

PREOPERATIVE CHARACTERISTICS

Patients undergoing EVAR tend to be older with more extensive comorbidities, and are more likely to be male (Table 15–3).[6]

TABLE 15-3. BASELINE DEMOGRAPHICS AND COMORBID CONDITIONS OF PATIENTS UNDERGOING ENDOVASCULAR AND OPEN REPAIR OF INTACT AORTIC ANEURYSMS. UNMATCHED MEDICARE BENEFICIARIES FROM SCHERMERHORN ET AL. APPEAR IN THE LEFT COLUMNS 2001–2004 AND THOSE FROM THE NSQIP SAMPLE FROM 2000–2003 APPEAR ON THE RIGHT.[6,14]

	Medicare (unmatched cohorts)			NSQIP		
	EVAR	Open	P value	EVAR	Open	P value
Sample size	29542	32056		460	582	
Male Gender	83.2%	74.6%	<.001	84.6%	79.6%	0.04
Age				74.0	71.2	<.001
67–69	11.9%	15.6%	<.001			
70–74	26.8%	32.0%	<.001			
75–79	35.7%	35.3%	0.41			
80–84	15.8%	12.2%	<.001			
>=85	9.8%	4.9%	<.001			
Comorbid Conditions						
Prior Myocardial Infarction within 6 months	1.9%	1.8%	0.73			
Myocardial Infarction within 6-24 months	9.1%	7.1%	<.001	1.8%	0.8%	.16
Valvular Heart Disease	12.2%	9.6%	<.001			
Congestive Heart Failure	16.1%	11.6%	<.001	2.8%	2.1%	.42
Peripheral Vascular Disease	21.2%	21.4%	0.53	8.0%	8.6%	
Cerebrovascular Disease	16.1%	16.8%	<.02			
Stroke with Deficit				7.4%	5.3%	.17
Hypertension	67.1%	65.0%	<.001	69.6%	74.5%	.10
Diabetes Mellitus	17.8%	14.3%	<.001	12.7%	11.0%	.42
Chronic Obstructive Pulmonary Disease	30.8%	28.9%	<.001	25.4%	17.9%	.003
Renal Disease	5.1%	4.1%	<.001			
End Stage Renal Disease	0.6%	0.3%	<.001	1.3%	1.2%	.88
Cancer History	23.6%	18.2%	<.001			
Obesity	2.4%	1.6%	<.001			
Pack-year smoking (years)				44.4%	40.0%	.07

NSQIP National Surgical Quality Improvement Program
EVAR Endovascular aortic aneurysm repair
Schermerhorn ML, O'Malley AJ, Jhaveri A, et al. Endovascular vs. Open Repair of Abdominal Aortic Aneurysms in the Medicare Population. *N Engl J Med* 2008;358:464–474.
Hua HT, Cambria RP, Chuang SK, et al. Early outcomes of endovascular versus open abdominal aortic aneurysm repair in the National Surgical Quality Improvement Program-Private Sector (NSQIP-PS). *J Vasc Surg* 2005;41:382–389.

Age

In the Medicare population, the percentage of patients 80 years and older was significantly higher for EVAR and conversely, the percentage of patients under 74 was greater for open repair (P <.001). There were two times as many patients 85 years and older in the EVAR cohort (P <.001). These proportions were consistent from 2001 to 2004.[6] Dillavou et al. also found that there have been an increasing percentage of Medicare patients over 84 years undergoing all repair for both intact and ruptured AAA repair from 1994 to 2003. Patients undergoing repair of ruptured aneurysms tend to be older than those with intact aneurysms. This trend is more prominent in females as shown in the Medicare population where females had a mean that was three years older in the ruptured AAA cohort versus males who were 1.4 years older.[12,13]

Gender

Males undergo the majority of elective AAA repairs, making up between 75–80% of repairs overall, yet 75% of open AAA repair and 83% of EVAR.[2,3,6-8,12,13,16] Additionally, women have a 40% higher likelihood of presenting with ruptured aneurysms and are older than men for both intact AAA repair and ruptured AAA repair.[7,12] The proportion of open repairs done in females has increased over time (20% to 26%), likely due to the rise of EVAR, which is more likely to be performed in males. The percentage of females undergoing repair of a ruptured AAA has also increased from 20% to 24%.[8]

Comorbidities

Almost all comorbidities are greater in the EVAR population.[2,3,6,17] There are limitations to most administrative databases in accurately identifying all comorbidities as it is difficult to differentiate pre-existing conditions from complications in a single hospitalization. Additionally, there are a limited number of diagnoses that can be recorded, and those that affect reimbursement may have a greater likelihood of being documented versus those that do not. In the Medicare population, we, therefore, looked at a two-year period of data for each patient prior to hospitalization for AAA repair, so comorbid conditions could be identified with greater accuracy than is allowed in pure cross-sectional data. We found that myocardial infarction within two years, valvular heart disease, congestive heart failure, cerebrovascular disease, hypertension, diabetes, chronic obstructive pulmonary disease, renal insufficiency, end-stage renal disease, cancer history, and obesity were more common in the EVAR cohort (Table 15–3).[6] Hua et al., using the NSQIP that has a specific designation for comorbidities and current symptoms, found similar trends for EVAR patients to have a greater comorbidity burden. However, the only difference to reach statistical significance was chronic obstructive pulmonary disease, present in 25% of EVAR patients but only 18% of open repair patients (Table 15–3).[14] In contrast to randomized controlled trials that are designed to have equivalent cohorts, these results are able to show the differences in the actual patient population receiving EVAR versus open aneurysm repairs. These differences should be taken into account when comparing outcomes.

PERIOPERATIVE OUTCOMES

Perioperative Mortality for Intact Aneurysm Repair

Prior to the introduction of EVAR, analysis of the National Hospital Discharge Survey data from 1979 to 1997 revealed a mortality rate of 5.6% for elective open AAA repair.[18] Randomized control trials showed EVAR to have a significantly lower perioperative mortality than open repair (EVAR I: 1.6% vs. 4.6%; DREAM: 1.2% vs. 4.6%).[4,5] Within the Medicare population, matching patients undergoing open repair and EVAR via propensity scoring was done in order to closely adjust for demographic and comorbidity differences, and create cohorts that could be more comparable as with RCT data. This resulted in 22,830 patients within each repair group from Medicare in 2001 to 2004. The perioperative mortality after EVAR was 1.2% and after open repair was 4.8%, with a relative risk of 4.0 (95% CI, 3.5 to 4.7; P < .0001). Before propensity scoring to match groups, there were 61,598 patients with a mortality of 1.7% after EVAR and 4.6% after open repair, highlighting the older age and greater comorbidity of the EVAR population.[6] Other work using NIS data and statewide data have also demonstrated a lower mortality with EVAR.[2,3,7,8] The NIS, which includes all ages from 2001 to 2005, has shown a mortality of 1.3% after EVAR and 4.5% after open repair. Overall mortality for intact aneurysm repair for the years after EVAR introduction (2001–2005) was 3.1% while mortality in the years 1993–1998 was 4.7% (P < .0001) due to the lower mortality with EVAR and its increasing utilization.[8]

Predictors of Perioperative Mortality

Most population-based studies have found that predictors of mortality after intact AAA repair are increasing age, female gender, and open surgery. Odds ratios for the increased mortality risk with open surgery versus EVAR have ranged from 1.7–3.8.[3,7,13,14,16,19] A multivariate analysis using matched cohorts from the Medicare population showed that open repair carried a 3.2-fold risk of mortality (Table 15–4). For either type of repair, the strongest predictors of mortality were a history of hemodialysis or renal insufficiency. Weaker predictors were female gender, congestive heart failure and vascular disease.[19]

TABLE 15-4. MULTIVARIATE PREDICTORS OF PERIOPERATIVE MORTALITY AMONG MEDICARE PATIENTS UNDERGOING REPAIR OF INTACT ABDOMINAL AORTIC ANEURYSMS.[19]

Variable	OR	95%	CI	P-value
Open Repair	3.2	2.7	3.8	< .0001
Age (vs 67–69yrs)				
71–75 years	1.2	0.9	1.6	.34
76–80 years	1.9	1.4	2.5	< .0001
> 80 years	3.1	2.4	4.2	< .0001
Female	1.5	1.3	1.8	< .0001
Dialysis-dependent end-stage renal disease	2.6	1.5	4.6	< .001
Chronic renal insufficiency	2.0	1.6	2.6	< .0001
Congestive heart failure	1.7	1.5	2.1	< .0001
Vascular disease (Peripheral arterial or cerebrovascular disease)	1.3	1.2	1.6	< .0001

Giles KA, Schermerhorn ML, O'Malley AJ, et al. Risk prediction for perioperative mortality of endovascular versus open repair of abdominal aortic aneurysms using the Medicare population. In submission to *J Vasc Surg*.

In a younger cohort from the NSQIP database, Hua et al. found open repair to have a 2.5-fold increased risk of mortality (OR, 95%CI: 2.4, 1.03-5.8, P < .05) while other predictors included dialysis (51.4, 10.0-264, P < .0001), poor functional status (5.8, 2.2-14.9, P < .001), weight loss (7.4, 2.0-28, P < .01), and a history of angina (5.5, 1.6-19.6, P < .01).[14]

Age Differences

Mortality differences are most prominent in older age groups. Age stratification in matched Medicare cohorts revealed that patients 85 years and older had an absolute mortality benefit of 8.5% (EVAR 2.7%, open repair 11.2%) while those under 70 had an absolute mortality benefit of 2.1% (EVAR 0.4%, open repair 2.5%) (Table 15–5).[6]

Gender Differences

Just as females are more likely to present with rupture, they are more likely to fare worse with AAA repair, whether EVAR or open repair. This holds true for elective repair as well as ruptured AAA repair with females having a 25% to 60% higher mortality.[7,12,16]

Perioperative Complications

Open repair has traditionally been associated with high morbidity. Huber et al. found that 32.4% of the patients experienced complications after open repair using data from the 1994–1996 NIS.[20] EVAR has been associated with a lower medical complication rate compared to open repair in the perioperative period including myocardial infarction, pneumonia, and acute renal failure. Most surgical complications were also found to be lower after EVAR (Table 15–6).[6]

Length of Stay and Discharge Destination

Length of stay is much longer after open repair compared to EVAR. The mean LOS in Medicare patients was 9.3 days after open repair and 3.4 days after EVAR (P < .001). Similarly, NIS data shows a mean stay of 8.8 days after open repair and 3.6 days after EVAR (P < .001).[3] Discharge to home also favors EVAR. Up to 95% of surviving patients are discharged home after EVAR whereas only 82% are discharged home after open repair.[6] The NIS has shown similar proportions.[3,8]

TABLE 15-5. MORTALITY BY AGE GROUP AFTER ENDOVASCULAR AND OPEN ABDOMINAL AORTIC ANEURYSM REPAIR IN MEDICARE BENEFICIARIES 2001–2004.[6]

Perioperative Outcomes	EVAR (n=22,830)	Open (n=22,830)	p value	Relative risk	95% CI
Mortality					
All ages	1.2%	4.8%	<.001	4.00	3.51 to 4.56
Age 67–69	0.4%	2.5%	<.001	6.21	4.98 to 7.73
Age 70–74	0.8%	3.3%	<.001	4.12	3.51 to 4.84
Age 75–79	1.3%	4.8%	<.001	3.69	3.25 to 4.19
Age 80–84	1.6%	7.2%	<.001	4.49	4.02 to 5.02
Age >85	2.7%	11.2%	<.001	4.14	3.80 to 4.52

EVAR Endovascular aortic aneurysm repair

Schermerhorn ML, O'Malley AJ, Jhaveri A, et al. Endovascular vs. Open Repair of Abdominal Aortic Aneurysms in the Medicare Population. *N Engl J Med* 2008;358:464–474.

TABLE 15-6. PERIOPERATIVE COMPLICATIONS AFTER EVAR AND OPEN REPAIR OF ABDOMINAL AORTIC ANEURYSMS IN MEDICARE BENEFICIARIES 2001–2004.[6]

Perioperative Outcomes	EVAR (n=22,830)	Open (n=22,830)	p value	Relative risk	95% CI
Medical Complications					
Myocardial infarction	7.0%	9.4%	<.001	1.34	1.26 to 1.42
Pneumonia	9.3%	17.4%	<.001	1.89	1.79 to 1.98
Acute renal failure	5.5%	10.9%	<.001	2.00	1.87 to 2.14
Renal failure requiring dialysis	0.4%	0.5%	0.047	0.33	1.00 to 1.75
Deep vein thrombosis or pulmonary embolism	1.1%	1.7%	<.001	1.51	1.29 to 1.76
Surgical Complications					
Conversion to open repair	1.6%	**	**	**	**
Acute mesenteric ischemia	1.0	2.1%	<.001	2.19	1.87 to 2.56
Reoperation for bleeding	0.8%	1.2%	<.001	1.50	1.24 to 1.80
Tracheostomy	0.2%	1.5%	<.001	7.46	5.48 to 10.14
Thrombectomy	0.4%	0.2%	<.001	0.50	0.35 to 0.71
Embolectomy	1.3%	1.7%	<.001	1.29	1.11 to 1.50
Repair of infected graft or graft-enteric fistula	0.01%	0.09%	<.001	7.00	2.09 to 23.46
Major amputation	0.04%	0.13%	<0.01	3.00	1.47 to 6.14
Lysis of adhesions without resection	0.1	1.2%	<.001	13.05	8.37 to 20.33
Bowel resection	0.6%	1.3%	<.001	2.17	1.77 to 2.65
Ileus or bowel obstruction without resection or lysis of adhesions	5.1%	16.7%	<.001	3.25	3.05 to 3.46

EVAR Endovascular aortic aneurysm repair

Schermerhorn ML, O'Malley AJ, Jhaveri A, et al. Endovascular vs. Open Repair of Abdominal Aortic Aneurysms in the Medicare Population. *N Engl J Med* 2008;358:464–474.

Cost

Cost data are variable. Analysis of Medicare data from 2001 to 2003 showed that hospital charges for open repair and EVAR were not significantly different ($55,084 vs. $56,936, P =NS). Medicare reimbursements, however, were higher for open repair versus EVAR ($22,248 vs. $19,724, P < .002).[13] Conversely, NIS data for 2001 to 2005 have shown that median hospital charges for EVAR were significantly higher ($51,755, vs. $43,232 for open repair, P < .0001).[8]

FOLLOW-UP OUTCOMES

Long-term Mortality

The majority of population-based datasets do not have the ability to assess follow-up outcomes; however, with the Medicare denominator file, survival may be tracked and follow-up is possible. This allows a comparison to randomized-control-trial results that have shown that the perioperative mortality benefit of EVAR eventually diminishes and long-term survival for both repairs are similar after 18 months.[21,22] In the Medicare population, the survival benefit from EVAR persisted beyond three years. This effect was age dependent with increasing durability of the survival benefit with increasing age. This appeared to be largely driven by differences in operative mortality (Figure 15–1).[6]

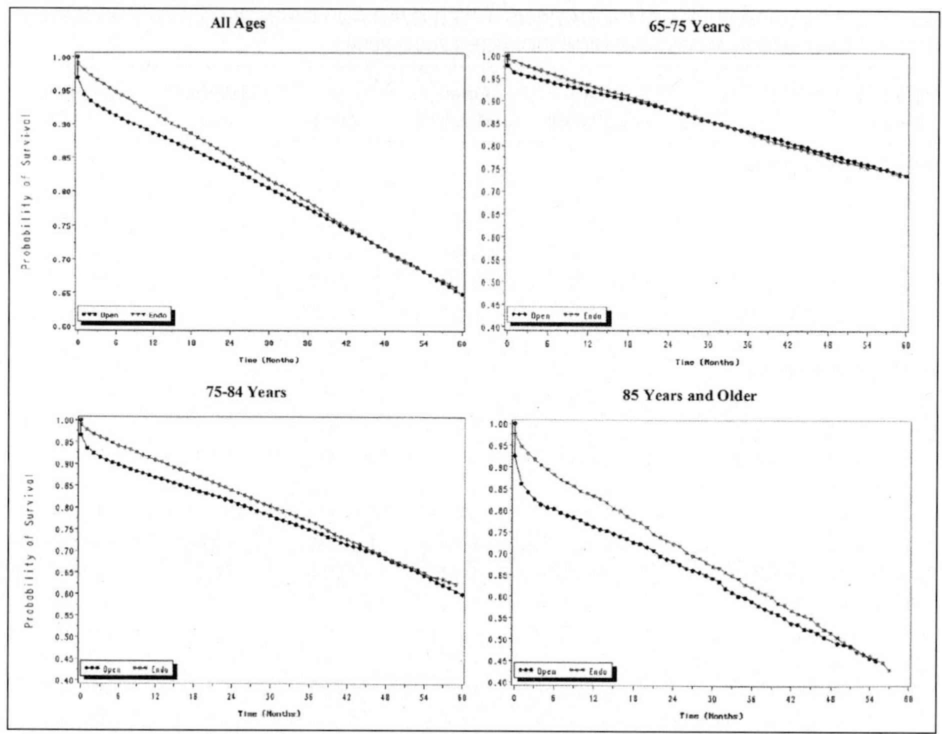

Figure 15-1. Survival of Patients Undergoing Endovascular Repair or Open Repair of Abdominal Aortic Aneurysms, Overall and According to Age.

Rupture/Reinterventions

In addition to the Medicare denominator files that allow survival to be followed, the unique patient identifier with Medicare Parts A and B allows rehospitalizations and re-interventions to be followed as well.

RCTs have shown that the need for postoperative reinterventions and late complications are higher than after open repair. In the Medicare analysis at four years, rupture rates were higher after EVAR than after open repair (1.8% vs. 0.5%, P < .001).[6] While this confirms there is some ongoing risk of rupture after EVAR, it demonstrates that there is some ongoing risk after open repair as well.

In EVAR 1, secondary interventions were performed in 20% after EVAR and 6% after open repair within four years.[22] However, they only considered aneurysm-related reinterventions, and did not take into account laparotomy related complications. Within Medicare patients, AAA-related reinterventions were also more common after EVAR (9.0% vs. 1.7%, P < .001); however, the majority of these were minor endovascular reinterventions such as placement of an extension cuff or coil embolization. Laparotomy related reinterventions, however, were more prevalent after open repair (9.7% vs. 4.1%, P < .001). These included repair of abdominal wall hernias, lysis of adhesions, and bowel resections. Hospitalization for bowel obstruction without operation was also greater after open repair (14.2%, vs. 8.1% after EVAR, P < .001) (Table 15–7).[6] This is likely an underestimation of the true differences since we did not control for prior laparotomy and these patients are more likely to undergo EVAR versus an open repair.

TABLE 15-7. POSTOPERATIVE AAA-RELATED AND LAPAROTOMY-RELATED REINTERVENTIONS AND HOSPITALIZATIONS FOLLOWING ENDOVASCULAR AND OPEN ABDOMINAL AORTIC ANEURYSM REPAIR IN MEDICARE BENEFICIARIES 2001–2004.[6]

	Year 1		Year 2		Year 3		Year 4		
	EVAR	Open	EVAR	Open	EVAR	Open	EVAR	Open	p value*
Rupture	0.32%	0.16%	0.65%	0.29%	1.26%	0.41%	1.79%	0.47%	<.001
Any AAA-related Reintervention	2.68%	0.54%	4.76%	0.83%	6.94%	1.21%	8.95%	1.72%	<.001
Major Reoperations	0.37%	0.19%	0.73%	0.26%	1.19%	0.34%	1.57%	0.57%	<.001
Conversion to open repair	0.08%	N/A	0.17%	N/A	0.27%	N/A	0.39%	N/A	N/A
Open AAA repair	0.27%	0.11%	0.52%	0.14%	0.89%	0.22%	1.14%	0.40%	<.001
Redo AAA repair or aorto-bifemoral bypass	0.14%	0.05%	0.35%	0.07%	0.70%	0.10%	0.92%	0.15%	<.001
Axillo-remoral or axillo-bifemoral bypass	0.12%	0.07%	0.17%	0.09%	0.19%	0.13%	0.22%	0.26%	0.40
Repair of infected graft or graft-enteric fistula	0.06%	0.12%	0.11%	0.16%	0.15%	0.19%	0.18%	0.31%	0.13
Minor Revisions	2.41%	0.37%	4.23%	0.61%	6.08%	0.92%	7.76%	1.25%	<.001
Revisions (endovascular)	1.88%	0.17%	3.46%	0.31%	5.19%	0.49%	6.74%	0.59%	<.001
Repeat endovascular AAA repair	0.17%	0.04%	0.40%	0.06%	0.80%	0.08%	1.16%	0.08%	<.001
Embolization	0.71%	0.04%	1.30%	0.08%	1.97%	0.17%	2.33%	0.19%	<.001
Angioplasty (aortic or iliac)	0.58%	0.10%	0.80%	0.17%	0.97%	0.27%	1.10%	0.32%	<.001
Extension cuff	0.78%	0.03%	1.62%	0.04%	2.71%	0.04%	3.82%	0.06%	<.001
Revisions (open)	0.57%	0.21%	0.87%	0.32%	1.06%	0.45%	1.17%	0.68%	<.001
Thrombectomy	0.12%	0.14%	0.17%	0.19%	0.24%	0.30%	0.29%	0.40%	0.61
Femoral-femoral bypass	0.47%	0.09%	0.73%	0.16%	0.86%	0.21%	0.91%	0.34%	<.001
Laparotomy-Related Reinterventions	1.36%	3.37%	2.39%	6.25%	3.46%	8.13%	4.12%	9.73%	<.001
Ventral hernia repair	0.33%	1.93%	0.64%	4.02%	0.90%	5.10%	1.08%	5.77%	<.001
Lysis of adhesions without bowel resection	0.17%	0.62%	0.26%	0.89%	0.42%	1.14%	0.52%	1.54%	<.001
Bowel resection	0.97%	1.11%	1.69%	1.87%	2.46%	2.65%	2.97%	3.41%	<0.05
Large bowel	0.84%	0.87%	1.44%	1.40%	2.05%	1.98%	2.46%	2.59%	0.57
Small bowel	0.20%	0.30%	0.34%	0.58%	0.54%	0.85%	0.67%	1.07%	<.001
Laparotomy-Related Hospitalizations without Bowel Resection/Lysis Of Adhesions	2.23%	4.87%	4.36%	8.80%	6.40%	11.67%	8.10%	14.19%	<.001

EVAR Endovascular aortic aneurysm repair

AAA Abdominal aortic aneurysm

Schermerhorn ML, O'Malley AJ, Jhaveri A, et al. Endovascular vs. Open Repair of Abdominal Aortic Aneurysms in the Medicare Population. *N Engl J Med* 2008;358:464–474.

CONCLUSION

Population data have been useful to confirm the perioperative benefits of EVAR seen in RCTs. They demonstrate that results in centers involved in RCTs are generalizable to the U.S. population. They also suggest that the benefit of EVAR may be more durable than that seen in RCTs. Perioperative and long-term benefits of EVAR increase with age and likely comorbidity due in most part to greater reduction in operative mortality. Population data also corroborate the increased AAA-related reinterventions after EVAR, as well as confirm the ongoing risk of rupture in both groups although higher after EVAR. Laparotomy-related complications, previously overlooked, must be considered in future comparisons.

REFERENCES

1. Parodi JC, Palmaz JC, Barone HD. Transfemoral intraluminal graft implantation for abdominal aortic aneurysms. *Ann Vasc Surg*. 1991;5:491–499.
2. Anderson PL, Arons RR, Moskowitz AJ, et al. A statewide experience with endovascular abdominal aortic aneurysm repair: Rapid diffusion with excellent early results. *J Vasc Surg*. 2004;39:10–18.
3. Lee WA, Carter JW, Upchurch G, et al. Perioperative outcomes after open and endovascular repair of intact abdominal aortic aneurysms in the united states during 2001. *J Vasc Surg*. 2004;39:491–496.
4. Prinssen M, Verhoeven ELG, Buth J, et al. A Randomized Trial Comparing Conventional and Endovascular Repair of Abdominal Aortic Aneurysms. *N Engl J Med*. 2004;351: 1607–1618.
5. Greenhalgh R. Comparison of endovascular aneurysm repair with open repair in patients with abdominal aortic aneurysm (EVAR trial 1), 30-day operative mortality results: randomised controlled trial. *Lancet*. 2004;364:843–848.
6. Schermerhorn ML, O'Malley AJ, Jhaveri A, et al. Endovascular vs. Open Repair of Abdominal Aortic Aneurysms in the Medicare Population. *N Engl J Med*. 2008;358:464–474.
7. McPhee JT, Hill JS, Eslami MH. The impact of gender on presentation, therapy, and mortality of abdominal aortic aneurysm in the United States, 2001–2004. *J Vasc Surg*. 2007;45: 891–899.
8. Giles KA, Pomposelli F, Hamdan A, et al. Decrease in total aneurysm related deaths in the era of endovascular aneurysm repair. In submission to *J Vasc Surg*.
9. American College of Surgeons National Surgical Quality Improvement Program. www.acsnsqip.org.
10. Healthcare Cost and Utilization Project. www.ahrq.gov/data/hcup.
11. Databases and Related Tools from HCUP. Fact Sheet. AHRQ Publication No. 06-P022. May 2006. Agency for Healthcare Research and Quality, Rockville, MD. .
12. Dillavou ED, Muluk SC, Makaroun MS. A decade of change in abdominal aortic aneurysm repair in the United States: Have we improved outcomes equally between men and women? *J Vasc Surg*. 2006;43:230–238.
13. Dillavou ED, Muluk SC, Makaroun MS. Improving aneurysm-related outcomes: Nationwide benefits of endovascular repair. *J Vasc Surg*. 2006;43:446–452.
14. Hua HT, Cambria RP, Chuang SK, et al. Early outcomes of endovascular versus open abdominal aortic aneurysm repair in the National Surgical Quality Improvement Program-Private Sector (NSQIP-PS). *J Vasc Surg*. 2005;41:382–389.
15. Bush RL, Johnson ML, Hedayati N, et al. Performance of endovascular aortic aneurysm repair in high-risk patients: Results from the Veterans Affairs National Surgical Quality Improvement Program. *J Vasc Surg*. 2007;45:227–235.

16. Leon J, Luis R., Labropoulos N, et al. To what extent has endovascular aneurysm repair influenced abdominal aortic aneurysm management in the state of Illinois? *J Vasc Surg*. 2005; 41:568–574.
17. Greco G, Egorova N, Anderson PL, et al. Outcomes of endovascular treatment of ruptured abdominal aortic aneurysms. *J Vasc Surg*. 2006;43:453.
18. Heller JA, Weinberg A, Arons R, et al. Two decades of abdominal aortic aneurysm repair: Have we made any progress? *J Vasc Surg*. 2000;32:1091–1101.
19. Giles KA, Schermerhorn ML, O'Malley AJ, et al. Risk prediction for perioperative mortality of endovascular versus open repair of abdominal aortic aneurysms using the Medicare population. In submission to *J Vasc Surg*.
20. Huber TS, Wang JG, Derrow AE, et al. Experience in the United States with intact abdominal aortic aneurysm repair. *J Vasc Surg*. 2001;33:304–311.
21. Blankensteijn JD, de Jong SECA, Prinssen M, et al. Two-Year Outcomes after Conventional or Endovascular Repair of Abdominal Aortic Aneurysms. *N Engl J Med*. 2005;352:2398–2405.
22. EVAR Trial Participants. Endovascular aneurysm repair versus open repair in patients with abdominal aortic aneurysm (EVAR trial 1): randomised controlled trial. *Lancet*. 2005;365: 2179–2186.

16

Sexual Dysfunction after Conventional and Endovascular AAA Repair: Results of the DREAM Randomized Trial

Monique Prinssen, M.D., Erik Buskens, M.D., Rudolf P. Tutein Nolthenius, M.D., Steven M.M. van Sterkenburg, M.D., Joep A.W. Teijink, M.D., and Jan D. Blankensteijn, M.D. on Behalf of the DREAM Trial Participants

Open abdominal aortic aneurysm (AAA) repair has been associated with impairment of sexual functioning. Sexual dysfunction after open repair (OR) of AAA is often attributed to autonomic nerve injury and changes in pelvic blood supply. As endovascular aneurysm repair (EVAR) does not require dissection in the area of the iliac bifurcation; it is expected not to affect sexual functioning. However, little is known about this subject. There is clinical evidence that sexual problems have a mixed etiology with physical, medical, social, and psychological components. So, it is not unlikely that other factors may be responsible for the sexual impairment after OR also.[1-2] Only a few studies have focused on sexual dysfunction after AAA repair, most in conjunction with conventional surgery.[3-5] The aim of our study was to assess sexual functioning in the first postoperative year after elective EVAR and OR in a randomized study.

METHODS

Study Design and Patient Samples

In the Dutch Randomized Endovascular Aneurysm Management (DREAM) trial, 153 patients (141 men; mean age 71 years, range 53–85) suitable for both treatments were randomly allocated to EVAR (n = 77) or OR (n = 76) between November 1999 and August

2002. There was one crossover from OR to EVAR, but the analysis was based on intention to treat. The study design has been described in detail elsewhere.[6] The Institutional Review Boards of all participating hospitals (Appendix) approved the study, and informed consent was obtained from each patient.

Sexual functioning was assessed on a scale adapted from the Medical Outcomes Study (MOS)[7], which consists of five questions concerning sexual functioning (Table 16–1). The questionnaire was sent to all patients preoperatively and at five time points in the first postoperative year (three, six, 13, 26, and 52 weeks). If the questionnaire was not filled out completely, questions were completed with a telephone call. For analysis purposes, a patient was considered to report sexual dysfunction for each of the items if any of the following answers were given: completely agree, partly agree, and partly disagree.

Statistical Analysis

Baseline characteristics (age, gender, SVS/AAVS [Society for Vascular Surgery/American Association for Vascular Surgery] risk score8, and medication) of patients in both trial arms were compared with the Student t and chi-square tests. The proportion of patients reporting sexual dysfunction on at least one of the five aspects, and the proportion for each individual aspect of sexual functioning, were calculated and compared between the EVAR and OR group using the Fisher's exact test. Changes in the magnitude of sexual dysfunction over time versus the preoperative value were analyzed with the Wilcoxon signed rank test. Analyses were performed using SPSS version 11.0 (SPSS Inc., Chicago, IL, USA). $P < 0.05$ was considered significant.

RESULTS

There were no differences in baseline characteristics between the EVAR and OR groups (Table 16–2). Both pre- and postoperatively, there were no significant differences between the trial arms in the number of patients using any β blockers, calcium channel blockers, digoxin, or diuretics. Preoperatively, 64% of the patients in the OR group used one or more of these medications compared to 51% in the EVAR group.

In the OR group, 47 patients received an aorto-aortic tube graft and 30 a bifurcated graft; in the EVAR group, all endografts were bifurcated except one tube graft. Internal iliac artery patency after surgery was unchanged in 72/77 (94%) patients

TABLE 16-1. MEDICAL OUTCOMES STUDY QUESTIONNAIRE ON SEXUAL FUNCTIONING

Do you agree or disagree with the following statements?	Completely agree	Partly agree	Partly disagree	Completely disagree
a. I'm not interested in sex	☐	☐	☐	☐
b. I have difficulties in relaxing and enjoying sex	☐	☐	☐	☐
c. I have difficulties in becoming sexually aroused	☐	☐	☐	☐
d. I have difficulties in having an orgasm	☐	☐	☐	☐
e. I have difficulties in getting and/or keeping an erection (for men only)	☐	☐	☐	☐

TABLE 16-2. BASELINE CHARACTERISTICS ACCORDING TO THE SVS/AAVS RISK FACTOR

	OR (N)	EVAR (N)
Male:Female	69/7	72/5
Median Age (yrs) (range)	70 (53-85)	70 (55-82)
Diabetes (%)		
not available	0	1 (1%)
none (0)	72 (95%)	71 (92%)
adult onset, diet (1)	3 (4%)	4 (5%)
adult onset, insuline (2)	1 (1%)	1 (1%)
Tabacco use (%)		
not available	1 (1%)	1 (1%)
none or > 10 yrs ago (0)	39 (51%)	28 (36%)
not current, < 10 yrs ago (1)	13 (17%)	17 (22%)
current, < 1 pack/day (2)	15 (20%)	28 (36%)
current, > 1 pack/day (3)	8 (11%) ·	3 (4%)
Hyperlipidemia (%)		
not available	7 (9%)	3 (4%)
normal levels (0)	37 (49%)	44 (57%)
mild elevation, diet (1)	7 (9%)	8 (10%)
strict dietary control (2)	1 (1%)	1 (1%)
dietary + drug control (3)	24 (32%)	21 (27%)
Hypertension (%)		
not available	0	2 (3%)
none (0)	40 (54%)	35 (45%)
single drug therapy (1)	23 (30%)	27 (35%)
2 drug therapy (2)	11 (14%)	11 (14%)
> 2 drugs or uncontrolled (3)	2 (3%)	2 (3%)
Carotid disease (%)		
not available	0	1 (1%)
no symptoms (0)	67 (88%)	67 (87%)
asymptomatic, but disease (1)	4 (53%)	1 (1%)
TIA or temporary stroke (2)	3 (39%)	5 (6%)
stroke/neurologic deficit (c)	2 (3%)	3 (4%)
Cardiac status (%)		
not available	0	1 (1%)
asymptomatic, normal ECG (0)	39 (51%)	44 (57%)
asympt., remote or occult MI (1)	33 (43%)	25 (32%)
stable AP, drug compensated CHF (2)	4 (5%)	7 (9%)
Renal status (%)		
not available	0	2 (3%)
no renal disease (0)	70 (92%)	69 (90%)
creatinine < 210 μmol/L (1)	5 (7%)	6 (8%)

(Continued)

TABLE 16-2. BASELINE CHARACTERISTICS ACCORDING TO THE SVS/AAVS RISK FACTOR (*Continued*)

	OR (N)	EVAR (N)
Pulmonary status (%)		
not available	0	2 (3%)
asympt., PFT >80% of predicted (0)	64 (84%)	51 (66%)
asympt., PFT 65-80% of predicted (1)	9 (12%)	21 (21%)
PFT 35-65% of predicted (2)	3 (4%)	3 (39%)
Medication affection sex. function (%)	49 (64%)	39 (51%)
Digoxin	5 (66%)	3 (4%)
Diurectics	12 (16%)	10 (13%)
Calcium-channel blockers	16 (21%)	14 (18%)
Beta-blockers	33 (43%)	26 (34%)

CHF: congestive heart failure, AP: angina pectoris, MI: myocardial infarction, PFT: pulmonary function test.

Reprinted by permission from: International Society of Endovascular Specialists from *J Endovasc Ther.* 2004 Dec;11(6):613-20.

assigned to the OR group and 61/76 (80%) patients assigned to the EVAR group ($p = 0.017$). One or bilateral patent internal iliac arteries were lost in five OR and in 14 EVAR patients; in addition, a single internal iliac artery (with preexistent contralateral occlusion) was sacrificed in one EVAR patient. Postoperatively, impaired sexual functioning was reported spontaneously at office visits by two patients in the OR group and by one in the EVAR patients.

The preoperative questionnaire response rate was 69% in the OR group and 87% in the EVAR group ($p = 0.007$). The postoperative response rates for OR and EVAR were 61% versus 66% ($p = 0.542$) at three weeks, 61% versus 66% ($p = 0.542$) at six weeks, 71% versus 70% ($p = 0.818$) at 13 weeks, 69% versus 68% ($p = 0.956$) at 26 weeks, and 69% versus 67% ($p = 0.819$) at 52 weeks.

The preoperatively reported sexual dysfunction rate (Table 16–3) was high in both groups; for the individual items, the proportions varied between 48% and 56% in the OR group and 53% and 60% in the EVAR group. Preoperatively, the percentage of patients reporting sexual dysfunction on any of the five aspects was 66% in OR group and 74% in the EVAR group ($p = NS$). There was no statistically significant difference

TABLE 16-3. PROPORTION OF PATIENTS REPORTING SEXUAL DYSFUNCTION

Sexual Dysfunction (aspect)	Pre % OR	EV	3 Weeks % OR	EV	6 Weeks % OR	EV	13 Weeks % OR	EV	26 Weeks % OR	EV	52 Weeks % OR	EV
Interest	48	53	67	77*	70	60	51	55	52	58	45	63
Pleasure	56	55	72	84*	74	65	62	59	58	71	51	70
Engagement	55	60	76	77	77*	58	61	53	66	63	53	64
Orgasm	53	57	72	78	77*	55	60	52	65	59	61	54
Erection	54	57	73	74*	72	58	58	56	60	57	60	54
Any aspect	66	74	79	82	77	68	69	70	76	71	66	69

*Significantly different from Pre at $p < 0.05$.

Reprinted by permission from: International Society of Endovascular Specialists from *J Endovasc Ther.* 2004 Dec;11(6):613–20.

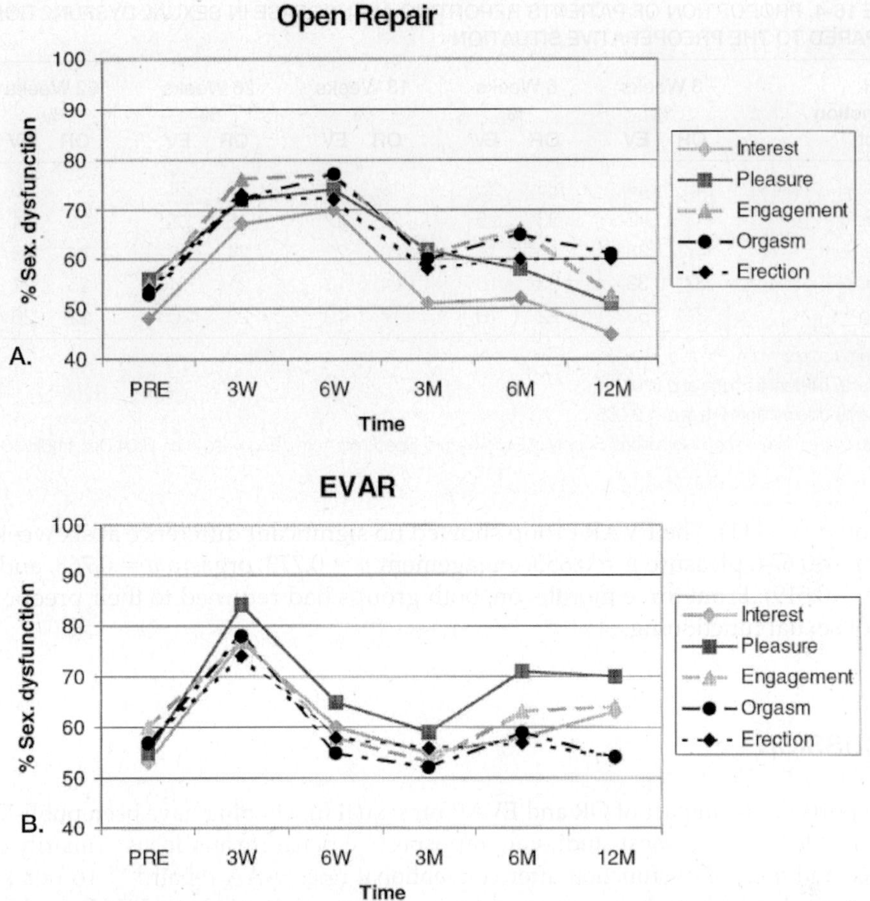

Figure 16-1. Proportion of sexual dysfunction for 5 aspects over time in the open **A.** and the EVAR **B.** groups. Reprinted by permission from: International Society of Endovascular Specialists from *J Endovasc Ther.* 2004 Dec;11(6):613–20.

in the proportion of patients reporting sexual dysfunction between the two groups for any of the five aspects at any time point or for sexual dysfunction in at least one aspect.

Nevertheless, surgery did have an impact on sexual functioning in both groups (Figure 16–1). Three weeks after surgery, the reported rate of sexual dysfunction on any of the five aspects increased to 79% in the OR group and 82% in the EVAR group. Looking at the reported changes in magnitude of sexual dysfunction at three weeks compared to preoperative values (Table 16–4), the OR group reported a significant increase on all five aspects (interest $p = 0.038$, pleasure $p = 0.009$, engagement $p = 0.006$, orgasm $p = 0.023$, and erection $p = 0.046$). In the EVAR group, there was an increased magnitude of sexual dysfunction on all aspects also, but only one (erection $p = 0.030$) reached statistical significance (other aspects not significantly increased: interest $p = 0.071$, pleasure $p = 0.065$, engagement $p = 0.054$, and orgasm $p = 0.112$). Six weeks postoperatively, the OR group still reported a significant increase in the magnitude of sexual dysfunction on three aspects (pleasure $p = 0.031$, engagement $p = 0.010$, and orgasm $p = 0.003$; other aspects not significantly increased were interest $p = 0.168$ and

TABLE 16-4. PROPORTION OF PATIENTS REPORTING AN INCREASE IN SEXUAL DYSFUNCTION COMPARED TO THE PREOPERATIVE SITUATION

Sexual Dysfunction (aspect)	3 Weeks %		6 Weeks %		13 Weeks %		26 Weeks %		52 Weeks %	
	OR	EV	OR	EV	OR	EV	OR	EV	OR	EV
Interest	45*	44	35	20	19	26	12	24	17	35
Pleasure	41†	42	33*	29	25	22	18	26	23	24
Engagement	47†	38	40*	17	24	22	24	26	24	38
Orgasm	37*	33	35‡	16	24	13	21	14	26	27
Erection	31*	53*	22	18	17	19	20	20	22	26

*Significantly different from Pre at $p < 0.05$.

†Significantly different from Pre at $p < 0.01$.

‡Significantly different from Pre at $p < 0.005$.

Reprinted by permission from: International Society of Endovascular Specialists from *J Endovasc* Ther. 2004 Dec;11(6):613–20.

erection $p = 0.111$). The EVAR group showed no significant difference at six weeks (interest $p = 0.674$, pleasure $p = 0.855$, engagement $p = 0.773$, orgasm $p = 0.768$, and erection $p = 0.519$). From three months on, both groups had returned to their preoperative level of sexual functioning.

DISCUSSION

Few reports on the impact of OR and EVAR on sexual functioning have been published. In the available literature, most studies are retrospective in nature and focus primarily on impotence and erectile dysfunction after conventional open AAA repair.[4-5,9] To our knowledge, no randomized study has compared sexual function after OR and EVAR until now.

Although surgery did not result in a significant difference in the proportion of patients reporting sexual dysfunction between the two groups, the impact of surgery on sexual function in the OR group was greater than in the EVAR group. This effect could be demonstrated despite a higher number of internal iliac arteries being lost or sacrificed in the EVAR group, which underscores the multifactorial pathogenesis of sexual dysfunction after surgery.

The preoperative rate of sexual dysfunction on any aspect was ~70% in our study, which may appear high compared to other reports[34], but there are several possible explanations for this difference. First, we had a better rate of response to our questionnaire than some other investigators have reported.[3-4,10] The prospective study design and the willingness of participants to enroll in a randomized trial were factors in favor of compliance. In a retrospective setting, patients who already have sexual dysfunction are probably less likely to respond to a questionnaire assessing sexual functioning. This bias leads to an underestimation of the percentage of patients having sexual dysfunction.

Another explanation for the high sexual dysfunction rate in our study could be that the questionnaires were sent after randomization. The knowledge of having a potentially life-threatening disease and awaiting an operation may have had an impact on quality of life and sexual functioning. Furthermore, the incidence of sexual dysfunction increases with age and the presence of comorbidities.[11-13] Vascular disease, smoking, ischemic heart disease, hypertension, and diabetes are known to have an impact on sexual function.[10,14-15]

Xenos et al.[3] and Lee et al.[4] both performed retrospective studies by sending questionnaires to all AAA patients who underwent OR and asked them to recall their sexual function preoperatively and three months postoperatively. As shown in other studies and also in ours, the impact of the operation on the quality of life has faded three months after the procedure. As such, this seems an acceptable time frame to assess sexual functioning. Furthermore, it does not seem likely that sexual function will change or improve after three months, as also shown in our data, so the reported postoperative sexual dysfunction rate at three months appears reliable. However, as Lee et al.[4] also stated, the incidence of preoperative sexual dysfunction may be clouded by recall bias in retrospective studies. Many responders probably remember their sexual function to be better than it really was prior to the operation. Accordingly, the true prevalence of sexual dysfunction likely will be underestimated in these studies. Mulligan and Katz[16] examined libido and erectile function in elderly men and found that only 15% had sexual intercourse, mostly due to erectile failure. Also, other studies reported sexual dysfunction rates in the same range as we found in our study.[17-18]

Xenos et al.[3] compared erectile function after OR and EVAR in a retrospective study design. They found significantly decreased sexual functioning after OR and no deterioration after EVAR. In our study, no differences where found between OR and EVAR. A likely explanation for this may be that Xenos' study was not randomized. Despite the fact that baseline characteristics did not differ significantly between their groups, this retrospective study may have been flawed by bias.

A potential shortcoming of our study is that we did not record information about the opportunities for sexual activity; that is, of having a spouse or a partner, which might have had an effect on the results. Another issue may be the medication taken by patients with AAA. Apart from the vascular disorder and other risk factors, some types of medication are known to possibly impair sexual function.[19] However, the relationship to a specific type of medication can be difficult to determine because existing comorbidities affect sexual function also.

Sexual functioning would appear to be an integral part of quality of life (QoL), which the DREAM trial also assessed.[20] The preoperative QoL scores of the study group were lower on several domains of the Short Form-36 questionnaire but did not significantly differ from the scores of the age-matched general Dutch population. At the three-week interval, both trial arms reported a significantly decreased QoL, but the OR group had significantly lower scores than the EVAR group. At six weeks, both groups showed a (partial) recovery of the QoL. Three months after surgery, both trial arms had regained their preoperative level. However, as the reported sexual dysfunction in this study is high, this might indicate that sexual activity in this population does not play an important role.

Another limitation in evaluating sexual dysfunction is that there are no validated questionnaires available on the issue. The Medical Outcomes Study evaluation we have used was selected as the most appropriate from several nonvalidated questionnaires.[7] Better tools need to be developed to study sexual function after surgery.

Very few patients reported sexual dysfunction spontaneously at office visits. The high rate of preoperative sexual dysfunction makes it impossible for this study to analyze sexual dysfunction in patients who reported normal sexual function preoperatively. A much larger study would be needed to have enough power to detect differences between treatment groups. Taking into account that the preoperative rate of sexual dysfunction is > 65% in the target population and that randomized studies like these are increasingly hard to conduct, it is unlikely this type of evidence will ever be available. Nevertheless, reanalysis of the DREAM data will be performed after all the questionnaires are available up to the 24-month follow-up.

In conclusion, sexual dysfunction rates are high in this population, even at the outset. Endovascular and open elective AAA repair both have an impact on sexual functioning in the early postoperative period. After EVAR, recovery to preoperative levels is faster than after open repair, but at three months, sexual dysfunction levels are similar in both groups.

This article is based on an earlier publication: *J Endovasc Ther* 2004;11(6):613–20

APPENDIX

Centers participating in the DREAM trial:

The Netherlands: Catharina Hospital, Eindhoven: J. Buth, A.V. Tielbeek; University Hospital Groningen: E.L.G. Verhoeven, T. Prins; St. Elisabeth Hospital, Tilburg: J.F. Hamming, L.E.H. Lampmann; University Medical Center Maastricht: G.W.H. Schurink, M. de Haan; Academic Medical Center Amsterdam: R. Balm, J.A. Reekers; Maxima Medical Center, Veldhoven: M.H.M. Bender, H. Pasmans; University Medical Center Leiden: M.J.T. Visser, E. van der Linden; University Medical Center Utrecht: J.D. Blankensteijn, W.P.Th.M. Mali; Medical Center Rijnmond Zuid, Rotterdam: A.A.E.A. de Smet, D. Vroegindeweij; Rijnstate Hospital, Arnhem: S.M.M. van Sterkenburg, G.B. ten Haken; Martini Hospital, Groningen: J.H.B. Boomsma, H.R. van Dop; Medical Center Haaglanden, Westeinde, 's-Gravenhage: J.C.A. de Mol van Otterloo, T.P.W. de Rooij; Erasmus Medical Center, Rotterdam: M.R.H.M. van Sambeek, P. Pattynama; Leyenburg Hospital, 's-Gravenhage: C.M.A. Bruijninckx, H. van Overhagen; University Medical Center St. Radboud, Nijmegen: J.D. Blankensteijn, L. Schulze Kool; St. Franciscus Gasthuis, Rotterdam: A.C. van der Ham, J.J.I.M. van der Velden; Academic Medical Center VU, Amsterdam: W. Wisselink, F.C. van den Berg; Albert Schweitzer Hospital, Dordrecht: R.P. Tutein Nolthenius, T.R. Hendriksz; OLVG, Amsterdam: A.C. Vahl, C. de Vries; Meander Medical Center, Amersfoort: A.J.C. Mackaay; Bronovo Hospital, 's-Gravenhage: H.J. Smeets; Vlietland Hospital, Schiedam: L.M.C. van Dortmont; Deventer Hospital: B.H.P. Elsman; Hospital Bernhoven, Oss: T.M. Smits; Jeroen Bosch Hospital, 's-Hertogenbosch: R.M.M. van Loenhout, M.J. Rutten; Atrium Medical Center, Heerlen: J.A.W. Teijink, H.F. Odink; Oosterschelde Hospital, Goes: E.N. Yilmaz; Maxima Medical Center Eindhoven: G. den Butter.

Belgium: University Hospital Antwerpen: J. Poniewierski; University Medical Center Gent: F.E.G. Vermassen; St. Jozef Hospital, Turnhout: P. Stabel; St. Trudo Hospital, St. Truiden: F. van Elst.

REFERENCES

1. Dunn KM, Croft PR, Hackett GI. Association of sexual problems with social, psychological, and physical problems in men and women: a cross sectional population survey. *J Epidemiol Community Health*. 1999;53:144–148.

2. Morales A. Erectile dysfunction: an overview. *Clin Geriatr Med*. 2003;19:529–538.
3. Xenos ES, Stevens SL, Freeman MB, et al. Erectile function after open or endovascular abdominal aortic aneurysm repair. *Ann Vasc Surg*. 2003;17:530–538.
4. Lee ES, Kor DJ, Kuskowski MA, et al. Incidence of erectile dysfunction after open abdominal aortic aneurysm repair. *Ann Vasc Surg*. 2000;14:13–19.
5. Sabri S, Cotton LT. Sexual function following aortoiliac reconstruction. *Lancet*. 1971;2:1218–1219.
6. Prinssen M, Buskens E, Blankensteijn JD. The Dutch Randomized Endovascular Aneurysm Management (DREAM) trial. Background, design and methods. *J Cardiovasc Surg* (Torino). 2002;43:379–384.
7. Brorsson B, Ifver J, Hays RD. The Swedish Health-Related Quality of Life Survey (SWEDQUAL). *Qual Life Res*. 1993;2:33–45.
8. Chaikof EL, Fillinger MF, Matsumura JS, et al. Identifying and grading factors that modify the outcome of endovascular aortic aneurysm repair. *J Vasc Surg*. 2002;35:1061–1066.
9. Dewar ML, Blundell PE, Lidstone D, et al. Effects of abdominal aneurysmectomy, aortoiliac bypass grafting and angioplasty on male sexual potency: a prospective study. *Can J Surg*. 1985;28:154–6, 159.
10. Wandell PE, Brorsson B. Assessing sexual functioning in patients with chronic disorders by using a generic health-related quality of life questionnaire. *Qual Life Res*. 2000;9:1081–1092.
11. Bacon CG, Mittleman MA, Kawachi I, et al. Sexual function in men older than 50 years of age: results from the health professionals follow-up study. *Ann Intern Med*. 2003;139:161–168.
12. Wespes E. Erectile dysfunction in the ageing man. *Curr Opin Urol*. 2000;10:625–628.
13. Montorsi F, Briganti A, Salonia A, et al. The ageing male and erectile dysfunction. *BJU Int*. 2003;92:516–520.
14. Hsueh WA. Sexual dysfunction with aging and systemic hypertension. *Am J Cardiol*. 1988;61:18H–23H.
15. Dey J, Shepherd MD. Evaluation and treatment of erectile dysfunction in men with diabetes mellitus. *Mayo Clin Proc*. 2002;77:276–282.
16. Mulligan T, Katz PG. Erectile failure in the aged: evaluation and treatment. *J Am Geriatr* Soc. 1988;36:54–62.
17. Kinsey AC, Pomeroy WR, Martin CE. Sexual behavior in the human male. 1948. *Am J Public Health*. 2003;93:894–898.
18. Feldman HA, Goldstein I, Hatzichristou DG, et al. Impotence and its medical and psychosocial correlates: results of the Massachusetts Male Aging Study. *J Urol*. 1994;151:54–61.
19. Thomas DR. Medications and sexual function. *Clin Geriatr Med*. 2003;19:553–562.
20. Prinssen M, Buskens E, Blankensteijn JD on behalf of the DREAM trial participants. Quality of life after endovascular and open AAA repair. Results of a randomized trial. *Eur J Vasc Endovasc Surg*. 2004;27:121–127.

Debate—EVAR Gold Standard For Good Risk Patients

17

Endovascular Repair of Abdominal Aortic Aneurysms: The New Gold Standard

Rabih A. Chaer, M.D., and Michel S. Makaroun, M.D.

Elective repair of abdominal aortic aneurysms (AAA) currently represents the standard of care to avoid the sequalae of progressive expansion and rupture, which result in considerable morbidity and mortality as well as significant cost to society.[1] Standard open repair has been associated with significant morbidity and mortality, prolonged hospital stay, and perioperative complications.[2] With the advent of catheter-based technologies, the first reports of AAA stent graft repair in 1991 have set the stage for a widespread application of endovascular aneurysm repair (EVAR). Minimally invasive endovascular techniques for the treatment of AAA have significantly reduced the morbidity of this procedure compared with standard surgical repair. In addition, patients with extensive comorbid medical illnesses in whom standard operative repair is contraindicated may be successfully treated using endovascular means.

The purpose of this chapter is to review the general principles governing the use of endovascular devices for the repair of AAA, and the clinical trial results that led to the approval and marketing of the current devices, as well as to review the current evidence in support of EVAR as the new gold standard for AAA repair.

EVAR CLINICAL TRIAL OVERVIEW

After the initial success of homemade endovascular stent grafts, commercially manufactured devices were developed and are currently increasingly utilized as a minimally invasive alternative to open repair. Four have received approval from the U.S. Food and Drug Administration (FDA), the AneuRx (Medtronic, Inc., Minneapolis, MN), Excluder (W.L. Gore and Associates, Flagstaff, AZ), Zenith (Cook, Inc., Bloomington, IN), and PowerLink (Endologix, Irvine, CA). A fifth, the Ancure, was approved and marketed for three years before being withdrawn for regulatory issues. Other devices that have received approval for use in the European Union or Canada remain at the clinical trial stage in the United States.

AneuRx Trials Overview

The AneuRx graft is a modular, bifurcated, woven polyester graft supported with a nitinol exoskeleton. The graft was approved based on FDA comparisons of 1,193 patients, 1,019 of whom received the device configuration currently marketed. The AneuRx graft was associated with a significant reduction in operative blood loss, decreased transfusion requirements, decreased intensive care unit (ICU) days, earlier return of gastrointestinal function, and earlier time to discharge. Two intraoperative ruptures were reported (0.17%) and three patients suffered from postoperative aneurysm rupture. Major complications were reduced in the stent graft group when compared to the open group including reoperation, secondary procedures, and medical complications (myocardial infarction, stroke, arrhythmia, renal failure). Overall major complication rate was 23% for the standard open repair and 12% for the endograft repair group (P < .03). Kaplan-Meier analysis of the endograft group revealed a freedom from all-cause rupture of 99.5% at one year, 98.5% at two years, 98.4% at three years, and 8.4% at four years. Freedom from surgical conversion was 98.5% at one year, 96.9% at two years, 94.2% at three years, and 90.4% at four years. Overall four-year survival rate of the endovascular group was low at 62.4%, reflecting the significant comorbidities of this high risk group of patients.[3,4]

Zenith Trial Overview

The Zenith endograft is a bifurcated, modular, three-component system. It is made from woven dacron sutured to stainless steel Z-stents, with a suprarenal stent component with positive fixation at the aortic attachment site. FDA approval was based on a comparison among four groups of patients: a control group, a standard-risk (SR) group, a high-risk group, and a roll-in group. In total, 352 patients were prospectively enrolled. Eighty concurrent controls were enrolled with the intent of comparing them to the standard repair endovascular group. Three hundred and fifty-one of the 352 patients (99.7%) underwent successful implantation of the endograft. Significantly decreased cardiac (P < .02), pulmonary (P < .001), and renal (P < .01) morbidities were noted at 30 days in the endograft group. Furthermore, EVAR patients had fewer transfusion requirements, diminished blood loss, shorter hospital stay, decreased ICU stay, and quicker return to daily activities. Mortality within 30 days was 0.5% in the EVAR group and 2.5% in the open surgical control group. All-cause mortality at 12 months was 3.5% in the standard risk EVAR group and 3.8% in the control group. Kaplan-Meier analysis demonstrated no difference in all-cause mortality and aneurysm-related death between the SR EVAR group and the control group. No acute conversions occurred in the study. Three late conversions were reported: one for endoleak, one for a rapidly expanding supraceliac pseudoaneurysm, and one for rupture at 222 days postoperatively. Eleven percent of the SR endograft group required secondary interventions compared to 2.5% of the control group at 12 months. The risk of endoleak (mostly Type II) was 7.4% at 12 months and 5.4% at 24 months. Migration was not seen in any patients over 12 months. The majority of the aneurysms were smaller at one and two years. The Zenith endograft, therefore, demonstrated a reduction in morbidity, mortality, and recovery time, as well as a high rate of aneurysm shrinkage.[5]

Excluder Trials Overview

The Excluder device is a modular bifurcated two-component system made from expanded polytetrafluoroethylene (ePTFE) graft material bonded to a nitinol exoskeleton by an ePTFE/fluorinated ethylene propylene composite film. The pivotal phase II trial was a prospective nonrandomized trial that enrolled 334 patients (235 test and 99 open control patients) in 19 different centers.[6] Compared to the control group, the test group had less blood loss, shorter hospital stay, and decreased recovery time. At one- and two-year follow-up, the freedom from major complications was significantly different among the two groups (36% control group versus 67% test group, p<0.0001). There was no significant difference in survival rate over the two-year follow-up. The long term results were recently published.[7] At five years, there were 10 open conversions, most frequently for enlarging sacs without endoleak. Including reinterventions and complications of reinterventions as adverse events, there was a significant, persistent long-term reduction in major adverse events. Also reported were 0% limb narrowing, 0% trunk migration, 0% component migration, 0% fracture, endoleak in 3% (two type II/68), and aneurysm growth (>5 mm compared to baseline) in 38% (30/78) of the test group. There were no aneurysm ruptures in either test or control group. The majority of patients who experienced aneurysm sac enlargement had no demonstrable endoleak throughout the 60-month follow-up. Based on explant analysis, information gathered from surgical conversion procedures, and in vitro animal studies, transudation of serum and fibrin components through the ePTFE graft material used in this device seemed to be the predominant contributing factor to the fluid accumulation and sac enlargement. This phenomenon had led the company to release an updated version of the Excluder device in July 2004. The new device incorporates an additional low-permeability layer to reduce fluid flow across the graft material. At one year, significant aneurysm sac regression and minimal sac expansion were noted after endovascular repair of abdominal aortic aneurysms with the new device.[8]

Endologix Trials Overview

The Endologix PowerLink system is a one-piece bifurcated graft comprised of PTFE supported by nitinol. A prospective multicenter trial using this device was conducted at 15 sites. Between 2000 and 2003, 258 patients were enrolled (192 test and 66 open control patients). Mean follow-up at 36 months was available.[9] Technical success was achieved in 97.9% of patients. Patients treated with this device had significantly decreased perioperative mortality, blood loss, operative time, and ICU and hospital stay as compared to the open control group. There were no reported type I, III, or IV endoleaks at the 48 months follow-up, nor were there any ruptures, graft fabric defects, or wire fractures. Aneurysm sac regression was noted in 83% of patients. The authors concluded that the PowerLink device is safe and protects treated patients from rupture, with longer follow-up needed to determine the durability of such repairs.

RANDOMIZED TRIALS OF OPEN VERSUS ENDOVASCULAR AAA REPAIR

The DREAM Trial

This was a multicenter, randomized trial comparing open with endovascular repair in 351 patients with an abdominal aortic aneurysm of at least 5 cm in diameter, and who were considered suitable candidates for both techniques. The 30-day outcomes showed that the operative mortality rate was 4.6% in the open-repair group and significantly reduced to 1.2% in the endovascular repair group.[10] However, two years after randomization, the cumulative survival rates were 89.6% for open repair and 89.7% for endovascular repair. The cumulative rates of aneurysm-related death were 5.7% for open repair and 2.1% for endovascular repair. The advantage of endovascular repair over open repair was, therefore, entirely accounted for by events occurring in the perioperative period, with no significant difference in subsequent aneurysm-related mortality.[11]

The EVAR Trials

EVAR 1 Trial.   Between 1999 and 2003, 1,082 elective patients were randomized to receive either endovascular (n = 543) or open AAA repair (n = 539). Patients deemed fit enough for open surgical repair were recruited for the study at 41 centers in the United Kingdom. The 30-day mortality in the EVAR group was 1.7% versus 4.7% in the open repair group (odds ratio 0.35 [95% CI 0.16-0.77], p = 0.009). The intention-to-treat analysis showed that 30-day and in-hospital mortality were two-thirds lower in the EVAR group than in the open repair group, and adjustment for baseline covariates did not alter the benefit of EVAR. The authors concluded that treatment by EVAR reduced the 30-day operative mortality by two-thirds compared with open repair, but that any change in clinical practice should await durability and longer term results.[12]

EVAR 2 Trial.   The goal of this trial was to identify whether EVAR improves survival compared with no intervention in patients unfit for open repair of aortic aneurysm. Three hundred thirty-eight patients aged 60 years or older who had aneurysms of at least 5.5 cm in diameter were randomized to either EVAR (n = 166) or no intervention (n = 172). Overall, a total of 197 patients underwent aneurysm repair (47 initially assigned to no intervention). The 30-day operative mortality in the EVAR group was 9% (13 of 150, 95% CI 5-15) and the no intervention group had a rupture rate of 9.0 per 100 person years (95% CI 6.0-13.5). By end of follow-up, 142 patients had died, 42 of aneurysm-related factors. There was no significant difference between the EVAR group and the no intervention group for all-cause mortality (hazard ratio 1.21, 95% CI 0.87-1.69, p = 0.25), or for aneurysm-related mortality. The authors concluded that EVAR did not improve survival over no intervention in patients already unfit for open aneurysm repair.[13] This study has been heavily criticized for long delays prior to treatment after randomization and a significant number of crossovers with many randomized to "no treatment" actually receiving aneurysm repair with acceptable mortality and morbidity.

CONTEMPORARY PERIOPERATIVE OUTCOMES
OF OPEN REPAIR

The outcomes of open infrarenal AAA repair have certainly improved over the past several decades, and have stabilized since the early 1990s, likely secondary to improvement in anesthetic and surgical technique, and advances in perioperative care. The reported rate of morbidity and mortality is still, however, significant when compared to endovascular repair in recent series. Although the reported early postoperative mortality is less than 3% in centers of excellence, it uniformly approaches 5–6% in reports from collective series, reflecting "real world" surgical outcomes. When subsets of high-risk patients are evaluated, the 30-day mortality is even higher, and is in the order of 8–10%. Similarly, the reported morbidity of open repair varies considerably among the reported series, and ranges from 3.9% to as high as 35%. and seems to increase with age. This include respiratory (8–16.5%), major cardiac (3.1–8%), renal (2–10%), visceral (<3%), sexual (erectile dysfunction in up to 83% of patients, retrograde or absent ejaculation in 9%), and wound-related complications. Although late graft related complications are unusual, they are associated with a high mortality and include anastomotic pseudoaneurysms (1–3% proximally, 8–9% distally), graft infection (0.3–1.3%), aortoenteric fistula (0.3–1.6%), limb thrombosis (1.6–5.3%), and aneurysm formation in the residual aorta (5%).[14] These complications are, however, likely to be underreported and underdiagnosed in the community because of the less rigid follow-up regimens following open repair as compared to EVAR.

LONG TERM FOLLOW-UP

EVAR has been clearly shown to be associated with improved short-term outcomes in perioperative morbidity and mortality when compared with open surgical repair. The concern, however, was initially raised about whether these early benefits will persist in the long term because of the higher reintervention rates with EVAR. Although prosthetic aortic replacement is highly durable with a low rate of reintervention, the need for secondary procedures 30 days after open repair can be as high as 6%, and addresses wound-related complication such as abdominal wall herniation, as well as vascular complications such as pseusodoaneurysms, aortoenteric fistulae, graft limb thrombosis, and anastomotic stenoses.[14] Only a minority of these complications seem to be amenable to endovascular repair, underscoring the morbidity of these reinterventions. Alternatively, most reinterventions required following EVAR are endovascular in nature, and reported long term outcomes seem to indicate that the requirement for secondary interventions decreases with time, suggesting that the improved design of modern stent grafts is more durable. This is indeed supported by two recent EVAR series looking at long-term follow-up. At a maximum follow-up of seven years, patients who undergo EVAR utilizing a variety of grafts show lower perioperative and late aneurysm-related mortality compared with a younger and substantially healthier group of patients with aneurysms treated with open repair. The higher need for secondary procedures in the endovascular group did not seem to affect the superiority of the overall performance of EVAR in the early and late intervals.[15] Similarly, the long-term report of the Excluder trial seems to indicate that the initial advantage of EVAR persists at five years. A concern that reinterventions may result in loss of the early benefits of EVAR was not sustained. Patients followed out to five years postprocedure had persistent benefit of reduced major adverse events with EVAR compared with standard open repair of AAA, with a similar overall survival and aneurysm-related survival.[7] Moreover, a large percentage of reinterventions after EVAR have been related to an aggressive stance on treating type II endoleaks, a position that is undergoing major reassessment with current strategies recommending treatment only in the few patients who show evidence of sac enlargement in the presence of type II endoleaks.

QUALITY OF LIFE

Quality of life (QOL) analysis has been performed in several studies of EVAR versus open repair. The perceived morbidity of open repair and its prolonged recovery has been clearly documented in several trials.[16,17] Although patients treated with EVAR or open repair show significant reductions in mean scores at one week postoperative as compared to baseline in four dimensions (physical function, social function, role-physical, and vitality), the decline was more pronounced in patients having open repair.[16] EVAR patients returned to their baseline scores by the fourth postoperative week, whereas complete recovery to baseline in the conventional patients was delayed to the eighth week. These results indicate that patients treated with EVAR exhibit better physical and functional scores as early as one week after discharge, and return to baseline status significantly earlier than patients treated with open surgery.[16] This clearly confirms the perceived advantage of EVAR over conventional AAA treatment. This has also been demonstrated in a randomized study comparing the comparing the impact of EVAR and open repair on the QOL.[17] In the early postoperative period, there was a significant QOL advantage for EVAR compared to OR. Nevertheless, this advantage was not sustained at six months and beyond. The intensive surveillance of EVAR did not seem, however, to result in an impaired QOL since follow-up protocols following open repair and EVAR were the same.

CONCLUSIONS

Although the operative risk for conventional open repair of elective infrarenal AAAs has steadily declined during the past several decades, this seems to apply only to tertiary referral centers where a low mortality rate can be achieved. Nevertheless, population-based studies suggest that the mortality rate for open AAA repair continues to exceed 5% in many communities, and the rate of overall morbidity remains high, even in recent modern series. Indeed, the low operative mortality does not seem to offset a significant set of other associated complications including wound-related complications, bowel obstruction, incisional hernias, colonic ischemia, and sexual dysfunction, which might have a more significant impact in the younger age group. EVAR, on the other hand, has been associated with significant overall reductions in the operative mortality rate in statewide and national audits, and this early advantage seems to persist for several years as reported in two recent trials. As analyzed from the 2003 Medicare database, EVAR uniformly results in lower perioperative mortality when compared to open repair, and this seems to occur at all age groups, even in younger patients.[18] Similarly, analysis of the outcomes of elective admission for nonruptured AAA treated with open or endovascular repair from the New York State discharge dataset Statewide Planning and Research Cooperative System (SPARCS) indicates that EVAR was being performed in a patient population with a higher frequency of comorbidities.[19] However, EVAR was still associated with significantly lower in-hospital mortality, fewer postoperative complications, and a dramatically shorter length of stay. These results suggested that, despite the rapid diffusion of this new technique, early perioperative outcomes may be superior to those with conventional open repair in the community setting.[19] Moreover, current evidence suggests that the higher incidence of secondary interventions and related expenses does not seem to affect the initial advantage of EVAR on long-term follow-up. This, along with the clearly documented superior quality of life in EVAR patient, sets EVAR as the new gold standard for AAA repair in patients with suitable anatomy, regardless of their age or other comorbidities.

REFERENCES

1. Reilly JM, Tilson MD: Incidence and etiology of abdominal aortic aneurysms. *Surg Clin North Am.* 1989;69:705–711.
2. Hertzer NR, Mascha EJ, Karafa MT, et al. Open infrarenal abdominal aortic aneurysm repair: the Cleveland Clinic experience from 1989 to 1998. *J Vasc Surg.* 2002;35(6):1145–54.
3. Zarins CK, the AneuRx Clinical Investigators. The US AneuRx clinical trial: 6-year clinical update 2002. *J Vasc Surg.* 2003;37:904–908.
4. Zarins CK, White RA, Moll FL, et al: The AneuRx stent graft: Four-year results and worldwide experience 2000. *J Vasc Surg.* 2001;33:S135–S145.
5. Greenberg RK, Chuter TA, Sternbergh WC 3rd, Fearnot NE. Zenith Investigators. Zenith AAA endovascular graft: intermediate-term results of the US multicenter trial. *J Vasc Surg.* 2004;39(6):1209–18
6. Matsumura JS, Brewster DC, Makaroun MS, Naftel DC. A multicenter controlled clinical trial of open versus endovascular treatment of abdominal aortic aneurysm. *J Vasc Surg.* 2003;37: 262–71.
7. Peterson BG, Matsumura JS, Brewster DC, Makaroun MS. Excluder Bifurcated Endoprosthesis Investigators. Five-year report of a multicenter controlled clinical trial of open versus endovascular treatment of abdominal aortic aneurysms. *J Vasc Surg.* 2007;45(5):885–90.
8. Haider SE, Najjar SF, Cho JS, et al. Sac behavior after aneurysm treatment with the Gore Excluder low-permeability aortic endoprosthesis: 12-month comparison to the original Excluder device. *J Vasc Surg.* 2006;44(4):694–700.
9. Carpenter JP. The Powerlink bifurcated system for endovascular aortic aneurysm repair: four-year results of the US multicenter trial. *J Cardiovasc Surg* (Torino). 2006;47(3): 239–43.
10. Prinssen M, Verhoeven EL, Buth J, et al. Dutch Randomized Endovascular Aneurysm Management (DREAM)Trial Group. A randomized trial comparing conventional and endovascular repair of abdominal aortic aneurysms. *N Engl J Med.* 2004;351(16):1607–18.
11. Blankensteijn JD, de Jong SE, Prinssen M, et al. Dutch Randomized Endovascular Aneurysm Management (DREAM) Trial Group.Two-year outcomes after conventional or endovascular repair of abdominal aortic aneurysms. *N Engl J Med.* 2005;352(23):2398–405.
12. EVAR trial participants. Endovascular aneurysm repair versus open repair in patients with abdominal aortic aneurysm (EVAR trial 1): randomized controlled trial. *Lancet.* 2005; 365 (9478): 2179–86.
13. EVAR trial participants. Endovascular aneurysm repair and outcome in patients unfit for open repair of abdominal aortic aneurysm (EVAR trial 2): randomized controlled trial. *Lancet.* 2005; 365 (9478):2187–92.
14. Millon A, Branchereau, A. Results of Open Surgery for Infrarenal Abdominal Aortic Aneurysms. In: Branchereau A, Jacobs A, eds. *Open Surgery Versus Endovascular Procedures,* Oxford: Paris Consultants; 2007:149–160.
15. Cao P, Verzini F, Parlani G, et al. Clinical effect of abdominal aortic aneurysm endografting: 7-year concurrent comparison with open repair. *J Vasc Surg.* 2004;40(5):841–8.
16. Aquino RV, Jones MA, Zullo TG, et al. Quality of life assessment in patients undergoing endovascular or conventional AAA repair. *J Endovasc Ther.* 2001;8(5):521–8.
17. Prinssen M, Buskens E, Blankensteijn JD. DREAM trial participants. Quality of life endovascular and open AAA repair. Results of a randomised trial. *Eur J Vasc Endovasc Surg.* 2004;27(2):121–7.

18. Dillavou ED, Muluk SC, Makaroun MS. Improving aneurysm-related outcomes: nationwide benefits of endovascular repair. *J Vasc Surg*. 2006;43(3):446–51; discussion 451–2

19. Anderson PL, Arons RR, Moskowitz AJ, et al. A statewide experience with endovascular abdominal aortic aneurysm repair: rapid diffusion with excellent early results. *J Vasc Surg*. 2004;39(1):10–9.

18

EVAR Gold Standard for Good Risk Patients: Con

Kenneth J. Cherry, M.D.

Although EVAR is used more and more frequently, and is touted as the gold standard for treatment of abdominal aortic aneurysms, one cannot help but wonder if that is truly the case. Suprarenal fixation, fenestrated grafts, branch grafts, and growing familiarity with the technique have led to a lessening of strict anatomic criteria for success. The long-term results are not in.

There are many compelling reasons why we should not regard EVAR as the gold standard for good risk patients:

1. Results of open surgery and EVAR

Major medical centers with true expertise is aortic surgery have elective mortality rates for infrarenal abdominal aortic aneurysms of 1% to 3%. Furthermore, population-based longitudinal studies have shown that these aortic grafts hold up. In contradistinction, the early results of EVAR are promising. Midterm results are probably close to those of open repair, but the long-term results are not known. To maintain this equivalency at the midterm, multiple reinterventions are necessary. Individual studies as well as meta-analyses have shown that the rate of reintervention is much greater for EVAR patients. In the EVAR-1 Trial, reinterventions were required three times as often in patients with endovascular repair as for those who had open repair. At four years, 20% of patients had reintervention. In the DREAM Trial and a smaller trial from Canada, twice as many patients having EVAR required reintervention.

2. Quality of Life

EVAR has not delivered a better quality of life at midterm.

3. Cost

A meta-analysis of all reports between 1999 and 2005 reporting the cost or cost effectiveness for nonruptured aneurysms was performed. These were studies involving 50 patients or more. All studies found that endovascular repair cost more than conventional surgery. Midterm cost for medically fit patients was greater for endovascular repair with no differences in overall survival or quality of life.

In summary, EVAR is not the gold standard for good risk patients, but an excellent option for higher risk and older patients.

REFERENCES

1. Hiramoto JS, Reilly LM, Schneider DB, et al. Long-term outcome and re-intervention after endovascular abdominal aortic aneurysm repair using the Zenith stent graft. *J Vasc Surg.* 2007;45.3:461-466.
2. Zarins CK, Bloch DA, Crabtree T, et al. Stent graft migration after endovascular repair: importance of proximal fixation. *J Vasc Surg.* 2003;38:1254-1272.
3. Hallett JW Jr, Marshall DM, Petterson TM, et al. Graft-related complications after abdominal aortic aneurysm repair: Reassurance from a 36-year-population based experience. *J Vasc Surg.* 1997;25:277-286.
4. Lederle FA, Kane RL, MacDonald R, Wilt TJ. Systematic Review: Repair of unruptured abdominal aortic aneurysm. *Ann Inter Med.* 2007;146(10):735-741.
5. Dutch Randomized Endovascular Aneurysm Management (DREAM) Trial Group. Two-year outcomes after conventional or endovascular repair of abdominal aortic aneurysms. *N Engl J Med.* 2005;352:2398-2405.
6. DREAM Trial Participants. Quality of life endovascular and open AAA repair. Results of a randomized trial. *Eur J Vasc Endovasc Surg.* 2004;27:121-127.
7. Prinssen M, Buskens E, Nolthenius RP, et al. Sexual dysfunction after conventional and endovascular AAA repair: results of the DREAM Trial. *J Endovasc Ther.* 2004;11:613-620.
8. EVAR Trial Participants. Endovascular aneurysm repair versus open repair in patients with abdominal aortic aneurysm (EVAR trial 1): randomised controlled trial. *Lancet.* 2005;365: 2179-2186.
9. Society for Vascular Surgery Outcomes Committee. Endovascular abdominal aortic aneurysm repair: long-term outcome measures in patients at high-risk for open surgery. *J Vasc Surg.* 2006;44:229-236.
10. Jonk YC, Kane RL, Lederle FA, MacDonald R, Cutting AH, Wilt TJ. Cost-effectiveness of abdominal aortic aneurysm repair: A systematic review. *Int J Tech Assess Health Care.* 2007;23: 205-215.
11. Peterson BG, Matsumura JS, Brewster DC, Makaroun MS and Excluder Bifurcated Endoprosthesis Investigators. Five-year report of a multicenter controlled clinical trial of open versus endovascular treatment of abdominal aortic aneurysms. *J Vasc Surg.* 2007;45;5:885-890.
12. Falkensammer J, Oldenburg WA, Biebl M, et al. Abdominal aortic aneurysm neck remodeling after open aneurysm repair. *J Vasc Surg.* 2007;45;5:900-905.
13. Statius van Eps RG, Leurs LJ, Hobo R, et al. on behalf of the EUROSTAR Collaborations. Impact of renal dysfunction on operative mortality following endovascular abdominal aortic aneurysm surgery. *British J Surg.* 2006;94;2:174-175.
14. Elkouri S, Gloviczki P, Mckusick MA, et al. Perioperative complications and early outcome after endovascular and open surgical repair of abdominal aneurysms. *J Vasc Surg.* 2004; 39:497-505.
15. Franks SC, Sutton AJ, Bown MJ, Sayers RD. Systematic review and meta-analysis of 12 years of endovascular abdominal aortic aneurysm repair. *Eur J Vasc Endov Surg.* 2007;33;2: 154-171.

Minimally Invasive Techniques For Treatment of Aortic and Iliac Aneurysms

19

Totally Laparoscopic Aortic Surgery: The North American Experience

*Andrew J. Olinde, M.D., Yves-Marie Dion, M.D.,
Albert D. Sam II, M.D., James W. McNeil, M.D.,
Stephen A. Hebert, R.N., and John D. Frusha, M.D.*

During the past decade, advancements in vascular surgery have focused on the development of less invasive treatment modalities. Balloon angioplasty and stenting have radically changed the therapy of aortoiliac occlusive disease. Rupture of abdominal aortic aneurysms can be prevented by insertion of endovascular grafts. Nonetheless, a significant number of patients with diffuse arterial inflow disease require open surgical bypass for restoration of blood flow. Likewise, aortic aneurysms with short angulated necks or small iliac arteries must be repaired by way of open laparotomy. The surgical trauma of large painful midline or flank abdominal incisions is associated with bowel dysfunction and extended hospital stays.

Laparoscopy has been accepted for years in the fields of general and gynecologic surgery. In fact, the open technique has become nearly obsolete in many operative procedures. The difficulties of aortic exposure and anastomosis have prevented vascular surgeons from embracing this innovative approach. Improved instrumentation, however, has made it another viable and less invasive means of treating both occlusive and aneurysmal disease of the aorta. As reported in our earlier study, laparoscopy appears to prevent postoperative adynamic ileus, decrease pain, and shorten hospital stay.[1] The following is the experience of the United States authors (AJO, ADS, JWM, SAH, JDF) in the totally laparoscopic bypass treatment of aortoiliac occlusive disease and the Canadian author (YMD) in the exclusion of abdominal aortic aneurysms.

HISTORICAL REVIEW

Following description of laparoscopic cholecystectomy in Germany by Muhe and in France by Mouret in the mid 1980s, the general surgery community quickly adopted this "minimally" invasive form of therapy. By 1991, other surgical techniques like antireflux procedures, colectomies, common bile duct explorations, and splenectomies had become commonplace. The same year, our Canadian author (YMD) recognized the benefits of laparoscopy and applied it in the laboratory, exposing the aorta in piglets.[2] Initially, a gasless approach was attempted with an abdominal lift device. It was felt this device would allow maximal exposure of the aorta and avoid potential air embolism associated with pneumoperitoneum. However, it was demonstrated that the danger of air embolism was very low with abdominal insufflation and a significant advantage of the pneumoperitoneum was actual further enlargement of the working cavity.[3] Further investigation found that retraction of the viscera within the peritoneal cavity was very difficult and tedious, impeding adequate aortic exposure. This led to the technique whereby a "peritoneal apron" is developed by dividing the peritoneum anterior to the left colon, tacking it to the midline, and thereby separating the small bowel from the retroperitoneal working space. The first aortic bypass was performed in a pig positioned in a 90-degree right lateral decubitus position. To translate this technique to a human application, it was necessary to mobilize the animal on the operative table in order to perform the femoral anastomoses. Four years of experience in the laboratory led to the first totally laparoscopic aortobifemoral bypass in man in June 1995. Subsequently, dedicated laparoscopic vascular instruments were developed including aortic cross-clamps, intracorporeal deployable clamps, tunnelers, on-line needleholders and heavy-duty scissors to cut calcified plaque. The stage was now set for the current described technique.

PATIENT SELECTION FOR OCCLUSIVE DISEASE

In this United States series, between January 2002 and September 2005, 38 patients were selected for totally laparoscopic aortobifemoral bypass (LABF) in the treatment of severe aorto-iliac occlusive disease. These patients had diffuse inflow disease not amenable to balloon angioplasty or stenting. Preoperative evaluation included an abdominal computed tomography scan, angiography, arterial Doppler study, and a cardiac stress test. CT scans were particularly important to detect venous anomalies such as a retroaortic left renal vein, horseshoe kidney, and to evaluate the degree of aortic calcification. Exclusion criteria were concentric infrarenal aortic calcification, morbid obesity, history of left hemicolectomy, and severe medical comorbidities. The average patient age was 61.7 years with 20 males and 18 females. Indications for surgery included disabling claudication in 27 patients (71%), ischemic rest pain in 10 patients (26%), and tissue loss in one patient (3%). Thirty-three patients (86%) were active heavy smokers, 30 (79%) were hypertensive, seven (18%) were diabetic, and nine (27%) had angina or a history of myocardial infarction (Table 19–1).

SURGICAL TECHNIQUE OF LABF

The technique of laparoscopic aortic surgery follows that first described by Dion and Gracia.[4] All patients receive general anesthesia. Epidural analgesia is not necessary during or after the procedure. The anesthesia team must avoid excessive hypercapnia, which can lead to cardiac depression. The patient is positioned with the left hip ele-

TABLE 19-1. DEMOGRAPHIC DATA AND RISK FACTORS IN 38 PATIENTS.

	n	%
Mean Age (y)	61.7	n/a
Male / Female Subjects	20/18	n/a
Tobacco Use	33	86
Hypertension	30	79
Diabetes	7	18
Coronary Disease	9	27
Claudication	27	71
Rest Pain	10	26
Tissue Loss	1	3

vated 30 degrees (Figure 19–1). A 2-cm incision is made just medial and superior to the anterior superior iliac spine, splitting the oblique muscles down to the preperitoneal space. This allows the surgeon to place his index finger into the retroperitoneum and feel the frequently calcified left external iliac artery. A 12-mm trocar is inserted to provide for insufflation of the retroperitoneum with CO_2 gas and visualization of the left external iliac artery and ureter. This ensures the proper dissection plane throughout the procedure. Both femoral bifurcations are exposed if an aortofemoral bypass (not tube graft) is planned. A pneumoperitoneum is then established and followed by placement of a periumbilical 10-mm trocar. Additional 5-mm and 10-mm trocars are placed between the pubis and umbilicus and umbilicus and xyphoid, respectively. With use of a 0-degree laparoscope, the peritoneum is divided from above the left inguinal ring to the costal margin anterior to the white line of Toldt. The assistant surgeon stands on the right side of the patient, creating an "apron" by separating the peritoneum from the underlying muscle and fascia with a spatula. Two working 10-mm ports are placed in the left flank by the lead surgeon. The peritoneal apron is suspended to the midline with 2-0 Prolene Keith needles, preventing the bowel from entering the retroperitoneum. Fan retractors are inserted through two of the midline

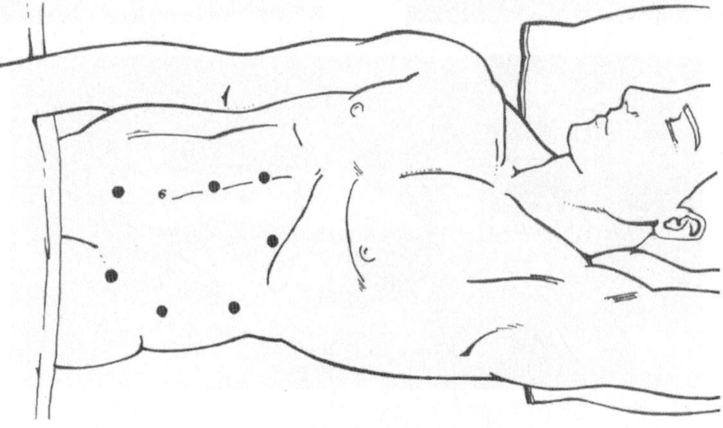

Figure 19-1. Patient positioning and trocar placement. Printed with permission from: Olinde AJ, McNeil JW, Sam A, Hebert SA, Frusha JD. Totally laparoscopic aortobifemoral. *J Vasc Surg*. 42:27–34.

trocars to retract the viscera medially, providing a working space to perform the bypass. The left kidney is left in its bed, not elevated by the fan retractors. The 30-degree laparoscope is placed into the middle left flank trocar, and the surgeon works with graspers through the two remaining flank trocars. The left ureter is identified as it crosses the psoas muscle and left in place, care taken not to lift it with the fan retractors. Just medial to the aorta lies the left gonadal vein. This landmark structure is followed from the psoas muscle to its drainage into the left renal vein. The pulsatile aorta is exposed from its bifurcation to the left renal vein. Next, the inferior mesenteric artery is clipped and divided, and posterior lumbar arteries are controlled. A seventh 10-mm trocar is placed in the subxyphoid area for insertion of the laparoscopic vascular clamp. A bifurcated dacron graft is placed through the 12-mm trocar into the abdominal cavity, and each limb is tunneled to the groins using a long Debakey aortic vascular clamp. Heparin is administered, and the infrarenal aorta is cross-clamped. The distal aorta is closed with a Multifire Endo GIA 30 3.5-mm stapler with knife removed (Auto Suture, Norwalk, Connecticut) (Figures 19–2A and 19–2B). A Powered Multifire Endo GIA 60 4.8-mm stapler with knife removed (Auto Suture) is used if the distal aorta has severe calcification. The aorta is divided with laparoscopic scissors and endarterectomized if necessary (Figure 19–2C). An end-to-end proximal aortic anastomosis is performed in a running fashion with two 18-cm 3-0 Prolene sutures attached to pledgets. This avoids the need for time-consuming intracorporeal knots at the beginning of the running sutures. The two sutures need only be tied together anteriorly, completing the anastomosis. An end-to-side aortic anastomosis can be performed to

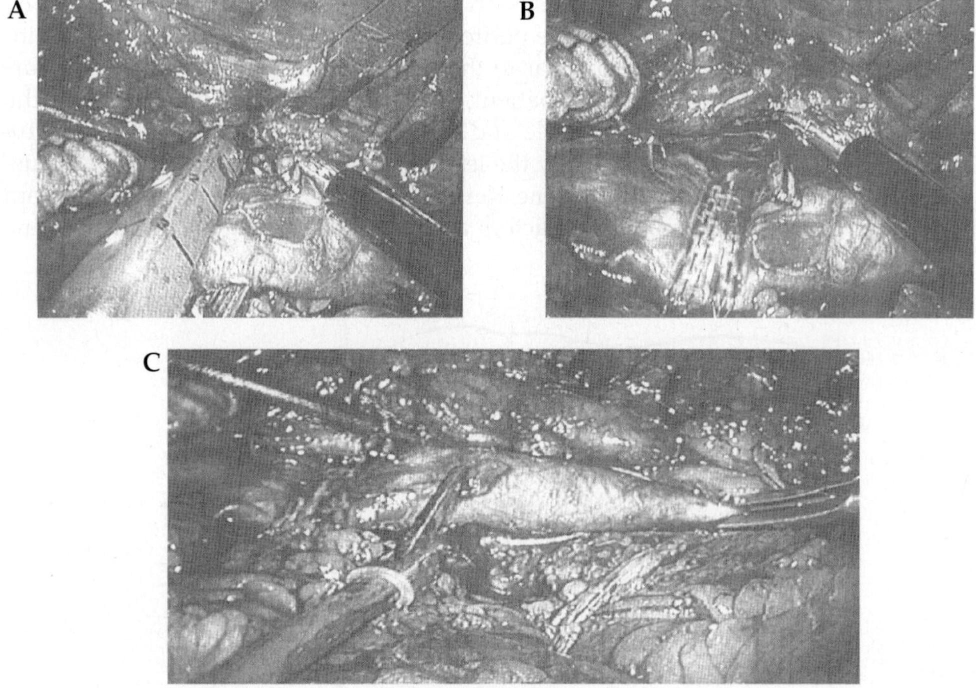

Figure 19-2. Closure of distal aorta with GIA stapler and division of aorta with laparoscopic scissors. Printed with permission from: Olinde AJ, McNeil JW, Sam A, Hebert SA, Frusha JD. Totally laparoscopic aortobifemoral. *J Vasc Surg.* 42:27–34.

preserve pelvic perfusion if there is significant bilateral external iliac artery occlusive disease. In this instance, an intracorporeal deployable vascular clamp is used to control the distal aorta instead of a GIA stapler. Likewise, deployable vascular clamps are necessary to occlude the iliac arteries when an aortic tube graft is placed to repair an abdominal aortic aneurysm. The aortic clamp is released, and the anastomosis is inspected for hemostasis. Interrupted Prolene sutures may be required with persistent bleeding. Femoral anastomoses are completed, and flow is restored to the legs. The retroperitoneum is again inspected for any bleeding, after which the sutures holding the peritoneal apron are cut, allowing the apron to cover the dacron graft. A custom-made laparoscopic Doppler probe (Parks Medical Electronics, Aloha, Oregon) is inserted through a trocar to be certain that the blood flow to the sigmoid colon is adequate. The groin and trocar sites are closed in the usual fashion.

RESULTS AND COMMENTS

Totally laparoscopic aortobifemoral bypasses were performed successfully in 33 of 38 patients. The failures included one patient with extensive adhesions, preventing creation of a peritoneal apron, and resulting in open conversion. Another patient had unexpected marked inflammation of the periaortic tissues, making laparoscopic dissection impossible and leading to laparotomy. One patient had generalized bleeding in the retroperitoneum prior to bypass and a decision was made to convert to an open procedure. The fourth unsuccessful case had a retroaortic left renal vein adherent to the aorta. We elected to make a short upper midline incision in order to free the left renal vein from the aorta and avoid catastrophic hemorrhage. The fifth patient had extreme calcification of the distal aorta and required a lower midline incision in order to close the aortic stump. By definition, the last two cases were laparoscopic-assisted aortobifemoral bypasses.

Operative time is defined as the time elapsed from the skin incision to closure of the skin. Median operative time for the LABF patients was 233 minutes (range, 179 to 365 minutes). Aortic cross-clamp time is defined as the time elapsed from placement of the proximal aortic clamp to completion of the femoral anastomoses. Median cross-clamp time was 78 minutes (range, 53 to 141 minutes) for the entire group of patients. Aortic anastomotic time is defined as the time elapsed during performance of the proximal aortic anastomosis only. Overall median aortic anastomotic time was 33 minutes (range, 14 to 56 minutes) (Table 19–2). We compared our first 20 LABF patients to a group of 18

TABLE 19-2. OPERATIVE AND POSTOPERATIVE RECOVERY TIMES (*N* = 33)

	Median	Range
Operative Time (minutes)	233	179-365
Aortic Cross-Clamp Time (minutes)	78	53-141
Aortic Anastomosis Time (minutes)	33	14-56
Intensive Care Unit Stay (days)	1	1-2
Hospital Stay (days)	4	2-24
Narcotic Infusion (days)	2	1-4
Began Liquid Diet (days)	1	1-2
Began Solid Diet (days)	3	2-7

open aortobifemoral bypass patients during the same time period in an earlier study.[1] As expected, the operative, aortic cross-clamp, and anastomotic times were longer in the laparoscopic group than the open surgical group. With experience, all times decreased in the latter part of our series, demonstrating a significant learning curve.

Median intensive care unit stay was one day (range, one to two days) and median hospital stay was four days (range, two to 24 days). None of the patients in the LABF group received epidural analgesia. Median duration of patient-controlled intravenous narcotics was two days (range, one to four days). A liquid diet was begun at a median time of one day (range, one to two days) and a solid diet commenced at three days (range, two to seven days) (Table 19–2). Nasogastric tubes were not used in LABF patients in the postoperative period. As reported in our earlier study, intensive care and hospital stays were shorter in the LABF group than patients with open aortobifemoral bypasses.[1] Additionally, both liquid and solid diets were begun earlier in the LABF group.

All totally laparoscopic aortobifemoral bypass grafts remain patent, although three patients have been lost to follow-up. One patient did require dacron patch revision of her right femoral anastomosis and deployment of a stent in the left limb of her graft six months after surgery. Both stenotic areas appeared to be secondary to intimal hyperplasia. Patency is determined by palpable femoral pulses and satisfactory ankle/arm indices during follow-up office visits. The majority of complications occurred early in our experience. There was a 2.6% mortality due to a mesenteric infarction, possibly secondary to excessive retraction. Other complications included a postoperative pelvic abscess, hydronephrosis, and two early graft limb occlusions requiring thrombectomies and revisions. One patient developed a small bowel obstruction from an incarcerated trocar site hernia, necessitating operative reduction.

Most aortobifemoral bypasses today are performed through large generous transperitoneal midline or retroperitoneal flank incisions. Although exposure is ample, open procedures are accompanied by prolonged bowel dysfunction, significant pain, and extended hospital stays. Attempts have been made to reduce the surgical trauma by limiting the length of the incision as described by Turnipseed.[5] Hybrid laparoscopic-assisted bypass grafts have also been championed by several authors using hand ports or small flank incisions.[6-8] The least invasive procedure of all is the totally laparoscopic aortobifemoral bypass. This procedure has a significant learning curve but can be mastered by vascular surgeons. The necessary intracorporeal anastomotic skills can be refined by intensive practice on a standard pelvic trainer or the newer simulator. With experience, it has been demonstrated that operative, aortic cross-clamp, and anastomotic times can all be reduced to times marginally longer than open aortobifemoral bypass. Attachment of pledgets to each suture avoids time-consuming knot-tying and decreases anastomotic time. Laparoscopy minimizes bowel dysfunction, leading to earlier resumption of liquid and solid diets. In addition, reduction in postoperative pain results in shorter intensive care and hospital stays. Ileus is reported to be decreased with the retroperitoneal approach, but it still requires the generous debilitating incision.[9] Incisional hernias have been reported to occur in 11% of patients at six months after open surgery for aortoiliac occlusive disease.[10] Laparoscopy should lower the incidence of hernias dramatically due to the small size of trocar insertion sites. Likewise, small bowel obstruction has been reported in 2.9% of patients with open abdominal aortic procedures, with 41% requiring surgical enterolysis.[11] Paradoxically, we did have one early small bowel obstruction due to an unrecognized trocar site hernia in our series. Laparoscopy may be a means to reduce the significant number of gastrointestinal complications found with open aortic surgery. Finally, the respiratory compromise associated with long painful upper midline incisions is lessened by the use of laparoscopy, as demonstrated with cholecystectomy.[12]

Our experience indicates that the laparoscopic approach does not reduce the mortality of aortic surgery. This has been described in other series of laparoscopic vascular surgery patients.[13,14] Severe comorbidities are a contraindication to aortobifemoral bypass whether performed with the open or laparoscopic technique. This subset of patients with severe cardiac, pulmonary, or renal diseases would benefit from the lower risk axillobifemoral bypass. The complication rate of LABF must be proven over time to be equivalent to open surgery before this technique can be generally recommended. Complication rates of 14.8% to 24% have been reported in recent laparoscopic vascular surgery series.[15-17] Morbidity rates should decrease with experience as demonstrated in our earlier series.

Abdominal Aortic Aneurysms

The experience with the totally laparoscopic repair of abdominal aortic aneurysms (AAA) is early and is primarily with our Canadian author (YMD).[18] From 1995 to the present, he has performed over 100 laparoscopic aortobifemoral bypasses for occlusive disease and 31 laparoscopic AAA repairs. Patients must have at least one centimeter of aortic neck and have no aneurysmal involvement of the iliac arteries. Exclusion criteria are similar to that of patients evaluated for laparoscopic bypass of aortoiliac occlusive disease. Marked angulation of the aortic neck or small iliac arteries are not exclusions for laparoscopic repair, unlike with endograft deployment. Dissection of large AAAs can be difficult, especially if there is an inflammatory component (Figure 19–3). Routine clipping of the inferior mesenteric artery, lumbar arteries, and the middle sacral artery ensure a shorter clamping time and minimal back-bleeding when the aneurysm is opened (Figure 19–4). Intracorporeal deployable vascular clamps are used

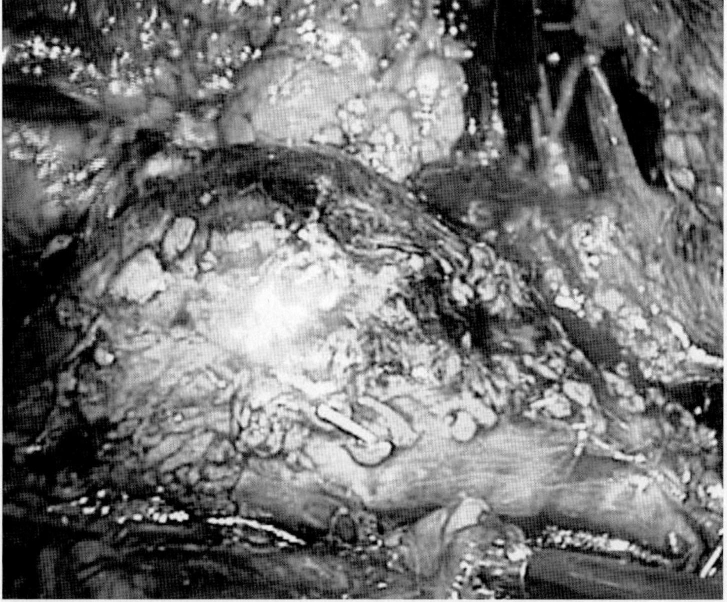

Figure 19-3. Completed laparoscopic dissection of abdominal aortic aneurysm.

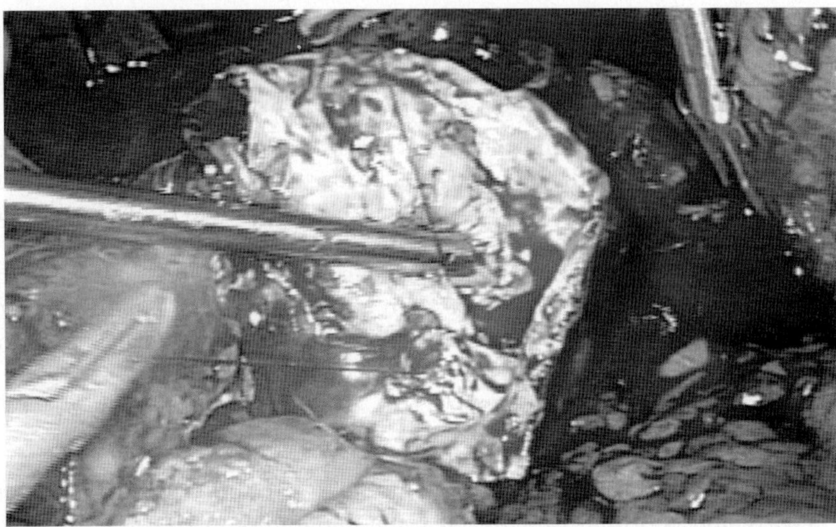

Figure 19-4. Aortic neck clamped and aneurysm opened. A lumbar artery orifice is closed with polypropylene suture.

to control the iliac arteries without occupying trocar sites. Because of concern with clamping time, it is not presently recommended to perform more than two intra-abdominal anastomoses. AAAs are best repaired laparoscopically with tube grafts, not aortobiiliac bypasses (Figure 19–5). If the procedure appears difficult, one should not hesitate to convert to an assisted technique or a laparotomy.

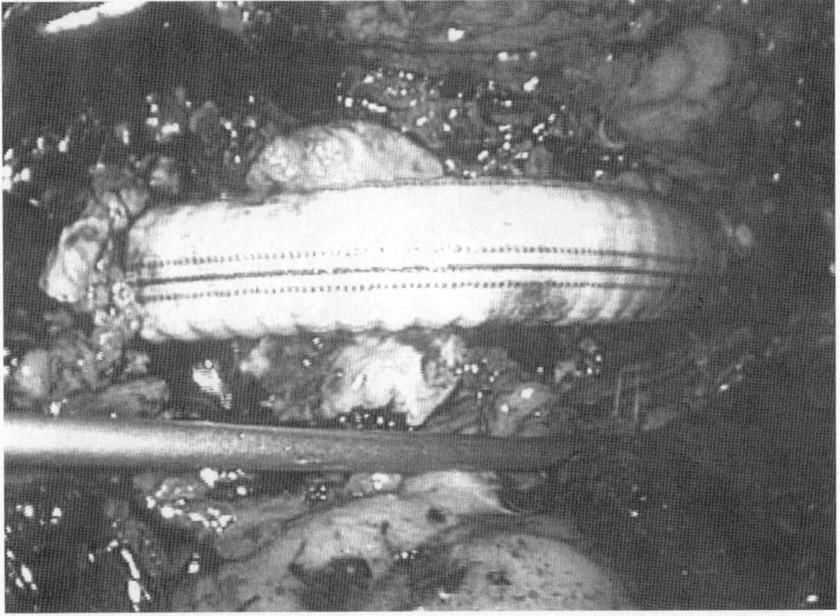

Figure 19-5. Abdominal aortic aneurysm repaired totally laparoscopic with tube graft.

THE FUTURE

Laparoscopy is a less invasive approach in the treatment of occlusive and aneurysmal disease of the aorta. Vascular surgeons can master the techniques of exposure and anastomosis, although it requires extensive practice on a pelvic trainer or simulator. It may be beneficial to form a surgical team with the assistance of a physician with substantial laparoscopic experience or one with a postgraduate fellowship in advanced laparoscopy. Attendance at a course in laparoscopic vascular surgery is highly recommended. A proctor also may be helpful in the initiation of a laparoscopic vascular surgery program. Development of an automated aortic stapling instrument could replace the difficult handsewn anastomosis and enable most vascular surgeons to perform LABF. Robotics also may allow surgeons to more safely and securely perform the intracorporeal anastomosis.[17,19] These technologic advances may allow laparoscopy to become part of the vascular surgeon's armamentarium in the treatment of abdominal aortic aneurysms and occlusive disease.

REFERENCES

1. Olinde AJ, McNeil JW, Sam A II, et al. Totally laparoscopic aortobifemoral bypass: A review of 22 cases. *J Vasc Surg.* 2005;42(1):27–34.
2. Dion YM, Chin AK, Thompson A. Experimental laparoscopic aortobifemoral bypass. *Surg Endosc.* 1995;9(8):894–897.
3. Dion YM, Levesque C, Doillon CJ. Experimental carbon dioxide pulmonary embolization after vena cava laceration under pneumoperitoneum. *Surg Endosc.* 1995;9(10):1065–1069.
4. Dion YM, Gracia CR. A new technique for laparoscopic aortobifemoral grafting in occlusive aortoiliac disease. *J Vasc Surg.* 1997;26(4):685–692.
5. Turnipseed WD. A less invasive minilaparotomy technique for repair of aortic aneurysm and occlusive disease. *J Vasc Surg.* 2001;33:431–434.
6. Kolvenbach R, Da Silva L, Deling O, et al. Video-assisted aortic surgery. *J Am Coll Surg.* 2000;190:451–457.
7. Arous ES, Nelson PR, Yood SM, et al. Hand-assisted laparoscopic aortobifemoral bypass grafting. *J Vasc Surg.* 2000;31:1142–1148.
8. Alimi YS, DeCaridi G, Hartung, et al. Laparoscopy-assisted reconstruction to treat severe aortoiliac occlusive disease: Early and mid term results. *J Vasc Surg.* 2004;39:777–783.
9. Sicard GA, Reilly JM, Rubin BG, et al. Transabdominal versus retroperitoneal incision for abdominal aortic surgery: report of a prospective randomized trial. *J Vasc Surg.* 1995;21(2):174–181.
10. Raffeto JD, Cheung Y, Fisher JB, et al. Incision and abdominal wall hernias in patients with aneurysm or occlusive aortic disease. *J Vasc Surg.* 2003;37:1150–1154.
11. Siporin K, Hiatt JR, Treiman RL. Small bowel obstruction after abdominal aortic surgery. *Am Surg.* 1993;59(12):846–849.
12. Frazee RC, Roberts JW, Okeson GC, et al. Open versus laparoscopic cholecystectomy. A comparison of postoperative pulmonary function. *Ann Surg.* 1991;213(6):651–654.
13. Goeau-Brissonniere O. What is the future for laparoscopic aortic surgery? *Ann Vasc Surg.* 2004;8(4):393–394.
14. Edoga JK, Asgarian K, Singh D, et al. Laparoscopic surgery for abdominal aortic aneurysms. Technical elements of the procedure and a preliminary report for the first 22 patients. *Surg Endosc.* 1998;12(8):1064–1072.
15. Coggia M, Javerliat I, DiCenta J, et al. Total laparoscopic bypass for aortoiliac occlusive lesions: 93-case experience. *J Vasc Surg.* 2004;40(5):899–906.

16. Remy PH, Deprez AF, D'hont CH, et al. Total laparoscopic aortobifemoral bypass. *Eur J Vasc Endovasc Surg.* 2005;29:22–27.
17. Kolvenbach R, Schwierz E, Wasilljew S, et al. Total laparoscopically and robotically assisted aortic aneurysm surgery: a critical evaluation. *J Vasc Surg.* 2004;39:771–776.
18. Dion YM, Gracia C, Ben El Kadi H. Totally laparoscopic abdominal aortic aneurym repair. *J Vasc Surg.* 2001;33:181–185.
19. Wisselink W, Cuesta MA, Gracia C, et al. Robot-assisted laparoscopic aortobifemoral bypass for aortoiliac occlusive disease: a report of two cases. *J Vasc Surg.* 2002;36:1079–1082.

20

Endovascular Management of Isolated Iliac Artery Aneurysms

Graham W. Long, M.D., F.A.C.S.
Charles J. Shanley, M.D., F.A.C.S.

Isolated iliac artery aneurysms are extremely rare, occasionally catastrophic, and potentially lethal clinical entities. The deep pelvic location of these aneurysms makes detection on routine physical examination or the development of local compressive symptoms unlikely until the aneurysms have reached considerable size. These factors help explain why the vast majority of isolated iliac artery aneurysms are detected incidentally on radiographic studies performed for other indications, as well as the high incidence of symptomatic and ruptured aneurysms in reported clinical series.[1] Challenging pelvic anatomical and technical considerations also contribute to increases in reported morbidity and mortality for open surgical repair of isolated iliac artery aneurysms, especially when compared to aortoiliac aneurysm disease.[2,3] Considered together, these observations make endovascular strategies particularly attractive for isolated iliac artery aneurysms. Not surprisingly, recent series from a number of experienced centers recommend endovascular repair as a safe and effective alternative to open repair in appropriately selected patients.[4-7] Moreover, the low prevalence of isolated iliac artery aneurysms in the context of rapidly evolving endovascular technologies make large scale prospective, randomized trials comparing endovascular to conventional open repair extremely unlikely in the modern era. For this reason, it is likely that vascular specialists caring for patients with isolated iliac artery aneurysm will continue to make treatment recommendations based on sound clinical judgment honed by experience and iteratively refined over time through careful study of an evolving literature.

EPIDEMIOLOGY

Isolated iliac artery aneurysms are extremely rare. Population-based studies suggest that their prevalence may be as low as 0.03% based on autopsy findings.[8] The common iliac artery is involved nearly three times as frequently as the internal iliac artery, and the external iliac artery is almost always spared in patients presenting with isolated iliac artery aneurysm. Multiple and bilateral aneurysms are not uncommon.[3,9,10]

In contradistinction, iliac artery aneurysms are frequently observed in patients with abdominal aortic aneurysm (up to 20%) and the clinical risk factors (i.e., male gender, hypertension, advanced age, systemic atherosclerosis, and so on) are essentially identical; therefore, it is incumbent on the vascular specialist to maintain a high index of suspicion if diagnostic and therapeutic delays are to be avoided.[3,10-13] Less frequent etiologies include systemic bacteremia (mycotic), history of pelvic trauma, pregnancy, and connective tissue disorders (i.e., cystic medial necrosis, Takayasu arteritis, Kawasaki disease, Marfan's disease, Ehlers-Danlos syndrome, and others).

NATURAL HISTORY

The presentation of isolated iliac artery aneurysms is highly variable. Delay in diagnosis is the most important factor contributing to the historically high reported incidence of symptomatic and ruptured aneurysms, and undoubtedly contributed to the attendant increases in operative morbidity and mortality.[1,14,15] Most patients with isolated iliac artery aneurysms are asymptomatic and come to the attention of the vascular specialist only as a result of detection on radiographic studies performed for other indications. In symptomatic patients, the deep pelvic location of these aneurysms contributes to nonspecific and insidious clinical signs and symptoms secondary to local compression of adjacent pelvic structures, or to continued occult expansion ultimately leading to catastrophic rupture. While most patients are asymptomatic, patients with larger aneurysms often describe a history of vague hypogastric, flank, or groin pain. Expansion can also result in a variety of local compressive signs and symptoms including hydronephrosis or hematuria (ureteral obstruction), large bowel obstruction, limb swelling due to iliac vein compression or thrombosis, and a variety of neurogenic symptoms due to peripheral nerve compression including pain, paresthesias, and lower extremity neurologic deficits.

As is the case with aortoiliac aneurysm disease, as aneurysm size increases, the associated risk of rupture and the attendant morbidity and mortality also increase. For this reason, all good-risk patients with clearly documented iliac artery aneurysms should be considered for repair. Prospective evidence is lacking to recommend a specific diameter threshold above which repair of isolated iliac artery aneurysm is clearly indicated. The current consensus is that aneurysms greater than 3.0 to 3.5 cm in maximal diameter should be considered for elective repair in otherwise good-risk patients and in all patients with local compressive symptoms.[16] The advent of safe and effective endovascular strategies may support a more aggressive approach to these aneurysms in the future.

DIAGNOSTIC EVALUATION

The vast majority of iliac artery aneurysms are discovered incidentally on routine imaging for other conditions. Physical examination is notoriously unreliable owing to the deep pelvic location of these aneurysms, but occasionally a large aneurysm can be palpated in the hypogastrium or on careful rectal or vaginal examination. Plain abdominal radiography demonstrating the "eggshell" calcification of the aortic wall as classically described for abdominal aortic aneurysm is noted only occasionally.

Color-flow duplex ultrasound of the abdomen and pelvis is an inexpensive, noninvasive, and painless screening tool in patients with suspected aortoiliac aneurysm disease. Ultrasound has the obvious advantage of avoiding ionizing radiation with the attendant disadvantages of being highly user-dependent and of limited utility in the morbidly obese and patients with excessive bowel gas. The latter limitations are particularly relevant with respect to isolated iliac artery aneurysms located deep in the pelvis, and it is incumbent on the vascular specialist to consider these limitations in any recommendations.

Computed tomography remains the gold standard for characterization of aortoiliac aneurysms, and is particularly important for accurate determination of aneurysm size, extent, vascular calcification, and local visceral, vascular, or neural compression. The addition of contrast angiography (CTA) to computed tomography has markedly facilitated treatment planning for endovascular aneurysm repair. The authors employ a standardized protocol for CTA to include 3 mm axial slice thickness and postprocessing for three-dimensional reconstruction. The principles of image analysis for endovascular treatment planning are identical to those employed for aortoiliac aneurysms. Detailed axial and 3-D images are especially helpful when there is considerable tortuosity involving the aorta and iliac vessels, and to assess the caliber and constitution of the access vessels as well as the proximal and distal landing zones in the aneurysmal artery. Meticulous procedural planning to anticipate contingencies facilitates choice of the most appropriate endograft.

Drawbacks to CTA for treatment planning (and longitudinal follow-up) include the potential for nephrotoxic and allergic reactions to the intravenous contrast and the use of ionizing radiation. The latter is particularly important for CTA as it has been estimated that each scan carries with it the equivalent radiation dose of approximately 1,000 chest radiographs. The implications over the lifetime of a young patient are undoubtedly significant and should be discussed preoperatively.[17]

Magnetic resonance imaging (MRI) and angiography (MRA) are suitable substitutes for CTA. Initially, these modalities were advocated as an alternative to CTA in patients with chronic renal insufficiency, but the recent discovery of gadolinium-induced nephrogenic systemic fibrosis has all but removed this from the diagnostic and planning armamentarium for this group. Furthermore, it is recommended that patients with implanted pacemakers, defibrillators, orthopaedic prosthetics, and even certain endografts not undergo MRI studies, factors that constitute significant limitations in this elderly patient population.

TREATMENT STRATEGIES

Endovascular approaches to isolated iliac artery aneurysm vary with the site of the aneurysm. Isolated aneurysms involving the common iliac artery with appropriate proximal (>10 mm) and distal (>20 mm) landing zones can be safely treated using an appropriately sized covered stent or stent-graft (Figure 20–1). In patients with an inadequate proximal landing zone, or for patients with bilateral common iliac artery aneurysm, a bifurcated aortoiliac endograft is required (Figure 20–2). Interestingly,

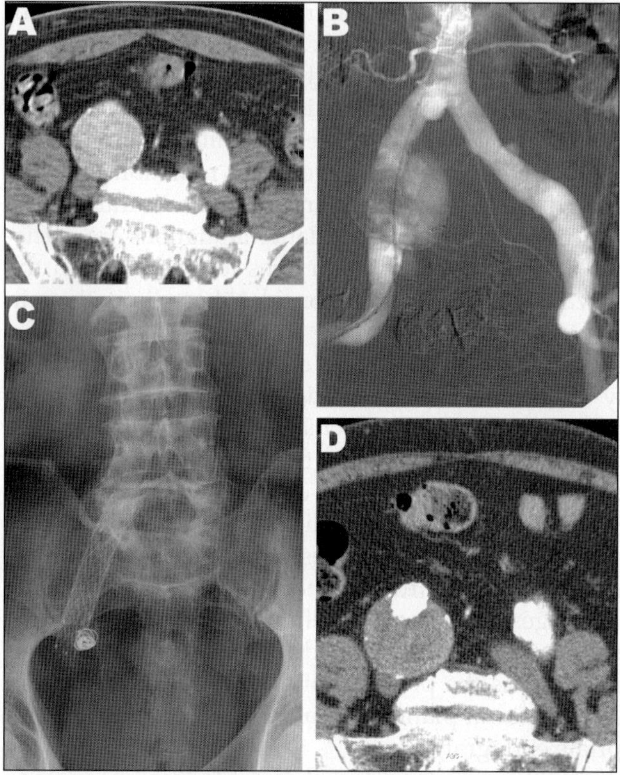

Figure 20-1. (A) Preoperative computed tomographic image of a 4.7cm diameter right common iliac artery aneurysm. **(B)** Digital subtraction angiogram demonstrating aneurysm with 2cm proximal neck and right hypogastric artery embolization coils. **(C)** Plain abdominal radiograph after placement of endografts from the proximal right common iliac artery into the external iliac artery. **(D)** Thirty-six month postoperative computed tomographic image demonstrating 4.3cm aneurysm sac without endoleak.

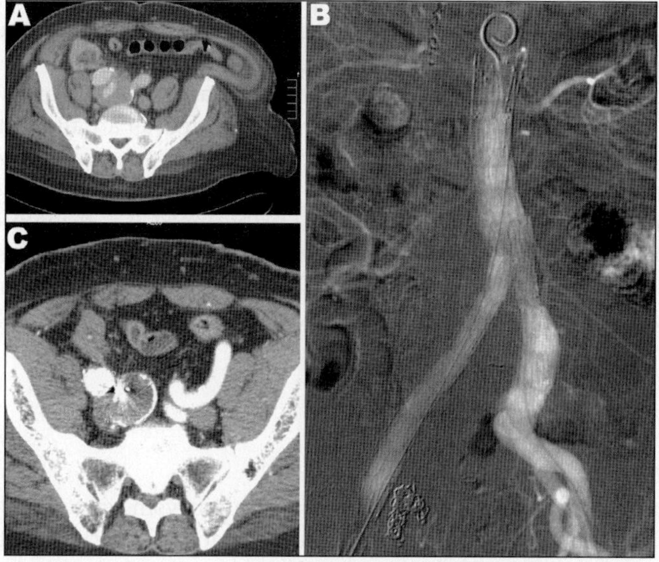

Figure 20-2. (A) Computed tomographic image of a 5.6cm right common iliac artery aneurysm involving the aortic and iliac bifurcations. **(B)** Completion digital subtraction angiogram after placement of a bifurcated aortic endograft and right hypogastric artery embolization coils. **(C)** Twenty-seven month postoperative computed tomographic image demonstrates 3.7cm residual aneurysm sac and embolization coil artifact.

TABLE 20-1. CLASSIFICATION OF TREATMENT STRATEGIES FOR ISOLATED ILIAC ARTERY ANEURYSMS PROPOSED BY FAHRNI ET AL.

Location: type	Neck Characteristics	Treatment Strategy
Common iliac artery: Ia	Adequate proximal neck	Common to external iliac endograft Internal iliac coil embolization
Common iliac artery: Ib	Inadequate proximal neck	Bifurcated aortoiliac endograft Internal iliac coil embolization
Internal iliac artery: IIa	Inadequate proximal neck	Common to external iliac endograft Internal iliac coil embolization of anterior and posterior divisions and main trunk
Internal iliac artery: IIb	Adequate proximal neck	Coil embolization of internal iliac neck, sac, anterior and posterior divisions No endograft required

Saratzis et al.[18] report promising results on mid-term follow-up of seven patients using a commercially available endograft limb containing a bare proximal stent extending into the aortic bifurcation for use in patients with common iliac neck lengths less than 10 mm. In patients with an inadequate distal landing zone, the endograft limb should be extended approximately 20 to 25 mm into the proximal external iliac artery.

Endovascular management of the internal iliac artery is based, in part, on the presence or absence of aneurysmal changes involving the common iliac bifurcation. A classification system of isolated iliac artery aneurysms and treatment strategies for each type, based on aneurysm location and neck characteristics, has been proposed by Fahrni (Table 20–1).[6]

If the common iliac artery bifurcation is not aneurysmal, then it may be reasonable to simply extend the endograft limb into the external iliac artery, covering the internal iliac artery ostium. If the common iliac artery bifurcation is aneurysmal and the internal iliac artery is normal, then endovascular placement of embolization coils to occlude the main trunk of the internal iliac artery is recommended from either an ipsilateral or contralateral femoral approach. In these cases, an effort is made to prevent placement of embolization coils into the anterior and posterior divisions, as this increases the incidence of ipsilateral buttock claudication. An alternative to coil placement in the main trunk is placement of a proprietary endovascular plug. Placement of a single endovascular plug may provide a modest economic advantage over the use of embolization coils.[19,20] If the hypogastric artery is aneurysmal and requires treatment, the anterior and posterior divisions are intentionally occluded with endovascular coils along with the aneurysm sac. In selected cases of isolated internal artery aneurysm with a proximal neck of at least 10 to 15 mm, thrombosis is achieved by placement of coils into the anterior and posterior divisions, aneurysm sac, and the proximal neck without placement of an endograft. This approach is often reserved for patients too ill for open repair or those with a hostile abdomen, since buttock claudication may result and can be disabling. This is also true for patients with bilateral common or internal iliac artery aneurysms for whom an endovascular approach is chosen. In the latter scenario, internal iliac artery embolization is often staged to allow collateral development and to decrease the incidence of pelvic ischemic complications, as well as to limit contrast-induced nephropathy.

During endovascular procedures in general, and procedures necessitating internal iliac artery occlusion in particular, preservation of common and profunda femoris ar-

TABLE 20-2. ISOLATED ILIAC ARTERY ANEURYSM: CONTEMPORARY ENDOVASCULAR RESULTS

Series	Boules et al.	Pitoulias et al.	Chaer et al.
Number of patients (aneurysms)	45 (61)	32 (33)	52 (52)
Mean follow-up (months)	22	35±21	17±2
Age (mean ± SD)	75±9	64±8	73±2
Male gender (%)	42 (93)	30 (94)	47 (90)
Aneurysm diameter, cm (mean ± SD)	4.2 +1.7	4.5+1.6	4.3-0.1
Technical success	100%	100%	100%
Hospital length of stay (mean, days)	1.3±1.0	2.1±0.6	1.3±1.0
Need for transfusion	–	0	3/52 (6%)
30-day morbidity	2/45 (4%)	6/32 (19%)	8/52 (15%)
30-day mortality	0	0	1/52 (2%)
Primary patency (24 months)	43/45 (95%)	32/33 (97%)	42/52 (81%)
Endoleak	9/33 (27%)	0	3.52 (6%)
Internal Iliac embolization	39/45 (87%)	13/33 (39%)	45/52 (86%)
Buttock claudication	9/39 (23%)	4/13 (30%)	34/52 (65%)

terial side branches during surgical exposure is particularly important to assist in maintaining pelvic collateral flow. Other options include reimplantation or bypass of the internal iliac artery using the external iliac artery as inflow source in order to maintain antegrade flow into the internal iliac artery.[21]

There are a number of recent reports comparing institutional experiences with open and endovascular repair of isolated iliac artery aneurysms (Table 20–2).[4,22,23] In general, the results for elective endovascular repair of isolated iliac artery aneurysm parallel those observed for endovascular aortoiliac aneurysm repair. Operative and 30-day mortality rates were low and similar for open and endovascular repair of nonruptured iliac artery aneurysms. Not unexpectedly, operative time, transfusion, and postoperative length of stay were significantly less in patients undergoing endovascular repair. Mid-term graft patency and freedom from secondary intervention were excellent in both groups.

Endograft thrombosis, endoleak, kinking, and migration were uncommon following endovascular repair, and graft-related complications were managed using standard endovascular principles and techniques. Coil embolization of the internal iliac arteries was associated with a variable incidence of buttock claudication that in the vast majority of cases was short lived. Colon ischemia was extremely rare. There were few cases of subsequent aneurysm sac expansion or late rupture following endovascular repair. Few cases of endovascular repair of ruptured iliac artery aneurysms were reported, and those reported cases undoubtedly reflect a selection bias. Nevertheless, consistent with recent reports for ruptured aortoiliac aneurysm, endovascular repair in selected patients appears to have a lower reported mortality rate.[24] It is noteworthy that the aneurysm sac appears to remain stable on midterm follow-up in a significant number of patients undergoing endovascular repair for isolated iliac artery aneurysm. Therefore, patients presenting with significant local compressive symptoms (i.e., limb swelling from venous outflow obstruction, hydronephrosis, or nerve compression) should probably not be treated with endovascular repair.

Finally, the available literature clearly supports occlusion of the internal iliac artery in most patients undergoing endovascular repair of isolated iliac artery aneurysm. Recently developed side branch technology is a potential strategy to maintain antegrade perfusion of the ipsilateral internal iliac artery in anatomically appropriate patients. This approach has the putative advantage of preventing buttock claudication and decreasing the risk of colon ischemia. Serracino-Inglott et al. describe eight patients undergoing repair of aortoiliac of isolated iliac artery aneurysms.[25] These were technically successful in all eight patients and reported no endoleaks, no deaths, or no major complications. Median follow-up was six months. A single occlusion of a side branch device was observed in a patient with an internal iliac artery aneurysm. There were no episodes of colonic ischemia, new onset claudication, or erectile dysfunction. Malina et al. described the implantation of a branched endovascular graft that preserved antegrade hypogastric flow in nine of 10 patients treated.[26] One occlusion of the external iliac artery occurred six months postoperatively in this series, and one death occurred 13 days postoperatively from myocardial infarction. Three graft-related endoleaks were treated with implantation of adjunctive stent-grafts (two intraoperative and one late). This promising side-branch technology is not yet available in the United States, but it is available in Canada, Europe, and Australia.

In the modern era, continued evolution and improvement in endovascular technologies have forever changed the management algorithm for isolated iliac artery aneurysm. Nevertheless, it is important to emphasize that open surgical repair by a competent vascular surgeon remains a safe, effective, and in most cases, permanent treatment option for this disease. Moreover, the indications, techniques, and outcomes for endovascular therapy will continue to evolve in the context of a growing body of evidence. In the current state of the art, it is incumbent on the vascular specialist to discuss the inherent uncertainties in addition to the putative benefits of endovascular therapy for isolated iliac artery aneurysm.

SUMMARY

Isolated iliac artery aneurysms are extremely rare. The majority is detected incidentally on radiographic studies performed for other indications. Challenging pelvic anatomical and technical considerations contribute to increases in morbidity and mortality for open surgical repair of isolated iliac artery aneurysms. While open surgical repair has clearly stood the test of time and is an entirely appropriate treatment approach in these patients, the weight of the current evidence suggests that endovascular repair is a safe, effective, and durable alternative in anatomically appropriate patients.

REFERENCES

1. Krupski WC, Selzman CH, Floridia R et al. Contemporary management of isolated iliac aneurysms. *J Vasc Surg.* 1998;28(1):1–11; discussion 11–13.
2. Plate G, Hollier LA, O'Brien P et al. Recurrent aneurysms and late vascular complications following repair of abdominal aortic aneurysms. *Arch Surg.* 1985;120(5):590–594.
3. Richardson JW, Greenfield LJ. Natural history and management of iliac aneurysms. *J Vasc Surg.* 1988;8(2):165–171.
4. Boules TN, Selzer F, Stanziale SF et al. Endovascular management of isolated iliac artery aneurysms. *J Vasc Surg.* 2006;44(1):29–37.

5. Caronno R, Piffaretti G, Tozzi M et al. Endovascular treatment of isolated iliac artery aneurysms. *Ann Vasc Surg.* 2006;20(4):496–501.

6. Fahrni M, Lachat MM, Wildermuth S et al. Endovascular therapeutic options for isolated iliac aneurysms with a working classification. *Cardiovasc Intervent Radiol.* 2003;26(5): 443–447.

7. Tielliu IF, Verhoeven EL, Zeebregts CJ et al. Endovascular treatment of iliac artery aneurysms with a tubular stent-graft: mid-term results. *J Vasc Surg.* 2006;43(3):440–445.

8. Brunkwall J, Hauksson H, Bengtsson H et al. Solitary aneurysms of the iliac arterial system: an estimate of their frequency of occurrence. *J Vasc Surg.* 1989;10(4):381–384.

9. Levi N, Schroeder TV. Isolated iliac artery aneurysms. *Eur J Vasc Endovasc Surg.* 1998;16(4): 342–344.

10. McCready RA, Pairolero PC, Gilmore JC et al. Isolated iliac artery aneurysms. *Surgery.* 1983;93(5):688–693.

11. Brunkwall J, Bergentz SE. Solitary iliac aneurysms. In: Yao JST and Pearce WH, eds. *Aneurysms: new findings and treatments.* Norwalk; Connecticut: Appleton & Lange; 1994:459.

12. Lawrence PF, Lorenzo-Rivero S, Lyon JL. The incidence of iliac, femoral, and popliteal artery aneurysms in hospitalized patients. *J Vasc Surg.* 1995;22(4):409–15; discussion 415–416.

13. Lowry SF, Kraft RO. Isolated aneurysms of the iliac artery. *Arch Surg.* 1978;113(11): 1289–1293.

14. Casana R, Nano G, Dalainas I et al. Midterm experience with the endovascular treatment of isolated iliac aneurysms. *Int Angiol.* 2003;22(1):32–35.

15. Katz DJ, Stanley JC, Zelenock GB. Operative mortality rates for intact and ruptured abdominal aortic aneurysms in Michigan: an eleven-year statewide experience. *J Vasc Surg.* 1994;19(5):804–15; discussion 816–817.

16. Kasirajan V, Hertzer NR, Beven EG et al. Management of isolated common iliac artery aneurysms. *Cardiovasc Surg.* 1998;6(2):171–177.

17. Einstein AJ, Henzlova MJ, Rajagopalan S. Estimating risk of cancer associated with radiation exposure from 64-slice computed tomography coronary angiography. *JAMA.* 2007; 298(3):317–323.

18. Saratzis N, Melas N, Saratzis A et al. EndoFit stent-graft repair of isolated common iliac artery aneurysms with short necks. *J Endovasc Ther.* 2006;13(5):667–671.

19. Ha CD, Calcagno D. Amplatzer Vascular Plug to occlude the internal iliac arteries in patients undergoing aortoiliac aneurysm repair. *J Vasc Surg.* 2005;42(6):1058–1062.

20. Resnick SA, Eskandari MK. Outcomes of Amplatzer Vascular Plugs for Occlusion of Internal Iliacs during Aortoiliac Aneurysm Stent Grafting. *Ann Vasc Surg.* 2008;22(5): 613–617.

21. Lee WA, Nelson PR, Berceli SA et al. Outcome after hypogastric artery bypass and embolization during endovascular aneurysm repair. *J Vasc Surg.* 2006;44(6):1162–8; discussion 1168–1169.

22. Chaer RA, Barbato JE, Lin SC et al. Isolated iliac artery aneurysms: a contemporary comparison of endovascular and open repair. *J Vasc Surg.* 2008;47(4):708–713.

23. Pitoulias GA, Donas KP, Schulte S et al. Isolated iliac artery aneurysms: endovascular versus open elective repair. *J Vasc Surg.* 2007;46(4):648–654.

24. Dix FP, Titi M, Al-Khaffaf H. The isolated internal iliac artery aneurysm—a review. *Eur J Vasc Endovasc Surg.* 2005;30(2):119–129.

25. Serracino-Inglott F, Bray AE, Myers P. Endovascular abdominal aortic aneurysm repair in patients with common iliac artery aneurysms—Initial experience with the Zenith bifurcated iliac side branch device. *J Vasc Surg.* 2007;46(2):211–217.

26. Malina M, Dirven M, Sonesson B et al. Feasibility of a branched stent-graft in common iliac artery aneurysms. *J Endovasc Ther.* 2006;13(4):496–500.

21

Selection and Choice of Endovascular Grafts for Abdominal Aortic Aneurysm

Richard M. Green, M.D.

The decision to recommend endovascular aneurysm repair (EVAR) and then to choose a specific device is critical to the individual patient, the surgeon, and the evolution of endovascular care. Fortunately there are over ten years of data that make this choice easier with the knowledge that the treatment will be effective and durable. The annual number of EVAR procedures has increased 600% since 2000, a reflection of the efficacy of this technology. EVAR, once under attack[1-3] is likely the main reason that the annual number of deaths in the United States from abdominal aortic aneurysms has significantly decreased.[4]

ASSESSING THE RISK OF CONVENTIONAL TREATMENT

It is still reasonable to take the position that conventional repair is the most reliable method of managing AAA particularly in young patients. I don't share that view and recommend open surgical repair only to those patients who request it and those with anatomic contraindications to EVAR. It is essential that the surgeon know his/her results with both types of repair as it is inappropriate to quote a mortality rate from a center of excellence that does not reflect a personal experience. It is also necessary to factor into the risk equation the medical status of the patient. I believe that when all these factors are taken into consideration EVAR becomes even more attractive as surgeons tend to underestimate the risks of open repair.

In 1992, the Society for Vascular Surgery/International Society for Cardiovascular Surgery defined age, cardiac function, pulmonary function, and renal function as the predictors of medical risk for elective aneurysm repair.[5] Other factors are now known to affect mortality rates, namely the experience of the surgeon and the hospital. Dardik et al. reviewed all patients undergoing elective aneurysm repair in the state of Maryland between 1990 and 1995.[6] There were 2,335 operations performed by 219 surgeons in 46 hospitals and the in-hospital overall mortality rate was 3.5%. A multivariate analysis of these data showed that patient age (0.0002), low hospital volume (0.039), and very low volume surgeons (0.01) were independent variables of mortality. Specifically, patients older than 80 years had a mortality rate of 7.3% after aneurysm repair as compared to a rate of 2.2% for patients less than 65 years. Furthermore, the mortality rates for hospitals with high volumes (>50 during study period) and surgeons with very high volumes (>100 during study period) were roughly one-half the rates of hospitals and surgeons with little experience in aneurysm repair. Data from the National Inpatient Sample on 16,540 patients undergoing elective conventional AAA repair between 1994 and 1996 indicate an in-hospital mortality rate of 4.2% and an overall complication rate of 32.4%.[7] None of these figures include the long-term problems of graft thrombosis, infection, anastomotic aneurysms, sexual dysfunction, incisional hernias and bowel obstructions from adhesions.[8]

Steyerberg et al. have identified seven factors that predict surgical death rates after AAA repair.[9] The information provided after a thorough meta-analysis of multiple series allows each surgeon to predict the mortality rate for any given patient using surgeon and hospital specific data. The factors that are included in the analysis are the average mortality rate for the hospital for a minimum of 25-50 similar procedures by the surgeon plus points for renal insufficiency (Cr>1.8mg-dl), congestive heart failure, EKG ischemia, FEV1<1 liter, older age and female gender. A score is tabulated (Table 21–1) and a risk calculated. For instance, an 80-year-old woman with a 6 cm AAA, a past history of CHF, and a creatinine of 2.2 mg-dl would have a specific mortality rate approaching 20% (assuming the surgeon has an operative mortality rate of 4%).[10] If this analysis is valid and there is no reason to think otherwise, the benefits of EVAR done in similar high risk patients is evident already.

TABLE 21-1. RISK CALCULATION OF MORTALITY FOLLOWING OPEN AAA RESECTION (AFTER STEYERBERG ET AL.[9]

Center Specific Average Operative Mortality Rates

%	3	4	5	6	8	12
Score	−5	−2	0	+2	+5	+10

Individual Prognostic Factors

Age (yr)	60	70	80
Score	−4	0	+4
Gender	Female		
Score	+4		
Cardiac co-morbidity	MI	CHF	ECG: ischemia
Score	+3	+8	+8
Renal co-morbidity (Cr>1.8)	Impairment		
Score	+12		
Pulmonary co-morbidity	Impairment		
Score	+7		

Estimated Individual Operative Mortality Rate

Sum score	(5)	0	5	10	15	20	25	30	35	40
Mortality rate %	1	2	3	5	8	12	19	28	39	51

EARLY RESULTS OF EVAR

Early concerns about EVAR relate to what happens after implantation Many of the original durability issues after EVAR occurred with devices that have already been withdrawn from the marketplace and are no longer germane. It is now well documented that EVAR can be performed safely with a variety of devices in patients with suitable anatomy. Technical success in well over 98% of patients is achievable with proper patient selection.[11-14] These patients have documented benefits that include decreased ICU utilization, decreased blood loss, shorter hospitalizations, and recovery times.[15] In addition, EVAR does not interfere with male potency. Despite device failures, endoleaks, remodeling, etc., EVAR has prevented rupture in 98–99% and prevented growth in 85–90% of patients treated over the last decade of clinical usage.[15] The decade of experience has reinforced the importance of the initial guidelines of mandatory, periodic follow-up.[16]

SELECTION FOR PATIENTS FOR EVAR

The selection of patients appropriate for EVAR is largely anatomical. The availability of a product that fits a patient's anatomy ultimately dictates the applicability of EVAR. No single device will accommodate every patient with an AAA. Ideally no device should be used outside of its recommended anatomic guidelines but significant co-morbidities may influence the surgeon to expand the anatomic indications for a patient that clearly requires AAA repair but has a prohibitive operative risk for the open procedure. One must accept the increased likelihood of more device-related problems when selecting patients with poor anatomy or significant medical co-morbidities for EVAR. The reluctance to use EVAR technology in less than ideal anantomic situations is mitigated by the availability of ancillary products that facilitate the management of endoleaks and access problems.

Data do not support the natural temptation to lower the threshold for aneurysm repair with EVAR because of the reduced morbidity and mortality rates of the lesser procedure. Markov models examining whether the optimal diameter for elective aneurysm repair in average and high-risk patients should be different for the two treatment modalities.[17] Assumptions were made from published reports and were as follows: the annual rupture rates for infrarenal aortic aneurysms <4cm, 4.5 cm, 5.5 cm, and 6.5 cm were 0%, 1%, 11%, and 26% respectively; the mortality rates were 1% for EVAR and 3.5% for conventional repair (age 70 years); the immediate conversion rate from EVAR to open repair was 5% and was 1% per year thereafter. The benefit of EVAR increased with increasing patient age disappeared with procedural mortality rates exceeding 3.5% and long-term endovascular grafts failure rates exceeding 6% per year. These failure and conversion estimates are higher than those observed during the first decade of the EVAR experience. While the authors concluded that lowering the threshold for EVAR is not justified at this time with the exception of patients >80 years in poor health where the data support reducing the diameter threshold from 8.1 cm to 5.7 cm., another look at real data might change their conclusion.

Support for an aggressive endovascular approach in patients unfit for open operation can be found in the literature. Conway and colleagues from Cardiff, Wales[18] prospectively maintained a registry of 106 patients with AAA >5.5 cm in diameter over a 10-year period that were turned down for elective repair. The mean age of the study population was 78.4 years. The actuarial survival rates for the 106 patients at

1, 2, and 3 years was 54%, 40%, and 17%. They concluded that the risk of dying from the AAA versus the risk of dying from a non-AAA cause was not different as long as the AAA was less than 6 cm. As the size of the AAA increased, an increased risk of death from rupture was noted. The largest cohort in this series was a group of 31 patients who refused operation. Twenty of these patients died, 12 secondary to their AAAs. Those patients who met the size criteria for operation in the UK Small Aneurysm Trial but were medically unfit had a mortality rate of 22% at 10 months and 50% at 2 years.[19] Buth et al. analyzed EUROSTAR data and found that patients unfit for open AAA repair had higher morbidity and mortality rates after EVAR when compared to patients with normal operative risk.[20] These older, sicker patients who underwent EVAR had a cumulative survival of 58% at 3 years suggesting limited advantage for repair in this high risk group of patients. They concluded that a patient must have a life expectancy of at least one year before any meaningful benefit in life expectancy after EVAR could be realized.

ANATOMIC CONSIDERATIONS

Important anatomic factors that affect device selection include the diameter, length, shape, and angulation of the infrarenal neck, any involvement of the common iliac arteries with either aneurysmal or occlusive disease, occlusive disease or marked tortuosity of the ilio-femoral access vessels, or intrinsically small iliac arteries. It is critical that the device fit the patient's anatomy as opposed to making a patient fit a specific device. Anatomic factors are best evaluated with thin-cut (1.5 mm) CT scans. Reformatted spiral CT scans can be used to accurately measure lengths and angles that are more difficult to assess with standard imaging. These reformatted axial studies have drastically reduced the need for arteriography in the evaluation of a patient for EVAR.

Stable fixation is the key to long-term durability. The ability of a device to maintain its position over time is dependent on the balance between the displacement and the stabilizing forces. The displacement forces on the proximal attachment site are related to the diameter and curvature of the aorta. Stabilization factors include the radial force upon the proximal and distal attachment sites from stents, columnar support and penetrating components such as hooks and barbs. As the angulation increases, the attachment area must lengthen as increasing angulation of the proximal neck is associated with significant Type I endoleaks and migration. A length of 15 mm is sufficient in the absence of proximal angulation. Patients with angulation rxceeding 45 degrees are not anatomically ideal and should receive an endograft only when other options are even less desirable.

Greenberg at al examined EVAR in 55 patients with short proximal necks (<15mm) using the Talent graft.[21] 13 of these patients had necks less than 10 mm. Endoleaks were more frequent in patients with larger aneurysms and were not correlated with the length of the proximal neck. Further validation and longer follow-up periods will be required, however, before EVAR for short necks can be recommended. An unexplained finding in this series was a striking increase in the proximal neck diameter of 0.9 mm over 30 days. These grafts were all oversized as a matter of policy and are designed with self-expanding stents. Data from Juan Parodi suggest that dilatation of the proximal neck does not happen to the same degree when balloon-expandable proximal attachments are used. He found that after 5 years that there was no dilatation of the proximal anastomoses in his original series of patients.[22]

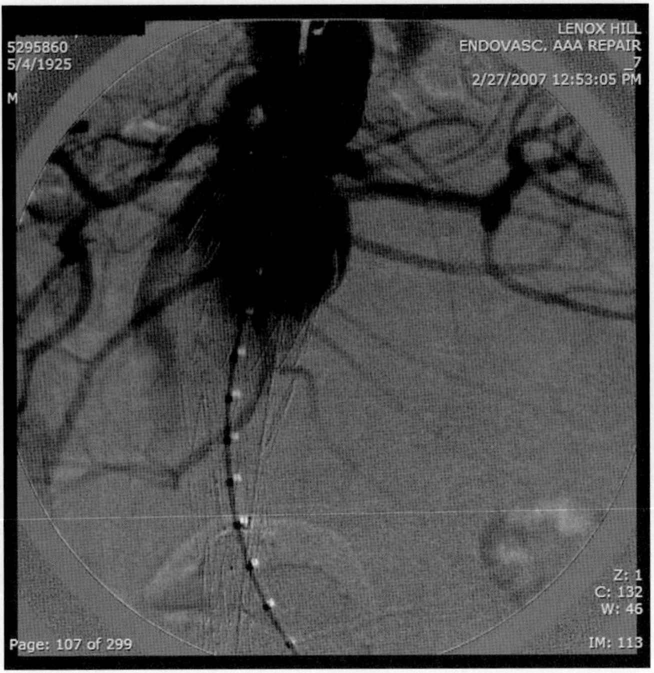

Figure 21-1. 81 year old man with recent MI and painful aneurysm. Proximal neck 7mm from lowest renal artery. Zenith endograft placed with demonstration of large Type I endoleak.

Achieving a permanent seal at an attachment site is dependent upon the apposition of graft material to a segment of the normal vessel. Devices are designed to function in cylindrical vessels and may not achieve a satisfactory seal in a conical vessel. The CT image in Figure 21–1 shows a Type I endoleak in a critically ill patient with a symptomatic AAA with a short proximal neck. We obviously knew that this anatomic configuration was not ideal for EVAR. We were able to deploy large balloon expandable stent (Figure 21–2) and the patient is alive and well without an endoleak at 3.5 years.

Currently available devices include those with infrarenal fixation and suprarenal fixation. There is a great deal of subjectivity in choosing which of the types of devices to use in an individual patient. I prefer suprarenal fixation in most cases unless there is a significant angle between the suprarenal aorta and the infrarenal neck. There are two devices currently available with suprarenal fixation-Talent (Medtronic) and Zenith (Cook). There are no data that suggest any adverse outcomes specifically related to the suprarenal stent component. One difficulty I have encountered however is accessing diseased renal arteries following graft deployment and now treat severe renal ostial lesions prior to deploying the suprarenal graft. This is a very helpful technique especially when the neck is short as the stent provides an accurate marker of the lower border of the renal artery.

The Talent device has been reconfigured to the Aneuryx delivery system which is a tremendous improvement over the original deployment system. Cook is currently testing a modification of the Zenith device that has fewer deployment steps and a smaller insertion sheath. I believe that both devices perform well in the properly selected patient and both allow some compromise on the proximal neck length. I also feel that the Talent device in its new delivery apparatus is easier to accurately deploy

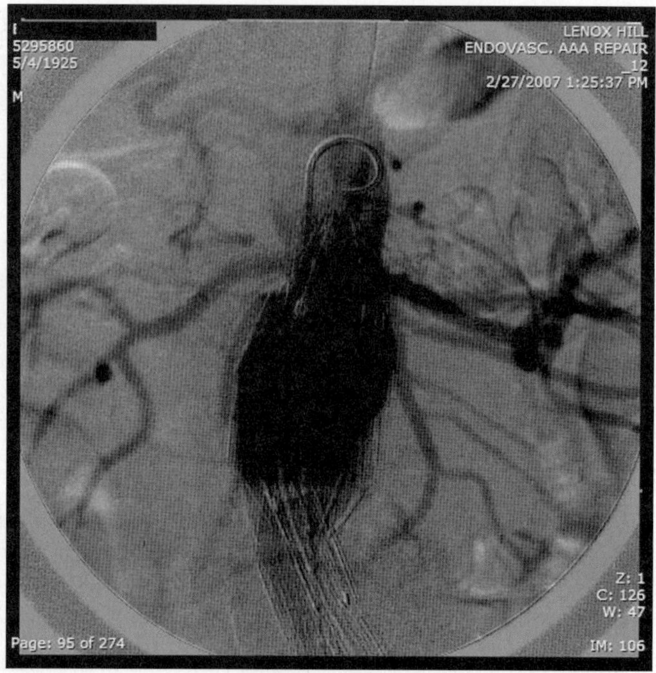

Figure 21-2. Patient in Figure 21-1 after placement of Palmaz stent. Endoleak reduced. CT scan 2 days later showed no further leak. Patient alive and well without endoleak 3 $^{1}/_{2}$ years later.

in a compromised proximal neck. Zenith has other advantages however (longer common trunk and more flexibility to adjust for length) and I use the two grafts with confidence interchangeably.

Endografts with infrarenal fixation should be used when the proximal neck length exceeds 15mm, the proximal diameter is less than 32 mm, and the angulation is less than 60 degrees. Currently available devices are Medtronic Aneuryx (Santa Rosa CA), Gore Excluder (Flagstaff AZ and Endologic Powerlink (Irvine CA). Whereas each of these devices is quite different they all provide secure repair and freedom from rupture. The choice among the three is operator dependent. I do feel that the Aneuryx device allows more precise control of the proximal deployment. This attribute is most significant in a patient with a severely angululated proximal neck where the Excluder graft may jump distally leaving a gap between the lowest renal artery and the beginning of the fabric. I have no personal experience with the Powerlink graft.

Heavily calcified, narrow aortic bifurcations may not provide sufficient room for a bifurcated graft and limb compression and graft thrombosis may occur. Alternatively, the contralateral limb may be difficult to deploy. For this reason, maintaining wire access to the sac is critical prior to cannulation of the contralateral iliac limb. Once both limbs have been deployed, the distal aorta can be dilated with angioplasty balloons in the iliac limbs. Modular, fully supported devices are easier to deploy in a narrow aortic bifurcation. Two limbs up to 16 mm each can fit into a 20 mm aorta depending on the degree of angulation. It should be noted that the long-body modular designs are not ideal in this setting and if for other reasons one must be used the body should be left shorter than usual. Unibody bifurcated devices are particularly difficult to manipulate when the aortic bifurcation is small and severely calcified. The availability of an

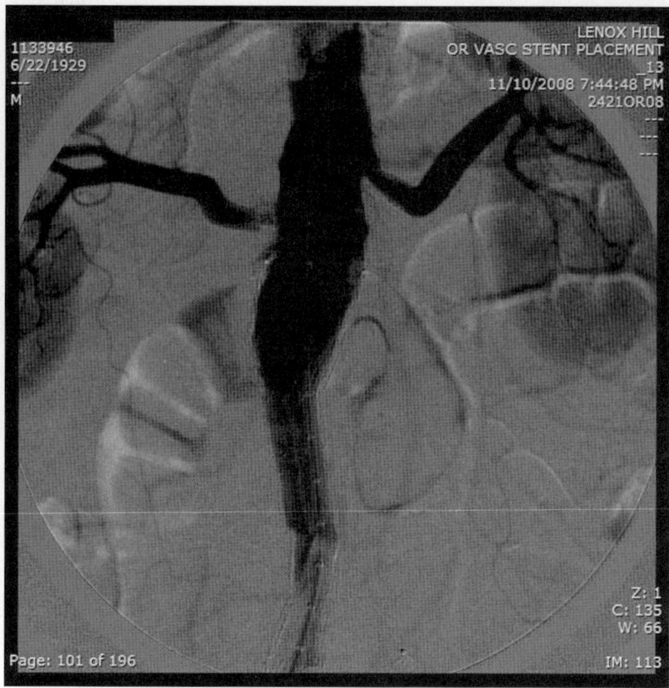

Figure 21-3. Use of the Zenith ReNu graft in a limited 16 mm distal domain. An alternative technique would involve use of a bifurcated graft and balloon angioplasty of the domain. I chose the former because of the severe calcification at the distal aorta.

aorto-uni-iliac (AUI) device (Cook ReNu, Bloomington IN) is a useful tool in this setting and rather than struggle with a compromised domain I prefer the AUI with a femoral femoral bypass and contralateral iliac artery occlusion. (Figure 21–3)

The iliac arteries must be of sufficient diameter to allow access to the aneurysm yet still provide suitable deployment sites within the size ranges of the available devices. The combination of significant calcification and tortuosity should raise a red flag regarding access and consideration of alternatives such as iliac conduits or endoconduits with covered stents such as Bard Fluency (C.R. Bard, Murray Hill NJ) or the Gore Viabahn (Flagstaff AZ). The distal attachment sites should not interfere with the existing internal iliac arteries and there should be a landing zone at least 2 cm in length. Iliac aneurysms can be excluded by deploying the endograft in the external iliac artery and occluding the ipsilateral hypogastric artery. I prefer to coil the hypogastric artery prior to endograft deployment so I can be certain that occlusion has actually occurred. Our experience suggests an increased incidence of limb occlusion after deployment in the external iliac artery with both Talent and Zenith endografts. Recommendations to avoid this are (1) when using a Talent graft use the Aneuryx iliac limbs because they are more flexible than the Talent and (2) when using a Zenith place a self-expanding stent within the iliac limb and extend it for a few centimeters onto the external iliac artery. Figures 21-4a and b show two examples of endoconduits for EVAR access.

The purpose of hypogastric embolization and occlusion is twofold: first and most important, to provide a secure distal landing zone and avoid a Type Ib endoleak and second, to prevent retrograde filling of the sac to prevent a Type II endoleak. Buttock claudication and erectile dysfunction occur in up to 40% of patients after

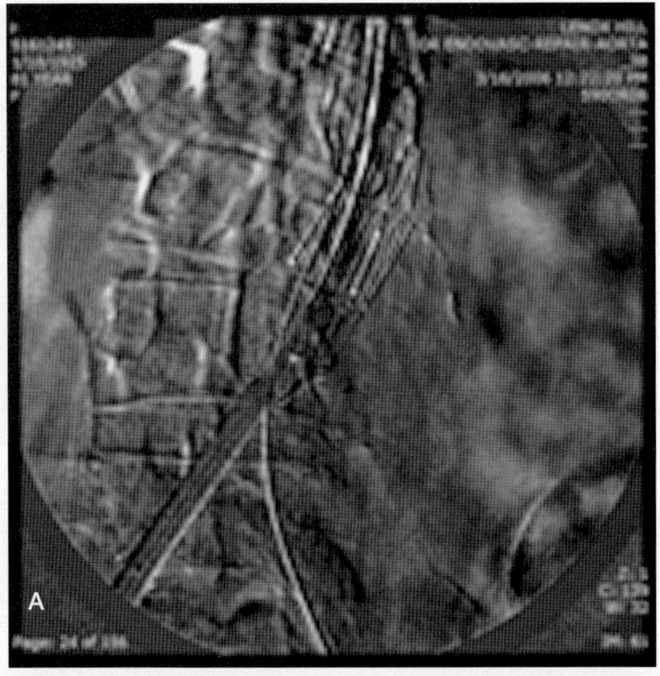

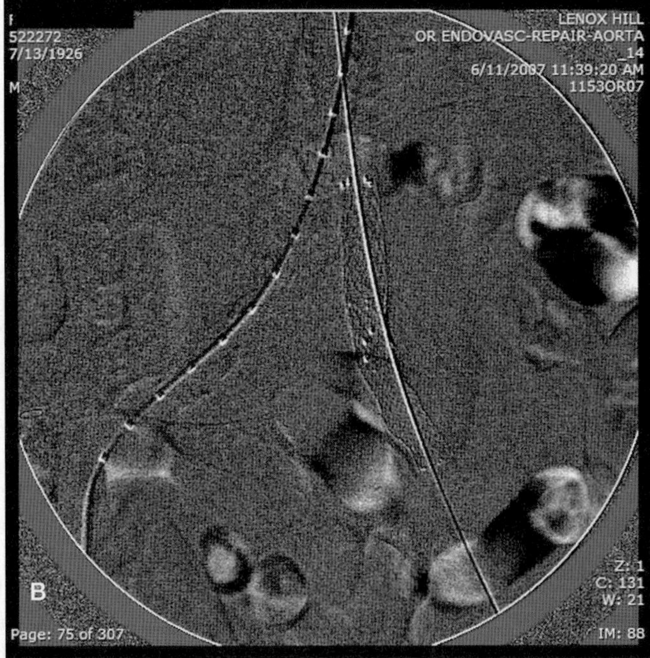

Figure 21-4. A. 81 year old lady with CHF and symptomatic 7 cm AAA. Zenith endograft could not be advanced beyond common iliac artery due to both tortuosity and calcification. An endoconduit was created with a Bard Fluency graft (8mm) that allowed easy passage of endograft and completion of EVAR. Patient alive at 3½ years without any aneurysm related issues. **B.** shows an endoconduit prior to insertion of the device.

hypogastric occlusion. While most of the time improvements are noted 11-12% of patients will have persistent claudication and 9% to 13% will have persistent erectile dysfunction.[23-24] Specific anatomic situations seem to be associated with a higher incidence of ischemic problems: bilateral hypogastric embolization, unilateral embolization with stenosis on the contralateral side, and pre-existing or iatrogenic interruption of collateral pathways from the external iliac and common femoral circulation. (25) Although the pelvis has one of the best collateral networks in the body, these patients have multiple pathways interrupted simultaneously (lumbar, IMA, hypogastric, and in some cases common femoral), which may result in ischemic symptoms postoperatively. While buttock claudication and impotence seem to be clearly attributable to interruption of these pathways, acute ischemic complications such as colonic infarction or soft tissue necrosis are much more likely due to distal embolization of atheromatous debris at the time of surgery.

It had been suggested that more proximal coil occlusion (Figure 5a) of the hypogastric artery is much less likely to cause claudication than branch embolization, which is logical in that it preserves communication between the anterior and posterior divisions of the hypogastric collateral pathway. If so, occlusion of the IIA orifice with a vascular plug (nonselective embolization) may be the optimal method of control of backbleeding into the sac and maintenance of the pelvic circulation. Certain embolic devices, such as the Amplatzer Plug, (AGA Medical Corporation, Golden Valley, MN) have the advantage of achieving rapid occlusion with a single device, as well as permitting repositioning prior to release. (Figure 21-5b) Our experience with bilateral IIA embolization is limited and we do so with great trepidation. Our preference when both IIA require embolization is to create a hypogastric artery bypass distal to the coils prior to EVAR deployment. Several other approaches have been employed to preserve pelvic collateral flow when both hypogastrics would need to be occluded to accomplish endovascular repair of an aneurysm. One suggested approach is staged embolization, in which each hypogastric artery is embolized at a separate procedure over a period of weeks to months, followed by the EVAR procedure itself.[25] Others stress the importance of the preservation of the deep femoral artery collateral vessels and recommend profundoplasty at the time of EVAR. Since the incidence of ischemic complications remains unpredictable, it is unclear whether isolated case reports of a successful outcome provides evidence that the theoretical advantage of giving collaterals time to develop is valid. It also leaves the patient at risk with an untreated aneurysm for a considerable period of time.

DESIGN CONSIDERATIONS

There are unibody and component devices. There are fully supported and unsupported grafts. Some attachments are with balloon-expandable stents, others are with self-expanding stents. Some stents are barbed, others are not. Some devices allow for partial deployment and movement prior to engagement, others do not. Some have longer common trunks than others. Some grafts are made of polyester, others are made of polytetrafluorethylene. Some stents are stainless steel, others are made of nitinol. Some stents are attached to the graft fabric by sutures, others are attached chemically. Some devices cross the renal arteries with uncovered stents, others do not. Some of these design factors may ultimately prove superior others but at this time conclusions are conjectural and individual preferences are based on operator bias and device availability.

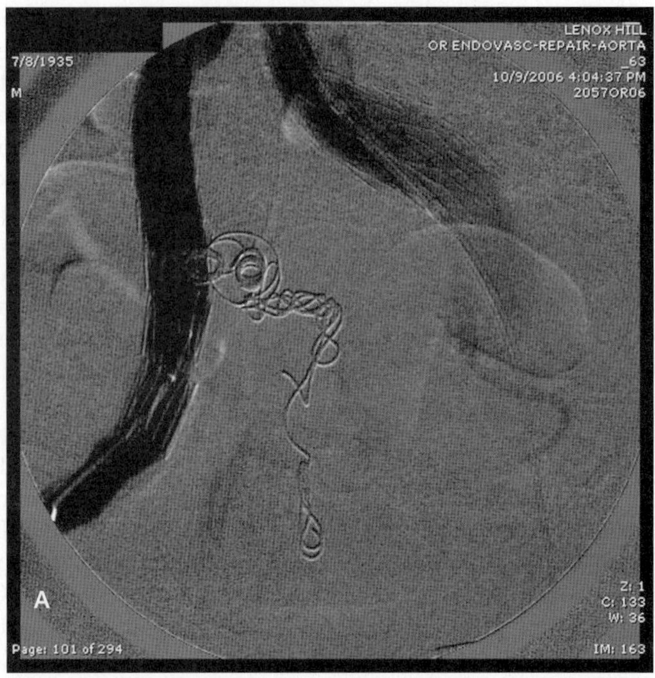

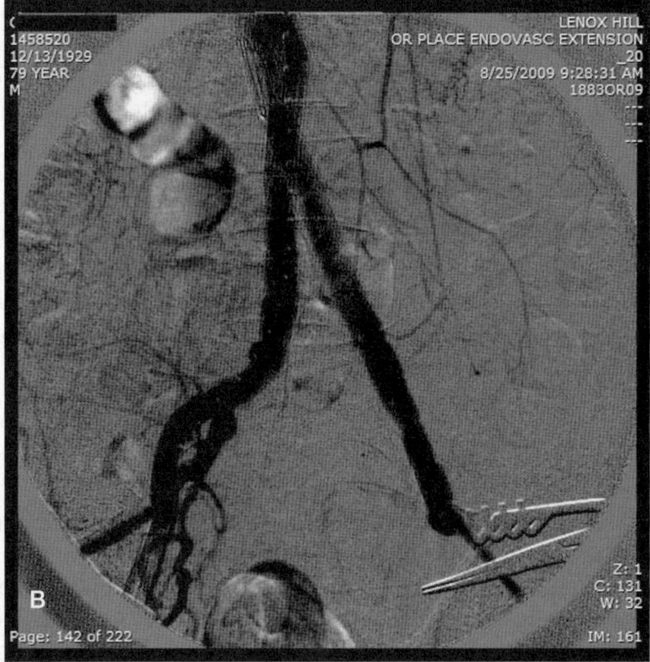

Figure 21-5. A. Post-deployment of a Zenith endograft following coil occlusion of the internal iliac artery. We no longer use coils but rather an Amplatz plug **B.** whenever feasible both for time and cost savings

Modular systems offer flexibility in the size and length of the iliac attachments but have the disadvantage of component separation (Type III endoleak). Unibody constructs cannot develop Type III endoleaks and have a lower risk of distal attachment migration. The disadvantage of the unsupported unibody design is an increased risk of twisting and/or kinking during deployment and compression from stenotic iliac artery lesions. The pull-out force increases in a proportional relationship to the number of barbs and/or hooks and whether a balloon-expandable or a self-expanding stent is utilized. There does not appear to be any significant adverse effects of suprarenal fixation.[26] There is however a problem with suprarenal stent fixation when there is angulation of the suprarenal aorta. Opposing angulations can result in displacement of the sealing stent and a Type I endoleak. There are some data that suggest that Type II endoleaks are less frequent with devices whose main body is both long and supported as compared to shorter body configurations.[27] Another advantage of the long-bodied graft is the potential to straddle the aortic bifurcation, provide greater longitudinal support and therefore less of a tendency to migrate. Some of the characteristics of the approved devices are listed in Table 21–2. I have included some of the issues related to each graft largely based upon my own bias. Each of these grafts appears to successfully and safely provide protection against AAA rupture.

TABLE 21-2. DEVICE CHARACTERISTICS

	Design	Fixation	Problems	Advantages

AneuRx[1]
Main body
  20–28 mm; limbs
  12–16 mm
	Polyester, modular fully supported device with metal rings sutured to fabric	Radial force from self-expanding stents	None with improved delivery system. Not For large necks	Simple deployment-Can use aortic extension to "bell-bottom" large iliac

PowerLink 2	Unibody, bifurcated ePTFE with metal support	Has advantage of Unibody columnar Support	Learning curve for Unbody system	Can treat neck up to 32 May have advantage in Short angulated necks

Talent[3]
Main body up to
  36 mm with limbs
  up to 20 mm.
  Each graft is
  customized
	Modular, fully supported polyester with suprarenal stent fixation	Self-expanding without hooks or barbs	Delivery system is prone to kinking in tortuous anatomy and unsheathing device can be problematic	Simple deployment, excellent customer service. Can accommodate large and short proximal neck

Excluder[4]
Main body
  20–31 mm; limbs
  taper from 16 mm
  anywhere to
  10 mm
	Exoskeleton of nitinol with PTFE graft material without sutures. Modular.	Self-expanding and fully supported. Can be configured as both cylinder and tapered graft.	Deployment less controlled than with devices that allow for some adjustments after upper stents released	Flexible delivery reduces chance of access vessel injury. Flexible, supported limbs likely to reduce incidence of occlusion.

Zenith[5]
Main body size
  up to 36 mm and
  limbs up to 20 mm
	Modular exoskeleton of stainless steel self-expanding stents with a barbed suprarenal stent.	Radial force and suprarenal barbs. Main body designed to terminate 15 mm from aortic bifurcation.	More difficult deployment sequence to master because of the neec to recapture the cap holding the suprarenal stent.	Excellent quality delivery system in setting of access vessel tortuosity.

[1]Medtronic, Santa Rosa CA
[2]Endologix, Irvine CA
[3]Medtronic, Santa Rosa CA
[4]W.L. Gore & Associates, Flagstaff, Arizona
[5]Cook, Bloomington, Indiana

CONCLUSIONS

The decision to recommend one type of aneurysm repair over another varies from institution to institution and is governed by a number of factors including anatomy, medical co-morbidity, operator skills, and access to the devices. Since most patients, if given a choice, would opt for the less invasive procedure, the fundamental question each of us must ask is how to select those most suitable for EVAR given the increasing but limited long-term data available. There is compelling evidence that in properly selected patients, EVAR appears to be comparable to conventional repair using rupture and death as endpoints within the first year following deployment. One only has to discharge a patient with a symptomatic AAA on home oxygen on the second post-operative day to appreciate the giant step forward endoluminal therapy has made.

It is now appropriate to offer EVAR to anatomically suitable patients with significant medical co-morbidities and/or hostile abdomens. A truly informed opinion however requires each of us to examine our results with both techniques in both healthy and compromised patients. The decision to liberalize the usage of EVAR should only occur when results are superior to the other choices including observation.

Increasing choice of devices over the past decade allows the surgeon to fit the device to the patient and not vice versa. Some patients will require suprarenal fixation, some will not. Others will require small insertion sheaths, others will not. Some patients will require supported iliac limbs, others will not. I anticipate that adjusting to the patient's anatomy will lessen the stresses on the devices and improve long-term performance.

REFERENCES

1. Ohki T, Veith FJ, Lipsitz R, et al. Increasing incidence of mid- and long-term complications after endovascular graft repair of AAAs: A word of caution based on an 8-year experience with 212 cases. *Ann Surg.* 2001.
2. Collins J, Murie JA. Endovascular treatment of abdominal aortic aneurysms: a failed experiment. *Brit J Surg.* 2001;88:1281–1282.
3. Nowygrod R, Egorova N, Greco G et al. Trends, complications, and mortality in peripheral vascular surgery. J Vasc Surg 2006;43:205–216.
4. Giles GA, Pomposelli F, Hamdan A et al. Decrease in total aneurysm-related deaths in the era of endovascular repair. J Vasc Surg 2009;49:543–50.
5. Chaikoff E.L. editor. The Care of Patietns with an Abdominal Aortic Aneurysm: The Society for Vascular Surgery Guidelines. J Vasc Surg 2009:50; Supplement 8S;128–9.
6. Dardik A, Lin JW, Gordon TA, Williams M, Perler B. Results of elective abdominal aortic aneurysm repair in the 1990s: a population based alaysis of 2335 cases. *J Vasc Surg.* 1999; 30:985–995.
7. Huber TS, Wang J, Derrow DE, et al. Experience in the United States with intact abdominal aortic aneurysm repair. *J Vasc Surg.* 2001;33:304–311.
8. Hallett JW Jr, Marshall DM, Petterson TM, et al. Graft-related complications after abdominal aortic aneurysm repair: Reassurance from a 36 year population-based experience. *J Vasc Surg.* 1997;25:277.
9. Steyerberg EW, Kievit J, Otterloo JC, et al. Perioperative mortality of elective abdominal aortic aneurysm: A clinical prediction rule based on literature and individual patient data. *Archives Int Med.* 1995;155:1998–2004.

10. Hallett JW Jr. What are the realistic expectations for standard open abdominal anrtic aneurysm repair in contemporary practice: The gold standard. *Vascular Surgery 2002: New approaches to old problems.* Department of Continuing Education, Harvard Medical School, Boston Mass May 9–11, 2002.
11. Zarins CK, White RA, Schwarten D, et al. AneuRx stent graft versus open surgical repair of abdominal aortic aneurysms: Multicenter prospective clinical trial. *J Vasc Surg.* 1999;29: 292–308.
12. Moore W, Kashyap V, Vescer C, et al. Abdominal aortic aneurysm: A 6-year comparison of endovascular versus transabdominal repair. *Ann Surg.* 1999;230:298–306.
13. Greenberg Rk, Chuter TAM, Lawrence-Brown M, et al. Analysis of renal function after aneurysm repair with a device using supra-renal fixation (Zenith AAA endovascular graft) in contrast to open surgical repair. J Vasc Surg 2004;39:1219–28.
14. Sapirstein W, Chandeeysson P, Wentz C. The Food and Drug Administration approval of endovascular grafts for abdominal aortic aneurysm: An 18-month retrospective. *J Vasc Surg.* 2001;34:180–183.
15. May J, White GH, Yu W, et al. Concurrent comparison of endoluminal versus open repair in the treatment of abdominal aortic aneurysms: Analysis of 303 patients by life table method. *J Vasc Surg.* 1998;27:213–221.
16. Sapirstein W, Chandeeysson P, Wentz C. The Food and Drug Administration approval of endovascular grafts for abdominal aortic aneurysm: An 18-month retrospective. *J Vasc Surg.* 2001;34:180–183.
17. Finlayson S, Birkmeyer J, Fillinger M, Cronenwett J. Should endovascular surgery lower the threshold for repair of abdominal aortic aneurysms? *J Vasc Surg.* 1999;29:973–985.
18. Conway KP, Byrne J, Townsend M, Lane IF. Prognosis of patients turned down for conventional abdominal aortic aneurysm repair in the endovascular and sonographic era: Szilagyi revisited? *J Vasc Surg.* 2001;33:752–757.
19. The UK Small Aneurysm Trial: design, methods, and progress. The UK Small Aneurysm Trial participants. *Eur J Vasc Endovasc Surg.* 1995;9:42–48.
20. Buth J, van Marrewijk CJ, Harris P, et al. Outcome of endovascular abdominal aortic aneurysm repair in patients with conditions considered unfil for an open procedure: A report on the EUROSTAR experience. *J Vasc Surg.* 2002;35:211–221.
21. Greenberg R, Fairman R, Srivastava S, et al. Endovascular grafting in patients with short proximal necks: an analysis of short-term results. *Cardiovasc Surg.* 2000;8:350–354.
22. Personal communication. Dr. Juan Parodi, Buenos Aires, Argentina.
23. Leyden S, Sternbach Y, Green RM. Clinical implications of internal iliac artery embolization in endovascular repair of aortoiliac aneurysms. *Ann Vasc Surg.* 2001;15(5):539–43.
24. Lin, PH, Bush RL, et al. A prospective evaluation of hypogastric artery embolization in endovascular aortoiliac aneurysm repair. *J Vasc Surg.* 2002;36:500–506.
25. Mehta M, Veith F, Ohki T et al. Unilateral and bilateral hypogastric artery interruption during aortoiliac aneurysm repair in 154 patients. J Vasc Surg 2001;33:S27–32.
26. Greenberg RK, Lawrence-Brown M, Bhandari M, et al. An update of the Zenith endovascular graftfor abdominal aortic aneurysms: initial implantation and mid-term follow-up data. *J Vasc Surg* 2001;33:S157–64.
27. Fairman RM, Velazquez OC, Carpenter JP, Baum RA. How are Type II endoleaks related to graft design. Presented at the VEITH Symposium, New York City, November 2001.Hollier LH, Taylor LM Jr, Ochsner J. Recommended indications for operative treatment of abdominal aortic aneurysms. *J Vasc Surg.* 1992;15:1046–1056.

Hybrid Procedures For Complex Aortic Aneurysms

22

Pararenal and Type IV Thoracoabdominal Aortic Aneurysm Repair Utilizing Visceral Reconstruction with Endovascular Stent Graft Exclusion

Margaret H. Walkup, M.D., Robert R. Mendes, M.D., and Blair Keagy, M.D.

A pararenal aneurysm (PRA) or a type IV thoracoabdominal aortic aneurysm (TAAA) may involve all or a large majority of the abdominal aorta, and may include any combination of the celiac, superior mesenteric, or renal arteries. Currently, these types of aneurysms are not an indication for endovascular repair. The conventional repair of these aneurysms may require an aortic cross-clamp suprarenally or above the celiac trunk, which is associated with significant perioperative mortality. Derrow et al. have reported mortality rates approaching 20%[1] for repair of all types of TAAAs combined. This increased risk is related to visceral and renal ischemia. As well, there is a great deal of physiologic stress placed on the heart during the technically difficult repair with a bypass graft and vessel reimplantation. Morbidity of TAAA repair is also significant with spinal cord ischemia occurring as frequently as 15%, pulmonary complications in up to 40%, and renal impairment in up to 30% of patients.[2-5] Patients with multiple comorbidities are often at high risk for the conventional approach. However, the mortality rate of observation approaches 76% at two years with aneurysm rupture responsible for half of these deaths.[6]

Advances in endovascular techniques have made it possible to approach these challenging cases differently without aortic cross-clamping. Patients can undergo visceral and renal reconstruction prior to endovascular exclusion of the aneurysm. stent graft exclusion with visceral vessel reconstruction has very encouraging early term results, demonstrating no paraplegia in several studies.[7,8] For some groups, this repair has become preferable to the open technique.[7] In this chapter, we will describe techniques for the endovascular repair of pararenal and type IV TAAAs with adjunctive visceral vessel reconstruction in which initial reports have described promising results. [8-14]

PREOPERATIVE CONSIDERATIONS

Providing adequate proximal and distal fixation sites to accomplish aneurysm exclusion with an appropriate sealing region is the most challenging task in many patients. Commercially available stent grafts require a minimal aortic neck length of 15 mm both proximal and distal to the aneurysmal portion of the abdominal aorta and iliac arteries, respectively, and a neck angle less than 45 degrees to provide an adequate seal zone.[15-17] Given the larger size of the thoracic aorta, additional length is needed, and 20 to 30 mm is generally thought to be necessary. While it is crucial that the aortic walls be fairly parallel and free from significant calcification and thrombus, implanting the device in a region where significant angulation exists can also jeopardize the durability of the endovascular repair.

To provide a more favorable anatomy, it may be required to reconstruct the celiac, superior mesenteric, or renal arteries. Occasionally, a complete abdominal aortic debranching may be necessary. However, before performing visceral procedures, it is important to evaluate the anatomic and hemodynamic status of the visceral section including both renal arteries. A preoperative spiral computed tomography angiogram (CTA) or magnetic resonance angiogram (MRA) with 2 to 3 mm intervals combined with sagital and coronal reconstructions of the aorta provide the most thorough evaluation of the aneurysm, the aorta, and its branches. If any questions about the anatomy arise, visceral angiography can be performed. For hemodynamic evaluation, we have relied on duplex ultrasonography, which has a high degree of accuracy when performed in experienced peripheral vascular laboratories.

Multiple factors are involved in the determination of which vessels need to be revascularized. These include prohibitive abdominal surgical risks, aberrant vasculature, or an occluded target vessel. For example, patients who have a replaced right hepatic artery originating from the superior mesenteric artery (SMA) or patients with an occluded celiac artery may have adequate collateral flow to the liver. The potential source of inflow must also be determined from the preoperative imaging. Patients with significant aortoiliac disease may be better suited with an antegrade inflow source from either the thoracic aorta, hepatic, or splenic arteries. If the hepatic or splenic arteries are to provide the inflow source for the bypass, careful evaluation of the celiac axis is essential to ensure it is free of significant disease. Patients with favorable iliac vessels may undergo retrograde bypasses, many of which can be performed under a regional anesthesia.

Visceral and renal reconstruction must be performed prior to endovascular exclusion of the aneurysm. Reconstruction may be done concomitantly with the endovascular repair. However, complex cases involving complete debranching of the abdominal aorta or reconstruction using the thoracic aorta as the donor vessel can be done in a staged procedure. In all cases of vessel bypass and debranching, ligation of the native vessel at its origin must be performed to prevent type II endoleaks.

OPERATIVE CONSIDERATIONS

Pararenal Aneurysms

Patency rates have been assessed in bypass grafting for chronic mesenteric ischemia and renal artery stenosis, and have been reported at 90% to 95% at 36 months in some series.[18,19] While this is encouraging, no long-term data currently exist to document the patency of bypass grafts for the purpose of aortic debranching.

Unilateral Renal Artery Bypass. This is typically used when one kidney is nonfunctional or the patient has one renal artery that is located more caudal than the other. When this is required, the ipsilateral external iliac vessel is typically chosen as the donor vessel. Be sure to choose a donor site distal to the anticipated placement of an endovascular stent graft. This allows for a retroperitoneal approach with regional anesthesia. Typically, an oblique retroperitoneal incision is made. Dissection is performed through the muscular layers of the abdominal wall, the intact peritoneum is retracted medially, and the retroperitoneal space is entered laterally. Both the renal artery and the external iliac artery can be exposed from this approach. The bypass may need to originate from either the very distal common iliac or external iliac artery, depending on their individual lengths, the extent of aneurysmal disease involvement, and the planned landing zone of the endograft. Proximal and distal control of the target vessels is then obtained, and a 6–8 mm polytetrafluoroethylene (PTFE) graft is used for the bypass (Figure 22–1). After confirmation of the graft patency with a continuous wave doppler, the proximal renal artery is ligated. Placement of large hemoclips to mark the iliac anastamotic site will prove useful for future endovascular interventions.

Hepatorenal Bypass. Designed primarily to treat renal occlusive disease before endovascular techniques, the bypass procedure can be used to provide an extra-anatomical bypass to either the right renal artery or the celiac artery when used in "reverse" fashion.

This is utilized for revascularization of the right renal artery in a patient with severe aortoiliac occlusive disease involving the external iliac artery. Most procedures are performed through a subcostal incision, although a midline celiotomy can be used if necessary. The hepatic artery is identified through the lesser omentum. Control of,

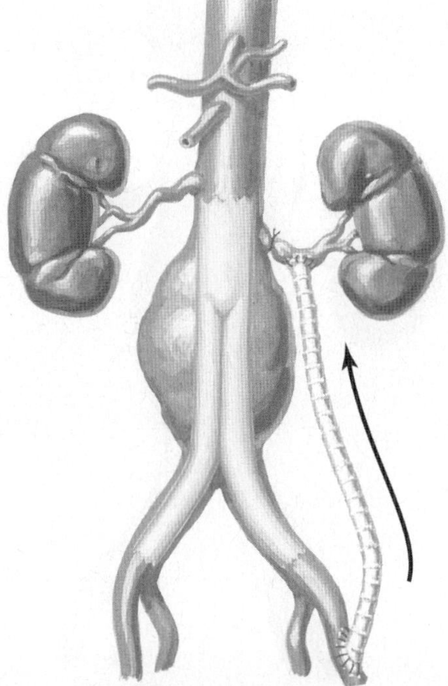

Figure 22-1. Ileorenal bypass

and anastamosis to, the hepatic artery proximal to the gastroduodenal artery (GDA) is ideal but not always possible. The duodenum is mobilized medially using a Kocher maneuver, the renal vein is identified, and the right renal artery is controlled by vessel loops. An appropriate conduit, either autologous or synthetic, should be chosen to match the target vessel diameters. Some surgeons prefer autologous saphenous vein when treating patients with occlusive renal disease because it may impart a greater long-term patency. This, however, has not been documented in the treatment of patients without occlusive disease. After systemic heparinization, the end-to-side renal anastomosis is usually performed first, followed by the hepatic artery reconstruction in an end-to-side fashion. Generally, the bypass follows a gentle curved "C" configuration (Figure 22–2). If needed, an end-to-end anastomosis can be performed to the GDA. Caution should be taken when the GDA is used because it provides important mesenteric collateral flow. Again, ligate the proximal right renal artery to avoid the potential for subsequent type II endoleak.

Splenorenal Bypass.   Similar to the hepatorenal bypass, the splenorenal bypass may be utilized in patients requiring left renal revascularization without an acceptable external iliac donor artery. A midline celiotomy or a left subcostal incision may be used for vascular exposure. In either case, the posterior pancreas is mobilized by cephalad reflection of its inferior border. The splenic artery is mobilized from the left gastroepiploic artery to its distal branching point. The left adrenal vein is divided, which allows for the caudal retraction of the left renal vein. At this point, the splenic artery is divided, spatulated, and anastomosed to the left renal artery in an end-to-end manner.

The procedures above all include endovascular abdominal aortic aneurysm repair to completely exclude the aneurysm in a single stage repair. Access to the abdominal aorta is commonly via bilateral common femoral artery exposure or through the

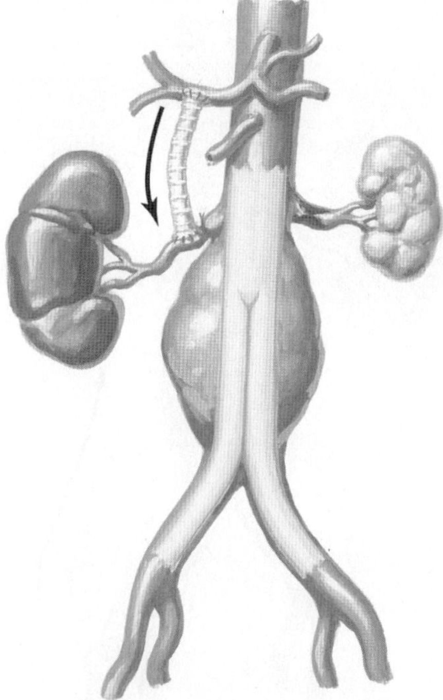

Figure 22-2. Hepatorenal bypass

retroperitoneal exposure used for the iliorenal bypass. If necessary, the endovascular exclusion can be performed in a second stage procedure.

Type IV Thoracoabdominal Aneurysms (Complete Aortic Debranching)

In a large number of patients, the celiac and SMA are located in proximity to one another, and both vessels must be relocated to ensure adequate neck length. The choice of inflow source is usually determined by either previous aortic surgery or the extent of aneurysmal or occlusive disease. Our studies demonstrate that antegrade revascularization to the mesenteric vessels from the descending thoracic aorta has a low morbidity and excellent patency rates (100%) at 34 months.[20] In this procedure, the descending thoracic aorta is controlled with a side-biting clamp, which allows for continual perfusion to the abdominal viscera and the spinal cord. We believe the reduction in visceral ischemia time is important as is the stability of blood pressure throughout the operation due to the maintenance of aortic blood flow.

In a comparison of mesenteric bypasses, studies have not found any significant difference in patency between antegrade and retrograde bypass grafts.[21,22] It is important to note, however, that the supraciliac aorta and not the descending thoracic aorta was used as the inflow for the antegrade bypasses in these studies. In general, we have found the descending thoracic aorta to have less incidence of atherosclerotic disease, and it may provide a more consistent inflow source for the antegrade bypass graft.

Thoracoceliac with Thoracomesenteric-left Renal Bypass (Antegrade Bypass). This is utilized when patients require a complete aortic debranching prior to the placement of the endovascular exclusion device. The patient is intubated with a double lumen endotrachial tube to allow for intraoperative deflation of the left lung to ease in exposure of the distal descending thoracic aorta. The patient is then positioned in a right lateral decubitus position, often with the aid of an axillary roll and beanbag for patient stabilization. The thoracoabdominal incision is made through the ninth rib interspace for best exposure of the distal thoracic and upper abdominal aorta.

The peritoneal contents are bluntly dissected from the undersurface of the diaphragm retracting anteriorly while the left kidney remains posterior in the retroperitoneum to facilitate the exposure of the mesenteric vasculature. The diaphragm is then incised in a curvilinear fashion 2 cm from its costal edge to preserve its innervation. Suture markers are placed as the diaphragm is taken down to ease reapproximation. The inferior pulmonary ligament and the crus are divided. The mesenteric vessels are exposed to a suitable bypass site.

The descending thoracic aorta is clamped with a single side-biting clamp during the proximal anastomosis of both bypasses to allow for continued perfusion to the viscera and minimize trauma to the aorta. Prosthetic bypass graft conduits are used and routed through the diaphragmatic hiatus to their respective vessels in an end-to-side fashion to establish antegrade flow. We typically use two separate grafts for mesenteric bypass. In our opinion, this allows greater freedom in graft orientation, although a bifurcated graft is an acceptable alternative. Revascularization of the left kidney is accomplished with a bypass graft from the thoracomesenteric graft to the left renal artery (Figure 22–3). On completion of all bypass grafts, the proximal celiac, superior mesenteric, and left renal arteries are ligated. Caution is advised in this situation: if a type II endoleak from the celiac, mesenteric, or renal artery occurs after the deployment of the stent graft, access is extremely limited, if not impossible, via

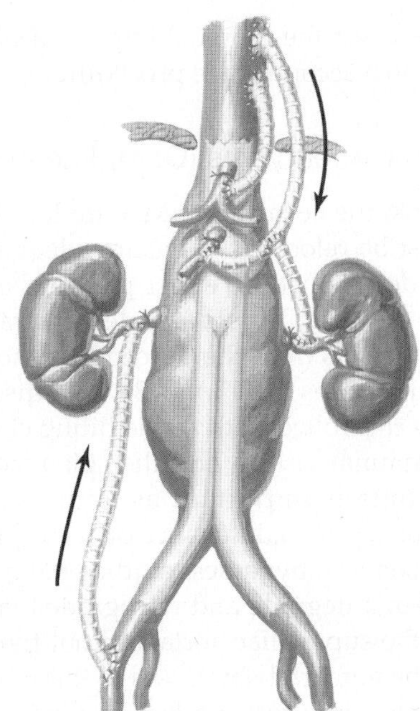

Figure 22-3. Thoracoceliac with thoracomesenteric-left bypass, right ileorenal bypass

endovascular means. The inferior border of the thoracic anastomosis is marked with a large clip to aid in identification for future endovascular interventions.

The second stage of the repair consists of a bypass graft from the right external iliac artery to the right renal artery through a retroperitoneal exposure, as described above. Endovascular abdominal aortic aneurysm repair completes the exclusion of the aneurysm.

Iliomesenteric Reconstructions (Retrograde Bypass).   A transperitoneal abdominal approach is used to expose the abdominal aorta and the origins of the renal arteries, the celiac axis, and the SMA. Once again, the location of the iliac donor site is critical. The bypass may need to originate from either the very distal common iliac or external iliac artery. Either the left or right iliac artery may be used as an inflow source for the bypass. Currently, we prefer to use individual ringed PTFE grafts, but bifurcated grafts may also be used as a conduit. The graft to the SMA is placed in a "lazy C" configuration as the graft lays better with less potential to kink. The limb to the celiac axis is tunneled anterior to the renal vein through the loose tissue in the retropancreatic space (Figure 22–4). The anastomosis is performed to the inferior aspect of the common hepatic artery just distal to the left gastric artery.

The celiac artery may also be revascularized via a right iliohepatic bypass that courses along the right retroperitoneum (Figure 22–5), taken off a right iliorenal bypass, or have a hepatorenal bypass supplied by an iliac inflow source (Figure 22–6). Ligation of vessel origins completes the debranching of the abdominal aorta prior to endovascular exclusion.

Complete Visceral Revascularization (Retrograde).   Each renal artery should be considered separately. For the left renal artery, three options exist: splenorenal bypass, il-

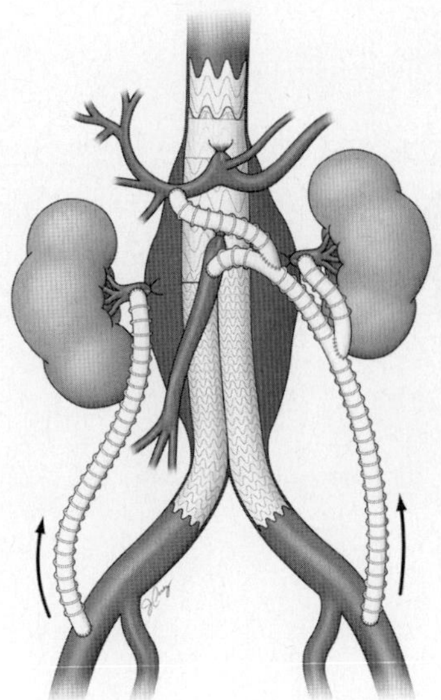

Figure 22-4. Ileomesenteric and left renal reconstructions with retrograde bypass, right ileorenal bypass

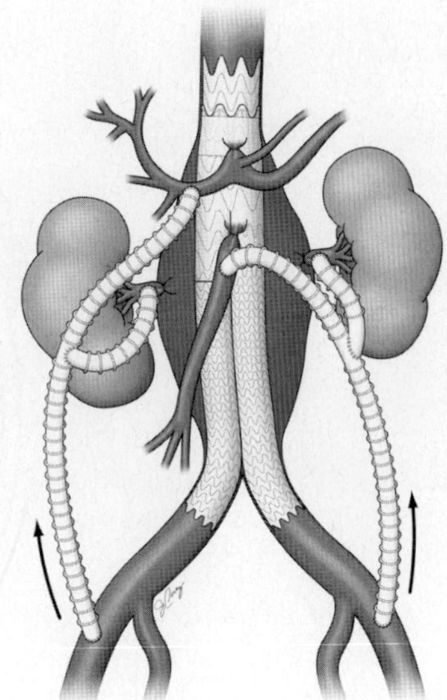

Figure 22-5. Right ileohepatic-right renal bypass, left ileomesenteric-left renal bypass

iorenal bypass (Figure 22–1), or attachment to one limb of the celiac or SMA reconstruction (Figure 22–6). The right renal artery similarly can be managed with an iliorenal bypass (Figure 22–1), hepatorenal bypass (Figure 22–2), or attachment to the visceral reconstruction limb (Figure 22–5).

Numerous configurations exist for the revascularization of the abdominal aortic branches. As was previously stated, the patient's anatomy, prior surgeries, and the location of aneurysmal and occlusive disease will often dictate your intraoperative strategies for aortic debranching.

Endograft Devices.   As endovascular technologies improve, more devices will become available for use in repairing type IV TAAA. Graft selection remains dependent on patient anatomy.

POSTOPERATIVE CONSIDERATIONS

An analysis of Crawford's experience with 346 type IV TAAA repairs demonstrated a mortality of 6%, renal failure of 24%, and a paraplegia/paraparesis rate of 4%.[23] The Cleveland Clinic examined their outcomes when placing a cross-clamp suprarenally or supravisceral in 138 juxtarenal aneurysms, and found their overall mortality rate to be similar at 5.1%. They also discovered that clamp placement above the visceral arteries, as opposed to suprarenal, was a significant predictor of mortality (11.6% vs. 2.1%) and postoperative renal insufficiency (41.9% vs. 22.1%).[24] Other studies also support that clamping above the renal arteries significantly increases the incidence of postoperative renal dysfunction, requiring dialysis compared with infrarenal clamping.[25,26]

In the hybrid procedure, the aorta is never cross-clamped, allowing for continual perfusion to the abdominal viscera and the spinal cord. Both Fulton et al. and Black et al. reported no incidents of paraplegia following their hybrid procedures.

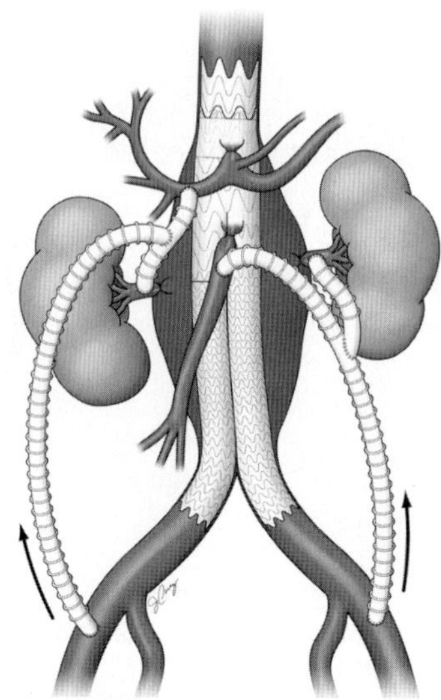

Figure 22-6. Left ileomesenteric-left renal bypass, right ileohepatorenal bypass

Additionally, the mortality for the hybrid procedure in pararenal and type IV TAAAs was 0%.[7,8] In our series, we had one endoleak (type I) that was sealed with the placement of a proximal cuff. No endoleak has been identified in the type IV repair reported by Black et al. after 12 months follow-up. No renal impairment requiring dialysis was reported by Fulton et al., while 2 out of 26 patients required temporary renal support in the patient population reported by Black et al. Graft patencies of visceral bypasses for the hybrid procedures are excellent at 100% and 98% for Fulton et al. and Black et al., respectively. These initial results suggest that similar to infrarenal AAA endovascular repair, visceral bypass combined with endovascular repair of pararenal and type IV TAAAs reduces the morbidity and mortality of open repair.

FUTURE CONSIDERATIONS

Customized, fenestrated stent grafts emerged in 1999 as a possible solution to many of the problems limiting endovascular aneurysm repair (EVAR) in the anatomically unfavorable patients described above. Since that initial report, fenestrated EVAR devices have become commercially available, obtaining the CE mark in Europe and currently undergoing clinical trials in the United States. In addition to fenestrated endografts, branched techniques have been introduced for the treatment of juxtarenal and suprarenal aneurysms.[27–30] Technical and short-term results have been promising with both fenestrated and branched techniques. Recent intermediate studies[31,32] demonstrate safe and effective outcomes in preventing aneurysm rupture while maintaining branch vessel patency.

CONCLUSION

The hybrid procedure presents an attractive alternative to open repair because potential benefits could be gained by the avoidance of supraceliac aortic cross-clamping. Currently, complicated devices that allow for fenestration or branched designs are lacking in the United States or are only in the initial phases of development.[33] Until branched and fenestrated endograft devices become widely distributed, hybrid procedures will be necessary to reduce the major morbidity and mortality associated with pararenal and thoracoabdominal aneurysm repair. In this patient population, the complexity of the disease and comorbid conditions encountered demand that the approach to each patient be individualized. The risks and benefits of all options, including open surgical repair, observation, and hybrid procedures, should be carefully and thoroughly evaluated.

REFERENCES

1. Derrow AE, Seeger JM, Dame DA, et al. The outcome in the United States after thoracoabdominal aortic aneurysm repair, renal artery bypass, and mesenteric revascularization. *J Vasc Surg*. 2001;34:54–61.
2. Cox GS, O'Hara PJ, Hertzer NR, et al. Thoracoabdominal aneurysm repair (a representative experience). *J Vasc Surg*. 1992;15:780–787.
3. Dardik A, Perler BA, Roseborough GS, Williams GM. Aneurysmal expansion of the visceral patch after thoracoabdominal aortic replacement (an argument for limiting patch size?). *J Vasc Surg*. 2001;34:405–409.
4. Vaccaro PS, Elkhammas E, Smead WL. Clinical observations and lessons learned in the treatment of patients with thoracoabdominal aortic aneurysms. *Surg Gynecol Obstet*. 1988;166:461–465.
5. Schepens MA, Defauw JJ, Hamerlijnck RP, et al. Surgical treatment of thoracoabdominal aortic aneurysms by simple crossclamping: Risk factors and late results. *J Thorac Cardiovasc Surg*. 1994;107:134–142.
6. Crawford ES, DeNatale RW. Thoracoabdominal aortic aneurysm (observations regarding the natural course of the disease). *J Vasc Surg*. 1986;3:578–582.
7. Black SA, Wolfe JHN, Clark M, et al. Complex thoracoabdominal aortic aneurysms: Endovascular exclusion with visceral revascularization. *J Vasc Surg*. 2006;43:1081–1089.
8. Fulton JJ, Farber MA, Marston WA, et al. Endovascular stent-graft repair of pararenal and type IV thoracoabdominal aortic aneurysms with adjunctive visceral reconstruction. *J Vasc Surg*. 2005;41:191–198.
9. Rimmer J, Wolfe JH. Type III thoracoabdominal aortic aneurysm repair (a combined surgical and endovascular approach). *Eur J Vasc Endovasc Surg*. 2003;26:677–679.
10. Kotsis T, Scharrer-Pamler R, Kapfer X, et al. Treatment of thoracoabdominal aortic aneurysms with a combined endovascular and surgical approach. *Int Angiol*. 2003;22:125–133.
11. Watanabe Y, Ishimaru S, Kawaguchi S, et al. Successful endografting with simultaneous visceral artery bypass grafting for severely calcified thoracoabdominal aortic aneurysm. *J Vasc Surg*. 2002;35:397–399.
12. Lundbom J, Hatlinghus S, Odegard A, et al. Combined open and endovascular treatment of complex aortic disease. *Vascular*. 2004;12:93–98.
13. Quinones-Baldrich WJ, Panetta TF, Vescera CL, Kashyap VS. Repair of type IV thoracoabdominal aneurysm with a combined endovascular and surgical approach. *J Vasc Surg*. 1999;30:555–560.
14. Chiesa R, Melissano G, Civilini E, et al. Two-stage combined endovascular and surgical approach for recurrent thoracoabdominal aortic aneurysm. *J Endovasc Ther*. 2004;11:330–333.
15. Chaikof EL, Fillinger MF, Matsumura JS, et al. Identifying and grading factors that modify the outcome of endovascular aortic aneurysm repair. *J Vasc Surg*. 2002;35:1061–1066.
16. Dillavou ED, Muluk SC, Rhee RY, et al. Does hostile neck anatomy preclude successful endovascular aortic aneurysm repair? *J Vasc Surg*. 2003;38:657–663.

17. Sternbergh WC, Carter G, York JW, et al. Aortic neck angulation predicts adverse outcome with endovascular abdominal aortic aneurysm repair. *J Vasc Surg*. 2002;35:482–486.

18. Moawad J, McKinsey JF, Wyble CW, et al. Current results of surgical therapy for chronic mesenteric ischemia. *Arch Surg*. 1997;132:613–618.

19. McMillan WD, McCarthy WJ, Bresticker MR, et al. Mesenteric artery bypass (objective patency determination). *J Vasc Surg*. 1995;21:729–740.

20. Farber MA, Carlin RE, Marston WA, et al. Distal thoracic aorta as inflow for the treatment of chronic mesenteric ischemia. *J Vasc Surg*. 2001;33:281–288.

21. Kansal N, LoGerfo FW, Belfield AK, et al. A comparison of antegrade and retrograde mesenteric bypass. *Ann Vasc Surg*. 2002;16:591–596.

22. Park WM, Cherry KJ, Chua HK, et al. Current results of open revascularization for chronic mesenteric ischemia: A standard for comparison. *J Vasc Surg*. 2002;35:853–859.

23. Svensson LG, Crawford ES, Hess KR et al. Experience with 1509 patients undergoing thoracoabdominal aortic operations. *J Vasc Surg*. 1993;17:357–368.

24. Sarac TP, Clair DG, Hertzer NR, et al. Contemporary results of juxtarenal aneurysm repair. *J Vasc Surg*. 2002;36:1104–1111.

25. Green RM, Ricotta JJ, Ouriel K, DeWeese JA. Results of supraceliac aortic clamping in the difficult elective resection of infrarenal abdominal aortic aneurysm. *J Vasc Surg*. 1989;9: 124–134.

26. Jean-Claude JM, Reilly LM, Stoney RJ, Messina LM. Pararenal aortic aneurysms (the future of open aortic aneurysm repair). *J Vasc Surg*. 1999;29:902–912.

27. Faruqi RM, Chuter TA, Reilly LM, et al. Endovascular repair of abdominal aortic aneurysm using a pararenal fenestrated stent-graft. *J Endovasc Surg*. 1999;6:354–358.

28. Adam DJ, Berce M, Hartley DE, Anderson JL. Repair of juxtarenal para-anastomotic aortic aneurysms after previous open repair with fenestrated and branched endovascular stent grafts. *J Vasc Surg*. 2005;42:997–1001.

29. Anderson JL, Adam DJ, Berce M, Hartley DE. Repair of thoracoabdominal aortic aneurysms with fenestrated and branched endovascular stent grafts. *J Vasc Surg*. 2005;42:600–607.

30. Verhoeven EL, Zeebregts CJ, Kapma MR, et al. Fenestrated and branched endovascular techniques for thoraco-abdominal aneurysm repair. *J Cardiovasc Surg (Torino)*. 2005;46: 131–140.

31. O'Neil S, Greenburg RK, Haddad F, et al. A prospective analysis of fenestrated endovascular grafting: Intermediate-term outcomes. *Eur J Vasc Endovasc Surg*. 2006;29:1–9.

32. Muhs BE, Verhoeven ELG, Zeebregts CJ, et al. Mid-term results of endovascular aneurysm repair with branched and fenestrated endografts. *J Vasc Surg*. 2006;44:9–15.

33. Saito N, Kimura T, Odashiro K, et al. Feasibility of the Inoue single-branched stent-graft implantation for thoracic aortic aneurysm or dissection involving the left subclavian artery (short- to medium-term results in 17 patients). *J Vasc Surg*. 2005;41:206–212.

23

Abdominal Aortic Debranching

Robert R. Mendes, M.D.
Mark A. Farber, M.D.

Current therapy for aortic aneurysmal disease is in a state of flux. While endovascular devices have been approved to treat thoracic aortic aneurysms (TAA) and abdominal aortic aneurysms (AAA), branched and fenestrated technology has not yet been approved by the FDA. As a result, debranching techniques have arisen to enable treatment of pararenal aneurysms (PRA) and thoracoabdominal aortic aneurysms (TAAA) in many patients who were deemed untreatable with conventional methods. The conventional repair of these aneurysms requires an aortic crossclamp, either suprarenal, above the celiac trunk, or in the thoracic aorta, which is accompanied by significant physiologic changes, and is associated with increased perioperative morbidity and mortality. Derrow et. al. have reported mortality rates approaching 20%[1] for repair of all types of TAAAs combined. This increased risk is related to visceral and renal ischemia. Morbidity of TAAA repair is also significant with spinal cord ischemia occurring as frequently as 15%, pulmonary complications in up to 40%, and renal impairment in up to 30% of patients.[2-5] Patients with multiple comorbidities are often at high risk for the conventional approach. Some clinicians may advocate a conventional approach; however, the mortality rate of observation approaches 76% at two years with aneurysm rupture responsible for half of these deaths.[6]

Advances in endovascular techniques have made it possible to approach these challenging cases differently without aortic crossclamping. Patients can undergo visceral and renal reconstruction prior to endovascular exclusion of the aneurysm. Stent-graft exclusion with visceral vessel reconstruction has very encouraging early term results, demonstrating no paraplegia in several studies.[7,8] For some groups, this repair has become preferable to the open technique.[7] In this chapter, we will describe techniques for the endovascular repair of pararenal and TAAAs with adjunctive visceral vessel reconstruction in which initial reports have described promising results.[8-14] Whether this approach serves as only a bridge until improved techniques and devices can be developed, or becomes an established method of therapy, remains to be seen.

PREOPERATIVE CONSIDERATIONS

The most common reason for not recommending an endovascular repair of an abdominal aortic aneurysm is an inadequate proximal implantation site. Commercially available stent grafts require a minimal aortic neck length of 15 to 17 mm and an neck angle less than 45 degrees to provide an adequate seal zone.[15,16] While it is crucial that the aortic walls be fairly parallel and free of significant calcification and thrombus, implanting the device in a region where significant angulation exists can also jeopardize the durability of the endovascular repair.

When adverse neck anatomy is present, visceral reconstruction can be used, providing a more favorable implantation site. Often, it may require reconstruction of the celiac, superior mesenteric, and/or renal arteries. Occasionally, a complete abdominal aortic debranching may be necessary. The benefit of complete visceral debranching has been questioned by several authors (personal communication), but does have a role in selected patients with severe CHF in whom aortic crossclamping would not be tolerated.

It should be noted that before performing visceral procedures, it is important to evaluate the anatomic and hemodynamic status of the visceral section including both renal arteries. A preoperative spiral computed tomography angiogram (CTA) or magnetic resonance angiogram (MRA), with 2 to 3 mm intervals combined with sagital and coronal reconstructions of the aorta, provides the most thorough evaluation of the aneurysm, the aorta, and its branches. Occasionally, visceral angiography is necessary when adequate noninvasive imaging cannot be obtained. For hemodynamic evaluation, we have relied on duplex ultrasonography, which has a high degree of accuracy when performed in experienced peripheral vascular laboratories. In addition, it provides baseline information to which postreconstruction evaluations can be compared.

Multiple factors are involved in the determination of which vessels need to be revascularized. Inspection of the aorta and determining where an appropriate landing zone exists is paramount. Once these have been established, the vascular specialist can then determine which vessels need to be reconstructed. Additional factors also play a role and include prohibitive abdominal surgical risks, aberrant vasculature, and occluded target vessels. The most variable is probably the celiac artery. Results with celiac artery ligation have been variable, ranging from no complications to severe liver failure and death. Some individuals believe that pre-existing celiac stenosis or a replaced right hepatic artery arising from the superior mesenteric artery are good indicators that sufficient collateral flow to the liver exists, and the celiac artery revascularization does not need to be performed.

The potential source of inflow must also be determined from the preoperative imaging. Patients with significant aorto-iliac disease may be better suited with an antegrade inflow source from either the thoracic aorta, hepatic, or splenic arteries. If the hepatic or splenic arteries are to provide the inflow source for the bypass, careful evaluation of the celiac axis is essential to ensure it is free of significant disease, which is often determined by duplex ultrasound as mentioned previously. Patients with favorable iliac vessels may undergo retrograde bypasses, some of which can be performed under a regional anesthesia.

Visceral and renal reconstruction should be performed prior to endovascular exclusion of the aneurysm. Reconstruction may be done either concomitantly or sequentially with the endovascular repair. While some reports have shown a higher incidence of complications with concomitant repair, this is a very controversial area. However, when complex cases involving complete debranching of the abdominal aorta or reconstruction using the thoracic aorta as the donor vessel are done, it is important to evaluate the patients at the completion of the first stage to ensure stability before proceeding with the second portion of the simultaneous procedure. In all cases, ligation of the native vessel at its origin must be performed to prevent type II endoleaks.

OPERATIVE CONSIDERATIONS

Pararenal Aneurysms

Patency rates have been assessed in bypass grafting for chronic mesenteric ischemia and renal artery stenosis, and have been reported at 90% to 95% at 36 months in some series.[18,19] While this is encouraging, no long-term data currently exist to document the patency of bypass grafts for the purpose of aortic debranching.

Unilateral renal artery bypass.   This is typically used when one kidney is non-functional or the patient has one renal artery that is located more caudal than the other. Revascularization options for this configuration include the ipsilateral external iliac vessel or the hepatic or splenic artery for a right and left approach, respectively. If a retrograde approach is desired, then the donor site location is typically chosen as the external iliac artery because it is almost always spared in aneurysmal disease. In addition, this technique ensures an adequate distal seal site can be achieved, either in the common iliac artery, or in cases with concomitant common iliac disease, in the external iliac, proximal to the bypass. Additionally, ilio-renal bypasses can be performed using regional anesthesia if desired. Typically, an oblique retroperitoneal incision is made. Dissection is performed through the muscular layers of the abdominal wall, the intact peritoneum is retracted medially, and the retroperitoneal space is entered laterally. Both the renal artery and the external iliac artery can be exposed from this approach. The bypass origin site is determined by the presence of occlusive disease, aneurysmal involvement, and the planned landing zone of the endograft. Proximal and distal control of the target vessels is then obtained and a 6-8 mm polytetrafluoroethylene (PTFE) graft is used for the bypass (Figure 23–1). While we have typically chosen PTFE to construct our bypasses, others have obtained excellent success with dacron-based conduits. After confirmation of the graft patency with a continuous wave doppler, the proximal renal artery is ligated. Placement of large hemoclips to mark the iliac anastamotic site can prove useful for future endovascular interventions.

Hepatorenal bypass.   Designed primarily to treat renal occlusive disease before endovascular techniques, the bypass procedure can be used to provide an extra-anatomical bypass to either the right renal artery or the celiac artery when used in "reverse" fashion.

This option is often chosen when small external iliac or aorto-iliac occlusive disease exists. Most procedures are performed through a subcostal incision, although a midline celiotomy can be used if necessary. The hepatic artery is identified through the lesser omentum. Control of, and anastamosis to, the hepatic artery proximal to the gastroduodenal artery (GDA) is ideal but not always possible. The duodenum is mobilized medially using a Kocher maneuver, the renal vein is identified, and the right renal artery is controlled by vessel loops. An appropriate conduit, either autologous or synthetic, should be chosen to match the target vessel diameters. Some surgeons prefer autologous saphenous vein when treating patients with occlusive renal disease because it may impart a greater long-term patency. This, however, has not been documented in the treatment of patients without occlusive disease. We have found SVG to be easier to manipulate and handle in these circumstances.

After systemic heparinization, the end-to-side renal anastomosis is usually performed first, followed by the hepatic artery reconstruction in an end-to-side fashion. Generally, the bypass follows a gentle curved "C" configuration (Figure 23–2). If needed, an end-to-end anastomosis can be performed to the GDA. Caution should be taken when the GDA is used because it provides important mesenteric collateral flow. Again, ligation of the proximal right renal artery should be performed to avoid the potential for subsequent type II endoleak.

Splenorenal bypass.   Similar to the hepatorenal bypass, the splenorenal bypass may be utilized in patients requiring left renal revascularization without an acceptable external iliac donor artery. A midline celiotomy or a left subcostal incision may be used for vascular exposure. In either case, the posterior pancreas is mobilized by cephalad reflection of its inferior border. The splenic artery is mobilized from the left gastroepiploic artery to its distal branching point. The left adrenal vein is divided, which allows for the caudal retraction of the left renal vein. At this point, the splenic

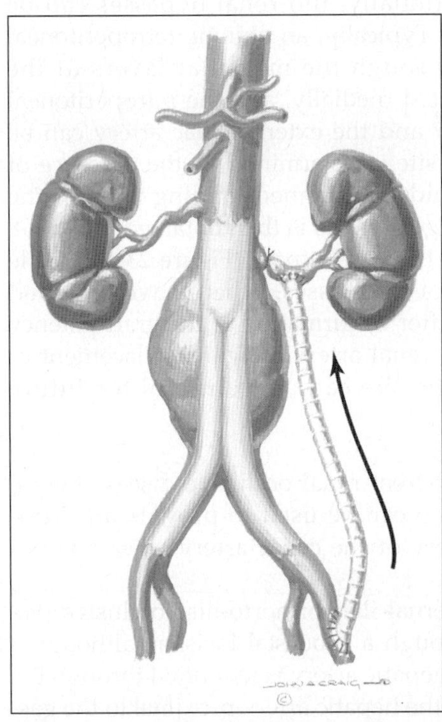

Figure 23-1. Pararenal aortic aneurysm excluded by performing a left iliorenal bypass and EVAR.

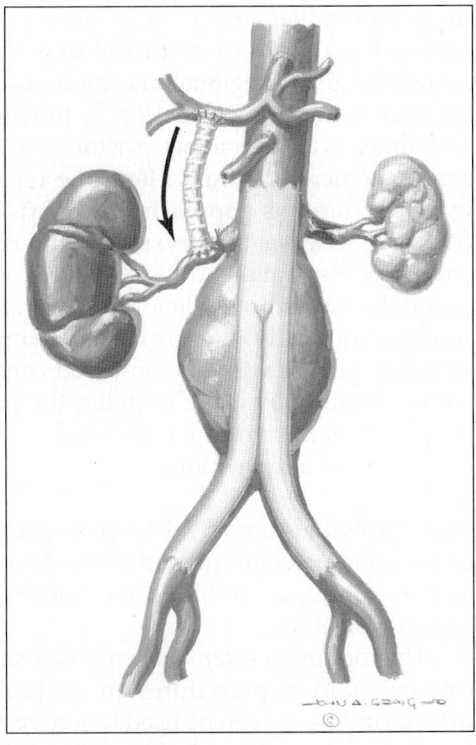

Figure 23-2. Hybrid repair of a pararenal aortic aneurysm utilizing a hepatorenal bypass to provide adequate neck length and an infrarenal device.

artery is divided, spatulated, and anastomosed to the left renal artery in an end-to-end manner. In certain situations, an interposition bypass can be utilized, and if the renal artery is exceptionally close, a direct end-to-side anastomosis can be performed to the splenic artery without dividing it.

The procedures above all include endovascular abdominal aortic aneurysm repair to completely exclude the aneurysm in a single stage repair. Access to the abdominal aorta is commonly via bilateral common femoral artery exposure or through the retroperitoneal exposure used for the iliorenal bypass. If necessary, the endovascular exclusion can be performed in a second-stage procedure. In cases where the external iliac artery has been chosen as a donor vessel, careful consideration should be given to the primary access site. Since most endovascular device have a main component system that is larger than the secondary components, the main body should be inserted on the iliac side, which has not been selected as a donor vessel, to avoid damage to the bypass from the delivery catheter and temporary occlusion of the bypass during endovascular exclusion.

THORACOABDOMINAL AORTIC ANEURYSMS (COMPLETE AORTIC DEBRANCHING)

In a large number of patients, the celiac and SMA are located in proximity to one another, and both vessels must be relocated to ensure adequate neck length. The choice of inflow source is usually determined by either previous aortic surgery or the extent of aneurysmal or occlusive disease. Our studies demonstrate that antegrade revascularization to the mesenteric vessels from the descending thoracic aorta has a low morbidity and excellent patency rates (100%) at 34 months.[20] In this situation, the descending thoracic aorta is controlled with a side biting clamp, which allows for continual perfusion to the abdominal viscera and the spinal cord. We believe the avoidance of visceral ischemia and spinal cord ischemia from complete aortic clamping is important in limiting potential complications.

In a comparison of mesenteric bypasses, studies have not found any significant difference in patency between antegrade and retrograde bypass grafts.[21,22] It is important to note, however, that the supraciliac aorta, and not the descending thoracic aorta, was used as the inflow for the antegrade bypasses in these studies. Generally speaking, the descending thoracic aorta is relatively free of atherosclerotic disease, and it may provide a more consistent inflow source for the antegrade bypass graft.

Thoracoceliac with thoracomesenteric-left renal bypass (antegrade bypass). This is utilized in highly selected patients who require a complete aortic debranching prior to the placement of the endovascular exclusion device. The patient is intubated with a double lumen endotrachial tube to allow for intraoperative deflation of the left lung to ease in exposure of the distal descending thoracic aorta. The patient is then positioned in a right lateral decubitus position, often with the aid of an axillary roll and bean bag for patient stabilization. The thoracoabdominal incision is made through the ninth rib interspace for best exposure of the distal thoracic and upper abdominal aorta.

The peritoneal contents are bluntly dissected from the undersurface of the diaphragm, retracting anteriorly, while the left kidney remains posterior in the retroperitoneum to facilitate the exposure of the mesenteric vasculature. The diaphragm is then incised in a curvilinear fashion 2 cm from its costal edge to preserve its innervation. Suture markers are placed as the diaphragm is taken down to ease reapproximation. If necessary, the diaphragm can be left intact and the bypasses tunneled next to the aorta. The inferior pulmonary ligament and the crus are often divided to facilitate exposure. The mesenteric vessels are exposed for 5 to 7 cm to provide a suitable bypass site.

The descending thoracic aorta is clamped with a single side biting Beck clamp during the proximal anastomosis of both bypasses to allow for continued perfusion to the viscera and minimize trauma to the aorta. Prosthetic bypass graft conduits are used and routed through the diaphragmatic hiatus to their respective vessels in an end-to-side fashion to establish antegrade flow. We typically use two separate grafts for mesenteric bypass. In our opinion, this allows greater freedom in graft orientation, although a bifurcated graft is an acceptable alternative. Revascularization of the left kidney is accomplished with a bypass graft from the thoracomesenteric graft to the left renal artery (Figure 23–3). After completion of all bypass grafts, the proximal celiac, superior mesenteric, and left renal arteries are ligated. Caution is advised in this situation. If a type II endoleak from the celiac, mesenteric, or renal artery occurs after the deployment of the stent graft, access is extremely limited, if not impossible, via endovascular means. The inferior border of the thoracic anastomosis is marked with a large clip to aid in identification for future endovascular interventions.

The second stage of the repair consists of a bypass graft from the right external iliac artery to the right renal artery through a retroperitoneal exposure, as described above. Endovascular abdominal aortic aneurysm repair completes the exclusion of the aneurysm.

Iliomesenteric reconstructions (retrograde bypass).   A transperitoneal abdominal approach is used to expose the abdominal aorta and the origins of the renal arteries, the celiac axis, and the SMA. Once again, the location of the iliac donor site is critical. The bypass may need to originate from either the very distal common iliac or external iliac artery. Either the left, right, or both iliac arteries may be used as an inflow source for the bypasses. Currently, we prefer to use individual ringed PTFE grafts, but bifurcated grafts may also be used as a conduit. The graft to the SMA is placed in a "lazy C" configuration as the graft lays better with less potential to kink. The limb to the celiac axis is tunneled anterior to the renal vein through the loose tissue in the retropancreatic space (Figure 23–4). The anastomosis is performed to the inferior aspect of the common hepatic artery or splenic artery, based on the best orientation and anatomy.

The celiac artery may also be revascularized via a right iliohepatic bypass that courses along the right retroperitoneum (Figure 23–5), taken off a right iliorenal bypass, or have a hepatorenal bypass supplied by an iliac inflow source (Figure 23–6). Ligation of vessel origins completes the debranching of the abdominal aorta prior to endovascular exclusion. When concomitant renal artery reconstruction is required, the renal arteries can be divided and directly anastomosed to the SMA on the left, and the ilioceliac bypass on the right.

Complete visceral revascularization (retrograde).   Each renal artery should be considered separately. For the left renal artery, three options exist: splenorenal bypass, iliorenal bypass (Figure 23–1), or attachment to one limb of the celiac or SMA reconstruction (Figure 23–6). The right renal artery can be managed similarly with an

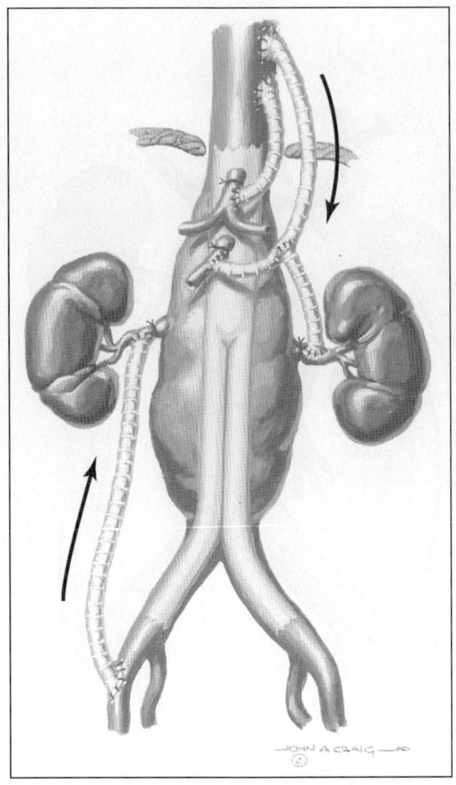

Figure 23-3. Type IV TAAA repair using a thoracoceliac, thoracomesenteric, thoraco-left renal and right iliorenal bypass in conjunction with EVAR.

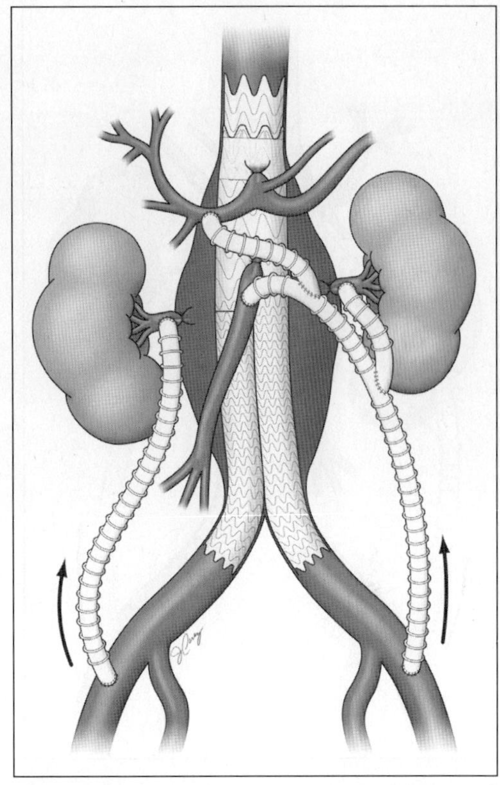

Figure 23-4. Repair of a type IV TAAA using retrograde right iliorenal bypass, left ilio-SMA, celiac, and left renal bypasses and EVAR.

iliorenal bypass (Figure 23–1), hepatorenal bypass (Figure 23–2), or attachment to the visceral reconstruction limb (Figure 23–5).

Numerous configurations exist for the revascularization of the abdominal aortic branches. As was previously stated, the patient's anatomy, prior surgeries, and the location of aneurysmal and occlusive disease will often dictate the intraoperative strategies for aortic debranching.

Endograft devices.   As endovascular technologies improve, more devices will become available for use in repairing pararenal and TAAA. Graft selection remains dependent on patient anatomy, instruction for use, and a surgeon's experience.

POSTOPERATIVE CONSIDERATIONS

An analysis of Crawford's experience with 346 type IV TAAA repairs demonstrated a mortality of 6%, renal failure of 24%, and a paraplegia/paraparesis rate of 4%. The Cleveland Clinic examined its outcomes when placing a crossclamp suprarenally or supravisceral in 138 juxtarenal aneurysms and found the overall mortality rate to be

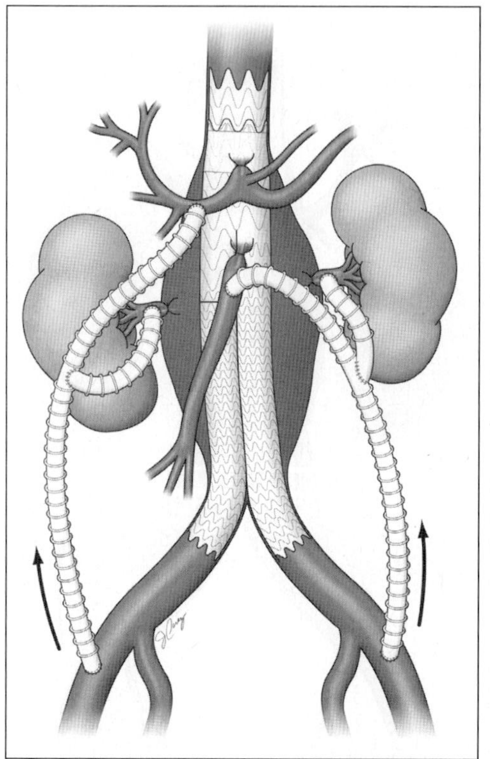

Figure 23-5. Complete visceral debranching using right iliorenal and celiac bypass, and left ilio-SMA and left renal bypass, along with an infrarenal device.

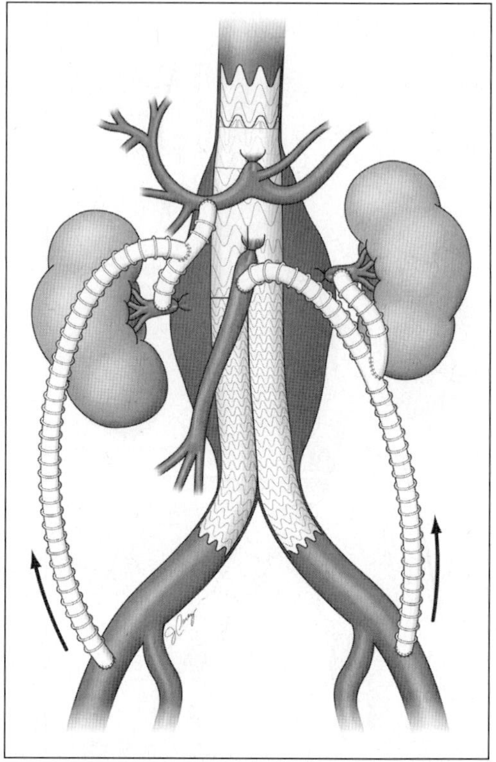

Figure 23-6. Type IV TAAA hybrid repair performed via hepatorenal bypass used in conjunction with a right iliac-based inflow.

similar at 5.1%.[23] The Cleveland Clinic also discovered that clamp placement above the visceral arteries, as opposed to suprarenal, was a significant predictor of mortality (11.6% versus 2.1%) and postoperative renal insufficiency (41.9% versus 22.1%).[24] Other studies also support that clamping above the renal arteries significantly increases the incidence of postoperative renal dysfunction, requiring dialysis, compared with infrarenal clamping.[25,26]

In the aforementioned hybrid procedures, the aorta is never crossclamped, allowing for continual perfusion to the abdominal viscera and the spinal cord. Both Fulton et. al. and Black et. al. reported no incidents of paraplegia following their hybrid procedures. Additionally, the mortality rate for the hybrid procedure in pararenal and type IV TAAAs was 0%.[7,8] In our series, we had one endoleak (type I) that was sealed with the placement of a proximal cuff. No renal impairment requiring dialysis was reported by Fulton et. al., while two out of 26 patients required temporary renal support in the patient population reported by Black et. al. Graft patency of visceral bypasses for the hybrid procedures are excellent at 100% and 98% for Fulton et. al. and Black et. al., respectively. These initial results suggest that similar to infrarenal AAA endovascular repair, visceral bypass combined with endovascular repair of pararenal and TAAAs reduces the morbidity and mortality of open repair.

FUTURE CONSIDERATIONS

Customized, fenestrated stent grafts emerged in 1999 as a possible solution to many of the problems limiting endovascular aneurysm repair (EVAR) in the anatomically unfavorable patients described above. Since that initial report,[27] fenestrated EVAR devices have become commercially available, obtaining the CE mark in Europe, and are currently undergoing clinical trial in the United States. In addition to fenestrated endografts, branched techniques have been introduced for the treatment of juxtarenal, suprarenal aneurysms, and TAAAs.[28,29] Technical and short-term results have been promising with both fenestrated and branched techniques.[30] Recent intermediate studies[31,32] demonstrate safe and effective outcomes in preventing aneurysm rupture while maintaining branch vessel patency. However, certain anatomic situations may arise that prohibit all branches from being revascularized by this method. For this reason, it is important for the vascular specialist to be familiar with the above techniques to provide all possible options for their patients.

CONCLUSION

The hybrid procedure presents an attractive alternative to open repair because potential benefits could be gained by the avoidance of aortic crossclamping. Currently, complicated devices that allow for fenestration or branched designs are not approved in the United States or are only in the initial phases in clinical trials.[33] Until branched and fenestrated endograft devices become widely distributed, hybrid procedures will be necessary to reduce the major morbidity and mortality associated with pararenal and thoracoabdominal aneurysm repair in high-risk patients. In this patient population, the complexity of the disease and comorbid conditions encountered demand that the approach to each patient be individualized. The risks and benefits of all options, including open surgical repair, observation, and hybrid procedures, should be carefully and thoroughly evaluated.

REFERENCES

1. Derrow AE, Seeger JM, Dame DA, Carter RL, Ozaki CK, Flynn TC, et al. The outcome in the United States after thoracoabdominal aortic aneurysm repair, renal artery bypass, and mesenteric revascularization. *J Vasc Surg.* 2001; 34: 54–61.
2. Cox GS, O'Hara PJ, Hertzer NR, Piedmonte MR, Krajewski LP, Beven EG. Thoracoabdominal aneurysm repair (a representative experience). *J Vasc Surg.* 1992; 15:780–787.
3. Dardik A, Perler BA, Roseborough GS, Williams GM .Aneurysmal expansion of the visceral patch after thoracoabdominal aortic replacement (an argument for limiting patch size?). *J Vasc Surg.* 2001; 34:405–409.
4. Vaccaro PS, Elkhammas E, Smead WL. Clinical observations and lessons learned in the treatment of patients with thoracoabdominal aortic aneurysms. *Surg Gynecol Obstet.* 1988; 166: 461–465.
5. Schepens MA, Defauw JJ, Hamerlijnck RP, De Geest R, Vermeulen FE. Surgical treatment of thoracoabdominal aortic aneurysms by simple crossclamping. Risk factors and late results .*J Thorac Cardiovasc Surg.* 1994; 107: 134–142.

6. Crawford ES, DeNatale RW .Thoracoabdominal aortic aneurysm (observations regarding the natural course of the disease). *J Vasc Surg*. 1986; 3: 578–582.

7. Black SA, Wolfe JHN, Clark M, Hamady M, Cheshire NJW, Jenkins MP. Complex thoracoabdominal aortic aneurysms: Endovascular exclusion with visceral revascularization. *J Vasc Surg*. 2006; 43:1081–1089.

8. Fulton JJ, Farber MA, Marston WA, Mendes R, Mauro MA, Keagy BA. Endovascular stent-graft repair of pararenal and type IV thoracoabdominal aortic aneurysms with adjunctive visceral reconstruction. *J Vasc Surg*. 2005; 41: 191–198.

9. Rimmer J, Wolfe JH. Type III thoracoabdominal aortic aneurysm repair (a combined surgical and endovascular approach). *Eur J Vasc Endovasc Surg*. 2003; 26: 677–679.

10. Kotsis T, Scharrer-Pamler R, Kapfer X, Liewald F, Gorich J, Sunder-Plassmann L, et al.Treatment of thoracoabdominal aortic aneurysms with a combined endovascular and surgical approach. *Int Angiol*. 2003; 22: 125–133.

11. Watanabe Y, Ishimaru S, Kawaguchi S, Shimazaki T, Yokoi Y, Ito M, et al. Successful endografting with simultaneous visceral artery bypass grafting for severely calcified thoracoabdominal aortic aneurysm. *J Vasc Surg*. 2002; 35: 397–399.

12. Lundbom J, Hatlinghus S, Odegard A, Eide TO, Lange C, Aasland J, et al. Combined open and endovascular treatment of complex aortic disease. *Vascular*. 2004; 12: 93–98.

13. Quinones-Baldrich WJ, Panetta TF, Vescera CL, Kashyap VS. Repair of type IV thoracoabdominal aneurysm with a combined endovascular and surgical approach. *J Vasc Surg*. 1999; 30: 555–560.

14. Chiesa R, Melissano G, Civilini E, Setacci F, Tshomba Y, Anzuini A. Two-stage combined endovascular and surgical approach for recurrent thoracoabdominal aortic aneurysm. *J Endovasc Ther*. 2004; 11: 330–333.

15. Chaikof EL, Fillinger MF, Matsumura JS, Rutherford RB, White GH, Blankensteijn JD, et al. Identifying and grading factors that modify the outcome of endovascular aortic aneurysm repair. *J Vasc Surg*. 2002; 35:1061–1066.

16. Dillavou ED, Muluk SC, Rhee RY, Tzeng E, Woody JD, Gupta N, et al.. Does hostile neck anatomy preclude successful endovascular aortic aneurysm repair? *J Vasc Surg*. 2003; 38:657–663.

17. Sternbergh WC, Carter G, York JW, Yoselevitz M, Money SR. Aortic neck angulation predicts adverse outcome with endovascular abdominal aortic aneurysm repair. *J Vasc Surg*. 2002; 35:482–486.

18. Moawad J, McKinsey JF, Wyble CW, Bassiouny HS, Schwartz LB, Gewertz BL. Current results of surgical therapy for chronic mesenteric ischemia. *Arch Surg*. 1997; 132: 613–618.

19. McMillan WD, McCarthy WJ, Bresticker MR, Pearce WH, Schneider JR, Golan JF, et al. Mesenteric artery bypass (objective patency determination). *J Vasc Surg*. 1995; 21: 729–740.

20. Farber MA, Carlin RE, Marston WA, Owens LV, Burnham SJ, Keagy BA. Distal thoracic aorta as inflow for the treatment of chronic mesenteric ischemia. *J Vasc Surg*. 2001; 33: 281–288.

21. Kansal N, LoGerfo FW, Belfield AK, Pomposelli FB, Hamdan AD, Angle N, et al. A comparison of antegrade and retrograde mesenteric bypass. *Ann Vasc Surg*. 2002; 16: 591–596.

22. Park WM, Cherry KJ, Chua HK, Clark RC, Jenkins G, Harmsen WS, Noel AA, Panneton JM, Bower TC, Hallett JW, Gloviczki P. Current results of open revascularization for chronic mesenteric ischemia: A standard for comparison. *J Vasc Surg*. 2002; 35: 853–859.

23. Svensson LG, Crawford ES, Hess KR, Coselli JS, Safi HJ. Experience with 1509 patients undergoing thoracoabdominal aortic operations. *J Vasc Surg*. 1993; 17:357–368.

24. Sarac TP, Clair DG, Hertzer NR, Greenberg RK, Krajewski LP, O'Hara PJ, et al.. Contemporary results of juxtarenal aneurysm repair. *J Vasc Surg*. 2002; 36:1104–1111.

25. Green RM, Ricotta JJ, Ouriel K, DeWeese JA. Results of supraceliac aortic clamping in the difficult elective resection of infrarenal abdominal aortic aneurysm. *J Vasc Surg*. 1989; 9:124–134.

26. Jean-Claude JM, Reilly LM, Stoney RJ, Messina LM. Pararenal aortic aneurysms (the future of open aortic aneurysm repair). *J Vasc Surg*. 1999;29:902–912.

27. Faruqi RM, Chuter TA, Reilly LM, Sawhney R, Wall S, Canto C, et al.. Endovascular repair of abdominal aortic aneurysm using a pararenal fenestrated stent-graft. *J Endovasc Surg.* 1999;6:354–358.

28. Adam DJ, Berce M, Hartley DE, Anderson JL. Repair of juxtarenal para-anastomotic aortic aneurysms after previous open repair with fenestrated and branched endovascular stent grafts. *J Vasc Surg.* 2005;42:997–1001.

29. Anderson JL, Adam DJ, Berce M, Hartley DE. Repair of thoracoabdominal aortic aneurysms with fenestrated and branched endovascular stent grafts. *J Vasc Surg.* 2005;42:600–607.

30. Verhoeven EL, Zeebregts CJ, Kapma MR, Tielliu IF, Prins TR, van den Dungen JJ. Fenestrated and branched endovascular techniques for thoraco-abdominal aneurysm repair. *J Cardiovasc Surg* (Torino). 2005;46:131–140.

31. O'Neil S, Greenburg RK, Haddad F, Resch T, Sereika J, Katz E. A prospective analysis of fenestrated endovascular grafting: Intermediate-term outcomes. *Eur J Vasc Endovasc Surg.* 2006 Mar 29: 1–9.

32. Muhs BE, Verhoeven ELG, Zeebregts CJ, Tielliu IFJ, Prins TR, Verhagen HJM, van den Dungen JJAM. Mid-term results of endovascular aneurysm repair with branched and fenestrated endografts. *J Vasc Surg.* 2006; 44: 9–15.

33. Saito N, Kimura T, Odashiro K, Toma M, Nobuyoshi M, Ueno K, et al. .Feasibility of the Inoue single-branched stent-graft implantation for thoracic aortic aneurysm or dissection involving the left subclavian artery (short- to medium-term results in 17 patients). *J Vasc Surg.* 2005; 41: 206–212.

24

Debranching of the Thoracic Aortic

Alan B. Lumsden, M.D., Eric K. Peden, M.D.,
J.C. Walkes, M.D., Michael J. Reardon, M.D.

With the approval of the TAG, thoracic aortic endograft in April 2005, physicians treating thoracic aortic aneurismal disease were provided with an important new tool for managing patients with this challenging aortic problem. Although the FDA approval was specifically for descending aortic aneurysms, it has been increasingly used to treat aneurismal disease, which extends into and over the aortic arch and the thoracoabdominal segment, albeit supported by a variety of bypass procedures. These adjunctive bypass operations are simply designed to convert the aorta into a simple tube, which can be treated with the TAG device. Although the concept of hybrid procedures has been popularized for use in the thoracic aorta, we described its use for an unusually low left renal artery for an infrarenal abdominal aortic aneurysm, treated with a stent graft.[1] The concepts, then, are exactly the same: provide a seal zone of adequate length and diameter to permit placement of an endograft. In the discussion below, we have divided the "debranching procedures into the aortic arch and visceral aortic segment. In patients with extensive aortic disease, both segments might need to be addressed.[1,2] The considerations and technical challenges involved in these procedures is described below.

THE AORTIC ARCH

Preoperative evaluation. As with all endograft procedures, careful preoperative evaluation, in most cases with thin slice CT scanning, is the imaging technique of choice. Three-dimensional reconstruction is particularly of value in the aortic arch because of tortuosity, the fact that slices through the arch make cuts along the lumen of the arch in a variety of unpredictable directions. The role of the thoracic CT is to determine whether there is an adequate landing zone distal to the left subclavian artery. Although the

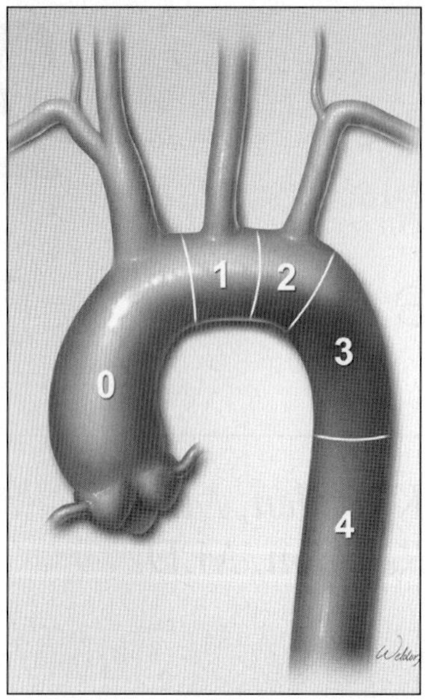

Figure 24-1. Zones of the aortic arch.

definition of a landing zone will be in flux as new devices become available, at the time of writing, this implies less than 38 mm diameter and 2 cams. length. To categorize endovascular repairs of TAAs, Criado and colleagues[4] mapped the thoracic aorta into five landing zones. Briefly, zone 0 involves the origin of the innominate artery, zone 1 involves the orifice of the left CCA, and zone 2 involves the origin of the left subclavian artery, whereas zones 3 and 4 include the descending thoracic aorta. More importantly, a stent graft landing in zone 1 will compromise the left CCA flow, and one landing in zone 0 compromises both the left CCA and innominate artery flows (Figure 24–1).

ZONE TWO DEPLOYMENTS

Any patient in whom an adequate landing zone is not available distal to the left subclavian artery is considered for subclavian coverage. This has been widely practiced, is even permitted in the many IDE trials, which have been completed and are currently underway. Indeed, sacrifice of the left subclavian artery was not even considered as part of the debranching concept until interventionalists began to consider extending endograft deployment to cover the common carotid artery. Similarly, as other aortic pathologies have begun to be treated, and much longer aortic segments covered than were permitted with the IDE trials, so has the potential role of the left subclavian artery, particularly in the blood supply of the spinal cord has been emphasized. The important role of the left vertebral artery—has been increasingly recognized. Revascularization of the left subclavian artery, by either carotid subclavian bypass or subclavian to carotid translocation, has consequently undergone evaluation and reevaluation as our experience has evolved.[5-9] Initially, our practice was to bypass all subclavian arteries in which planned coverage was anticipated. This was clearly an overuse of the procedure. This was followed by a period in which very few carotid

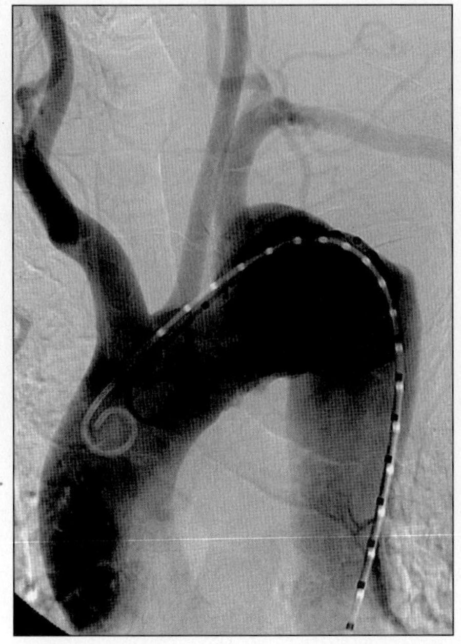

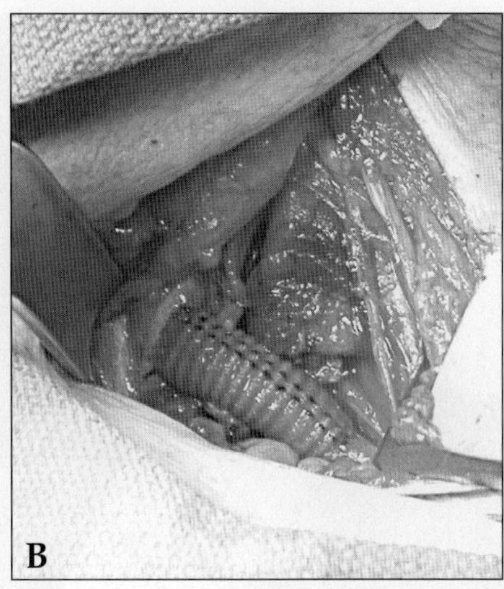

A

Figure 24-2. A Aneurysm which extends to the origin of the left subclavian artery. **B** Dacron graft used for left carotid to left subclavian artery bypass.

subclavian bypass procedures were performed. Contemporary practice involves selective subclavian revascularization:

Prior LIMA use for CABG
Critical left vertebral artery[10]
Atretic right vertebral artery
Absent right vertebral artery
Known left PICA syndrome
Extensive aortic coverage
Aortic dissections
Any patient in whom carotid-to-carotid bypass is performed for left CCA revascularization.

Although many advocate use of subclavian transposition over bypass, this has never been our practice for several reasons (Figures 24–2A and 24–2B). In the setting of a LIMA to LAD, transposition is contraindicated; bypass is preferable in order to maintain antegrade flow. Secondly, all of these patients have a large arch aneurysm, which can project up into the apex of the left chest and distort the mediastinum, complicating proximal exposure and ligation of the subclavian artery. In the future, single branched endografts or endovascualr techniques that preserve side branches might be available for perfusion of the subclavian artery[11] (Figure 24–3).

ZONE ONE DEPLOYMENT

When there remains an inadequate landing zone by deploying across the left subclavian artery using all of zone 2, it becomes necessary to deploy over the left common

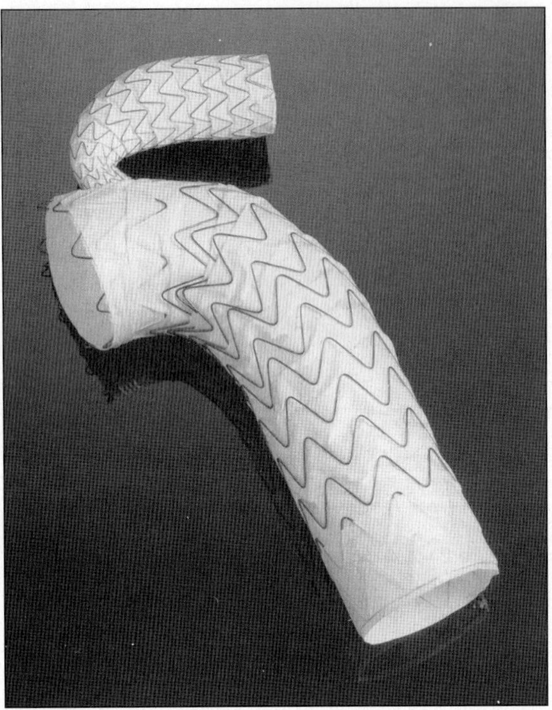

Figure 24-3. Proposed single branched thoracic aortic endograft under development from WL Gore.

carotid artery; that is, across all of zone 1. Although in diagrams such as ours, this looks appealing; in practice, it usually is very short and practically adds a minimum length to the landing zone (Figure 24–4). Another factor that affects the decision to perform a zone 1 deployment is anatomy of the common carotid origin (a wide fun-

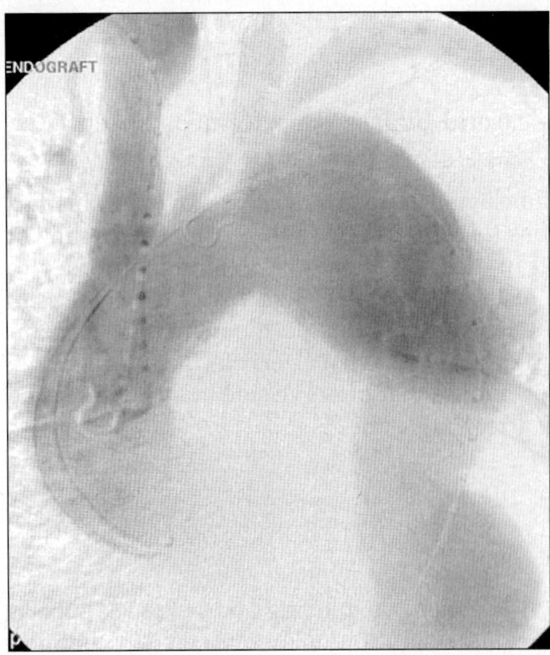

Figure 24-4. Complex aneurysm involving the left subclavian artery

neled origin may lead to displacement of the endograft up into the CCA origin. The presence of a vertebral artery arising form the arch between the left CCA and left subclavian artery must be carefully evaluated. There are, however, a few patients in whom this is appropriate. Consequently, common carotid-to-common carotid artery bypass is performed on any patient in whom the left CCA origin is to be covered, we routinely add carotid to left subclavian bypass as part of the procedure (Figures 24–5A and 24–5B).

The carotid-to-carotid bypass can be performed using either a looped subcutaneous graft or a retropharyngeal tunnel. Our preference is the subcutaneous route, but either is appropriate. When the interventionalist misjudges the adequacy of zone for endograft deployment, either partial coverage of the innominate origin occurs, or a persistent type I endoleak necessitates innominate bypass as described below in order to permit endograft extension.

ZONE ZERO DEPLOYMENT

When the aneurysm extends or is proximal to the innominate, then the complexity of the procedure increases dramatically.[2,3,12-14] Some of these patients have had segmental aortic replacement and this knowledge is very important in case planning. For example, prior descending thoracic aortic replacement in one case allowed us to debranch in standard fashion while using the descending thoracic aortic graft as inflow (Figures 24–6A and 24–6B). Prior ascending replacement provides a secure landing zone and safe clamp site for aorto-innominate bypass. Knowledge of the diameter of the implanted dacron graft is not very relevant as the graft dilates significantly. CT measurement of the graft diameter is always much greater than reported on an operation report. The quality of the ascending aorta is all important in performing aorto-innominate bypass: aneurysmal thinning was the cause on death in one of our patients, in whom we elected not to replace the ascending, and she died from suture line bleeding 24 hours postprocedure (Figures 24–7A and 24–7B). Heavy calcification likewise can result in catastrophic clamp complications.

The incision used to approach the ascending aorta is, in most cases, a median sternotomy (Figure 24–8). This is tolerated by even fairly sick patients, and provides excellent exposure to the ascending aorta and innominate and left common carotid arteries. In most cases, the left subclavian can be exposed, although this is completely dependent on arch and aneurysm anatomy.

When the aneurysm involves the ascending aorta, arch, and proximal descending aorta, our preference is one-stage open repair with deployment of an endograft through a side branch off the ascending aorta or aorto-innominate bypass graft. We have largely given up elephant trunks in favor of this one-stage repair, performing an end-to-end anastamosis in the distal arch followed by endograft deployment in antegrade fashion (Figures 24–9A and 24–9B).

ELEPHANT TRUNK ISSUES

There are several options for endograft placement during arch and descending aortic repair.

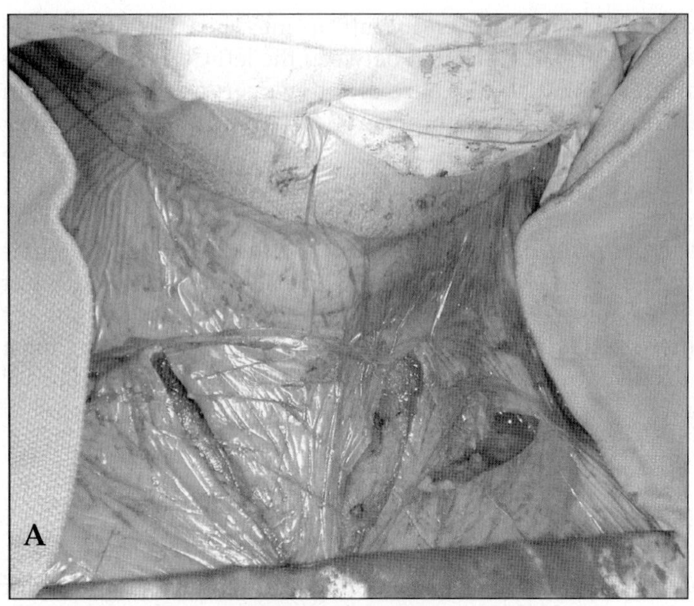

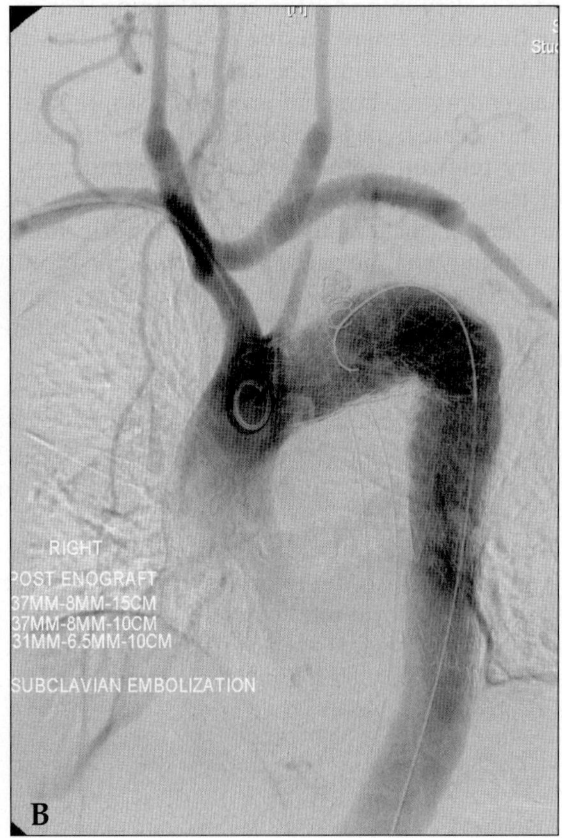

Figure 24-5. (A) Cervical incisions used to create a carotid-to-carotid bypass and left carotid-to-subcalavian bypass graft. **(B)** Completion angiogram demonstrating end-to-side (right common carotid-to-end left common carotid) bypass. Second dacron graft arises from the CCA to CCA graft, and is end to side into the left subclavian. The proximal stump of the Left CCA still fills with contrast while embolization coils occlude the origin of the left subclavian artery. A TAG thoracic endograft has been deployed flush with the origin of the left CCA.

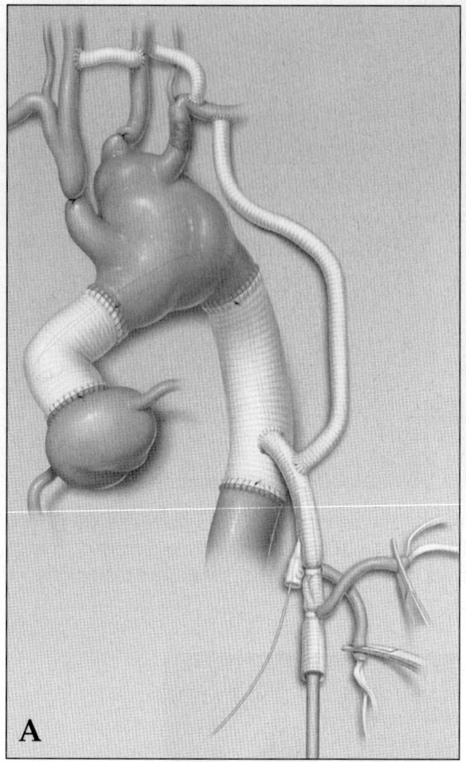

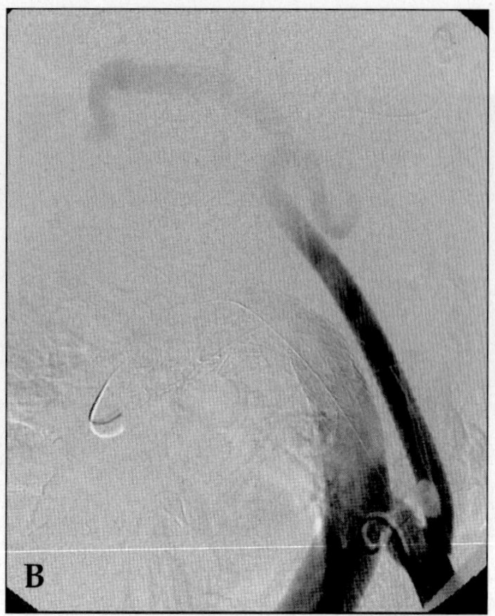

Figure 24-6. (A) Diagram of the debranching technique used in a patient who had a prior short ascending repair and repair of the descending thoracic aorta. It was felt that originating a graft from the ascending graft would have resulted in inadequate length for a seal zone. (B) Completion angiogram showing how the stent graft had been deployed through a conduit sewn to the descending thoracic aortic dacron graft.

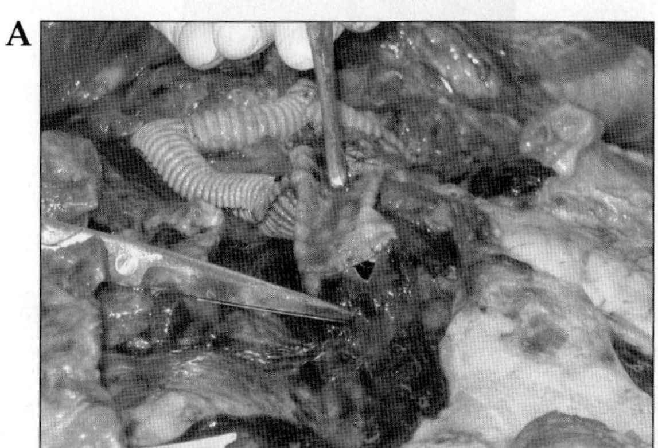

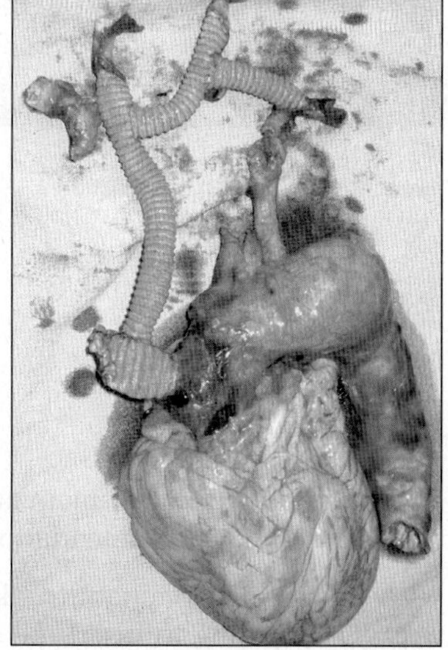

Figure 24-7. (A) Site of postopertive bleeding, a torn suture line in a thin ascending aorta. (B) Autopsy picture from the same patient demonstrating the configuration of the graft arrangement for total arch debranching.

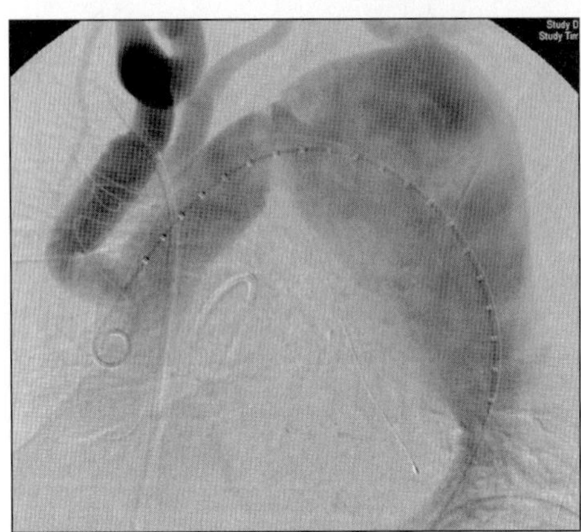

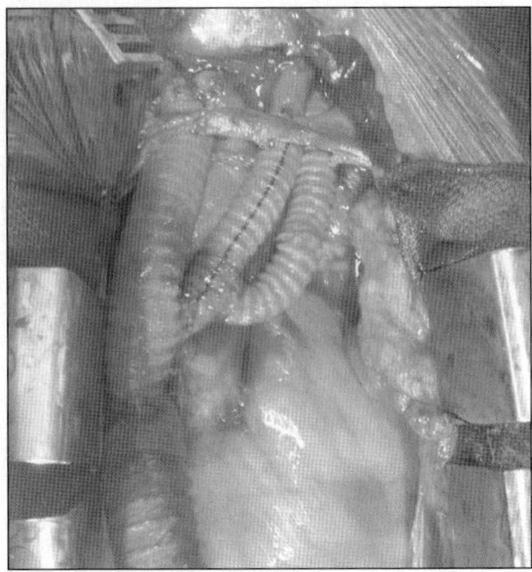

Figure 24-8. A median sternotomy provides excellent exposure of the ascending aorta, innominate artery, and left common carotid. In most cases, it is possible as in this illustration, to reach the left subclavian artery. It is divided close to the aorta and end-to-end anastomosis is created. This provides direct revascularization of the left vertebral artery.

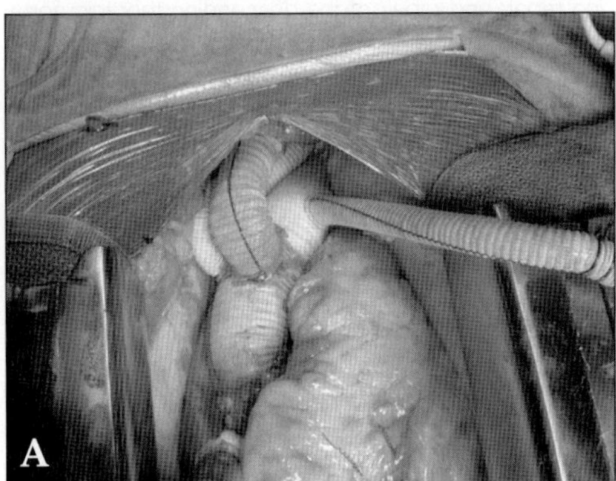

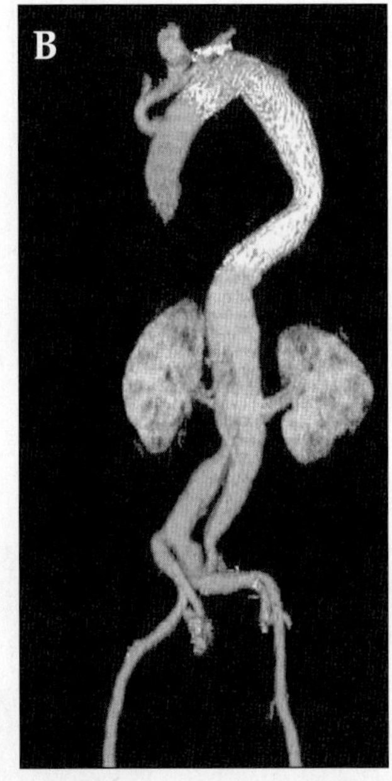

Figure 24-9. (A) and (B). Elephant trunk.

Standard arch replacement and elephant trunk with delayed retrograde endograft placement.[15] Our recommendations are:

1. Shorten the elephant trunk so that it does not flop around inside the aneurysm when trying to insert the endograft in retrograde fashion (Figures 24–10A and 24–10B).
2. Mark the end of the elephant trunk, either with large ligaclips or by sewing on the radio-opaque wren from a lap pad around the circumference of the graft.

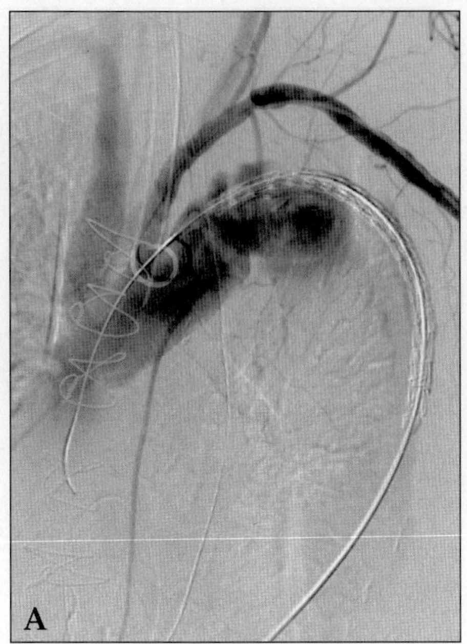
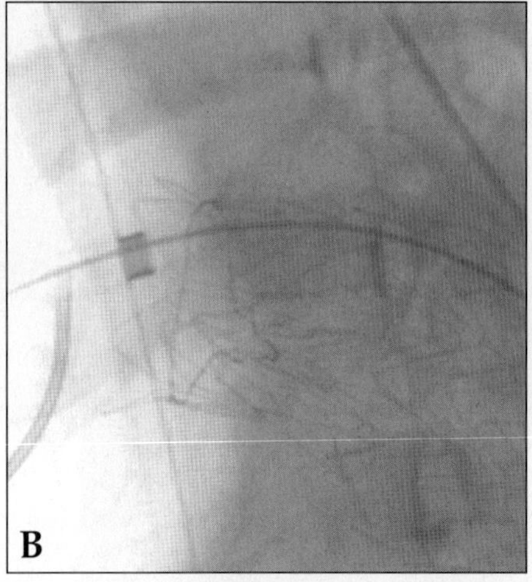

Figure 24-10. **A** The TAG device is catching on the elephant trunk and could not be advanced to the level of the left subclavian artery. The device was deployed in this position resulting in graft deformation shown in Figure 24–10B. **(B)** The gold ring representing the proximal end of the endograft shows some folding due to similar folding in the loose Dacron of the elephant trunk. This is worrying for severalreasons as it can increase the likelihood of stent fracture or proximal endoleak.

3. The concept of a frozen elephant trunk, stabilized with a balloon expandable stent, has been used as an option outside the United States.
4. Bypass the supra-aortic vessels rather than sew them on as a patch while moving the anastamosis proximally on the ascending aorta. This provides a much longer landing zone and might minimize the risk of stroke.
5. Hypothermic circulatory arrest is necessary for arch replacement. Nitinol-based endografts deploy minimally in a patient who has been cooled, although when ballooned into place will adapt to the aortic dimension and stay in situ during rewarming. Our preference, however, is to rewarm the patient first prior to endograft placement to avoid these issues.

We prefer to use a bifurcated hemashield graft in end-to-side fashion, arising from the ascending aorta, and end to end to the innominate artery and left common carotid artery. A presewn side limb to the left subclavian artery arises from the common carotid artery. If the subclavian artery is difficult to expose, then a standard cervical carotid subclavian bypass is performed. When carotid subclavian bypass is performed, we embolize the subclavian proximal to the origin of the vertebral artery using either coils or an Amplatzer vascular occluder device. It is very important that the pericardium investing the ascending aorta is opened and that the proximal bypass anastmosis is placed as far proximally as technically safe. The clamp and the anastamosis use about 3 cm. of the ascending aorta, which is then lost as a seal zone. We place a large clip at the distal margin of the anastamosis as a radio opaque marker delineating the proximal extent of the landing zone (Figure 24–11).

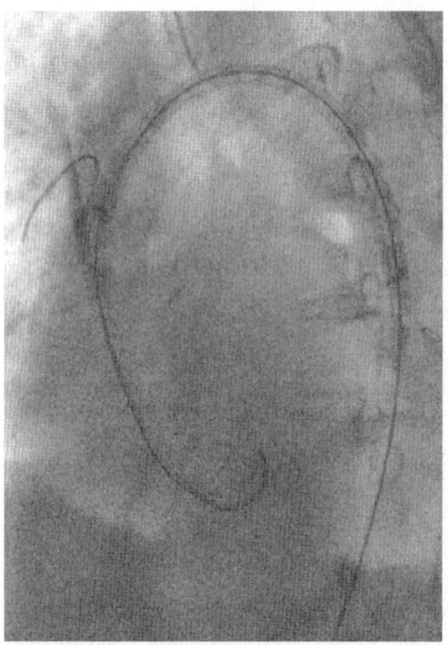

Figure 24-11. The radio-opaque band from a laparotomy pad has been sewn around the anastomosis on the ascending aorta. This allows the stent graft to be aligned very accurately.

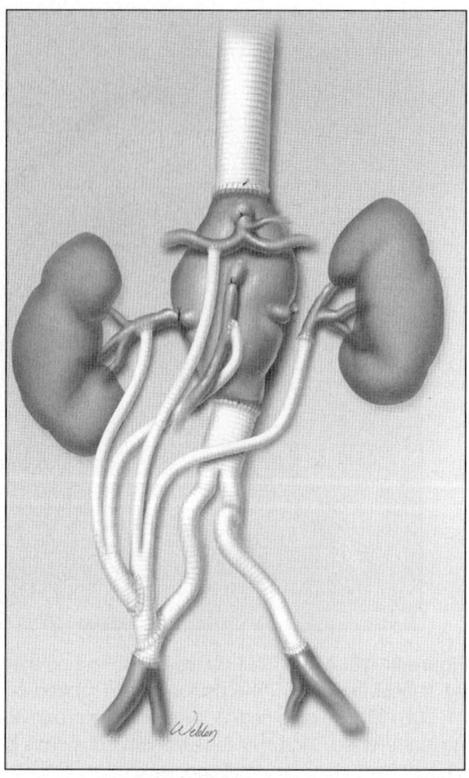

Figure 24-12. In this diagram, two bifurcated grafts project in retrograde fashion from the single iliac limb of an aortoiliac graft.

ANEURYSMS INVOLVING THE VISCERAL SEGMENT

Aneurysms, which extend to involve the visceral segment of the aorta, also have to be carefully evaluated in order to determine the extent and configuration of abdominal debranching required. In most cases, a decision must be made whether to cover the origins of the celiac and SMA or both of these vessels in conjunction with the renal arteries.[16,17] This location, like the ascending aorta, is one of the few situations in vascular surgery where a prior operation, namely replacement of the infrarenal aorta, is technically beneficial once it has been exposed. Again, provide a secure clamp and anastamotic site for the debranching bypasses as well as a secure landing zone for the stent graft.

That the celiac artery can be covered, without direct revascularization, when there are adequate collaterals from the SMA is likely; however, the judgment of adequacy of collateral is an imperfect science.[18] Demonstration of the presence of a patent pancreaticoduodenal arcade, with celiac filling via retrograde flow in the gastroduodenal artery is the best predictor of adequacy of the collaterals.[18] There are few situations, however, where simply covering the celiac alone provides sufficient additional length for sealing. Consequently, in most cases, the SMA orifice must also be covered, in which case we always bypass to both the SMA and the common hepatic artery. Typical configurations for retrograde bypasses are shown in (Figures 24–12, 24–13, and 24–14).

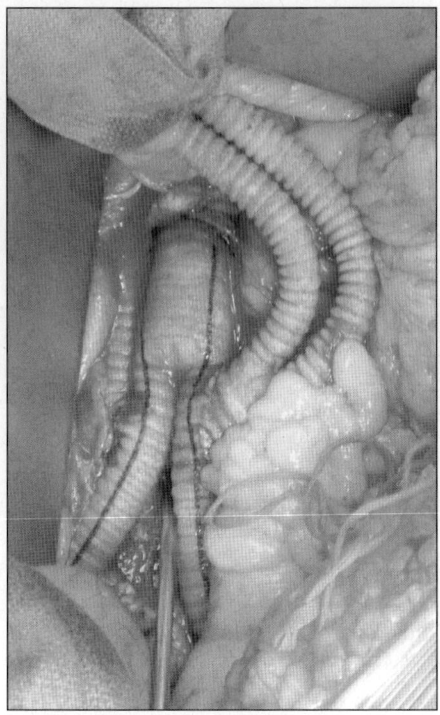

Figure 24-13. In our practice, the most typical arrangement is to place two separate bifurcated grafts from each iliac limb. The left graft runs to the left renal and superior mesenteric artery. The right-sided graft goes to the right renal and common hepatic artery.

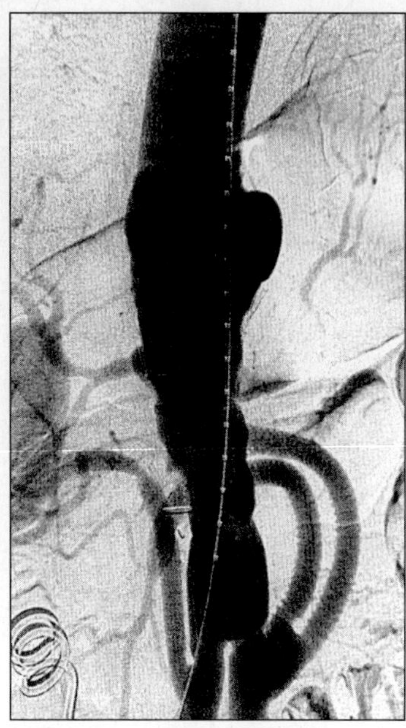

Figure 24-14. This patient had an occluded left renal artery. The angiogram reveals bypass grafts to the right renal, SMA, and common hepatic artery.

There are again some key technical issues worth highlighting.

The aortic component of a bifurcated graft used to replace the infrarenal aorta should be cut longer than usual in order to maximize the seal zone.

The aortic graft diameter should be increased to accommodate the distal end of the stent graft, the minimal diameter of which is 26 mm.

We typically originate two bifurcated dacron grafts (12 × 6mm) from each limb of the aortic graft. Those from the left limb go to the left renal artery and superior mesenteric artery. Those from the right go to the right renal and common hepatic artery.

Both the celiac artery and SMA must be legated as close to their aortic origins as possible.

When staged abdominal debranching followed by endograft placement is performed, it is essential to faciltate endograft placement during the intial procedure. Make sure the iliac limbs are fully stretched out, ideally place a graft down to the groin, and upsize the graft so that at least a 10 mm diameter limb is brought down to the femoral artery.

We have also used the ascending aorta as an inflow source for not only the supra-aortic trunks, but also for the celiac and SMA. The latter is relatively easy through a median sternotomy extended down to the umbilicus. The ascending aorta can easily support these bypass grafts (Figure 24–15).

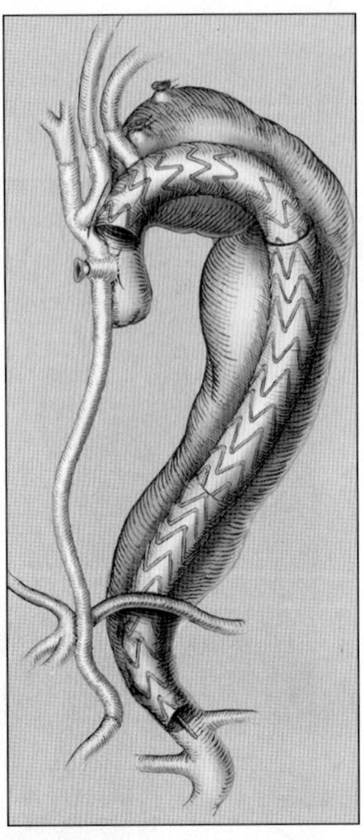

Figure 24-15. This diagram show the utility of the ascending aorta to provide inflow to the supra aortic trunks and the celiac/superior mesenteric artery.

REFERENCES

1. Brueck M, Heidt MC, et al. Hybrid treatment for complex aortic problems combining surgery and stenting in the integrated operating theater. *J Interv Cardiol.* 2006;19(6):539–43.
2. Zhou W, Reardon ME, et al. Hybrid approach to complex thoracic aortic aneurysms in high-risk patients: surgical challenges and clinical outcomes. *J Vasc Surg.* 2006;44(4):688–93.
3. Zhou W, Reardon ME, et al. Endovascular repair of a proximal aortic arch aneurysm: a novel approach of supra-aortic debranching with antegrade endograft deployment via an anterior thoracotomy approach. *J Vasc Surg.* 2006;43(5):1045–8.
4. Criado F J, Clark NS, et al. Stent graft repair in the aortic arch and descending thoracic aorta: a 4-year experience. *J Vasc Surg.* 2002;36(6):1121–8.
5. Gravereaux EC, Faries PL, et al. Risk of spinal cord ischemia after endograft repair of thoracic aortic aneurysms. *J Vasc Surg.* 2001;34(6):997–1003.
6. Moore RD, Brandschwei F. Subclavian-to-carotid transposition and supracarotid endovascular stent graft placement for traumatic aortic disruption. *Ann Vasc Surg.* 2001;15(5):563–6.
7. Chiesa R, Melissano G, et al. Spinal cord ischemia after elective stent-graft repair of the thoracic aorta. *J Vasc Surg.* 2005;42(1):11–7.
8. Peterson BG, Eskandari MK, et al. Utility of left subclavian artery revascularization in association with endoluminal repair of acute and chronic thoracic aortic pathology. *J Vasc Surg.* 2006;43(3):433–9.
9. Riesenman P J, Farber MA, et al. Coverage of the left subclavian artery during thoracic endovascular aortic repair. *J Vasc Surg.* 2007;45(1):90–4; discussion 94–5.
10. Woo EY, Bavaria JE, et al. Techniques for preserving vertebral artery perfusion during thoracic aortic stent grafting requiring aortic arch landing. *Vasc Endovasv Surg.* 2006;40(5):367–73.
11. Wang ZG, Li C. Single-branch endograft for treating stanford type B aortic dissections with entry tears in proximity to the left subclavian artery. *J Endovasc Ther.* 2005;12(5):588–93.

12. Melissano G, Civilini E, et al. Hybrid endovascular and off-pump open surgical treatment for synchronous aneurysms of the aortic arch, brachiocephalictrunk, and abdominal aorta. *Tex Heart Inst J*. 2004;31(3):283–7.
13. Schumacher H, Von Tengg-Kobligk H, et al. Hybrid aortic procedures for endoluminal arch replacement in thoracic aneurysms and type B dissections. *J Cardiovasc Surg* (Torino) 2006;47(5):509–17.
14. Neale ML, Hemli JM, et al. Ct16 hybrid open and endovascular procedures for complex aortic pathology in the high-risk surgical patient. *ANZ J Surg*. 2007;77 Suppl 1:A11.
15. Greenberg RK, Haddad F, et al. Hybrid approaches to thoracic aortic aneurysms: the role of endovascular elephant trunk completion. *Circulation*. 2005;112(17):2619–26.
16. Resch TA, Greenberg RK, et al. Combined staged procedures for the treatment of thoracoabdominal aneurysms. *J Endovasc Ther*. 2006;13(4):481–9.
17. Lawlor DK, Faizer R, et al. The hybrid aneurysm repair: extending the landing zone in the thoracoabdominal aorta. *Ann Vasc Surg*. 2007;21(2):211–5.
18. Vaddineni SK, Taylor SM, et al. Outcome after celiac artery coverage during endovascular thoracic aortic aneurysm repair: preliminary results. *J Vasc Surg*. 2007;45(3):467–71.

25

Hybrid Procedures for Treatment of Complex Aortic Aneurysms

Ali Azizzadeh, M.D., Anthony L. Estrera, M.D.,
Martin A. Villa, M.D., Charles C. Miller, Iii, Ph.D.
Sheila M. Coogan, M.D., Hazim J. Safi, M.D.

HYBRID PROCEDURES IN AORTIC SURGERY

In the last decade and a half, endovascular surgery has made revolutionary changes in the way we think about surgical options for complex aortic surgery. It has opened new vistas for vascular surgeons that were unimaginable just a few years ago.

Aortic surgery was first performed in the late 1940s. Tremendous advances in technique occurred in the 1950s with the establishment of abdominal aortic aneurysm surgery, as well as femoral-popliteal bypasses, carotid endarterectomies, and lumbar sympathectomies. In the late 1970s and 1980s, surgical repair was being performed on ascending aortic aneurysms as well as aneurysm of the transverse arch, descending thoracic, and thoracoabdominal aorta. Each segment of the aorta presented a unique challenge to the vascular surgeon in treatment of these complex aneurysms. For repair of the ascending aorta and the transverse arch, a woven dacron graft was used from the ascending to descending. Bypass grafts were then placed to the brachiocephalic arteries in a sequential fashion. This procedure was cumbersome and required bilateral thoracotomies. It was associated with large amounts of bleeding and a prolonged operative time while producing modest results. Subsequent to this, cardiopulmonary bypass was used in addition to moderate hypothermia. To protect the cerebral circulation, a perfusion catheter was inserted into the left common carotid and innominate artery. Blood from the cardiopulmonary bypass was used to perfuse the cerebral circulation. This became the standard for the repair of ascending and arch aneurysms in the 1950s, '60s, and '70s. In the mid-70s, profound hypothermia and circulatory arrest, in addition to cardiopulmonary bypass, was reintroduced in the treatment of the ascending and arch aneurysm.[1] It obviated the clutter of tubes in the operative field and this became the mainstay method of choice in the 1980s. This was accompanied by intraoperative bleeding and neurological deficit. The biggest limitation of this procedure was brain ischemia. In patients with greater than 40 minutes' circulatory arrest, the incidence of stroke was much higher.[2] Naturally, this led to additional searches for a method to extend the tolerance of cerebral ischemia. Antegrade cerebral perfusion was reintroduced in addition to moderate hypothermia. Retrograde cerebral perfusion was also introduced to protect the brain from ischemia.[3] In our service, this is the main method that we use to protect the brain.[4,5] In the 1970s, the use of distal aortic perfusion (pulsatile-nonpulsatile) was reintroduced with varying degree of success.[6] With regard to the descending and thoracoabdominal aortic aneurysm, distal aortic perfusion was used with various degrees of success in limiting neurological deficit. In the 1980s, the crossclamp-and-sew technique became the dominant method in the treatment of these difficult aneurysms.[7]

The clamp-and-sew technique simplified surgical repair markedly but it depended on the expediency of the surgeon. In the 1990s, adjuncts were added to this technique, providing marked improvement in both morbidity (neurological deficit) and mortality. Thoracoabdominal aortic aneurysm repair paralleled that of descending thoracic aortic aneurysm repair.

In the last decade, the evolution of endovascular repair made this modality available for treatment of various aneurysms. Endovacular repair has been widely adopted for the treatment of infrarenal abdominal aortic aneurysms. Today, patients with descending thoracic aneurysms can be offered this minimally invasive repair. Hybrid procedures are performed to extend the reach of this technique to aneurysms that include major vessels in the chest or abdomen. Development of branched and fenestrated endovascular technology may make this technique available to a wider group of patients. The durability of such repairs, however, remains to be determined.

In this brief chapter, we will concentrate on our practice in the use of hybrid technique in patients with extensive aortic aneurysms; that is, involving the ascending aorta, the transverse arch, and the descending thoracic or the thoracoabdominal aorta. In addition, we will describe our hybrid procedure for repair of high-risk patients with thoracoabdominal aortic aneurysms.

EXTENSIVE AORTIC ANEURYSMS

As stated above, these are aneurysms involving the ascending, transverse arch, and descending or thoracoabdominal aorta. The etiology of these aneurysms is either a medial degenerative process or dissection or Marfan's Syndrome or connective tissue disorder. Our preferred method of treatment for these extensive aneurysms is a staged procedure.[8] The initial procedure is performed via a median sternotomy. First, we replace the ascending aorta and the transverse arch, leaving a redundant dacron graft dangling in the descending aorta. This eliminates dissection between the pulmonary artery and the transverse arch during the second procedure. In the past, this led to catastrophic bleeding. This technique is called the "elephant trunk procedure," developed by Professor Hans G. Borst of Germany.[9] Four to six weeks later, we repair the descending or thoracoabdominal aorta using the adjuncts of distal aortic perfusion and CSF drainage. We use the redundant dacron to achieve the proximal thoracic aortic control.

The four- to six-week period of convalescence following the first procedure carries the risk of death due to rupture of the remaining aortic aneurysm. Hybrid techniques used to repair the descending thoracic aorta during the same procedure or a few days postoperatively remove the danger of death from rupture. Despite improvements in surgical technique and the advantages provided by the elephant trunk technique, each stage is not without morbidity and mortality. With the use of endovascular repair of the second stage, the need for a prolonged waiting time ($\geq$ 4 weeks) between the two stages is obviated. Most ruptures occur during this waiting period. In addition to avoiding the risk of rupture, a simultaneous endovascular repair eliminates the risk, morbidity, and cost of a second operation. It is especially useful in patients with aorto-iliac disease when access for endovascular repair can be challenging. A simultaneous second stage repair is currently limited to patients with a descending thoracic aortic aneurysm. Patients with thoracoabdominal aortic aneurysms require an additional open or hybrid procedure at a later date.

THORACOABDOMINAL AORTIC ANEURYSMS

The second stage procedure for patients with thoracoabdominal aneurysms can be performed using a hybrid technique currently used in Great Britain by Hammersmith et. al. Of course, this technique is applicable to patients with de novo thoracoabdominal aneurysms who have not had a previous elephant trunk procedure. The abdomen is opened, either retroperitoneally or transabdominally, and bypasses are performed to the celiac axis, superior mesenteric artery, and both renal arteries, effectively excluding the abdominal aorta. At the present time, this carries lower morbidity or mortality, but the long-term results are not available. The hybrid second stage repairs after the elephant trunk procedure in extensive aortic aneurysms is specially suitable for high-risk patients. This includes patients with severe medical comorbidities including low ejection fractions (<30%), glomerular filtration rates less than 50 mL/minute, and COPD. Of course, the designation of "high-risk patient" is subject to interpretation. We will describe our application of endovascular technique in these subsets of patients.

OPERATIVE TECHNIQUE

Stage 1: The Elephant Trunk Procedure

We take the patient to the operating room and place him in a supine position (Figure 25–1). We administer general endotracheal anesthesia. Our anesthesiologist inserts intravenous lines, central and peripheral, as well as Swan-Ganz catheter for hemodynamic monitoring. In addition, TEE is used continuously to monitor the heart function in real time.

We used the left or right common femoral artery or the ascending aorta for arterial cannulation of cardiopulmonary bypass. This can be verified using the TEE to exclude the presence or absence of atheromatous plaque in the ascending or descending thoracic aorta, making femoral ascending aortic cannulation risky. In the presence of atheromatous plaque as mentioned above, we use the right axillary artery cannulation either directly or 8 mm woven dacron tube graft sewed end to side to the artery. Then, we perform a midline sternotomy incision (Figure 25–1). We place self-retaining retractors and we incise the pericardium. The patient is anticoagulated using sodium heparin 5 mg per kilogram of body weight

The ascending aorta and the transverse arch will be in full view. We cannulate the superior and inferior vena cava and then we start cardiopulmonary bypass and commence cooling (Figure 25–2A). With regard to myocardial protection, we use antegrade and retrograde cardioplegia. The septal myocardial temperature is kept below

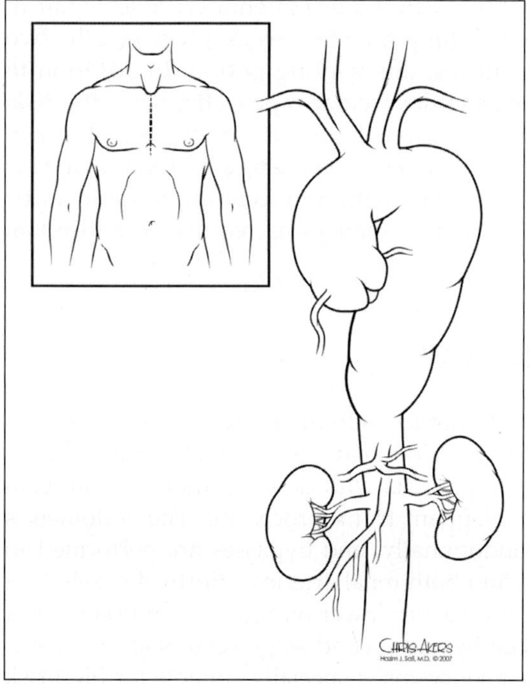

Figure 25-1. Median sternotomy exposure for extensive aortic aneurysm treated with the elephant trunk procedure.

20°C. We continue cooling until the EEG is isoelectric and the pupils are fixed and dilated. We place the patient in the head-down position. Then we stop cardiopulmonary bypass. We start retrograde cerebral perfusion of oxygenated blood via the superior

A   B

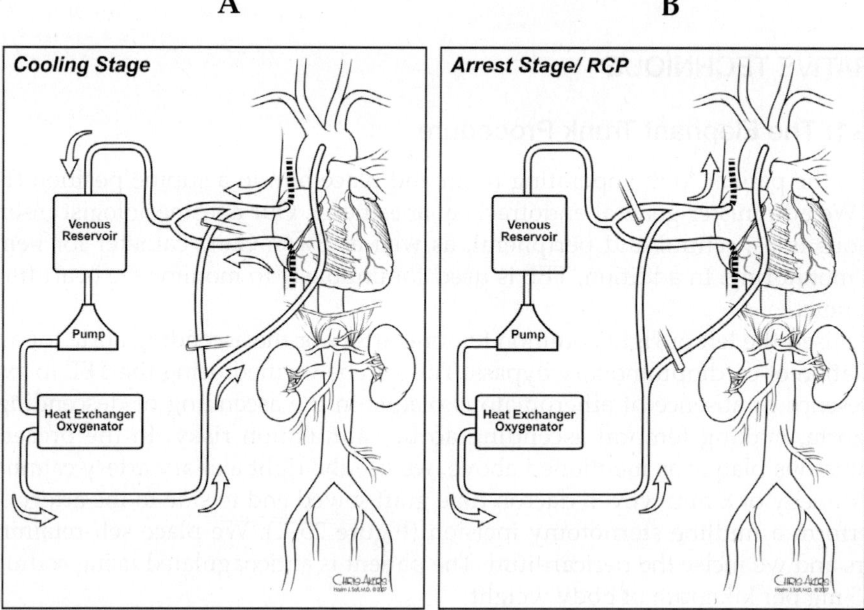

Figure 25-2. Cardiopulmonary bypass setup: **(A)** Cooling phase, ascending aortic cannulation with bicaval venous drainage. **(B)** On circulatory arrest, flow is reversed via the superior vena cava cannula to provide retrograde cerebral perfusion.

vena cava (Figure 25–2B). We open the ascending aortic aneurysm longitudinally (Figure 25–3). We use 3-0 polypropylene suture to retract the walls of the aneurysm. We proceed to excise the lesser curvature and two lateral walls of the transverse arch (Figure 25–4). At this time, the proximal descending aorta is in view. We use an appropriate size woven dacron tube graft impregnated with collagen or gelatin. We currently use woven dacron graft with a collar graft (Figure 25–5). The distal collared graft is inserted into the descending thoracic aorta (as an elephant trunk) (Figure 25–6).

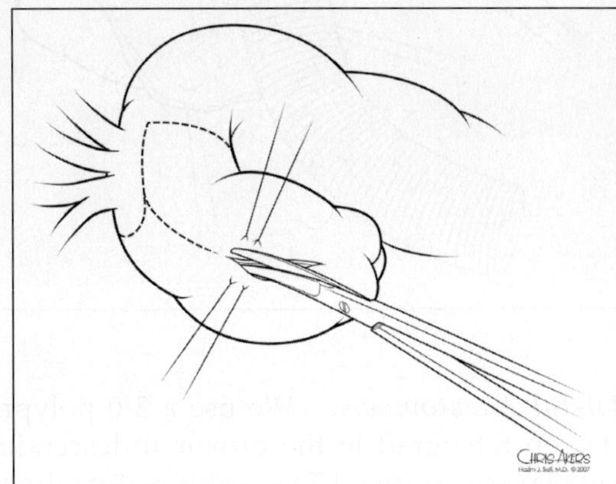

Figure 25-3. Exposure of ascending and transverse arch.

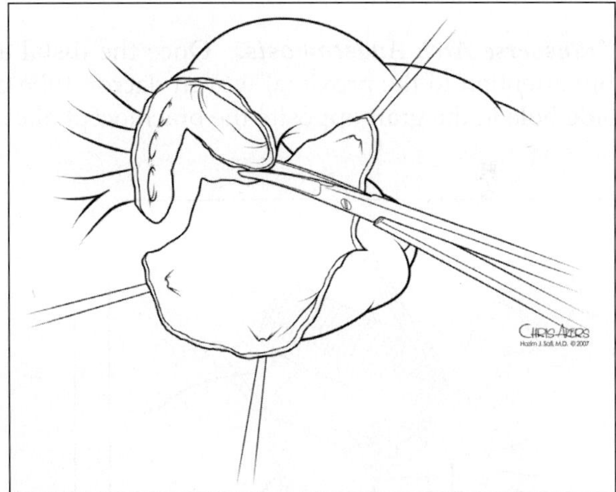

Figure 25-4. Resection of ascending and arch leaving patch for the great vessels (innominate, left common carotid, and left subclavian arteries).

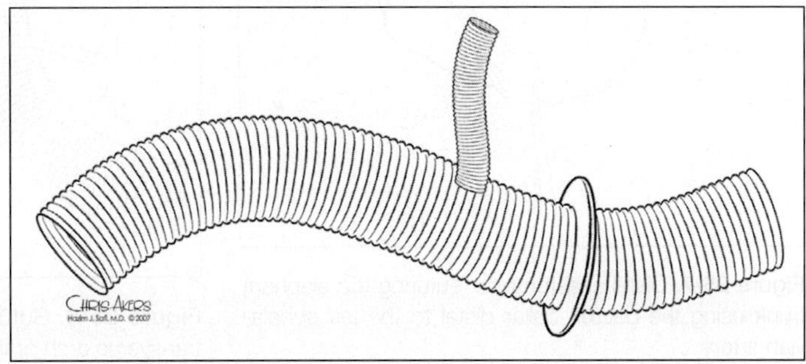

Figure 25-5. Commercially available collared dacron graft with attached side arm.

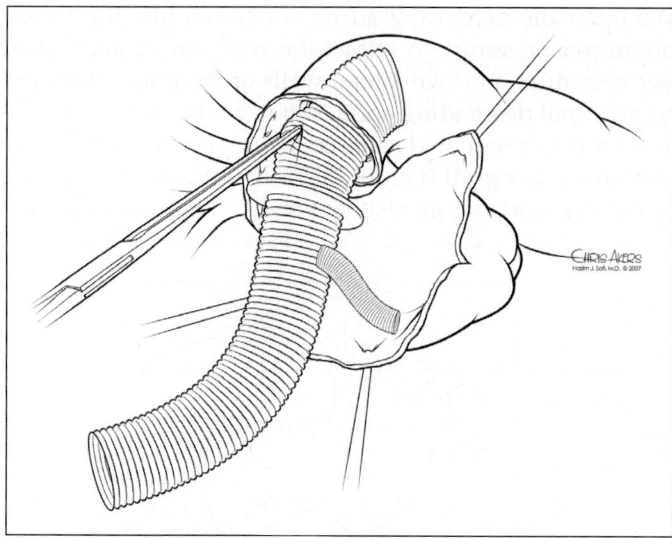

Figure 25-6. Insertion of the collared graft into the descending thoracic aorta.

Distal Anastomosis. We use a 3-0 polypropylene suture to sew the collar of the dacron tube graft to the proximal descending thoracic aorta at the level of the left subclavian or distal to it. This suture line is reinforced with 3-0 polypropylene pledgeted sutures (Figure 25–7).

Transverse Arch Anastomosis. Once the distal anastomosis is completed, we turn out attention to the proximal woven dacron tube graft. We make an elliptical-shaped side hole in the graft opposite the brachiocephalic arteries (Figure 25–8). The posterior

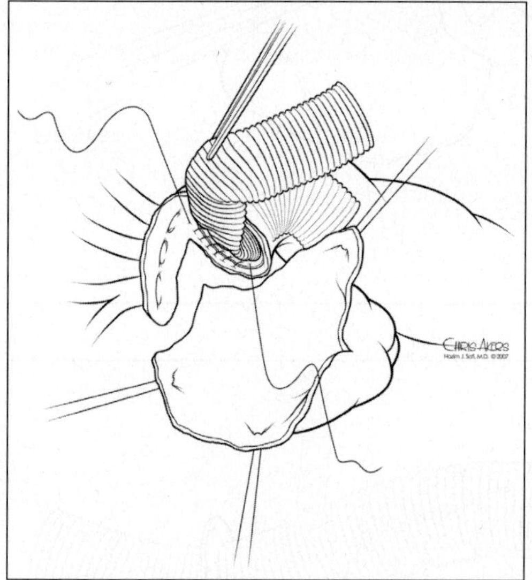

Figure 25-7. Distal anastomosis, suturing the elephant trunk using the dacron collar distal to the left subclavian artery.

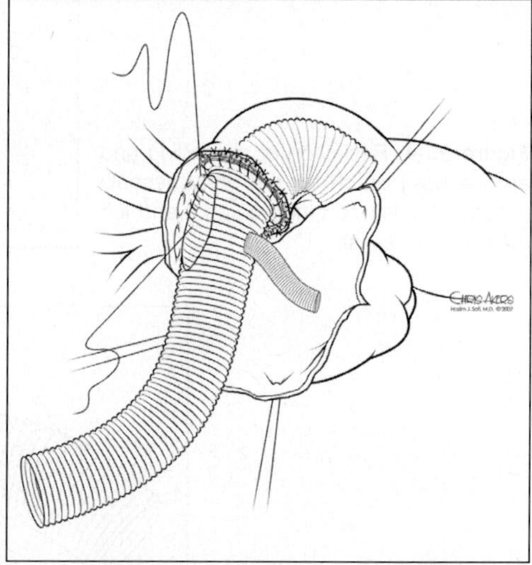

Figure 25-8. Suturing of the great vessels to the transverse arch graft.

anastomosis between the graft and the transverse arch commences at the level of the left subclavian, using 3-0 polypropylene suture to sew toward the innominate artery. Once the posterior row is finished, we commence the anterior row using the same 3-0 polypropylene sutures. On occasion, when the aortic wall is thin, we used a 4-0 or 5-0 polypropylene suture. We examine the anastomosis and reinforce it with polypropylene pledgeted sutures. Once the transverse arch anastomosis is completed, we use the arterial cannula of the cardiopulmonary bypass and connect it to the side arm of the dacron graft. Then, the cardiopulmonary is restarted. We flush all air and debris from the transverse arch. Then, we clamp the ascending aortic graft and elevate the head of the patient (Figure 25–9). Rewarming of the patient is begun until the nasopharyngeal temperature reaches 36.5°C. During this rewarming phase of cardiopulmonary bypass, we resect the tubular portion of the ascending aorta completely. Then our dacron graft is cut to appropriate length and sutured to the supracoronary ascending using 3-0 or 4-0 polyp sutures. This is reinforced with 3-0 pledgeted polypropylene sutures. In case the aortic valve is diseased, and/or the sinuses of Valsalva are dilated, then we perform aorta root replacement using composite valve graft prosthesis. We inspect the proximal anastomosis for bleeding points.

De-Airing of the Heart.   Once the above proximal aortic anastomosis is completed, we fill the heart with blood and de-air the ascending aorta via 18 gauge needles. Then, we place the patient in the head-down position and aspirate the left ventricle from any potential air and release the ascending aortic clamp, thus restoring the coronary flow via the native coronary arteries. We check the presence of air in the ascending aorta and left ventricle by transesophageal echocardiogram before the head is elevated. Once this is done, the head of the patient is elevated slowly.

We continue rewarming to 36°C nasopharyngeally. Once we reach that temperature and the patient is hemodynamically stable by demonstrating a good blood pressure, good cardiac output, and sinus rhythm, we begin weaning the patient from cardiopulmonary bypass. Once the patient is weaned successfully, all arterial and venous cannulae are removed. Hemostasis is achieved.

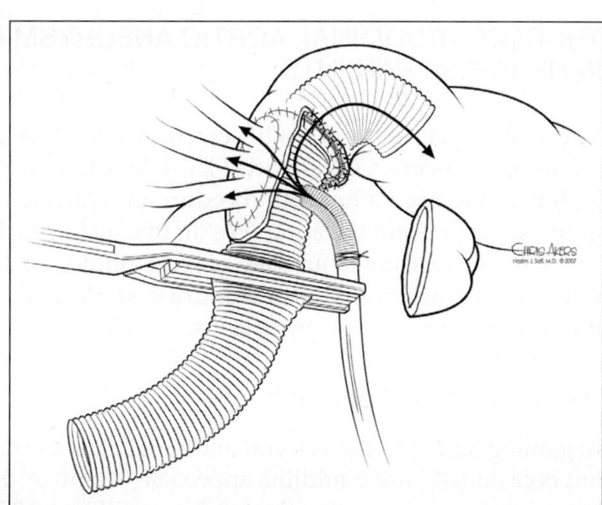

Figure 25-9. Reestablishing antegrade blood flow to systemic and cerebral circulation.

STAGE 2: Endovascular Repair of the Descending Thoracic Aorta

In properly selected patients, endovascular repair of the descending thoracic aorta can be performed simultaneously. The proximal landing zone is provided by the elephant trunk limb. We keep the elephant trunk limb short (10 cm) and mark the distal end with staples or stainless steel suture for easy identification under fluoroscopy. The distal landing zone above the celiac axis has to be of appropriate length and diameter to accommodate a commercially available thoracic device. All procedures are performed in a hybrid operating room equipped with fixed imaging capability. Intravascular ultrasound as well as TEE is used selectively when appropriate. The patient remains anticoagulated with the sternum open. Antegrade access to the descending thoracic aorta is obtained using the side arm graft. A large sheath (20-24 French) corresponding to the diameter of the stent graft is inserted (Figure 25–10). Retrograde access (5 French) is obtained from a femoral approach for angiography. The distal thoracic device is placed first. Additional devices are used to completely exclude the descending thoracic aorta. Appropriate overlap is allowed for proper sealing. The proximal and distal landing zones, as well as the overlapping segments, are angioplastied using a compliant balloon. A completion thoracic aortogram is performed to confirm the exclusion of the aneurysm. Additional intervention is performed for patients with a Type I or III endoleak in the proximal or distal landing zones or the overlapping segments. Patients with Type II endoleak, that is, due to a patent intercostal artery, are usually managed conservatively. At the conclusion of the procedure, the sheath is then removed from the ascending aortic side arm. We trim and oversew the graft with 4-0 polypropylene sutures. We close the median sternotomy incision in layers (Figure 25–11). We transfer the patient to the intensive care unit.[10]

We evaluate the patient neurologically for stroke, and paraparesis and paraplegia. We evaluate the patient's pulmonary status, and once the patient is stabilized, we extubate him. In the initial 24 hours after surgery, we monitor the patient for delayed neurological deficit. If there are any delayed effects, such as paraplegia, we don't hesitate to insert a CSF drainage catheter in L3-4 to drain freely for 72 hours. In the past, we have had an excellent response to delayed paraplegia with this management.

THORACOABDOMINAL AORTIC ANEURYSM REPAIR IN HIGH-RISK PATIENTS

In our practice, patients with ejection fractions less than 30%, GFR less than 50 ml/min, or severe COPD with FEV-1 less than 0.8 liters per second are considered high risk. We used a hybrid procedure in which we prepare the main visceral arteries from exclusion from the aorta. We do this by bypassing the celiac, superior mesenteric, and right and left renal arteries, either from the distal abdominal aorta or right or left common iliac arteries. This procedure is applicable to patients with Type II, III, and IV thoracoabdominal aortic aneurysms.

Retroperitoneal Approach

In gaining access to the visceral and renal arteries, we prefer a retroperitoneal incision, but occasionally use a midline approach. We place the patient in the right lateral decubitus position and we flex the left hip 60° (Figure 25–12). After we prepare and drape

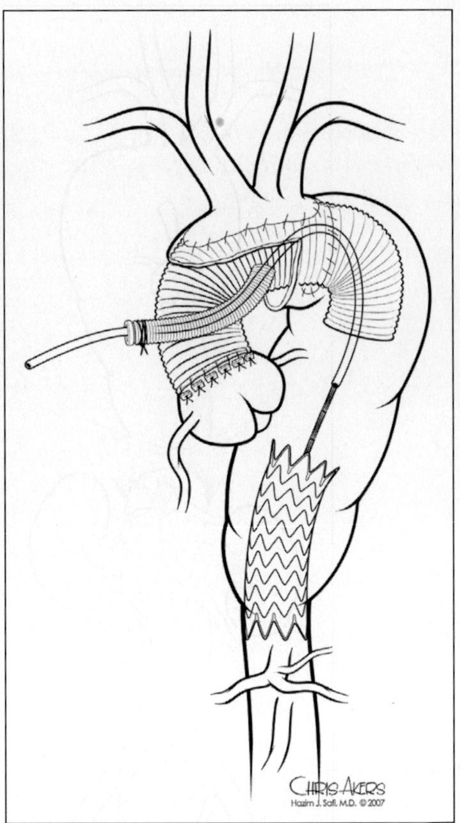

Figure 25-10. Endovascular stent deployment via the dacron side arm in an antegrade fashion. Deployment of the distal stent through the elephant trunk.

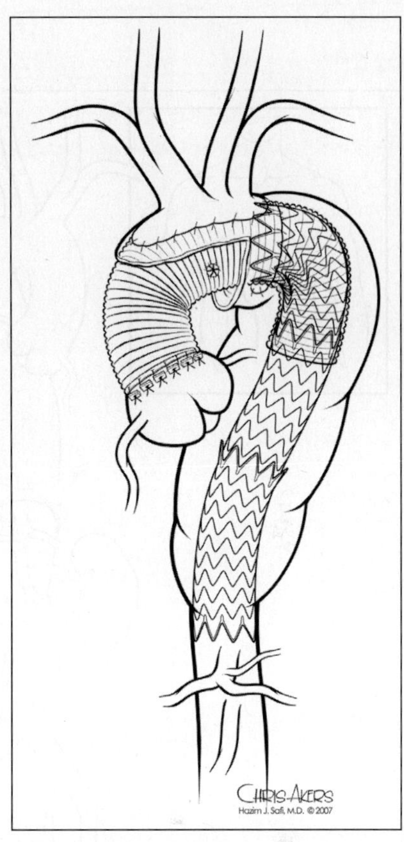

Figure 25-11. Complete repair of the hybrid elephant trunk.

the patient, we perform a thoracoabdominal incision where we retract the viscera medially, exposing the entire abdominal aorta from diaphragm to the iliac bifurcation. Then we place the self-retaining retractor, and we commence our dissection exposing the left common iliac, the left renal artery, the superior mesenteric, and the celiac axis. Once we establish that the left common iliac artery is suitable for anastomosis, we choose a 10 mm woven dacron tube graft impregnated with collagen or gelatin, and we suture it in end-to-side anastomosis. We prefer to do end-to-end anastomosis to the visceral arteries, so we transect the superior mesenteric artery from its origin and we oversew the abdominal aortic end of the superior mesenteric artery using polypropylene suture. The distal end of the superior mesenteric artery is sutured to the distal end of our dacron graft using 4-0 polypropylene suture. We then expose the celiac axis and transect it from the origin of the abdominal aorta, and we select an 8 or 10 mm woven dacron tube graft in end-to-end fashion using 4-0 polypropylene sutures. The other end will be sutured to the superior mesenteric artery graft in end-to-side fashion using 4-0 polypropylene suture. Another 8 mm graft is sutured to the SMA graft in end-to-side fashion using 4-0 polypropylene suture, and likewise is sutured end to end to the transected left renal artery (Figure 25–13). When this anastomosis is completed,

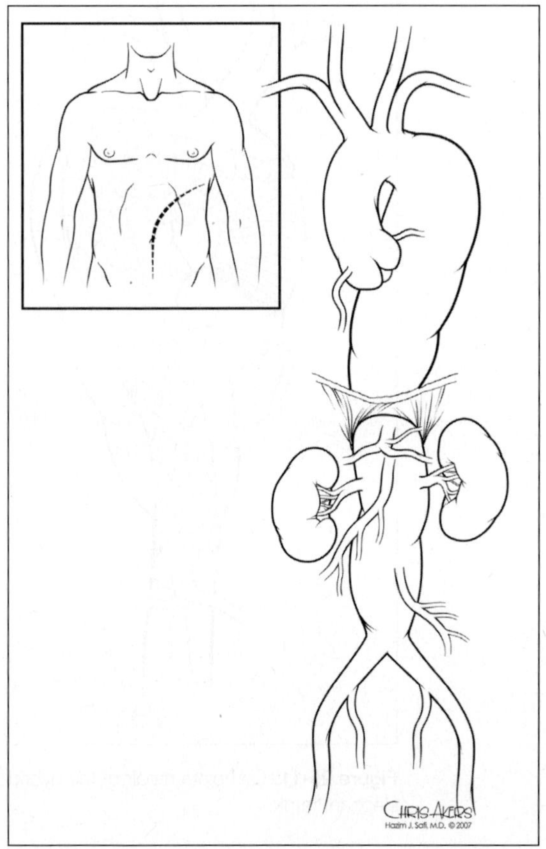

Figure 25-12. Hybrid thoracoabdominal aneurysm repair, exposure via left retroperitoneal incision or thoracoabdominal incision.

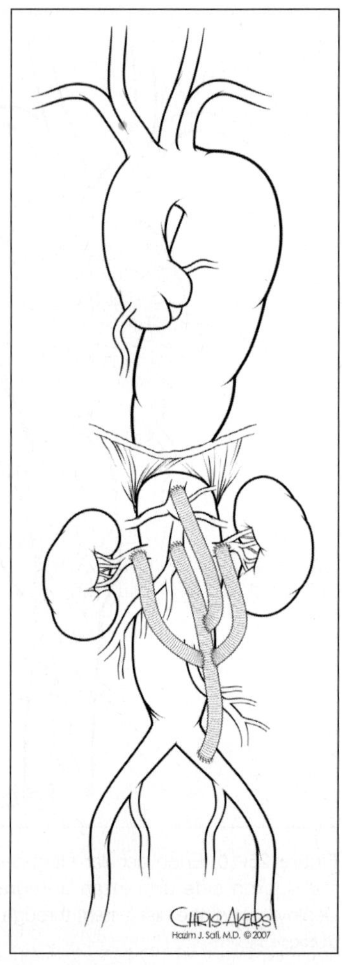

Figure 25-13. Debranching of the visceral and renal arteries for the first stage of the hybrid thoracoabdominal aneurysm repair.

attention is turned to the deployment of the endovascular stent graft. We prefer to use a side arm graft either connected to the above mentioned 10 mm dacron graft or to the left common iliac artery. A large sheath (20-24 French) corresponding to the diameter of the device is placed into the infrarenal aorta. The proximal device is usually deployed first. Additional devices are used with appropriate overlap to exclude the aneurysm. We seal the proximal and distal landing zones of the stent graft in the thoracic aorta and the distal abdominal aorta, respectively. The proximal and distal landing zones, as well as the overlapping segments, are angioplastied using a compliant balloon. A completion angiogram is performed to verify exclusion of the aneurysm and rule out an endoleak. At this point, the delivery sheath is removed. We then clamp the side arm graft and we prepare the right renal artery by transecting it from the abdominal aorta and suture it end to end to the side arm graft using 4-0 polypro-

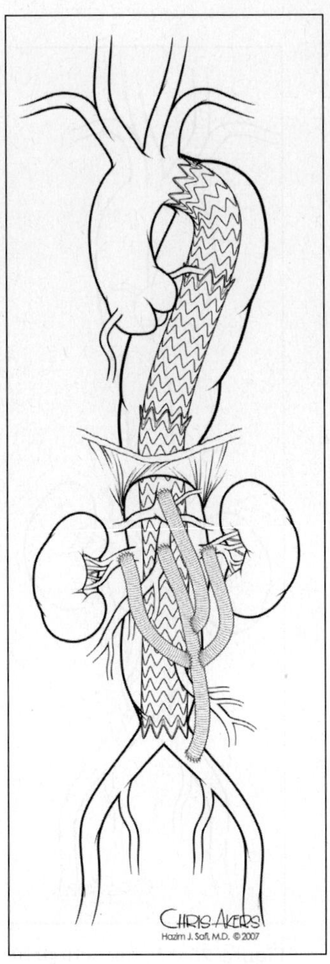

Figure 25-14. Second-stage hybrid thoracoabdominal aneurysm repair: complete endovascular stent exclusion of the TAAA.

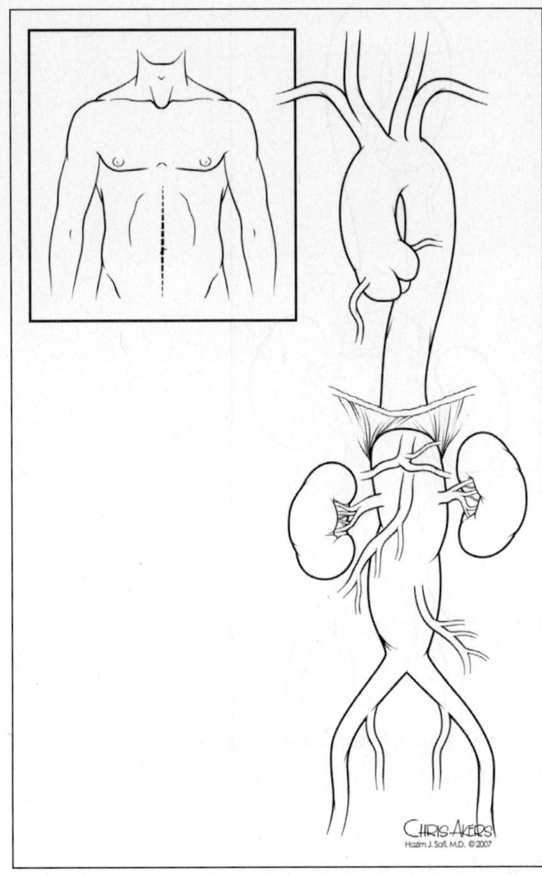

Figure 25-15. Hybrid thoracoab-dominal aneurysm repair, exposure via midline laparotomy incision.

pylene suture. Then we release the clamp, restoring flow to the right kidney (Figure 25–14). We close the thoracoabdominal incision in layers.

Transabdominal Approach

This procedure is performed through a standard midline approach (Figure 25–15). This incision is somewhat better tolerated in patients with low pulmonary reserve. The dissection, however, can be somewhat tedious in obese patients. Standard bypasses can be performed to bilateral renal arteries, as well as the superior mesenteric and celiac arteries (Figure 25–16). Depending on the patients' anatomy, a variety of different approaches can be used to revascularize the branches of the abdominal aorta. The endovascular exclusion is then performed using the same approach as above (Figure 25–17).

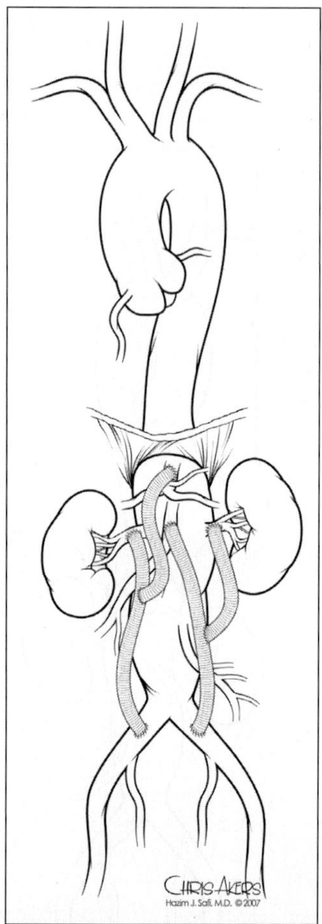

Figure 25-16. Debranching of the visceral and renal arteries for the first stage of the hybrid thoracoabdominal aneurysm repair. (Midline using both right and left iliac arteries.)

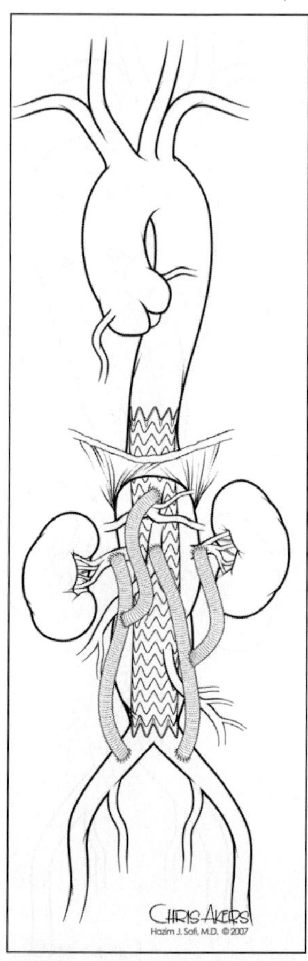

Figure 25-17. Second-stage hybrid thoracoabdominal aneurysm repair: complete endovascular stent exclusion of the TAAA. (Midline.)

CONCLUSION

The evolution and widespread adoption of endovascular techniques has revolutionized the modern practice of vascular surgery. Minimally invasive techniques have reduced the morbidity and mortality associated with open aortic surgery. Hybrid procedures extend the application of this approach to a wider group of patients. Further refinement of endovascular techniques including the introduction of branched and fenestrated technology, hold great promise for the future of vascular surgery.

ACKNOWLEDGMENT

We appreciate the editorial assistance of G. Ken Goodrick

REFERENCES

1. Griepp RB, Stinson EB, Hollingsworth JF, Buehler D. Prosthetic replacement of the aortic arch. *J Thorac Cardiovas Surg*. 1975;70:1051–63.
2. Svensson LG, Crawford ES, Hess KR, et al. Deep hypothermia with circulatory arrest. Determinants of stroke and early mortality in 656 patients. *J Thorac Cardiovas Surg*. 1993; 106:19–28.
3. Ueda Y, Miki S, Kusuhara K, et al. Surgical treatment of aneurysm or dissection involving the ascending aorta and aortic arch, utilizing circulatory arrest and retrograde cerebral perfusion. *J Cardiovas Surg*. 1990;31:553–8.
4. Safi HJ, Letsou GV, Iliopoulos DC, et al. Impact of retrograde cerebral perfusion on ascending aortic and arch aneurysm repair. *Ann Thorac Surg*. 1997;63:1601–7.
5. Estrera AL, Garami Z, Miller CC, 3rd, et al. Determination of cerebral blood flow dynamics during retrograde cerebral perfusion using power M-mode transcranial Doppler. *Ann Thorac Surg*. 2003;76:704–9.
6. Connolly JE, Wakabayashi A, German JC, et al. Clinical experience with pulsatile left heart bypass without anticoagulation for thoracic aneurysms. *J Thorac Cardiovas Surg*. 1971;62: 568–76.
7. Svensson LG, Crawford ES, Hess KR, et al. Experience with 1509 patients undergoing thoracoabdominal aortic operations. *J Vasc Surg*. 1993; 17: 357–68.
8. Safi HJ, Miller CC, 3rd, Estrera AL, et al. Staged repair of extensive aortic aneurysms: morbidity and mortality in the elephant trunk technique. *Circulation*. 2001;104:2938–42.
9. Borst HG, Walterbusch G and Schaps D. Extensive aortic replacement using "elephant trunk" prosthesis. *Thorac Cardiovas Surgeon*. 1983;31:37–40.
10. Azizzadeh A, Estrera AL, Porat EE, et al. The hybrid elephant trunk procedure: a single-stage repair of an ascending, arch, and descending thoracic aortic aneurysm. *J Vasc Surg*. 2006;44:404–7.

26

Branched Aortic Endografts: Techniques and Outcomes

Matthew J. Eagleton, M.D.
Roy K. Greenberg, M.D.

INTRODUCTION

Endovascular aneurysm repair (EVAR) is used commonly to treat large (5.5 cm) infrarenal abdominal aortic aneurysms (AAA). Compared to conventional open aneurysm repair, EVAR has been associated with a reduction in the 30-day mortality rate from 4.7% to 1.7%.[1,2] Successful long-term outcomes from EVAR depend on several factors including patient selection, technical expertise, endograft design, material construct, fatigue issues, and the ability of the device to remain in a stable and circumferentially apposed position with respect to the native vasculature above and below the aneurysmal segment. Ideally, the arterial segment providing a means of fixation and sealing is healthy, thus minimizing the potential for late dilation that could jeopardize device stability. Healthy vessels, in general, are cylindrical, have parallel walls, and are free of luminal debris and calcification.

Conventional EVAR defines the proximal neck as the region below the renal arteries to the beginning of the aneurysm sac. The distal neck is defined as the length of nonaneurysmal iliac artery the stent-graft will cover. The corresponding neck for thoracic aneurysms includes the isthmus of the aorta just distal to the subclavian artery (unless the subclavian artery will be covered) and the supraceliac aorta. Compromised necks have markedly limited the applicability of endovascular aneurysm repair, restricting the approach to patients who have acceptable healthy vessel distal to any critical aortic branches.[3] The residual patients (those not amenable to endovascular repair) are more complex to treat with conventional surgical techniques, have a higher incidence of complications, and thus have the most to gain from a less invasive approach.[4] Advanced endovascular technologies that allow treatment of more complex aneurysms that involve or abut the visceral segment using fenestrated and branched endovascular grafts offer alternative therapeutic options. These endovascular devices overcome problems with inadequate sealing zones by extending the sealing and fixation regions of the stent-graft proximally or distally without sacrificing branch vessels. Such repairs require a detailed understanding of imaging studies, adjunctive endovascular devices, interventional techniques, and high-level operative/interventional facilities.

IMAGING

Comprehensive aortic assessment and procedural planning using devices that incorporate branch vessels require an understanding of computed tomographic (CT) image acquisition and the ability to manipulate data on three-dimensional workstations. Endovascular device implantation requires skill in the orientation of three-dimensional devices based on two-dimensional angiographic imaging equipment. Such techniques differ drastically from the simpler longitudinal requirements necessary for success with a conventional infrarenal device. Longitudinal or rotational misalignment can result in critical end-organ ischemia with potentially disastrous complications. Additionally, posttreatment complications that have been reported with an alarming frequency with some infrarenal devices, such as migration or component separation, may prove fatal if combined with a fenestrated or branched device.[5] Currently, available spiral CT technology renders images of excellent quality that can be used to design devices that incorporate the visceral, renal, or internal iliac vessels. After image acquisition, however, image reconstruction must be done to allow accurate measurements of branch diameters, of lengths between the various vessels, and of the rotational relationship between the branches. After 1 mm reconstructions are performed with a smoothing algorithm, the studies are exported to an imaging workstation where multiplanar techniques can be used to evaluate the aorta and its branches. Renditions of aortic anatomy perpendicular to a centerline of flow allow accurate assessment of the proximal neck (Figure 26–1) and establish the diameter and length measurements. Not all reconstruction algorithms are entirely accurate, and in some situations, such an approach will not yield a properly designed graft.

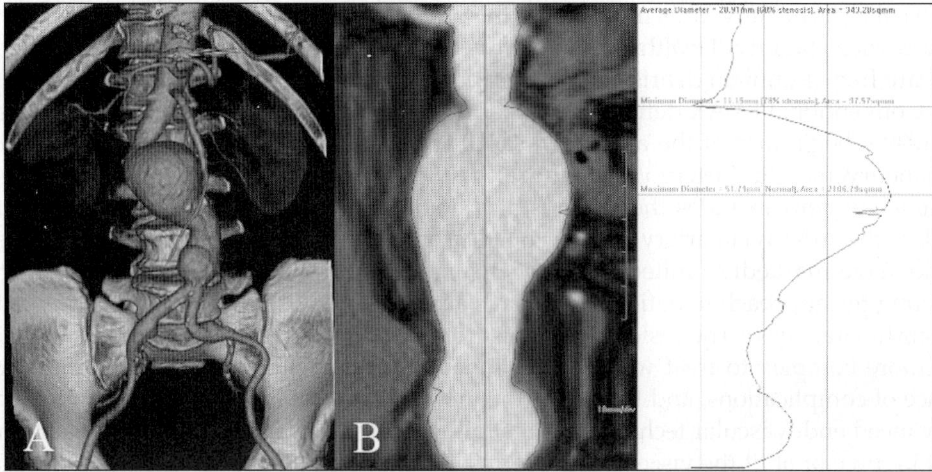

Figure 26-1. (A) Three-dimensional rendering of a patient with an infrarenal abdominal aortic aneurysm. **(B)** Renditions of aortic anatomy perpendicular to a centerline of flow. This allows for more accurate assessment of diameters and the locations and orientation of branch vessels.

FENESTRATED ENDOGRAFTING

Juxtarenal Abdominal Aortic Aneurysms

The most common reason for excluding patients from EVAR is the lack of a suitable proximal implantation site between the renal arteries and the aneurysm. Although commercially available devices provide a mechanism for supplementing fixation within the suprarenal aorta without detrimentally affecting renal function,[6,7] such a practice has not been advocated for the treatment of juxtarenal aneurysms. Despite evidence of short-term success with the treatment of short necks with devices intended to treat infrarenal aneurysms,[8] the risk of later failure remains high.[9] Early experiences with fenestrated devices were intended to address the short proximal neck,[10-13] while subsequent larger series have focused on patients who had short necks (<10mm) or proximal morphology (i.e., conical necks) that would not be well treated with conventional infrarenal devices.[14-16]

The devices used currently are hybrids of original abdominal devices. The primary goal of treating an aneurysm with a fenestrated graft is to move the sealing and fixation region of the repair into healthy aorta with a parallel neck and without wall defects. A fenestration (hole in the graft) allows the stent graft to occupy this more proximal location while providing for transgraft flow to the renal arteries (or other significant branches). It is designed to incorporate the minimum number of visceral vessels required to achieve fixation and seal within healthy aorta. The fenestrations are constructed to match the ostial diameter of the visceral vessels and maximize the sealing zone. Three types of fenestrations exist: scallops, large fenestrations, and small fenestrations (Figure 26–2). Anterior and posterior markers on the device assist with rotational alignments (Figure 26–3), and the edges of the fenestrations are demarcated to fine-tune alignment. Scallops are hemi-ovals 6 to 12 mm in height and typically are used for upper-targeted vessels such as the superior mesenteric artery. Large fenestrations are 8 to 12 mm in diameter and must be located at least 10 mm below the proximal fabric edge. Such fenestrations may or may not have a strut from an aortic stent crossing the opening, and thus are not designed to be combined with a branch stent. They simply are aligned with the intended vessel without additional stenting. Small fenestrations are 6 mm in width and 6 to 8 mm in height. These fenestrations must be at least 15 mm below the proximal fabric edge and are always strut-free. Balloon-expandable stents

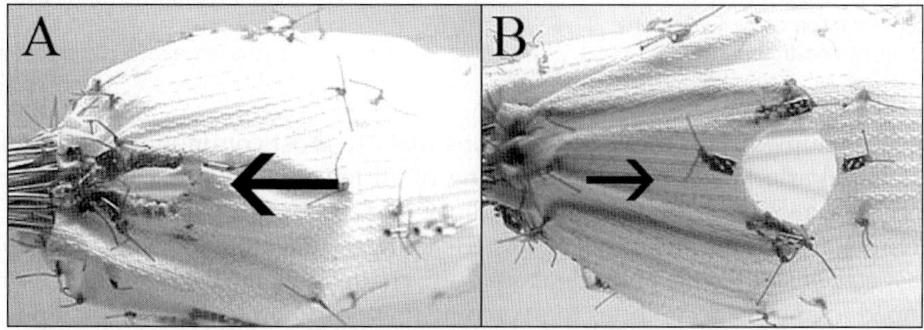

Figure 26-2. Aortic endograft that has **(A)** a proximal scallop (arrow) to allow continued flow to the superior mesenteric artery once placed, and **(B)** fenestrations (arrow) to allow continued flow to the renal arteries. Note the metal markers that have been sewn to the borders of the fenestration to assist in orientation of the device.

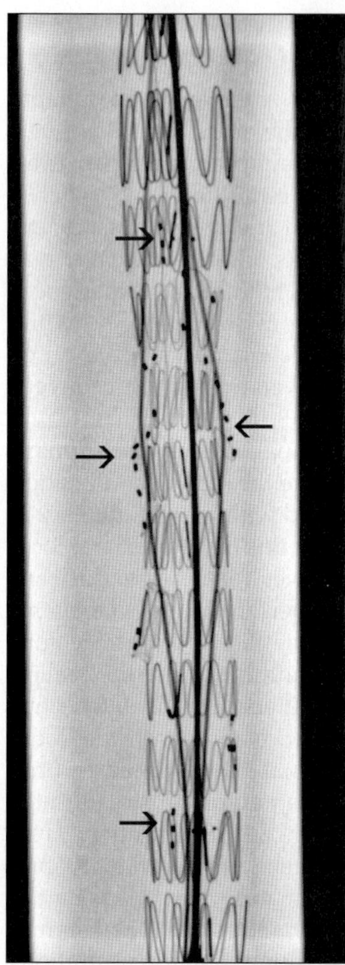

Figure 26-3. Fluoroscopic image of a branched aortic endograft depicting multiple markers (arrows) that have been placed on the device to assist in rotational orientation as well as outlining the sites of fenestrations.

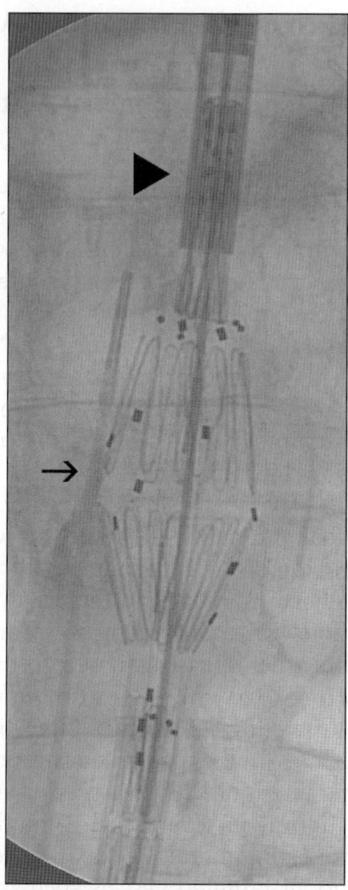

Figure 26-4. Fluoroscopic image of a fenestrated endograft that has been partially deployed. Note the markers that define the borders of the fenestration for the right renal artery (arrow). The top cap remains intact and the proximal aspect of the graft is constrained (triangle), allowing the device to be moved within the aneurysm for more precise placement with respect to the fenestrations and scallops.

are always coupled with these fenestrations that are most commonly used to incorporate the renal arteries. Accurate positioning of all fenestrations is mandatory, and the delivery system for the device has been adjusted to assist with positioning.

There are standard steps in fenestrated stent-graft insertion. Despite this, the technical aspects of stent-graft placement are quite challenging and experienced users have developed a range of techniques to overcome these difficulties. The basic steps include standard arterial access followed by insertion of the delivery system. Once orientation of the device is confirmed, the sheath is withdrawn to expand partially the fabric of the proximal tubular component (Figure 26–4). The fabric remains partially constrained by a tethering wire, and the uncovered stent with barbs remains affixed within the top cap

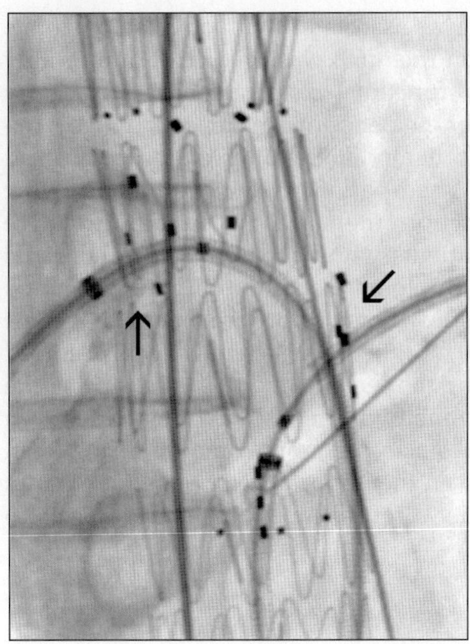

Figure 26-5. Fluoroscopic image of a fenestrated endograft with transgraft placement of sheaths into both the right and left renal arteries (arrows). The main body is then fully deployed and balloon-expandable stents are placed within the renal arteries with a short segment extending into the main body of the graft.

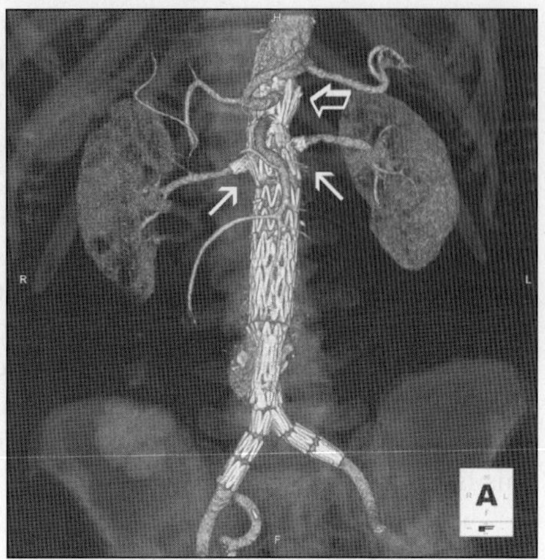

Figure 26-6. Three-dimensional rendering from a CT scan in a patient who had the placement of a fenestrated aortic endograft for the treatment of a juxtarenal AAA. Note the stents placed through the fenestrations into the renal arteries (arrows), as well as the maintained patency within the superior mesenteric artery (open arrow) that traverses a scallop.

until final positioning and access into the small fenestrations has been achieved. Next, catheterization of the target arteries is obtained, and this access is further supported by the placement of transgraft bridging sheath insertion (Figure 26–5). Then the tethering wire is released, and the top cap is deployed to allow engagement of the proximal fixation system with the aortic wall. Balloon-expandable stents then are placed into the desired fenestrations, the proximal (aortic) components of which are flared with sequentially larger balloons. The proximal tubular graft that contains the fenestrations then is coupled with a separate bifurcated system (Figure 26–6).

Several large series of fenestrated endograft deployments have been reported, demonstrating the mid-term safety and efficacy of fenestrated stent-grafting. O'Neill and colleagues[14] reported a series of 119 patients with mean follow up of 19 months. There was only one perioperative death, and survival at 12, 24, and 36 months was 92%, 83%, and 79%, respectively. The 30-day endoleak rate was 10%, and all endoleaks were type II in nature. Regression of the aneurysm sac was noted in 79% of the patients by 12 months. Complications related to the renal arteries was noted in 10 of the 231 stented renal arteries, and only one patient who did not have significant renal dysfunction preoperatively went on to require dialysis. Incorporation of the renal arteries raises questions about the effect of fenestrated stent-graft repair on long-term renal function. Haddad and colleagues[5] published a detailed analysis of renal function in 72 patients after fenestrated endovascular repair. These patients were divided into those who had underlying renal insufficiency before EVAR (n=23) and those who had normal baseline renal function (n=49). The study confirmed that, analogous to open surgical repair, preexisting renal dysfunction was associated with adverse outcome. Baseline renal dysfunction (glomerular filtration rate <60) was predictive of mortality (P=0.02; relative risk 8.52) and worsening renal function.[5] Baseline renal insufficiency also was independently associated with a higher incidence of renal events (P=0.04; relative risk 3.3). Four of the 72 patients required hemodialysis after the procedure; all had significant baseline renal insufficiency. When patients were evaluated for the longer term effect of the device on renal function, there was no apparent relative change in the glomerular filtration rate for patients who had no preoperative renal artery stenosis, whereas a slight improvement in glomerular filtration rate was noted in patients who had renal artery stenosis. This study noted improvements with respect to the device, procedure, and learning curve: 40% of the adverse renal events occurred during the first year of implantation, 26% during the second, and only 10% during the third year. Although renal issues are more common with fenestrated devices used in the setting of juxtarenal aneurysms, renal issues also are more common in the open surgical management of such situations.[17,18] Given the importance of renal function as an indicator for survival and late complications,[19] careful attention must be directed to this issue for the future.

Thoracic Aortic Aneurysms

The use of fenestrations has not been limited to treating infrarenal AAAs with unsuitable necks. There is limited experience in applying advanced endograft technology to the treatment of thoracic aortic aneurysms.[20] Although the left subclavian artery can be covered during the placement of a thoracic aortic stent-graft, this placement may be associated with upper extremity or cerebrovascular ischemic symptoms, and clearly cannot be done in the setting of coronary blood supply from the internal thoracic artery. More proximal fenestrations have been used to treat aneurysms that abut the carotid artery, covering the subclavian with and without prior carotid-subclavian bypass grafting. Fenestrations also can be incorporated into the distal aspect of a thoracic stent graft to extend the distal seal zone to the celiac artery proper. The devices used for proximal and distal fenestrations are more advanced versions of the Zenith (Cook, Inc. Bloomington, IN) thoracic device and require a modified delivery system to align the fenestrations properly. Additional studies on these devices are forthcoming.

BRANCHED GRAFTS

Thoracoabdominal Aortic Aneurysms

Thoracoabdominal aortic aneurysm repair is associated with significant morbidity (15–20%) and in particular, there is a risk of paraplegia (5–15%) and mortality (10–15%).[21-23] Aortic stent grafting may offer the ability to improve these outcomes. Initial attempts to provide a less invasive approach to treating these aneurysms involved hybrid techniques utilizing both open and endovascular surgery. Extra-anatomic bypass to the visceral and renal vessels was followed by subsequent aortic stent-graft repair of the aneurysm.[24,25] These procedures, however, still require major reconstructive surgery, and are far from minimally invasive. In order to apply solely endovascular technology for the treatment of thoracoabdominal aortic aneurysms, more complicated stent-graft designs are required to treat those more extensive lesions. One of the main differences with respect to stent-graft design in treating thoracoabdominal aortic aneurysms is that, in these aneurysms, the visceral vessels are not in proximity to the sealing zones. For this reason, branched endograft technology has been developed.[26]

While it would seem that the extent of the aneurysm should have little effect on outcome of endovascular success, the more extensive aneurysms are more difficult to treat.[27] Unlike fenestrated stent-grafting, treatment of these more extensive aneurysms typically require cannulation of all four branch vessels. The increased level of complexity mandates more intensive preoperative planning, more precise graft design, and allows for less margin of error during deployment. Delivery systems for these complex devices require equal attention to the implant design. It is critical for these grafts to be readily introduced from a femoral artery approach, have a method for precise deployment, and allow for postdeployment positional adjustments for accurate branch alignment and cannulation.

Unlike fenestrated grafts where a fenestration (a controlled hole) in the graft suffices, in these more complex aneurysms, the branch arteries arise from the aneurysm, and flow has to be carried across the aneurysm through the branches of the stent-graft. There are two modes by which this can be ensured. The first is the fenestrated branched stent-graft[27] or reinforced fenestrated graft.[28] In this style, the addition of a polytetrafluoroethylene covering to the bridging stents converts a fenestrated stent-graft into a form of branched stent-graft.[26] Sealing between the covered stent and the fenestration is tenuous because there is very limited overlap of material, simply the thickness of the vascular graft and the supporting nitinol ring outlining the fenestration. In addition, blood flow to the artery in question must traverse at a right angle to flow through the desired branch. This is not optimal from an engineering perspective but is currently necessary when working within a small lumen. The technique of deployment of this mode of "branched graft" is not significantly different than the conventional fenestrated grafts that require bare metal stents. These covered stents, however, are stiffer, bulkier, and have less trackability than the bare metal balloon-expandable stents.

The second mode of branched graft design is the cuffed branched stent-grafts[27] or directional branched stent-grafts (Figure 26–7).[28] These differ from fenestrated

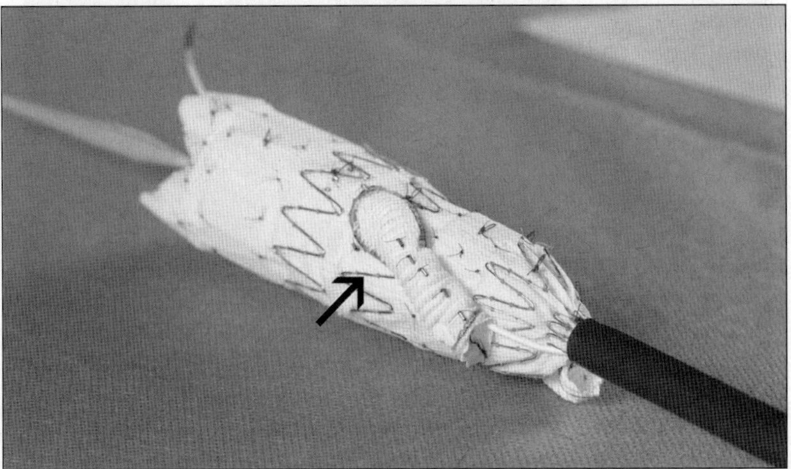

Figure 26-7. Partially deployed aortic stent-graft with a branch or cuff attached to the main body of the device. This particular branch represents a helical design. The longer body of the cuff allows for a longer seal zone with a self-expanding stent and orientation of the branch orifice in line with the direction of visceral vessel flow.

stent-grafts in a number of ways.[29] The cuff or branch creates an overlap zone between the stent-graft and the branch artery. It provides a segment of overlap that can be used to provide better sealing and fixation than the thin joint between a reinforced fenestration and mating visceral stent-graft. A longer overlap affords one the ability to utilize a self-expanding stent-graft rather than a balloon-expandable stent-graft. This may provide a means to better accommodate tortuosity and diameter discrepancies, and may limit type I endoleaks and component separation from this region.

Branch orientation and construction is a critical consideration when designing these endovascular grafts. Device design has seen the implementation of axial (caudally oriented) and helical (oriented directly toward the visceral ostium) branches. Other factors that need to be considered include flow direction (antegrade or retrograde) and branches attached to the inside or outside of the aortic component. Axial branches are relatively simple. The aortic device is deployed well above the target vessel, the branches are cannulated from a brachial approach, and mating self-expanding stent-grafts are deployed to join the target vessel and aortic graft (Figure 26–8). However, the length of the axial branch overlap segment is, by necessity, short (10 mm). Frequently, this joint must be reinforced with a balloon-expandable stent to prevent late component separation. A further issue exists with respect to flow direction. Stents exiting an axial branch are aligned with the aortic flow; however, the target vessel is not. Thus, the mating self-expanding stent-graft is forced to angulate to direct blood into the target organ and seal the aneurysm. This combination is of tenuous durability. Consequently, additional long self-expanding stents may be deployed to increase columnar support for the branch, thus limiting component separation and kinking. The durability of multiple layers of stents and stent-grafts stacked to create a channel is dubious, yet adverse results of this combination have not been reported.

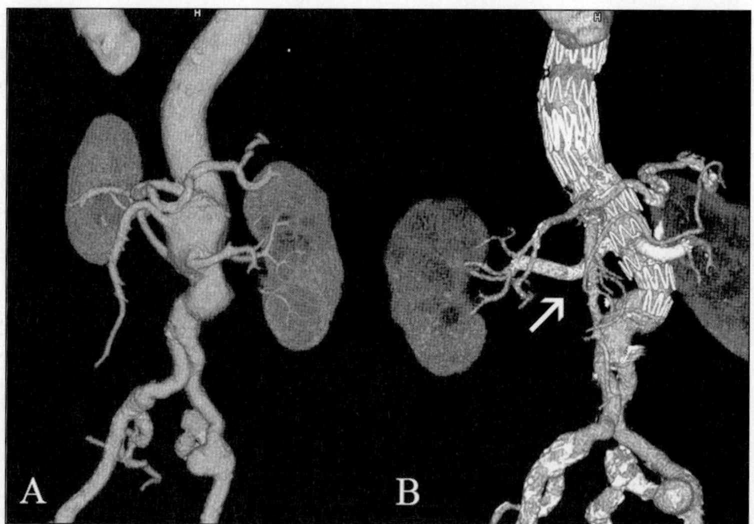

Figure 26-8. CT three-dimensional rendering of **(A)** an aortic aneurysm involving the visceral segment. The patient had previously undergone a conventional operative repair above and below this segment. **(B)** Axial branched graft repair was performed successfully with exclusion of the aneurysm. Note the nearly right-angled course the branches to the visceral vessels take, as well as the addition of both balloon- and self-expanding stents to the right renal artery (arrow) that were required to provide sufficient columnar support and prevent vessel kinking.

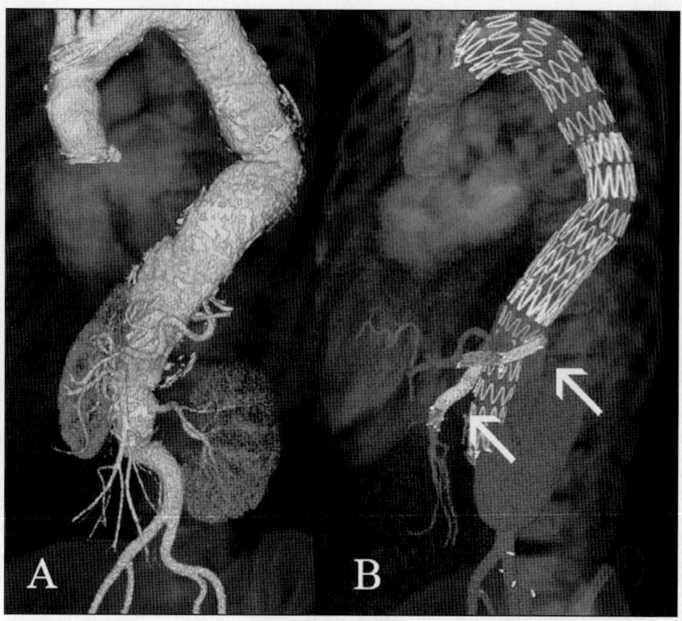

Figure 26-9. (A) Three-dimensional rendering from a CT scan of a patient with a thoracoabdominal aortic aneurysms treated with a branched endovascular graft utilizing a helical branch design. **(B)** Note on the postdeployment CT the location of the visceral branches arising from the posterior aspect of the graft (arrow). These branches are then mated with the visceral vessels with a self-expanding stent-graft. The helical design of the branch allows for a longer seal zone between the self-expanding stent and the cuff, and it allows for the orifice of the branch to be more in line with the ostia of its intended artery.

An alternative approach to branched grafting involves the use of helical branches. The development of helical branches was initiated to allow any angulation between the aorta and branch to be gently accommodated, avoiding the need to create steep angles that may inhibit blood flow and also detrimentally affect device durability. These branches exit the aortic component along its posterior aspect and traverse at a given pitch, terminating approximately 8 to 10 mm above the target vessel. The advantage of this design is the long overlap segment created (~30 mm) and the orientation of the branch orifice in line with the direction of visceral flow rather than aortic flow (Figure 26–9). This construct, when mated with a self-expanding stent-graft, may not require additional support from a balloon-expandable device or have a need for columnar support.

Stent-graft branches, however, are not without their complications. The branches take up space within the aneurysm as well as the delivery system. The devices are frequently bulky and typically require introduction using 20–22 F sheaths for delivery. The procedures, which require placement of an aortic device followed by one or more self-expanding covered stents into each of the visceral branch targets, require extensive fluoroscopy exposure, contrast dosing, and significant proficiency with catheter and wire techniques. The orientation of the cuff is determined by aneurysm morphology and the location and angle of the branch arteries. The site of access of these branches (femoral artery versus brachial artery) depends most on the orientation of the branch and the target artery. Covered stent delivery systems, however, are often bulky as well as sometimes stiff when attempting delivery from a left brachial artery approach without the use of stiff wires and kink resistant sheaths. A novel delivery

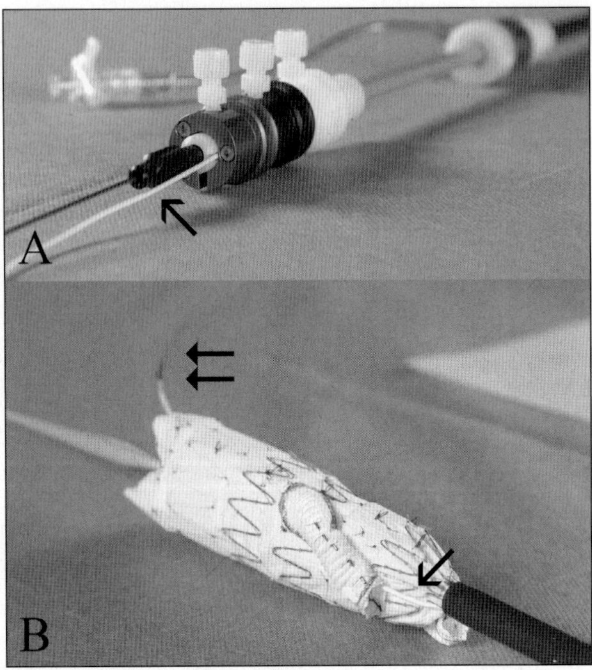

Figure 26-10. Demonstration of a novel delivery system that utilizes preloaded wires that allow for direct access into the branches of the endograft. The wires traverse the **(A)** delivery system (arrow) and exit the **(B)** branch (arrow), allowing for the distal aspect of the wire (double arrow) to be snared and easier access into the branch.

system utilizing wires preloaded through these directional branches has been developed, which greatly simplifies this process (Figure 26–10). In this setting, the initial graft would resemble a fenestrated device. However, preloaded wire(s) would be snared from a remote location to provide access directly into the branches and subsequently the target vessel. Such branch devices may optimally be combined with other forms of visceral vessel accommodation (fenestrated or reinforced fenestrated designs) to create a device that will reside appropriately within the anatomy at hand. Lastly, the creation of such complex implants requires customization, which may result in delays for such repairs and challenges with respect to production.

Investigators tend to pool results of both fenestrated branch grafts and cuffed branched grafts, with few series containing significant numbers of patients.[26,29-31] Chuter and colleagues recently published their series of branched stent-grafts for the treatment of complex aortic pathology.[31] In this series, 22 stent-grafts were placed with successful preservation of 81 visceral/renal branches. Perioperative mortality was 9.1%, and no cases of paraplegia, renal failure, stroke, or myocardial infarction were reported. One patient developed a type I endoleak that was successfully treated, while a second patient had a type II endoleak. At one month, branch graft patency was 98.75%. In Greenberg's series, in which 29 patients were treated, there was one perioperative death, and there were four late deaths (three of which were aneurysm related).[30] All patients were considered high risk for open surgical repair, mainly because of cardiopulmonary disease. Postoperative paralysis occurred in only one patient (.3%). No visceral branches were lost acutely or were occluded during follow-up. By 12 months follow-up, all patients experienced aneurysm sac diameter regression. These results demonstrate that endograft-branch vessel repair is clinically feasible with results that are comparable to, if not better than, those observed in conventional thoracoabdominal aortic aneurysm repair. A more extensive experience from the

Cleveland Clinic was recently reported by Roselli and colleagues who documented the results of branched endograft repair on 73 patients treated for thoracoabdominal aortic aneurysms.[32] Technical success occurred in 93% of the patients, and there were no conversions to open repair. Five technical failures were related to a death within 24 hours, and four patients in whom access into a single branch artery was not obtained. Major complications occurred 14% of patients and included paraplegia (2.7%), new onset dialysis (1.4%), prolonged ventilator support (6.8%), myocardial infarction (5.5%), and stroke (1.4%). Four early deaths occurred (prior to 30 days) and were secondary to myocardial infarction, worsening biventricular failure, mesenteric ischemia, and renal failure. Six patients died more than 30 days after surgery. Two patients died from complications related to spinal cord ischemia, one died of gastrointestinal hemorrhage, two deaths were cardiac in origin, and the sixth death was related to sepsis. There was an endoleak rate of 11%, of which there were three type I endoleaks and five type III endoleaks, all but one of which were treated before hospital discharge. The remaining endoleaks were type II. There were no reported aneurysm ruptures, sac expansion, graft migration, or component separations.

In an effort to assess outcomes of complex aortic endografting compared to conventional surgery, Greenberg performed a retrospective analysis on patients who underwent elective open surgical repair (N=372) or endovascular repair (N=352) of descending thoracic or thoracoabdominal aortic aneurysms.[33] The group of patients treated with endovascular repair was older and had more comorbid conditions than those undergoing open repair. Open repair, however, was more frequently applied to patients with type II or type III aneurysms and those that were associated with a chronic dissection. Despite the differences in patient age and comorbid conditions, mortality rates at 30 days (5.7% versus 8.3%) and 12 months (15.6% versus 15.9%) were not different between endovascular repair and surgical repair, nor was there a difference in the development of spinal cord ischemia (4% versus 8%, respectively, P=0.08). With the increasing application of endovascular techniques to treat complex aortic pathology, further analysis will become available to help us develop better branched devices and to determine which patient population would most benefit from their use.

Arch Aneurysms

In patients who have short proximal thoracic aortic necks or in aneurysms that involve the origin of the left subclavian artery or common carotid artery, EVAR typically has been accomplished by a two-staged approach combining both operative and endovascular repair. The first stage entails the placement of an "elephant trunk" through a median sternotomy. The subsequent second stage involves placement of a standard thoracic aortic stent-graft.[34] More advanced branched grafts have been used to treat thoracic aortic aneurysms that involve the aortic arch (Figure 26–11). A single-branched device, the Inoue single-branched stent-graft, has been used in 17 patients.[35] The devices, each custom made for specific patients, were placed distal to the left common carotid artery with the branch providing continued flow into the left subclavian artery. Inoue and his group[36] have placed more complex systems, involving multiple branches of the aortic arch, in a small number of patients. An alternative approach has been championed by Schneider and colleagues[37] and by Chuter and colleagues[38] who have described an extra-anatomic bypass after which a bifurcated stent-graft is placed through the right common carotid artery into the ascending aorta. The "contralateral limb" of the device, which is larger in diameter, then is cannulated from the descending

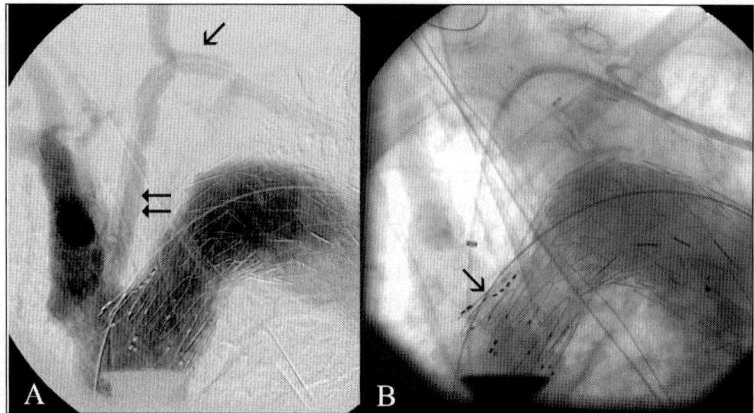

Figure 26-11. Fluoroscopic demonstration of a thoracic aortic endograft that involves the aortic arch. **(A)** This patient had a left carotid artery that arose from the inominate artery (bovine arch) (double arrow). In order to place it in a more ideal landing zone, the origin of the left carotid artery would be covered. To overcome this, a left carotid subclavian artery bypass was performed (arrow). **(B)** Subsequent to this, an endograft was placed that had a proximal scallop to allow partial coverage of the inominate artery (arrow). Note the sheath access that is maintained through the left carotid artery via the left brachial.

aorta where a mating thoracic stent-graft is used to complete the repair. While in its infancy, the use of branched aortic endografting will certainly revolutionize the current approach to arch, and possibly ascending, aortic aneurysm repair.

SUMMARY

The evolution of stent-graft technology will allow more widespread treatments of complex aortic aneurysmal disease. Such devices allow the treatment of the entire aorta in a manner intended to provide a long-term cure for aneurysmal aortic degeneration, regardless of the distribution of the biologic disease. Extensive experience with aortic endografting as well as renal, visceral, and arch vessel interventions, will be mandatory to ensure successful deployment of these complex devices. In addition, the surgeon must be familiar with the interpretation and processing of three-dimensional imaging modalities. Endovascular repair of complex aortic aneurysmal disease may lower the current and historically high morbidity and mortality rates associated with conventional repair. Continued improvement on these technologies will make current procedures, which can be quite complex, easier, and broaden the applicability of aortic endograft repair to regions of the aorta in which this is not currently the standard of care.

REFERENCES

1. Greenhalgh R, Brown L, Kwong G, et al. Comparison of endovascular aneurysm repair with open repair in patients with abdominal aortic aneurysm (EVAR trial 1), 30-day operative mortality results: randomized controlled trial. *Lancet.* 2004;364:843–848.
2. Prinssen M, Verhoeven E, Buth J, et al. A randomized trial comparing conventional and endovascular repair of abdominal aortic aneurysms. *N Engl J Med.* 2004;351:1607–1618.

3. Elkouri S, Martelli E, Gloviczki P, et al. Most patients with abdominal aortic aneurysm are not suitable for endovascular repair using currently approved bifurcated stent-grafts. *Vasc Endovascular Surg*. 2004;38:401–412.

4. Costin J, Watson D, Duff S, et al. Evaluation of the complexity of open abdominal aneurysm repair in the era of endovascular stent grafting. *J Vasc Surg*. 2006;43:915–920.

5. Haddad F, Greenberg R, Walker E, et al. Fenestrated endovascular grafting: the renal side of the story. *J Vasc Surg*. 2005;41:181–190.

6. Greenberg R, Chuter T, Sternbergh WI, et al. Zenith AAA endovascular graft: intermeidate-term results of the US multicenter trial. *J Vasc Surg*. 2004;39:1209–1218.

7. Greenberg R, Chuter T, Lawrence-Brown M, et al. Analysis of renal function after aneurysm repair with a device using suprarenal fixation (Zenith AAA endovascular graft (in contrast to open repair). *J Vasc Surg*. 2004;39:1219–1228.

8. Greenberg R, Fairman R, Srivastava S, et al. Endovascular grafting in patients with short necks: an analysis of short-term results. *J Cardiovasc Surg*. 2000;8:350–354.

9. Waasdorp E, de Vries J, Hobo R, et al. Aneurysm diameter and proximal aortic neck diamter influence clinical outcome of endovascular abdominal aortic repair: a 4-year EUROSTAR experience. *Ann Vasc Surg*. 2005;19:755–761.

10. Ouriel K, Clair D, Greenberg R, et al. Endovascular repair of abdominal aortic aneurysms: device-specific outcomes. *J Vasc Surg*. 2003;37:991–998.

11. Burks J, Faries P, Gravereaux E, et al. Endovascular repair of abdominal aortic aneurysms: stent graft fixation across the visceral arteries. *J Vasc Surg*. 2002;35:109–113.

12. Bove PG, Long GW, Shanley CJ, et al. Transrenal fixation of endovascular stent grafts infrarenal aortic aneurysm repair: mid-term results. *J Vasc Surg*. 2003;37:938–942.

13. Browne T, Hartley D, Purchas S, et al. A fenestrated covered suprarenal aortic stent. *J Vasc Endovasc Surg*. 1999;18:445–449.

14. O'Neill S, Greenberg R, Haddad F, et al. A prospective analysis of fenestrated endovascular grafting: intermediate-term outcomes. *Eur J Vasc Endovasc Surg*. 2006;32:115–123.

15. Greenberg R, Haulon S, Lyden S, et al. Endovascular management of juxtarenal aneurysms with fenestrated endovascular grafting. *J Vasc Surg*. 2004; 39:279–287.

16. Verhoeven E, Zeebregts C, Kapma M, et al. Fenestrated and branched endovascular techniques for thoraco-abdominal aneurysm repair. *J Cardiovasc Surg* (Torino). 2005;46: 131–140.

17. Sarac T, Clair D, Hertzer N, et al. Contemporary results of juxtarenal aneurysm repair. *J Vasc Surg*. 2002;36:1104–1111.

18. West C, Noel A, Bower T, et al. Factors affecting outcomes of open surgical repair of pararenal aortic aneurysm: a 10-year experience. *J Vasc Surg*. 2006;43:921–928.

19. Hertzer N, Mascha E. A personal experience with factors influencing survival after elective open repair of infrarenal aortic aneurysms. *J Vasc Surg*. 2005; 42:898–905.

20. McWilliams R, Murphy M, Hartley D, et al. In situ stent-graft fenestration to preserve the left subclavian artery. *J Endovasc Ther*. 2004;11:170–174.

21. Crawford E, Crawford J, Safi H, et al. Thoracoabdominal aortic aneurysms: operative and intraoperative factors determining immediate and long-term results of operations in 605 patients. *J Vasc Surg*. 1986;3:389–404.

22. Svensson L, Crawford E, Hess K, et al. Experience with 1,509 patients undergoing thoracoabdominal aortic operations. *J Vasc Surg* 1993;17:357–370.

23. Hollier L, Money S, Naslund T, et al. Risk of spinal cord dysfunction in patients undergoing thoracoabdominal aortic replacement. *Am J Surg*. 1992; 164:210–214.

24. Macierewicz J, Jameel M, Whitaker S, et al. Endovascular repair of perisplanchnic abdominal aortic aneurysm with visceral vessel transposition. *J Endovasc Ther*. 2000;7:410–414.

25. Fulton J, Farber M, Marston W, et al. Endovascular stent-graft repair of pararenal and type IV thoracoabdominal aortic aneurysms with adjunctive visceral reconstruction. *J Vasc Surg*. 2005;41:191–198.

26. Anderson J, Adam D, Berce M, et al. Repair of thoracoabdominal aortic aneurysms with fenestrated and branched endovascular stent grafts. *J Vasc Surg*. 2005;42:600–607.

27. Chuter T. Fenestrated and branched stent-grafts for thoracoabdominal, pararenal and juxtarenal aortic aneurysm repair. *Semin Vasc Surg.* 2007;20:90–96.
28. Greenberg R. Aortic aneurysm, thoracoabdominal aneurysm, juxtarenal aneurysm, fenestrated endografts, branched endografts, and endovascular aneurysm repair. *Ann NY Acad Sci.* 2006;1085:187–196.
29. Chuter T, Gordon R, Reilly L, et al. Multi-branched stent-graft for type III thoracoabdominal aortic aneurysm. *J Vasc Interv Radiol* 2001;12:391–392.
30. Greenberg R, West K, Pfaff K, et al. Beyond the aortic bifurcation: branched endovascular grafts for thoracoabdominal and aortoiliac aneurysms. *J Vasc Surg.* 2006;43:879–886.
31. Chuter T, Rapp J, Hiramoto J, et al. Endovascular treatment of thoracoabdominal aortic aneurysms. *J Vasc Surg.* 2008;47:6–16.
32. Roselli E, Greenberg R, Pfaff K, et al. Enodvascular treatment of thoracoabdominal aortic aneurysms. *J Thor Cardiovasc Surg.* 2007;133:1474–1482.
33. Greenberg R, Lu Q, Roselli E, et al. Contemporary analysis of descending thoracic and thoracoabdominal aneurysm repair. A comparison of endovascular and open techniques. *Circulation.* 2008;118:808–817.
34. Greenberg R, Haddad F, Svensson L, et al. Hybrid approaches to thoracic aortic aneurysms. *Circulation.* 2005;112:2619–2626.
35. Saito N, Kimura T, Odashiro K, et al. Feasibility of the Inoue single-branched stent-graft implantation for thoracic aortic aneurysm or dissection involving the left subclavian artery: short- to medium-term results in 17 patients. *J Vasc Surg.* 2005;41:206–212.
36. Inoue K, Hosokawa H, Iwase T, et al. Aortic arch reconstruction by transluminally placed endovascular branched stent graft. *Circulation.* 1999;100:316S–121S.
37. Schneider D, Curry T, Reilly L, et al. Branched endovascular repair of aortic arch aneurysm with a modular stent-graft system. *J Vasc Surg.* 2003;38:855.
38. Chuter T, Schneider D, Reilly L, et al. Modular branched stent graft for endovascular repair of aortic arch aneurysm and dissection. *J Vasc Surg* 2003;38:859–863.

Endovascular Graft for Ruptured Aortic Aneurysm

27

Impact of Endovascular Graft on Rupture of Abdominal Aortic Aneurysm (AAA)

James May, M.D. M.S., F.R.A.C.S.,
F.A.C.S., Geoffrey H. White, F.R.AC.S.,
and John P. Harris M.S., F.R.A.C.S., F.A.C.S.

IMPACT OF ENDOVASCULAR GRAFT ON RUPTURE OF AAA

The impact of endovascular graft on rupture of abdominal aortic aneurysm (AAA) is a multi faceted one. In many parts of the world, the ability to perform elective endovascular AAA repair in high-risk patients, considered unfit for open repair, has dramatically reduced the number of AAA patients presenting with rupture. Second, the endovascular method of aneurysm repair has found an increasing role in the treatment of ruptured AAA. This has had a favorable impact on the outcome of intervention for ruptured AAA. And third, and on the negative side, elective endovascular grafting of AAA has been followed by a small but steady proportion of patients whose aneurysms rupture unexpectedly, thus contributing to the pool of patients presenting with ruptured AAA. We have found, however, that when AAAs rupture in this situation, the outcome is significantly better than when AAAs rupture without any prior treatment. Thus, it can be seen that in three of the four interactions of endovascular grafting and rupture of AAA, the impact has been favorable. These interactions will be discussed sequentially.

Impact of Endovascular Graft on Reducing the Number of AAA Patients Presenting with Rupture

We undertook a study at Royal Prince Alfred Hospital to provide information on this topic. Our aim was to look at the proportion of patients undergoing urgent repair of ruptured AAA compared with those undergoing elective repair during two consecutive periods of time.

Between May 1992 and September 2003, 1,134 patients underwent repair of AAA. These were divided arbitrarily into two groups; 356 having their operation in the four-year period between May 1992 and May 1996 (Group 1), and 778 having their operation in the seven-year period between June 1996 and September 2003 (Group 2). In Group 1, 303 patients underwent elective repair of intact AAA while 53 (17.5%) underwent urgent repair of ruptured AAA. In Group 2,740 patients underwent elective repair of intact AAA while 38 (5.1%) underwent urgent repair of ruptured AAA. This difference in proportion of patients undergoing treatment for rupture in the two time periods was significant ($p < 0.01$) (Figure 27–1). Eighteen patients re-presenting with rupture following previous elective endovascular AAA repair in both periods of time were excluded to avoid counting the same patients twice. This group will be discussed further in the fourth interaction of endovascular grafting and rupture of AAA.

Of the 303 patients in Group 1 treated electively, 108 (35.6%) underwent endovascular repair while 195 underwent open repair. By comparison, of the 740 patients in Group 2 treated electively, 501 (67.7%) underwent endovascular repair while 239 underwent open repair. This difference in proportion between the two methods of treatment in the two time periods was significant ($p < 0.01$) (Figure 27–2). Forty-eight of 108 (44.4%) patients in Group 1 and 156 of 501 (31.3%) patients in Group 2 undergoing elective endovascular AAA repair were considered to be high risk and unfit for open repair.

There has been no change in our referral base nor any new providers of service in the area who could account for the reduction in the number of patients undergoing treatment for rupture from a mean of 13 per year to five per year. We believe this has resulted in large part from cumulative removal of high risk AAA patients by way of endovascular repair, from the pool of those who were previously denied treatment until rupture supervened. By this time, the mortality rate for repair was extremely high. The impact of endovascular graft on rupture of AAA via this mechanism, therefore, has been very favorable.

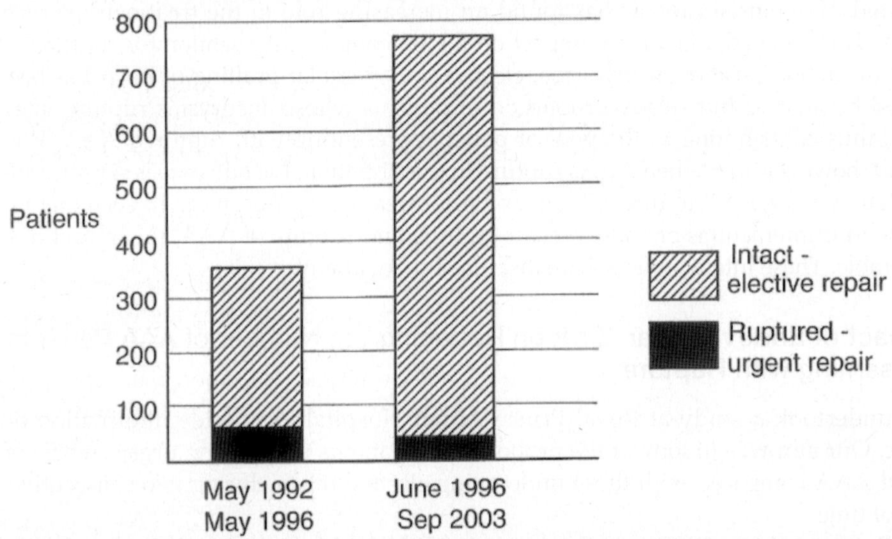

Figure 27-1. Graph showing proportion of patients undergoing urgent repair of ruptured AAA compared with elective repair of intact AAA for two consecutive periods of time.

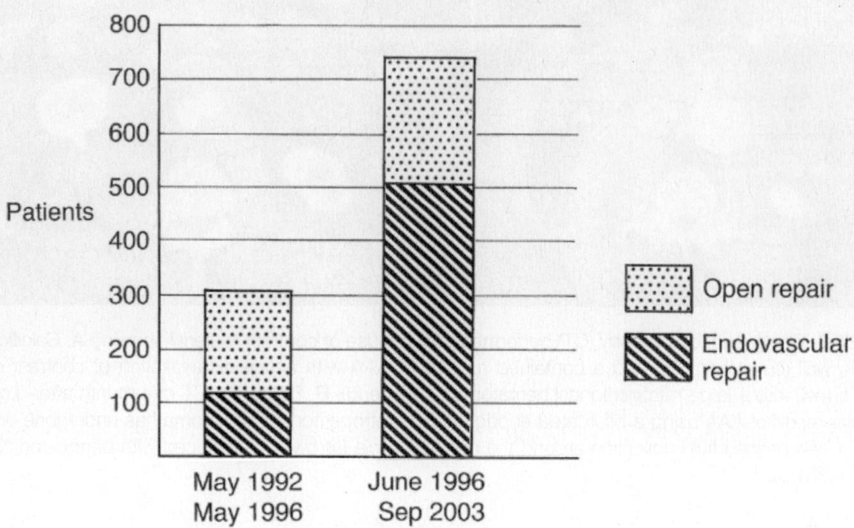

Figure 27-2. Graph showing proportion of patients whose AAAs were treated by open repair compared with endovascular repair for two consecutive periods of time.

Impact of Endovascular Repair on Early Outcome of Ruptured AAA

Elective endovascular repair of intact AAA has resulted in significant reduction in perioperative mortality and morbidity compared with open surgical repair.[1-3] Operative mortality rates for surgical repair of ruptured AAA range between 40%–50%[4] with an overall mortality of 75%–90% if account is taken of those who died before reaching hospital.[5] Vascular surgeons have felt intuitively, therefore, that the endovascular method of AAA repair should be capable of reducing the mortality of ruptured AAAs, given such a large margin for improvement. There are many theoretical benefits, which the endovascular method can bring to the management of ruptured AAA, including maintenance of retroperitoneal tamponarde with resulting reduction in blood loss (Figure 27–3), and avoidance of aortic cross-clamping with its resulting ischaemia reperfusion injury and minimizing hypothermia. From the first case report of endovascular repair of ruptured AAA by the Nottingham group in 1994[6] to the present time, it has not been easy to find objective evidence and statistical proof of the superiority of endovascular versus open repair for AAA rupture. The difficulty has been that not all AAAs are anatomically suitable for endovascular repair. It has not been possible, therefore, to report a series of consecutive patients with ruptured AAA, treated by the endovascular method, for historical or concurrent comparison with open repair. In an excellent review of the literature on endovascular repair of ruptured AAA, Hinchcliffe et al.[7] used a medline search of all English papers for the key words of endovascular aneurysm repair and ruptured AAA. Additional data were obtained from the published abstracts of international vascular and endovascular meetings. These reviewers noted that there have been reports from specialized vascular units, but these were limited to selected and stable patients.

Previous reports of anatomic eligibility for endovascular repair of ruptured AAA have ranged from 20%–40%.[8,9] This comparatively low rate of anatomical suitability is in keeping with previous reports that aneurysms that rupture are associated with

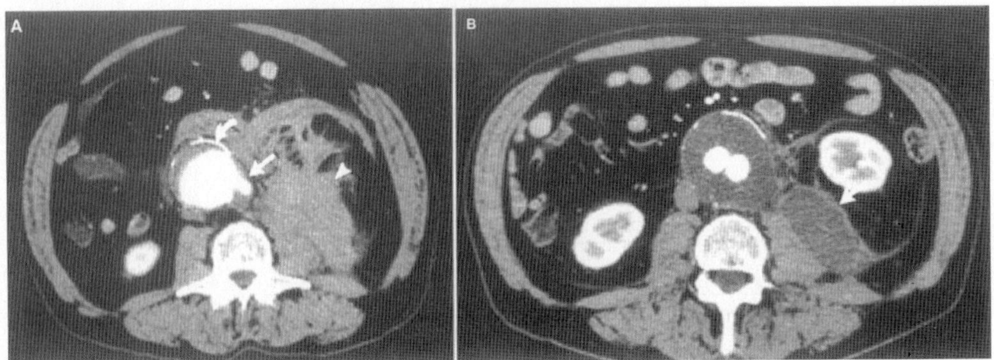

Figure 27-3. Computed tomography (CT) performed with the use of contrast material showing **A.** Calcification in the aortic wall (curved arrow), and a contained rupture of AAA with active extravazation of contrast material (straight arrow) into a large retroperitoneal hematoma (arrowhead). **B.** Follow-up CT one month after urgent endovascular repair of AAA using a bifurcated enodgraft. The retroperitoneal hematoma has undergone organization into a well-defined fluid collection around the psoas muscle (arrow). Reproduced with permission *N Engl J Med* 2004;351:12.

larger diameters than intact aneurysms,[10] and that larger aneurysms tend to have more adverse anatomical features that reduce the applicability of the endovascular method.[11] Despite the foregoing limitations, the Montefiore Medical Center group and the Florida College of Medicine, Gainesville group have reported much higher rates of anatomic eligibility of 83% and 76%, respectively.[12,13] Both groups have achieved this by using similar treatment algorithms for ruptured AAA. Patients at Montefiore with presumed rupture of aorto iliac aneurysm were treated with restricted fluid resuscitation (hypotensive hemostasis), transport to the operating room, and arteriography. Endovascular AAA repair was undertaken if aortoiliac anatomy was suitable. If the anatomy was unsuitable, conventional open repair was performed. Of 35 patients treated in this manner, 29 had endovascular AAA repair while six required open AAA repair. Supraceliac balloon placement and inflation, using a previously positioned guidewire, was required in 10 patients for circulatory collapse. Four patients died within 30 days, giving a very commendable perioperative mortality rate of 11%.

In the Gainesville group, all patients with a diagnosis of ruptured AAA who did not have a prior CT scan on arrival and who were hemodinamically stable (conscious with systolic blood pressure >80mmHg), underwent ultrafast contrast spiral CT for evaluation of anatomic suitability (Figure 27–4). In this algorithm, all patients who were unstable (unconscious or systolic blood pressure <80mmHg) were taken directly to the operating room for open AAA repair. The group reported 36 consecutive patients who underwent treatment of acute ruptured AAA. They were treated during two consecutive time periods. Nineteen of the 36 ruptured AAAs were repaired between January 1997 and December 2001 (early, before introduction of endovascular ruptured AAA program), and 17 were repaired between January 2002 and March 2004 (late, after introduction of endovascular ruptured AAA program)

All 19 ruptured AAAs in the early period were treated by conventional transperitoneal open repair under general anaesthesia. Of the 17 ruptured AAAs in the late period, 13 were treated by endovascular repair and four by open surgical repair.

Importantly, none of the four cases in which open surgery was performed in the late group was as a result of hemodynamic instability. All 13 endovascular patients

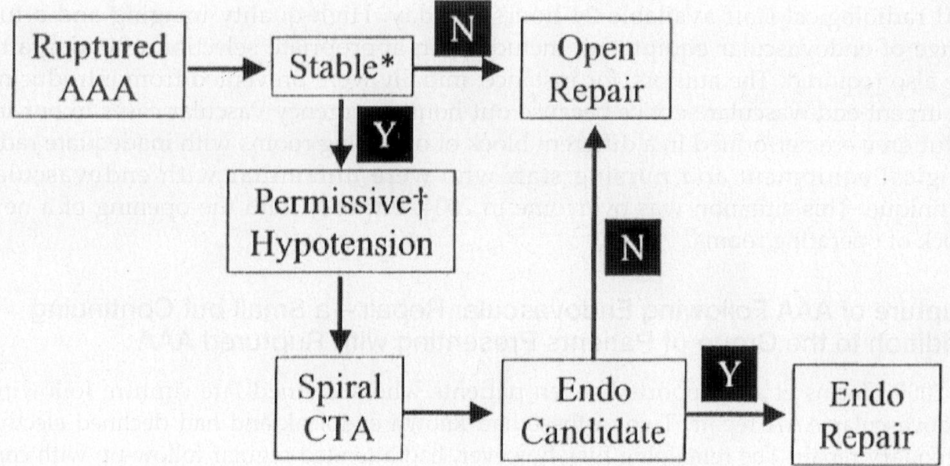

Figure 27-4. Algorithm of treatment of ruptured AAA at Florida College of Medicine Gainsville. *Stable: conscious with systolic blood pressure >80mmHg. All unstable patients treated by open repair. + Permissive hypotention: no fluid resuscitation unless systolic blood pressure <80mHg or decreased mentation. Reproduced with permission *J Vasc Surg* 2004;40:211–5 (Lee WA et al. Reference 13)

had technically successful implantation of bifurcated devices. The periopeartive mortality in the early and late periods was 37% versus 12%, respectively *(p* = 0.13). Median procedure times, blood loss, and length of stay were all significantly higher during the early period than in the late period.

Although the difference in perioperative mortality did not achieve statistical significance, the results are very encouraging, as are the results from the Montefiore group.

The above two reports differ in that the Gainsville group used commercially available bifurcated endografts exclusively while the Montefiore group used their own locally constructed aortouniiliac endograft. They also differed in their method of assessment of anatomical eligibility. The Montefiore group used on-table aortography. This has the advantage of speed and allows the patient to remain under the constant supervision of the surgical and anesthetic teams. The assessment of the proximal neck, however, is limited to the luminal profile rather than the full thickness of the aortic wall. The ultrafast contrast spiral CT scan used by the Gainsville group negates the time advantage of on-table aortography and has the additional benefit of excluding other pathology that may be responsible for the patient's symptoms. The differing configuration used by the two groups illustrates the widespread controversy that exists concerning endograft selection. The aortouniiliac device favored by the Montefiore group has the advantage of saving the time that would be required to cannulate the contralateral stump and deploy the contralateral limb in a bifurcated repair. It does, however, require coil embolization of the ipsilateral internal iliac artery and deployment of an occluding plug in the contralateral common iliac artery. Proponents of the bifurcated device point to elimination of both the cross-over graft and the vulnerability of the lower half of the body being dependent on one iliac limb.

One reason that endovascular grafting has not had a greater numerical impact on the treatment of ruptured AAA is the logistic requirements needed to set up an urgent endovascular service. Such a service requires experienced nursing, surgical, anesthetic and radiological staff available 24 hours per day. High-quality imaging and a full range of endovascular equipment, including an appropriate selection of endografts, are also required. The authors, for instance, initially were prevented from introducing an urgent endovascular service because out-hour emergency vascular cases in our institution were performed in a different block of operating rooms with inadequate radiological equipment and nursing staff who were unfamiliar with endovascular technique. This situation was overcome in 2004, but only with the opening of a new block of operating rooms.

Rupture of AAA Following Endovascular Repair—a Small but Continuing Addition to the Group of Patients Presenting with Ruptured AAA

In 2000, Zarins et al.[14] reported seven patients who sustained late rupture following endovascular AAA repair. Two of these had known endoleak and had declined elective secondary repair. The remaining five, however, had attended regular follow-up with contrast CT, confirming exclusion of their aneurysm sac from the circulation and no evidence of expansion of the sac. The endografts implanted in all patients were AneuRx, but similar unexpected cases of late rupture have been shown to occur with other types of endograft. Zarins attributed the rupture in five patients without known endoleak to instability of the devices at anchor zones and at points of modular connection. He advised close inspection of follow-up plain X-rays and CT scans to detect minor movements of radio-opaque parts.

Late rupture following endovascular AAA repair may occur in patients with endoleak, patients with endotension (sac expansion but no endoleak), and in patients with neither endoleak nor endotension. Zarins postulated that late rupture could be anticipated and prevented by secondary endovascular repair involving deployment of extension endografts at sites of instability in the primary endograft.

In a subsequent paper, Zarins[15] reported late rupture in 10 patients out of 1,193 patients undergoing previous endovascular repair with AneuRx devices, for a probability of rupture at four years of 1.6%. This small but continuing proportion of patients whose aneurysms rupture unexpectedly following endovascular repair impacts on rupture of AAA by contributing to the pool of patients presenting with ruptured AAA. There is the potential for this contribution to rise however, as demonstrated by Cho et al.[16] who reported a worrying probability of only 43% freedom from sac expansion (and presumed endotension) at four years following endovascular AAA repair with the Excluder (PTFE) device. Fortunately, there were no instances of rupture. Six months later, Thoo et al.[17] reported symptomatic sac enlargement and rupture due to seroma in five patients following open repair with Goretex (PTFE) grafts (Figure 27–5). Paradoxically, the clinical course of these patients was comparatively benign, with the authors suggesting that the most likely cause of the problem was fluid transfer through the graft material and recommending a circumspect rather than mandatory interventional approach to treatment, provided that communication between the arterial circulation and the aneurysm sac had been excluded.

Matsumura et al. reported that some of these unexpected ruptures were due to what they termed "transgraft microleaks".[18] These were small Type 3c endoleaks (due to fabric defect at sites of suture) that could not be imaged by conventional contrast CT or aortography. They demonstrated the endoleaks by using a combination of directed aortography and duplex ultrasound involving multiple oblique views.

Intermittent endoleak has also been reported and may account for some cases of unexpected late rupture. The intermittent nature of the type 3c endoleak has been shown to be due to changes in a patient's posture.

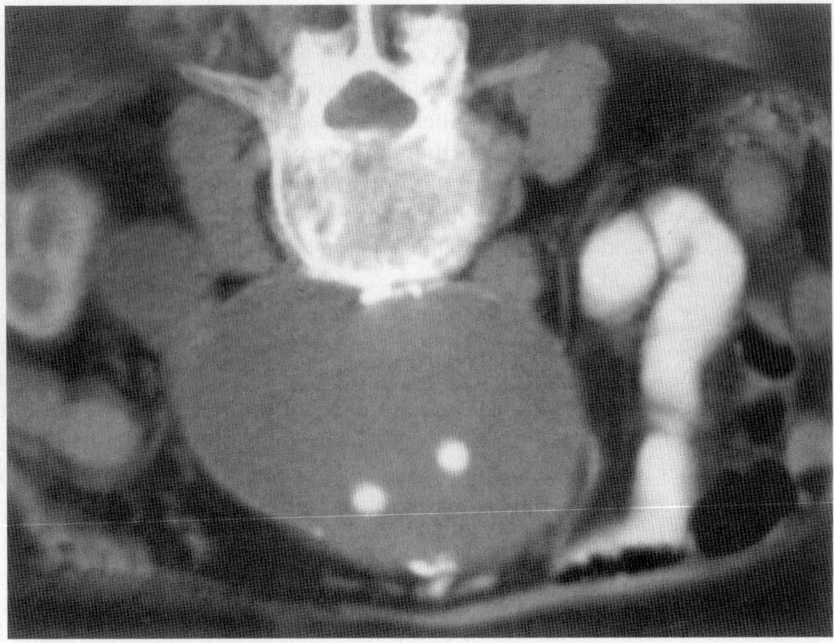

Figure 27-5. Figure CT performed with the use of contrast material demonstrating sac enlargement (10.5cm in diameter) due to seroma, 7 years after open repair of AAA with a bifurcated PTFE graft. There is a presumed rupture of sac contents into the left retroperitoneal tissues. No communication was demonstrated between the arterial circulation and the aneurysm sac, thus permitting conservative management without intervention. Reproduced with permission *J Vasc Surg* 2004;40:1090-5 (Thoo CHC et al Reference 17).

Endovascular Grafts Complicated by Late Rupture Impact on the Rupture Process by Having a Significantly Better Outcome Compared with Rupture of an Untreated AAA

We have previously reported unexpected survival in four patients at high risk who underwent open repair of late rupture of an AAA after previous enodvascular repair.[19] Our continuing experience of noting survival in patients at high risk in whom this outcome would not have been anticipated led to a subsequent concurrent comparison of outcome of ruptured AAA occurring after endovascular repair versus those occurring without prior treatment.[20] In this 11-year study (May 1992 to September 2003), 1,043 patients underwent elective repair of intact infrarenal AAAs. Endovascular repair was performed in 609 and open repair in 434 patients. Eighteen of 609 patients (3%) who underwent endovascular AAA repair required treatment because of rupture of the aneurysm at a mean of 29 months after their primary repair (Group 1). During the same 11-year period, another 91 patients without previous treatment required urgent repair of ruptured AAA (Group 2). Rupture was diagnosed by contrast CT or by the presence of extramural extravazation of blood at open repair. Hypotension (systolic blood pressure <100mmHg) was noted at presentation in four of 18 patients (22%) in Group 1 and 76 of 91 patients (84%) in Group 2. All patients underwent open repair by a transperitoneal approach, except for four patients in Group 1 and three patients in Group 2 who underwent endovascular repair of ruptured AAAs. The proportion of patients with hypotension at presentation in Group 1 (four of 18) was significantly less than in Group 2 (76 of 91; $p < .01$). The difference in perioperative (30 day) mortality rate in Group 1 (three of 18; 16.6%) compared with Group 2 (49 of 91; 53.8%) was also significant ($p < .01$). The outcome in Group 1 was, therefore, superior to that in Group 2. This study confirmed that endovascular AAA repair complicated by endoleak does not prevent rupture. The data suggests, however, that rupture, when it does occur in these circumstances, may not be accompanied by such major hemodynamic changes and high mortality as rupture of an untreated AAA. Further long-term follow-up and analysis in a larger group of patients are required to confirm this apparent intermediate level of protection afforded by failed endovascular repair, which does not prevent rupture but enhances survival after operation to treat rupture, possibly by ameliorating the hemodynamic changes associated with the ruptured process.

It seems that the most likely explanation for this better-than-expected survival in patients with ruptured AAA after endovascular repair is that these patients are in a relatively stable hemodynamic state at presentation. The findings at presentation and outcomes in patients in this study support our earlier hypothesis that seeks to explain these findings. By definition, all patients with rupture after endovascular AAA repair have an endoleak that enables communication between the aortic lumen and the exterior of the aneurysm sac. It is known that endoleak, whether previously known or not, enables systemic arterial pressure to be communicated to the sac of the AAA in the same way as would occur in an untreated AAA. The risk for rupture, therefore, remains the same in these patients as in those with untreated AAAs. Once rupture occurs, however, the quantity and rate of blood loss outside the aneurysm sac is limited by the endoleak chanel. Patients survive AAA rupture because of a combination of retroperitoneal pressurization and thrombosis-induced temporary hemostasis. These are more likely to be effective if the extravascular channel is long and narrow as a result of previous endovascular AAA repair. In the case of an untreated AAA, however, blood loss is limited by the defect in the ruptured sac, which has little chance to thrombose. In situations in which the endograft has migrated from the proximal neck of the aneurysm into the sac, it is clear that the preceding endovascular repair would have no effect on the outcome of the rupture.

In summary, the impact of endovascular graft on rupture of AAA is a complex one. It seems that elective endovascular AAA repair in high-risk patients is a major factor in reducing the number of AAA patients presenting with rupture. Such patients were previously denied treatment until rupture supervened, by which time the mortality rate for repair was extremely high. Second, specialized vascular units with a multidisciplinary urgent endovascular service have been able to increase the anatomic eligibility rate for endovascular repair of ruptured AAA to the 76%–83% range and reduce the overall perioperative mortality rate to the very commdable 11%–12% range in consecutively treated patients. Third, despite strict surveillance, elective endovascular AAA repair continues to be complicated by a 1%–3% incidence of late rupture, thus increasing the number of patients presenting with rupture. In the authors' experience, the mortality rate for treatment of rupture following previous endovascular AAA repair (16.6%), however, is significantly better than that occurring in patients without prior intervention (53.8%).

The overall impact of endovascular graft on rupture of AAA, therefore, has been a favorable one in which the mortality rate has been reduced. There is also the potential for a greater favorable impact with provision of staff and facilities enabling more widespread use of the technique beyond a limited number of specialized vascular centers.

REFERENCES

1. Lee WA, Carter BS Upchurch G, et al. Perioperative outcomes after open and endovascular repair of intact abdominal aortic aneurysms in the United States during 2001. *J Vasc Surg.* 2004;39:491–496.
2. Greenhalgh RM, Brown LC, Kwong GP, et al. Comparison of endovascular aneurysm repair with open repair in patients with abdominal aortic aneurysm (EVAR trial 1), 30-day operative mortality results: randomized controlled trial. *Lancet.* 2004;364 (9437):843–848.
3. Prinssen M, Verhoeven EL, Buth J, et al. A randomized trial comparing conventional and endovascular repair of abdominal aortic aneurysms. *N Engl J Med.* 2004;351(16):1607–1618.
4. Brown MJ, Sutton AJ, Bell PR, Sayers RD. A meta-analysis of 50 years of ruptured abdominal aortic aneurysm repair. *Br J Surg.* 2002;89:714–730.
5. Heikkinen M, Salenius JP, Auvinen O. Ruptured abdominal aortic aneurysm in a well-defined geographic area. *J Vasc Surg.* 2002;36:291–296.
6. Yusuf SW, Whitaker SC, Chuter TA et al. Emergency endovascular repair of leaking arotic aneurysm (letter). *Lancet.* 1994;344:1645.
7. Hinchliffe RJ, Braithwaite BD, Hopkinson BR. The endovascular management of ruptured abdominal aortic aneurysms. *Eur J Vasc Endovasc Surg.* 2003;25:191–201.
8. Hinchliffe RJ, Alric P, Rose D, et al. Comparison of morphologic features of intact and ruptured aneurysms of infrarenal abdominal aorta. *J Vasc Surg.* 2003;38:88–92.
9. Lee WA, Huber TS, Hirneise CM, et al. Eligibility rates of ruptured and symptomatic AAA for endovascular repair. *J Endovasc Ther.* 2002;9:436–442.
10. Szilagyi DE, Smith RF, DeRusso FJ et al. Contribution of abdominal aortic aneurysm within the catchment are a of a regional vascular surgical service. *Ann Surg.* 1966;164:678–699.
11. Armon MP, Yusuf SW, Whitaker SC et al. Influence of abdominal aortic aneurysm size on the feasibility of endovascular repair. *J Endovasc Surg.* 1997;4:279–283.
12. Veith FJ, Ohki T, Lipsitz EC et al. Treatment of ruptured abdominal aneurysms with stent grafts: a new gold standard? *Semin Vasc Surg.* 2003;16(2):171-175.
13. Lee WA, Hirneise CM, Tayyarah M, et al. Impact of endovascular repair on early outcomes of ruptured abdominal aortic aneurysms. *J Vasc Surg.* 2004;40:211–5.
14. Zarins CK, White RA Fogarty TJ. Aneurysm rupture after endovascular repair using the AneuRx stent graft. *J Vasc Surg.* 2000;31:960–70.
15. Zarins CK, & AneuRx Clinical Investigators. The US AneuRx Clinical Trial: 6-year clinical update 2002. *J Vasc Surg.* 2003;37:904–908.
16. Cho JS, Sillavou ED, Rhee RY, Makaroun MS. Late abdominal aortic aneurysm enlargement after endovascular repair with the Excluder device. *J Vasc Surg.* 2004;39:1236–1242.
17. Thoo CHC, Bourke BM, May J. Symptomatic sac enlargement and rupture due to seroma after open abdominal aortic aneurysm repair with polytetrafluoroethylene graft: implications for endovascular repair and endotension. *J Vasc Surg.* 2004;40:1090–1095.
18. Matsumura JS, Ryu RK, Ourier K. Identification and implications of transgraft microleaks after endovascular repair of aortic aneurysm repair. *J Vasc Surg.* 2003;34:190–197.
19. May J, White GH, Waugh R, et al. Rupture of abdominal aortic aneurysm: a concurrent comparison of outcome of those occurring after endoluminal repair versus those occurring de novo. *Eur J Vasc Endovasc Surg.* 1999;18:344–348.
20. May J, White GH, Stephen MS, Harris JP. Rupture of abdominal arotic aneurysm: Concurrent comparison of outcome of those occurring after endovascular repair versus those occurring without previous treatment in an 11-year single-center experience. *J Vasc Surg.* 2004;40:860–866.

28

Management Strategies, Adjuncts, and Technical Tips to Facilitate Endovascular Treatment of Ruptured Abdominal Aortic Aneurysms

Frank J. Veith, M.D.

This chapter deals with the endovascular management of ruptured infrarenal abdominal aortic aneurysms (RAAAs) and ruptured aortoiliac aneurysms. By definition, a RAAA is one in which the wall of the aneurysm contains a hole or a vent through which blood has leaked and is present outside the aneurysm wall. This article will not consider the treatment of so-called "acute aneurysms" that present with pain and even hypotension, but which show no evidence of blood outside the aneurysm wall, although some of the treatment methods presented can be used in this setting as well.

Unlike elective AAAs in which open surgery can be performed with a less than 5% operative mortality and a reasonably low morbidity, the open surgical treatment of RAAAs carries an operative mortality in the 45% range (35% to 55%).[1-6] This persists despite all the technical and other adjunctive improvements that have been suggested. Moreover, the morbidity of open surgery for RAAAs remains high. Thus, endovascular repair of ruptured aneurysms (EVRAR) offers considerable room for improvement.

In view of the poor results of open surgery for RAAAs, one may question why EVRAR has not been used more. One reason is that in the early days of endovascular aneurysm repair, it took time to take the measurements required for endografting, and it took additional time to procure the appropriate graft or grafts. The second reason is that all surgeons have traditionally advocated the need in RAAA patients to gain rapid aortic control, usually by clamp placement proximal to the aneurysm at the infrarenal or supraceliac level. This mandated emergency laparotomy.

It turns out that both these factors are not necessarily obstacles to EVAR. In 1994, we and others first began to treat RAAAs with endovascular grafts.[7-9] This was possible because the Montefiore and Nottingham groups had endografts that could be prepared rapidly and used to treat a wide variety of patients with RAAAs. It also was apparent in these early patient experiences that at least some RAAA patients remained stable or at least viable long enough for the endovascular grafting procedure to be successfully performed. EVRAR was proven feasible.

METHODS

Hypotensive Hemostasis

In the past, it has been noted that restricting blood transfusions and other fluid resuscitation was an effective way to control hemorrhage and improve treatment outcomes in patients who were bleeding. This was noted with patients who had upper gastrointestinal bleeding in the 1940s and subsequently, those who had a variety of other conditions including vascular trauma.[10-12] In the mid-1990s, we made the observation that restricting fluid resuscitation could also be effective in the ruptured aneurysm setting, and we coined the term "hypotensive hemostasis."[13-14] By that we mean aggressively restricting all fluid resuscitation in RAAA patients as long as they remain conscious and are able to talk and move. We accept a reduction in arterial systolic blood pressure to the 50–70 mm Hg range and still minimize fluid resuscitation, as difficult as that can sometimes be. However, by doing so, bleeding will temporarily cease and time will be available to perform an endovascular graft repair (Figures 28–1 and 28–2).

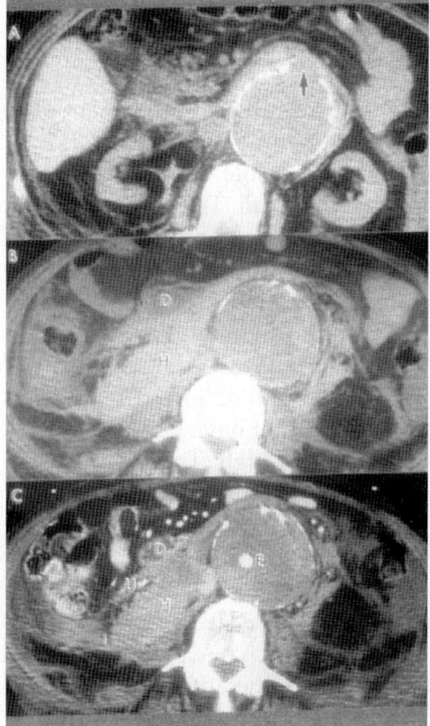

Figure 28-1. CT scan preoperatively (**A** and **B**) and four days after insertion of an aortounifemoral graft (MEGS) (**C**). Postoperatively, all contrast was contained within the graft and the RAAA was excluded. Note resolution of the retroperitoneal hemorrhage.

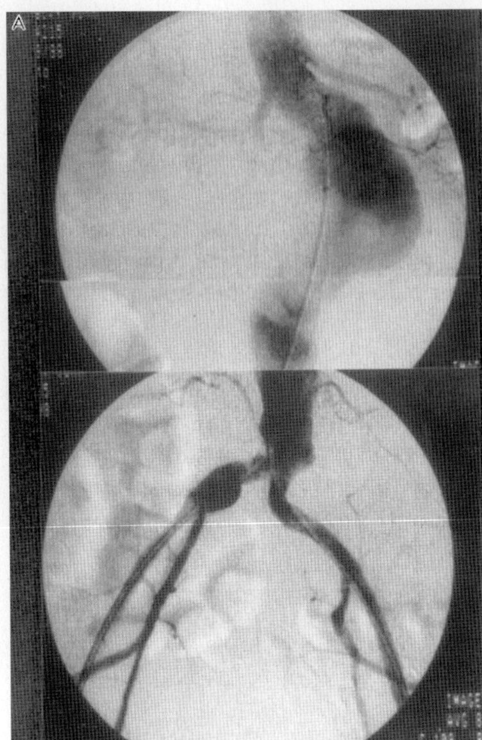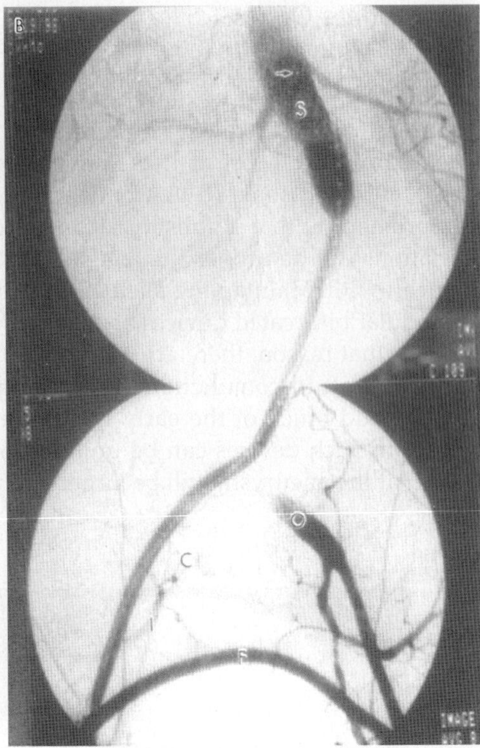

Figure 28-2. (A) Arteriogram in the operating room before placing the endograft in the patient shown in Figure 28-1. At this time, the patient's blood pressure was 50 mm Hg. Note there is no contrast outside the lumen of the aorta and the aneurysm because of the hypotension. **(B)** Completion arteriogram after placement of an aortounifemoral endovascular graft, an occluder (O) in the left common iliac artery, and coils (C) in the right hypogastric artery. A femorofemoral bypass (F) has also been performed. S is the proximal Palmaz stent. The arrow points to the top of the graft.

Supraceliac Balloon Control

Although hypotensive hemostasis can be an effective method to temporarily control bleeding in many RAAA patients, it can sometimes fail with cardiovascular collapse. Moreover, if patients are anesthetized with concomitant loss of their sympathetic nervous system compensation for a reduced blood volume, they frequently undergo cardiovascular collapse. In these circumstances, emergency aortic control proximal to the rupture site becomes mandatory. As detailed in the "Current RAAA Management Protocol" section that follows, placement under fluoroscopic control of a guidewire via a femoral or brachial access site in the supraceliac aorta should be carried out under *local* anesthesia. This enables angiographic evaluation of the patient's arterial anatomy to determine suitability for endovascular grafting. More importantly, this guidewire can be used to enable rapid placement of a large (14–16 Fr) sheath (Cook Inc.) through which a large compliant balloon can rapidly be inserted to occlude the supraceliac aorta.[13-18]

Appropriate Grafts

The original endovascular grafts that were used to treat RAAAs were fabricated or assembled by surgeons so that they could be quickly inserted in the ruptured aneurysm setting.[7-9,17,19,20] However, subsequently, a variety of commercially made grafts have been employed. Most of these have been of the modular bifurcated variety (Figure 28–3), although some RAAA patients have been treated with unibody devices. A key requirement is that a substantial inventory of devices be on hand so that anatomic variations can be properly managed and the adverse events that inevitably occur can be dealt with. Maintaining such an inventory of devices can be expensive, particularly if modular bifurcated devices are to be used.

For that reason, there are advantages to using a unilateral aortoiliac or aortofemoral endograft in conjunction with contralateral iliac occlusion and a femorofemoral bypass, and much of the early EVRAR experience employed devices with this configuration. Such devices can be unibody or modular. They offer the additional advantage that the aneurysm will be largely depressurized once the graft is deployed.

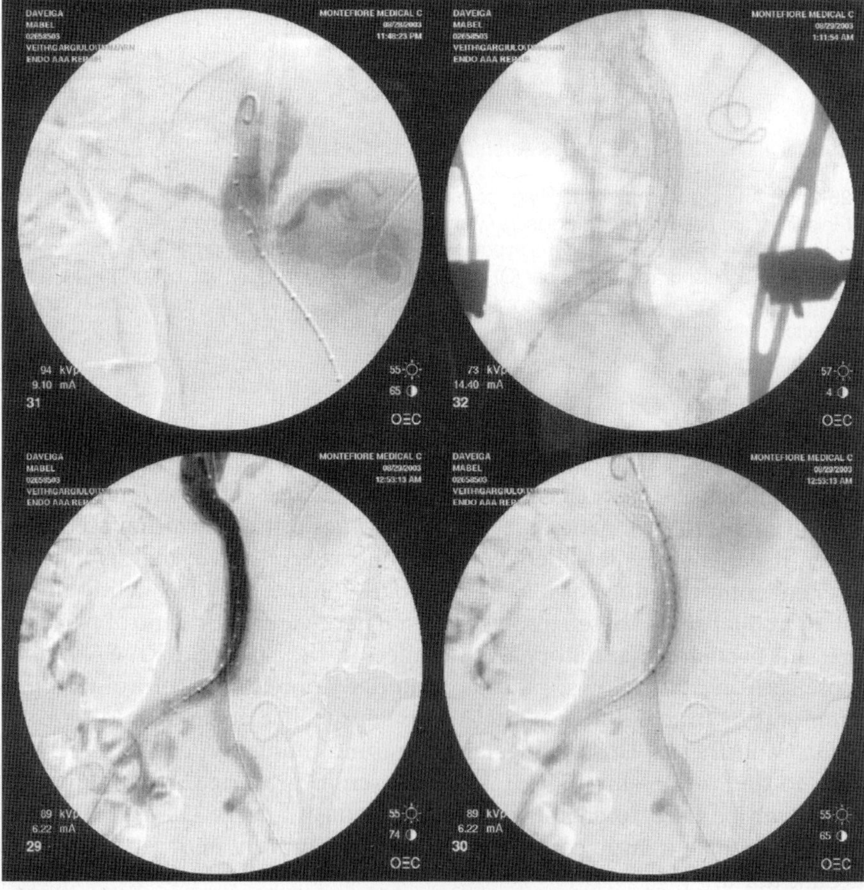

Figure 28-3. Intraoperative arteriograms in an 82-year-old Jehovah's Witness with a RAAA and unfavorable proximal neck anatomy. The patient had a blood pressure of 60 mm Hg and a hematocrit of 17%. Because she refused blood transfusions, an endovascular repair was attempted. The aneurysm was excluded with an AneuRx modular graft. She has survived over 5 years.

Current RAAA Management Protocol

Most centers require RAAA patients to be stable enough to undergo a computerized tomographic (CT) scan to confirm the rupture and allow a decision to be made whether or not patienta are suitable endovascular graft candidates. We do not adhere to that requirement although more than one-half of our RAAA patients have had a CT scan performed either in our own institution or elsewhere Our current RAAA management protocol is as follows. Once a presumed diagnosis of RAAA is made,[21] the patient is rapidly transported to the operating room, which must have full digital fluoroscopy capacity (OEC, model #9800), a radiolucent movable operating table, and a large inventory of endovascular supplies (catheters, guidewires, sheaths, stents, and endovascular grafts). As the patient is being prepared for the procedure, fluid is restricted as outlined above. Intravenous and intra-arterial lines are placed. Tubes are placed in the bladder and stomach. The patient is positioned, prepared, and draped with the right arm extended and the right antecubital fossa, lower chest, abdomen, and thighs exposed. The fluoroscope is placed on the patient's left side. Under local anesthesia, a 7 Fr sheath is placed in the femoral artery or a 5 Fr sheath is placed percutaneously in the right brachial artery. Through either of these sheaths a catheter and guidewire are manipulated into the supraceliac aorta. Using a pigtailed catheter in the suprarenal aorta, an abdominal aortogram is performed with posteroanterior and oblique views to define the aneurysm neck and iliac artery anatomy. A decision is made whether the patient is suitable for endovascular repair or will require an open repair. This decision is based on a number of factors including the patient's anatomy and the type of endograft available.

If an *open repair* is required, the guidewire is replaced in the supraceliac aorta. Anesthesia is induced and the open repair performed in a standard fashion. If the patient has cardiovascular collapse, a 14 or 16 Fr sheath is placed over the guidewire followed by a 33 or 40 cm compliant balloon (Meditech). Under fluoroscopic control, the balloon is placed and inflated in the infrarenal neck of the aneurysm if it is long enough. Balloon inflation is monitored fluoroscopically using dilute contrast to fill the balloon until the aorta is occluded. If the proximal neck is short, the balloon is placed and inflated in the supraceliac aorta. In this position, every effort must be made to minimize balloon inflation time and to obtain infrarenal clamp control as soon as possible. Systemic heparin is administered when the aorta is occluded.

If an *endovascular repair* is to be performed, it may, in some instances, be carried out under local anesthesia.[22] However, we have found that RAAA patients move about on the operating table, making accurate fluoroscopic localization and graft deployment difficult. We have, therefore, chosen general anesthesia in most of our RAAA patients. Large sheath and balloon placement is only carried out if required by the patient's cardiovascular collapse since these maneuvers can cause problems and the presence of the inflated balloon can complicate placement of the endograft. The large sheath must be left in place to support the balloon and to enable its removal.

EXPERIENCE WITH EVRAR

Since 1994, we have used endovascular techniques to treat 57 patients with RAAAs. In the first 12 cases, endovascular graft repair was performed only in patients who were considered prohibitive risks for open repair because of a hostile abdomen, medical comorbidities, or both. All these patients had preoperative CT scans although several were hemodynamically unstable at the time of their repair.[9,13]

In 1996, we adopted the current management protocol described above. With two exceptions—when staff and facilities were unavailable—all patients with RAAAs seen by our service between 1996 and the present were managed according to this protocol. These 45 patients plus the original 12 patients constitute our total experience.[13,14] Of these 45 patients, twelve were unsuitable for EVRAR. Eleven survived their open operation. Only three required suprarenal balloon control.

The remaining 45 patients (12 plus 33) were acceptable for EVRAR and had an endograft placed. Although 25 of these patients received a Montefiore Endovascular Grafting System (MEGS) aortounifemoral graft (Figure 28–2B),[9,13,14] the 20 remaining patients were treated with a commercially available graft. Of the 45 patients undergoing EVRAR, 39 survived and were discharged from the hospital with their aneurysm excluded. Only ten of the 45 patients undergoing EVRAR required balloon control during their procedure. Three of the 39 survivors required evacuation of their perianeurysmal hematoma because of abdominal compartment syndrome. One surviving patient developed a late (one year) type I endoleak that was successfully treated by placement of a second MEGS graft. There have been no other endoleaks although one patient required open conversion for endotension with an enlarging painful aneurysm.

Other Experience with EVRAR

Increasing numbers of EVRARs are being performed throughout the world using a variety of grafts, mostly commercially available. We are in the process of summarizing the results of these procedures.[23] Although there clearly is case selection in the performance of these procedures, the operative mortality of 21% is considerably below the 35% to 55% range reported for open RAAA repair. Clearly, EVRAR avoids many of the problems that are associated with open RAAA repair and contribute to the high mortality associated with this procedure. These problems include increased blood loss associated with release of tamponade, retroperitoneal dissection, and inadvertent venous injury, injury to other retroperitoneal structures including the duodenum and the ureters, hypothermia associated with hypotension and laparatomy, and the impaired blood coagulability common in the RAAA setting.

CONCLUSIONS

1. Hypotensive hemostasis with fluid restriction is effective in many patients with RAAA and is helpful in the management of this entity.
2. Fluoroscopically monitored proximal aortic balloon control can be obtained under local anesthesia. It is an advantageous method whether the definitive repair is performed open or with an endograft.
3. Proximal aortic control is only required in one-third of patients with RAAA provided hypotensive hemostasis is used.
4. EVRAR is feasible.
5. Preliminary results give promise that EVRAR will lower the morbidity and mortality rates of treatment for RAAA.
6. EVRAR will likely become the gold standard for treating the majority of patients with RAAA.

REFERENCES

1. Johansen K, Kohler TR, Nicholls SC, et al. Ruptured abdominal aortic aneurysm: The Harbor view experience. *J Vasc Surg.* 1991;13:240–247.
2. Gloviczki P, Pairolero PC, Mucha P. Ruptured abdominal aortic aneurysms: Repair should not be denied. *J Vasc Surg* 1992;15:851–859.
3. Marty-Ane CH, Alric P, Picot MC, et al. Ruptured abdominal aortic aneurysm: Influence of intraoperative management on surgical outcome. *J Vasc Surg.* 1995;22:780–786.
4. Darling RC, Cordero JA, Chang BB. Advances in the surgical repair of ruptured abdominal aortic aneurysms. *CardioVasc Surg.* 1996;4:720–723.
5. Dardik A, Burleyson GP, Bowman H, et al. Surgical repair of ruptured abdominal aortic aneurysms in the state of Maryland: Factors influencing outcome among 527 recent cases. *J Vasc Surg.* 1998;28:413–423.
6. Noel AA, Gloviczki P, Cherry KJ Jr., et al. Ruptured abdominal aortic aneurysms: The excessive mortality rate of conventional repair. *J Vasc Surg.* 2001;34:41–46.
7. Marin ML, Veith FJ, Cynamon J, et al. Initial experience with transluminally placed endovascular grafts for the treatment of complex vascular lesions. *Ann Surg.* 1995;222:1–17.
8. Yusuf SW, Whitaker SC, Chuter TA, et al. Emergency endovascular repair of leaking aortic aneurysm. *Lancet.* 1994;344:1645.
9. Ohki T, Veith FJ, Sanchez LA, et al. Endovascular graft repair of ruptured aorto-iliac aneurysms. *J Am Coll Surg.* 1999;189:102–123.
10. Andresen AFR. Management of gastric hemorrhage. NY State Med J 48:603–611, 1948
11. Shaftan GW, Chiu CJ, Dennis C, et al. Fundamentals of physiologic control of arterial hemorrhage. *Surgery.* 1968;58:851–856.
12. Bickell WH, Wall MJ Jr, Pepe PE, et al. Immediate versus delayed fluid resuscitation for hypotensive patients with penetrating torso injuries. *N Engl J Med.* 1994;331:1105–1109.
13. Veith FJ, Ohki T. Endovascular approaches to ruptured infrarenal aorto-iliac aneurysms. *J Cardiovasc Surg.* 2002;43:369–378.
14. Ohki T, Veith FJ. Endovascular grafts and other image guided catheter based adjuncts to improve the treatment of ruptured aortoiliac aneurysms. *Ann Surg.* 2000;232:466–479.
15. Hesse FG, Kletschka HD. Rupture of abdominal aortic aneurysm: control of hemorrhage by intraluminal balloon tamponade. *Ann Surg.* 1962;155:320–322.
16. Hyde GL, Sullivan DM. Fogarty catheter tamponade of ruptured abdominal aortic aneurysms. *Surg Gynecol Obstet.* 1982;154:197–199.
17. Greenberg RK, Srivastava SD, Ouriel K, et al. An endoluminal method of hemorrhage control and repair of ruptured abdominal aortic aneurysms. *J Endovasc Ther.* 2000;7:1–7.
18. Malina M, Veith FJ, Ivancev K, Sonesson B. Balloon occlusion of the aorta during endovascular repair of ruptured aortic aneurysm. *J Endovasc Ther.* 2005;12:556–559.
19. Yusuf SW, Whitaker SC, Chuter TAM, et al: Early results of endovascular aortic aneurysm surgery with aortouniiliac graft, contralateral iliac occlusion, and femorofemoral bypass. *J Vasc Surg.* 1997;25:165–172.
20. Yusuf SW, Hopkinson BR. It is feasible to treat contained aortic aneurysm rupture by stent-graft combination? In: Greenhalgh RM, ed. *Indications in Vascular and Endovascular Surgery.* London: WB Saunders; 1998:153–165.
21. Veith FJ. Emergency abdominal aortic aneurysm surgery. *Compr Ther.* 1992;18:25–29.
22. Lachat ML, Pfammatter T, Witzke HJ, et al. Endovascular repair with bifurcated stent-grafts under local anaesthesia to improve outcome of ruptured aortoiliac aneurysms. *Eur J Vasc Endovasc Surg.* 2002;23:528–536.
23. Veith FJ, Lachat M, Mayer D, et al. Collected world and single center experience with endovascular treatment of ruptured abdominal aortic aneurysms. *Ann Surg* 2009 (Nov); 250: In Press.

29

EVAR for the Treatment of Ruptured AAA

Mark D. Morasch, M.D.

ABSTRACT

Endovascular repair (EVAR) for ruptured AAA has been held out as a safer, less invasive alternative to open surgery with the potential to significantly reduce in-hospital mortality. Despite the inherent biases that accompany comparison of the two treatment modalities, there appears to be a clear role for EVAR for select patients in select centers. In order to successfully treat patients with ruptured AAA both open and endovascular modalities should be available and clear protocols using a team approach must be developed.

Open repair of ruptured abdominal aortic aneurysms (AAA) has been associated with high resultant mortality rates. Unfortunately, poor outcomes following open repair of AAA have been relatively consistent over the past few decades despite major improvements in health care delivery over that same period.[1-2] A consensus figure for in-hospital mortality following open repair of ruptured AAA could reach as high as 50%.

Endovascular repair (EVAR) for ruptured AAA has recently been held out as a safer, less invasive alternative to open surgery with the potential to, for the first time in decades, significantly reduce in-hospital mortality following the treatment of these abdominal catastrophies. In fact, some authors have reported mortality rates as low as the single digits.[3-4] These claims, however, have usually been made based upon the results of non-controlled and non-randomized, retrospectively-analyzed, case series.[5-10] Level one data is, at best, lacking. Furthermore, these positive results likely represent highly selective sets of data from large-volume expert centers and may not be truly representative of a more broad-based sample.

Realistically, the two therapies, open repair and EVAR cannot be fairly compared. In most studies, the patients ultimately chosen (and retrospectively analyzed) for EVAR are the most stable upon arrival to the treating hospital. Nearly all, in fact, are stable enough to undergo pre-operative evaluation with time consuming CT angiography in order to assess their candidacy for the minimally invasive alternative. Meanwhile, their unstable counterparts are taken immediately from the emergency room to open surgery in most instances. Furthermore, those patients stable enough to get a pre-operative CT but who are then ruled out for EVAR based upon anatomy have, by definition, the most challenging surgical neck and iliac anatomy. In another words, in most centers where EVAR is offered for ruptured AAA, the patients who ultimately receive the minimally invasive alternative treatment have been "cherry picked" based upon relative hemodynamic stability and upon favorable anatomy.

Despite the inherent biases, information is emerging to suggest that there is a clear role for EVAR for ruptured AAA in select patients who can be treated in select centers.[11–12] There are a number of clear advantages to the endovascular approach given patient suitability. Patients undergoing EVAR can usually be treated using local anesthesia which helps to avoid the hemodynamic changes associated with muscle relaxation and general anesthesia. The significant inflammatory response related to cytokine release may be blunted with EVAR. Large doses of heparin can be avoided as well. In addition, the morbidity associated with dissecting the aortic neck or following significant venous injury can be avoided. Understanding the ever present biases, the current literature has also suggested decreased procedure times, reduced blood loss, and improved overall and intensive care unit lengths of stay following EVAR for ruptured AAA when compared to open surgery.

The need for pre-operative CT imaging prior to EVAR for ruptured AAA continues to be debated. Most centers consider such screening to be mandatory both for purposes of confirming the diagnosis as well for morphological assessment. A few centers have developed protocols that provide for intra-operative assessment without CT delay using angiography or intravascular ultrasound. Realistically, time is usually available to send patients for CT evaluation with out undo risk. The majority of patients who are admitted to the hospital with ruptured AAA survive for a number of hours. In a study by Lloyd, the median time between rupture and death in a group of patients offered only palliation was nearly 11 hours with 88% surviving and remaining hemodynamically stable for longer than 2 hours.[13] In most centers, 2 hours is ample time to obtain a CT scan to assess suitability for EVAR. In the case of patients who presented with true hemodynamic instability, the decision must be made to either attempt to assess the morphology, and hence the candidacy for EVAR, without axial imaging using modalities available in the procedural suite or to commit to open reconstruction.

Conservative estimates regarding anatomic suitability for endovascular repair run around 50%.[14] If the selection criteria that have become standard for elective cases are relaxed for the treatment of ruptured AAA and patients with shorter and more angulated necks are accepted, it has been estimated that up to 80% of ruptures may be suitable for EVAR.[15] This number may even increase in the future with the development of new device technology. This has led a number of investigators to develop the concept of "endovascular damage control" which accepts a suboptimal radiographic result in exchange for temporizing the emergency. In the short term, some patients will still require laparotomy for failed EVAR or for the treatment of abdominal compartment syndrome.[16] The damage control approach can only be adopted provided patients consent to undergo vigilant late follow-up examination and understand the potential need for "preventive maintainance ".

As of 2006 only about 6% of patients with ruptured AAA were treated using EVAR techniques in the United States.[17] To put that number in some context, another recent study suggested that as many as 33% of men and 60% of women who present to the hospital in the UK receive no intervention at all for ruptured AAA.[18] There are several reasons for centers to be slow to adopt the endovascular approach. These reasons include limited availability of off-the-shelf devices on an urgent basis, lack of seasoned endovascular surgical expertise, and unavailability of dedicated operating room facilities and ancillary staff who are adequately equipped to perform these procedures. As such, many patients who would qualify for EVAR still undergo the open surgical alternative.

In order to successfully treat patients with ruptured AAA using endovascular means, a team approach must be developed. Like with any therapy, the team must practice. Strict protocols from the emergency room to discharge planning need to be put in place to streamline patient through-put. A dedicated team including trained interventional surgeons, anesthesiologists, nursing staff and radiology technicians are requisite to success.

By offering a combination of both open and endovascular repair options it may be possible to improve overall 30-day mortality results. Improved mortality may, in part, be the result of shifting infirmed patients who may be too high risk for open surgery to EVAR and there by improving the results for open surgery. We may also be able to reduce the numbers of patients offered palliative care as their only alternative since we now have EVAR as an alternative for the medically unfit patient who has favorable anatomy for endovascular repair. Long-term benefits are also possible but the data remains to be seen.

REFERENCES

1. Bown MJ, Sutton AJ, Bell PR, Sayers RD. A meta-analysis of 50 years of ruptured abdominal aortic aneurysm repair. *Br J Surg.* Jun 2002;89(6):714–730.
2. Sayers RD, Thompson MM, Nasim A, Healey P, Taub N, Bell PR. Surgical management of 671 abdominal aortic aneurysms: a 13 year review from a single centre. *Eur J Vasc Endovasc Surg.* Mar 1997;13(3):322–327.
3. Lee WA, Hirneise CM, Tayyarah M, Huber TS, Seeger JM. Impact of endovascular repair on early outcomes of ruptured abdominal aortic aneurysms. *J Vasc Surg.* Aug 2004;40(2): 211–215.
4. Brandt M, Walluscheck KP, Jahnke T, Graw K, Cremer J, Muller-Hulsbeck S. Endovascular repair of ruptured abdominal aortic aneurysm: feasibility and impact on early outcome. *J Vasc Interv Radiol.* Oct 2005;16(10):1309–1312.
5. Ockert S, Schumacher H, Bockler D, Megges I, Allenberg JR. Early and midterm results after open and endovascular repair of ruptured abdominal aortic aneurysms in a comparative analysis. *J Endovasc Ther.* Jun 2007;14(3):324–332.
6. Moore R, Nutley M, Cina CS, Motamedi M, Faris P, Abuznadah W. Improved survival after introduction of an emergency endovascular therapy protocol for ruptured abdominal aortic aneurysms. *J Vasc Surg.* Mar 2007;45(3):443–450.
7. Hinchliffe RJ, Braithwaite BD. Ruptured abdominal aortic aneurysm: endovascular repair does not confer any long-term survival advantage over open repair. *Vascular.* Jul-Aug 2007;15(4):191–196.
8. Kubin K, Sodeck GH, Teufelsbauer H, et al. Endovascular therapy of ruptured abdominal aortic aneurysm: mid- and long-term results. *Cardiovasc Intervent Radiol.* May-Jun 2008;31(3):496–503.
9. Mehta M, Taggert J, Darling RC, 3rd, et al. Establishing a protocol for endovascular treatment of ruptured abdominal aortic aneurysms: outcomes of a prospective analysis. *J Vasc Surg.* Jul 2006;44(1):1–8; discussion 8.
10. Wibmer A, Schoder M, Wolff KS, et al. Improved survival after abdominal aortic aneurysm rupture by offering both open and endovascular repair. *Arch Surg.* Jun 2008;143(6):544–549; discussion 550.

11. Peppelenbosch N, Geelkerken RH, Soong C, et al. Endograft treatment of ruptured abdominal aortic aneurysms using the Talent aortouniiliac system: an international multicenter study. *J Vasc Surg.* Jun 2006;43(6):1111–1123; discussion 1123.

12. Mastracci TM, Garrido-Olivares L, Cina CS, Clase CM. Endovascular repair of ruptured abdominal aortic aneurysms: a systematic review and meta-analysis. *J Vasc Surg.* Jan 2008; 47(1):214–221.

13. Lloyd GM, Bown MJ, Norwood MG, et al. Feasibility of preoperative computer tomography in patients with ruptured abdominal aortic aneurysm: a time-to-death study in patients without operation. *J Vasc Surg.* Apr 2004;39(4):788–791.

14. Towne JB. Endovascular treatment of abdominal aortic aneurysms. *Am J Surg.* Feb 2005; 189(2):140–149.

15. Dillon M, Cardwell C, Blair PH, Ellis P, Kee F, Harkin DW. Endovascular treatment for ruptured abdominal aortic aneurysm. *Cochrane Database Syst Rev.* 2007(1):CD005261.

16. Mehta M, Darling RC, 3rd, Roddy SP, et al. Factors associated with abdominal compartment syndrome complicating endovascular repair of ruptured abdominal aortic aneurysms. *J Vasc Surg.* Dec 2005;42(6):1047–1051.

17. Greco G, Egorova N, Anderson PL, et al. Outcomes of endovascular treatment of ruptured abdominal aortic aneurysms. *J Vasc Surg.* Mar 2006;43(3):453–459.

18. Filipovic M, Seagroatt V, Goldacre MJ. Differences between women and men in surgical treatment and case fatality rates for ruptured aortic abdominal aneurysm in England. *Br J Surg.* Sep 2007;94(9):1096–1099.

Management of Complications During And After Endovascular Repair

30

Management of Iliac Artery Injuries during Endovascular Abdominal and Thoracic Aortic Repair (EVAR-TEVAR)

Gale L. Tang, M.D., Jon S. Matsumura, M.D.

Iliac artery injuries during endovascular abdominal and thoracic aortic repair (EVAR and TEVAR) are largely the consequence of the need to pass large diameter delivery systems through iliac arteries that are too tortuous, narrow, calcified, or some combination thereof. Iliac injuries were the most frequent major adverse event in many of the endovascular aortic device clinical trials. This problem is magnified by the larger delivery systems required for TEVAR, as evidenced by the use of iliac conduits in 15%, 21%, and 9% of patients in the phase II multicenter trials of the TAG device, the Talent device, and the Zenith TX2 device, respectively.[1-3] Ischemia or hemorrhage from iliac artery rupture, avulsion, or dissection can add substantially to patient morbidity and mortality during EVAR and TEVAR.

Careful preoperative planning is the key to reducing the risk of iliac artery injury. This planning includes device selection, adjunctive strategies to deal with the unfavorable iliac-femoral segment, or the use of alternate delivery routes other than the common femoral artery. Intraoperative techniques to reduce risks include passing the large-diameter sheaths under direct fluoroscopic guidance, using an alternative strategy when significant resistance is encountered, and having bailout components available for the inevitable day when an injury does occur. When these unavoidable injuries occur, rapid recognition and appropriate management can sometimes limit morbidity to the patient.

CURRENT DEVICES

Current device delivery systems for EVAR and TEVAR have different deployment mechanisms, which vary in flexibility, tip configuration, coatings, need for a delivery

TABLE 30-1.

Device	Aortic Treatment Diameter (mm)	Graft Diameter (mm)	Sheath size ID (Fr)/Delivery system OD (Fr)	Crossing profile OD (mm)
AneuRx*	16-18	20	22/21.4	8.0/6.8
(cross once per	18-20	22	22/21.4	8.0/6.8
component if	20-22	24	22/21.4	8.0/6.8
sheathless)	22-24	26	22/21.4	8.0/6.8
	23-26	28	22/21.4	8.0/6.8
Excluder[†]	19-21	23	18 (16)[#]	7.0 (6.2)[#]
(cross once)	22-23	26	18	7.0
	24-26	28.5	18	7.0
Powerlink[†]	18-23	25	/21	8.0
(cross once per	23-26	28	/21	8.0
component)				
Zenith*	18-19	22	/18	7.0
(cross once	20-21	24	/18	7.0
on ipsilateral,	22	26	/18	7.0
once per	23-24	28	/20	7.6
component on	25-26	30	/20	7.6
contralateral)	27-28	32	/20	7.6
	29-32	36	/22	8.3

ID inner diameter; OD outer diameter; *measured from adventitia to adventitia; [†]measured from intima to intima; [#]Off-label sheath size

sheath, and overall size of system. Further, specific systems vary in the number of times a large-diameter device must traverse the access artery. The overall size of the delivery system is one of the more important factors. Tables 30–1 and 30–2 list the current devices, outer diameter (crossing profiles) of the various sizes of devices, and number of times a component must cross the access for EVAR (Table 30–1) and TEVAR (Table 30–2).

Some devices have the option to be delivered "bareback" or without the use of a larger sheath, but the tradeoff for this smaller size may mean that the difficult segment must be traversed multiple times. For example, in the VALOR trial using the Talent device for TEVAR required an average of 2.7 device components to treat thoracic aortic aneurysms.[2] In each of these patients, separate components could be individually introduced bareback with multiple passages through the iliac artery, or a larger sheath could be passed once into the aorta and each component placed through this sheath.

Delivery sheaths help shield the iliac luminal surface from damage from devices traversing the diseased intima. A progressively tapered dilator tip and hydrophilic coating are available in certain large-diameter systems. Visual inspection of a sheath that failed to cross a diseased segment may reveal damage to leading edge of the sheath, and this artery may be crossable with a new sheath of the same size.

EVALUATION OF AVAILABLE ACCESS

Tortuosity, size, and calcification are important characteristics to assess, but several additional factors may contribute to difficult iliac access. A careful history from the

TABLE 30-2.

Device	Graft Diameter (mm)	Sheath size ID (Fr)/Delivery system OD (Fr)	Crossing profile OD (mm)
Bolton Relay*^	18-19	22	/22-23	7.4, 7.7
(cross once per	20-21	24	/22-23	7.4, 7.7
component)	22-23	26	/22-23	7.4, 7.7
	24-25	28	/22-23	7.4, 7.7
	26-27	30	/22-23	7.4, 7.7
	28-29	32	/22-24	7.4, 7.7, 8.1
	30-31	34	/23-24	7.7, 8.1
	32-33	36	/23-24	7.7, 8.1
	34	38	/24-25	8.1, 8.4
	35-36	40	/24-25	8.1, 8.4
	37-38	42	/25	8.4
	39-40	44	/25	8.4
	41-42	46	/26	8.7
TAG†	23-24	26	20/22.8	7.6
(cross once)	24-26	28	20/22.8	7.6
	26-29	31	22/24.9	8.3
	29-32	34	22/24.9	8.3
	32-34	37	24/27.6	9.2
	34-37	40	24/27.6	9.2
Talent*	18-19	22	/22	7.0
(cross once per	20-21	24	/22	7.0
component)	22-23	26	/22	7.0
	24-25	28	/22	7.0
	26-27	30	/22	7.0
	28-29	32	/22	7.0
	30-31	34	/24	7.6
	32	36	/24	7.6
	33-34	38	/24	7.6
	35-36	40	/24	7.6
	37-38	42	/25	8.0
	39-40	44	/25	8.0
	41-42	46	/25	8.0
Zenith TX2*	24	28	20/23	7.5
(cross once per	25-27	30	20/23	7.5
component)	28-29	32	20/23	7.5
	30	34	20/23	7.5
	31-32	36	22/25	8.5
	33-34	38	22/25	8.5
	35-36	40	22/25	8.5
	37-38	42	22/25	8.5[J2]

ID inner diameter; OD outer diameter; *measured from adventitia to adventitia; ^ longer
length device for same diameter graft requires larger delivery system; †measured from intima to intima

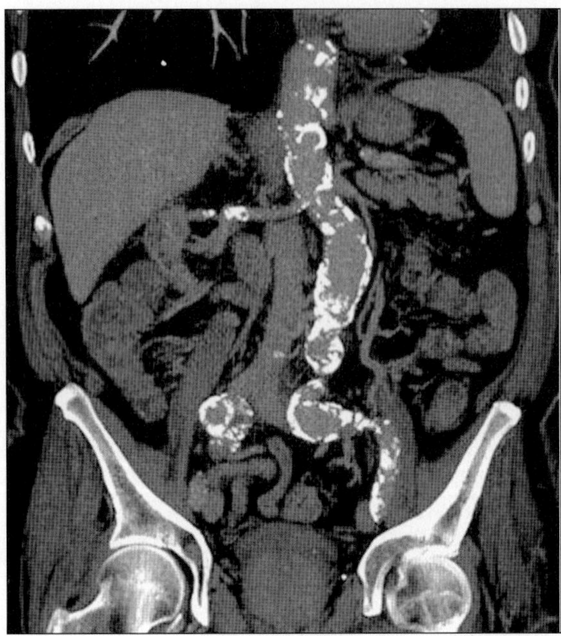

Figure 30-1. Significant iliac calcification and tortuosity on CT.

patient may reveal preexisting iliac stents, prior EVAR, previous radiation therapy, or prior retroperitoneal operation, which may make open conduit placement challenging (such as pelvic lymph node dissection or iliac artery operations). Sometimes, previous aortofemoral or aortoiliac bypass may facilitate subsequent access, but beware of older surgical bypass grafts that may become calcified or kinked, and note that the distal anastomosis is often a weak point for avulsion. Patients undergoing staged procedures such as open infrarenal AAA repair prior to TEVAR, or visceral debranching prior to TEVAR for thoracoabdominal repair, may benefit from a planned conduit being left in place at the time of their initial procedure.

Computed tomography angiography (CTA) is the current preferred method for the evaluation of access vessels for EVAR and TEVAR. Information regarding luminal diameter, calcification, degree of occlusive disease, and tortuosity is readily determined from examination of the preoperative CTA (Figure 30–1). Three-dimensional reconstructions, while not essential, can be especially useful to provide direct visualization of vessel tortuosity. In those patients whose renal insufficiency precludes use of CTA, a thin-cut noncontrast CT is still a useful preoperative planning tool to evaluate calcification and tortuosity. Magnetic resonance angiography (MRA) in those instances can be helpful to determine potential access vessels' luminal diameters. Preoperative contrast angiography is rarely required, but is helpful when available in determining luminal diameter and vessel tortuosity. In these cases, a stiff wire can be inserted during the diagnostic study to evaluate the response of vessel tortuosity to maneuvers that will facilitate sheath passage.

TORTUOSITY

Most degrees of vessel tortuosity can be overcome by using a stiff wire to "straighten" the artery prior to passing a large-diameter sheath or device delivery system

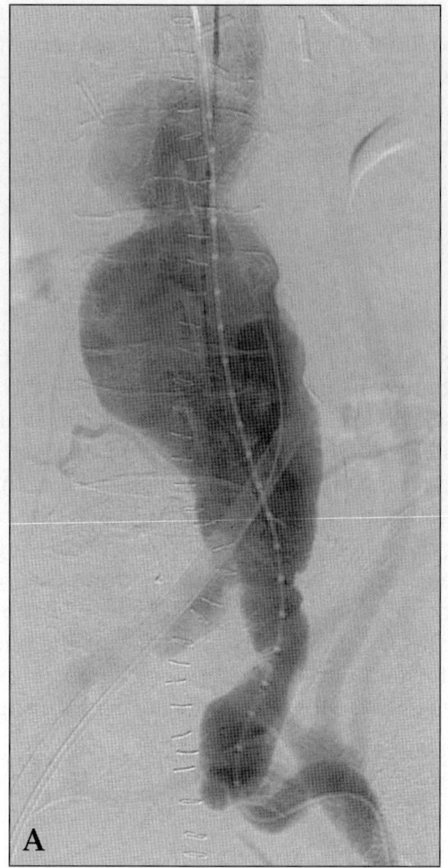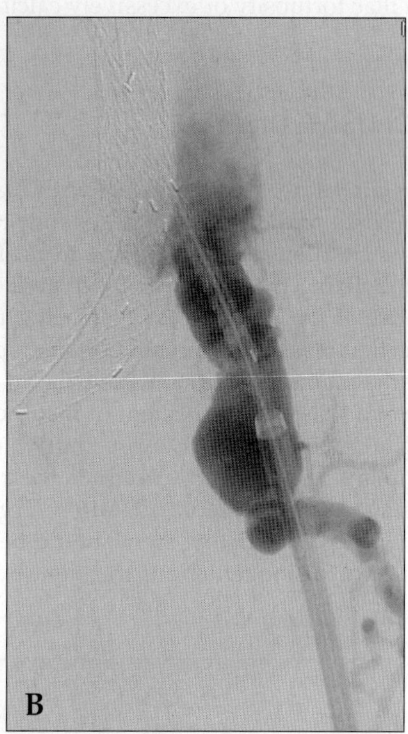

Figure 30-2. **(A)** Left external iliac artery tortuosity in patient with multivisceral debranching graft. **(B)** Tortuosity straightened after stiff wire and large-sheath passage.

(Figure 30–2A). Although this may result in an angiographic picture of "accordion" effect or pseudostenosis (Figure 30–2B), usually no permanent iliac damage results. A completion angiogram may be performed without the stiff wires and large sheaths to evaluate flow at the end of the procedure. Occasionally, manual external compression of the patient's abdomen may assist sheath passage.

Three additional wire techniques may be helpful to deal with excessive tortuosity in vessels that are not significantly calcified. A second stiff buddy wire passed adjacent to the original stiff wire may assist in straightening the tortuous vessel sufficiently to pass a sheath. Occasionally, tension held on both ends of a transfemoral buddy wire can provide significant assistance in straightening an excessively tortuous vessel. Tension held on both ends of a brachiofemoral or carotidfemoral wire is a useful adjunct, but does require an additional supradiaphramatic access.[4] These "body floss" techniques involve snaring the wire to bring it out through the second sheath. When using the body floss technique, a catheter may be left over the wire to reduce risk of arterial injury.

External iliac tortuosity can sometimes be overcome by open surgical straightening through a femoral cutdown. The proximal common femoral artery is retracted with the assistance of a circumferential vessel loop while the distal external iliac is exposed under the inguinal ligament using blunt dissection. If necessary, the inguinal ligament can be divided to provide more proximal iliac exposure. After delivery of the endograft, the excess redundancy may be excised if necessary, and an end-to-end anastomosis performed. This technique has limited effectiveness in straightening common iliac tortuosity or excessively calcified vessels.[4]

OCCLUSIVE DISEASE

The simplest technique to deal with iliac stenosis remains balloon angioplasty, either at the time of device insertion or four to six weeks preoperatively. Staging the procedure may allow the vessel time to heal in between procedures and decrease the risk of embolizing from the freshly dilated vessel. If possible, stenting should be avoided because of the risk of later displacing the stent. If a stent is required to treat an iliac dissection resulting from balloon angioplasty, it must be of sufficient size to accommodate the planned sheath. While balloon expandable stents can be overdilated, the presence of a self-expanding stent of insufficient diameter will preclude sheath crossing. In heavily calcified vessels, a preemptive covered stent, serving as an endoluminal conduit, may be preferred to reduce the risk of massive bleeding from an iliac rupture after aggressive balloon dilatation (Figure 30–3A and 30–3B). Passage of the sheath through any preexisting stent should be performed under direct fluoroscopic guidance to prevent dislodgement of the stent by the sheath. Movement of the stent during at-

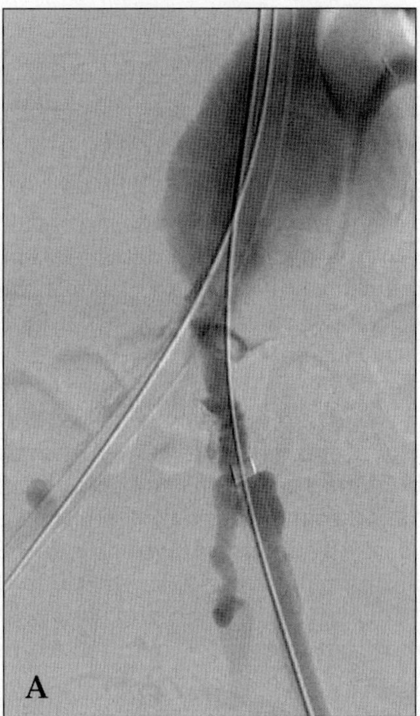
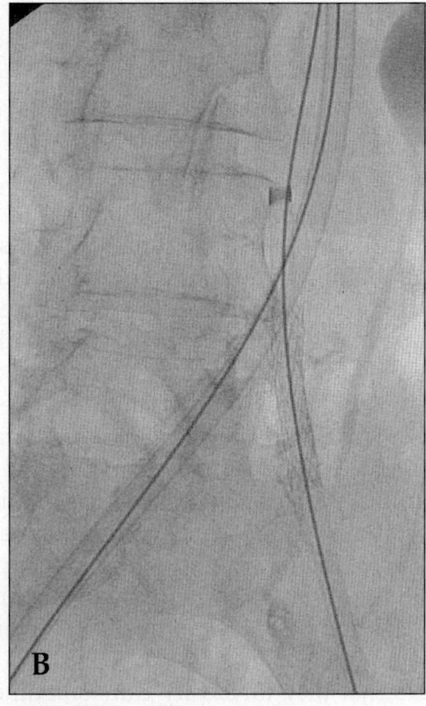

Figure 30-3. (A) Left common iliac artery calcification and stenosis prevented passage of 12Fr sheath. **(B)** Sheath passage successful after placement of 8 mm balloon expandable covered stent in left common iliac artery.

tempted sheath passage should prompt withdrawal of the sheath and use of a larger balloon for predilation of the stent or consideration of another option.

The hybrid procedure of remote balloon endarterectomy may be useful to deal with significant external iliac occlusive disease.[5] Serial balloon angioplasty of the external iliac artery is performed through an open femoral cutdown. Alternatively, a ring-stripper may be passed proximally to the iliac bifurcation to dissect the intima from the vessel wall. The atheromatous debris is removed using a clamp (like a Swedish Debakey) through the femoral arteriotomy. After completion of the stent-graft procedure, the external iliac artery should be evaluated and may require stenting of a residual flow-limiting dissection.[4]

SMALL ILIAC SIZE

Occasionally, serial dilation of the iliacs with hydrophilic dilators is sufficient to allow sheath passage. Von Segesser et. al. described a method of in situ balloon dilatation of a smaller caliber sheath to allow the passage of larger devices.[6] In their method, an 18Fr sheath is passed and the dilator removed. The entire length of the sheath is then dilated from within, using an 8 mm balloon to reach an internal diameter of 24Fr or a 9 mm balloon to reach an internal diameter of 27Fr. They did not experience any adverse events in their small five-case series, but caution that leaving a stiff wire in place during withdrawal of the balloon expanded sheath is prudent. An alternative strategy is to use an endoluminal or open conduit as described below.

CONDUITS

The presence of extensive calcification may make the above strategies hazardous. Circumferential calcification predisposes the iliacs to dissection or worse, rupture or complete avulsion. Occasionally, the femoral or iliac vessels may be too small to accommodate the planned device delivery system. In these cases, a planned conduit—either endoluminal or open surgical—may be the preferred strategy to deal with difficult iliac access.

The most commonly used technique involves placement of a 10 mm polyester or polytetrafluoroethylene (PTFE) graft. Control of the aorta and iliac arteries is obtained through a limited retroperitoneal exposure incision.[7] The graft is sutured end to side to the common iliac artery or directly to the infrarenal aorta (Figure 30–4). The sheath is inserted through the graft material (or though the end of the conduit using vessel loops or umbilical ties to control bleeding around the sheath) and passed through the surgical anastomosis under direct fluoroscopic guidance. The conduit may be tunneled through the retroperitoneal space parallel to the external iliac artery and brought out through a separate counter incision in order to assist in sheath passage. If the conduit was placed to bypass significant occlusive disease, at the end of the case, it can be converted into a surgical bypass and anastomosed to the femoral artery. Alternatively, it is transected and oversewn at the end of the procedure.

Instead of leaving the conduit in place, Eidt and Ali described a method of autogenous reconstruction.[8] This method also has the advantage of preserving flow through the internal iliac artery, and can be used when there is redundant external iliac artery causing difficult tortuosity. The iliac bifurcation is exposed through a limited retroperitoneal approach. The hypogastric artery is mobilized to the first branch, and the

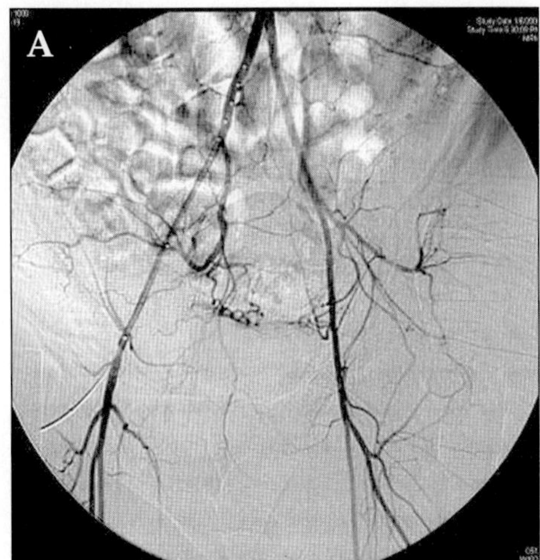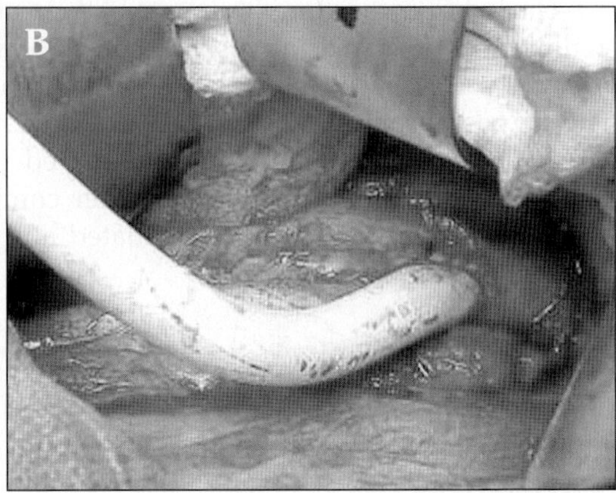

Figure 30-4. (A) Patient with small (5 mm iliac arteries bilaterally). **(B)** Open 10 mm ePTFE aortic conduit.

external iliac artery is mobilized to the inguinal ligament. After the distal hypogastric artery is clamped, the hypogastric artery is transected and oversewn flush at its origin from the common iliac artery. The external iliac artery is also transected distally, leaving 2-3 cm of proximal stump in continuity with the common iliac artery. The distal end of the external iliac artery is transposed onto the hypogastric artery using an end-to-end anastomosis. A prosthetic conduit is then anastomosed to the proximal transected stump of the external iliac artery and used to deliver the endograft. To complete the procedure, the conduit is removed and an end-to-side anastomosis is performed between the proximal external iliac artery stump and the distal external iliac artery.

Yano et. al. described an alternate "endoluminal" conduit to avoid the additional blood loss and procedure time required for the open placement of a conduit.[9] They sutured a stent to a prosthetic conduit and backloaded it into a sheath. The stent was deployed over the orifice of the internal iliac artery to anchor the endoluminal graft. The external iliac was then dilated from within the graft with a noncompliant balloon. At the completion of the procedure, the distal end of the endoluminal graft is anchored in the distal external iliac with a stent or brought down to the common femoral artery where a handsewn anastomosis with patch angioplasty is performed.[10] Commercially available covered stents and iliac graft limbs can be used instead of the homemade device, and these can even be placed percutaneously (endoconduit). In either method, a decision must be made about covering the origin of the internal iliac artery with extension over diseased common iliac artery to decrease the risk of sudden hemorrhagic shock. This must be balanced with the possible increased risk of pelvic and spinal cord ischemia.[11]

A planned conduit may be left in place during the first stage of a planned repair. Generally, this involves an extra 10 mm limb sutured to an aortic or debranching graft, or use of one of the limbs of a bifurcated graft. The planned conduit is tunneled through the retroperitoneal space and left oversewn and buried in the anterior abdominal wall. Large clips can be left on the oversewn end to facilitate locating the conduit. During the second procedure, the conduit is thrombectomized in segments and used to deliver the endograft. Again, passage of the large sheath through the conduit should be performed under direct fluoroscopic guidance as the conduit anastomosis with the main graft can be disrupted by passage of the sheath. At the end of the procedure, the conduit is trimmed back to the level of the fascia and oversewn.

ALTERNATE CANNULATION SITES

Occasionally, circumferential control of the iliac may be difficult such as in a reoperative field. Alternatively, a circumferentially calcified iliac that cannot be clamped safely may preclude the use of a conduit. In addition, the fresh anastomosis between a conduit and the native artery can be disrupted by large-sheath passage. The left common carotid artery has been described as an alternative cannulation site for TEVAR.[12] Carpenter et. al. described an alternative approach of directly cannulating the aorta, common iliac artery, or a preexisting aortic graft.[13]

The technique involves exposing the anterior surface of the distal aorta or proximal common iliac artery through a limited (usually left) retroperitoneal incision. A portion of the vessel free from calcification is chosen for cannulation. Two concentric subadventitial purse-string sutures are placed on opposite sides of the cannulation site. The artery is entered in the center of the purse string with an entry needle and guidewire, followed by exchange for a stiff wire through a catheter. The large sheath is then placed directly over the stiff wire and advanced under fluoroscopic guidance. Rumel tourniquets can be used to secure the purse strings around the sheath to provide hemostasis during the procedure. After endograft delivery, the inner purse string followed by the outer purse string are tied to close the arteriotomy. If necessary, additional pledgeted sutures can be used to reinforce the cannulation site.

MANAGEMENT OF ACCESS COMPLICATIONS

Focal dissection, embolization, iliac rupture, and iliac avulsion are the main types of iliac injuries during EVAR-TEVAR. Often, these injuries become manifest at the end of the case when the team may be relieved following a challenging deployment, and a high index of suspicion should be maintained. Performing a sheath injection during withdrawal of the large sheath may help identify an injury earlier, enabling more time for bailout maneuvers. If iliac rupture is likely, an occlusion balloon may be opened ahead of time just in case it is rapidly needed.

Focal dissection generally results in a diminished or absent femoral pulse. In patients with suspected iliac dissection, an iliac angiogram should be performed prior to removing wire access, but after the large sheath is removed so that flow characteristics can be evaluated. A stent may be required to tack down a significant intimal flap. The injury may actually be at the proximal common femoral artery level. If a femoral artery cutdown was performed, the intimal flap may be visualized within the arteriotomy and excised. Alternatively, if percutaneous access was obtained and the flap is detected in the femoral artery on retrograde angiogram, a cutdown and femoral endarterectomy may be required. Often, a patch closure of the femoral artery is useful.

Iliac rupture may occur after forceful balloon dilatation, especially if there is an eccentric calcified artery. To check for this possibility, an angiogram should be performed after balloon dilatation. If extravasation is seen, balloon reinflation for a

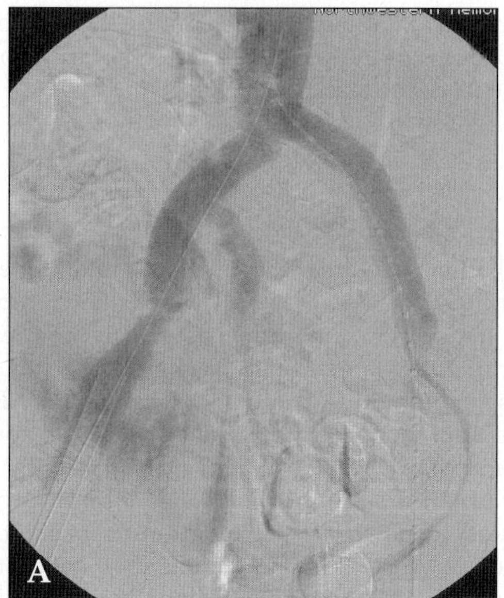

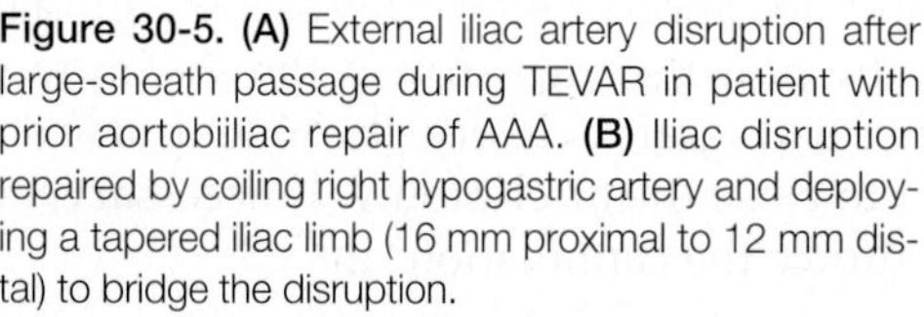

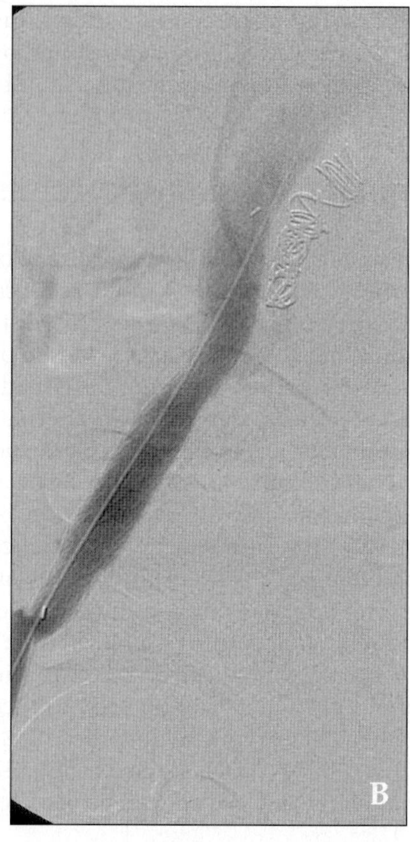

Figure 30-5. (A) External iliac artery disruption after large-sheath passage during TEVAR in patient with prior aortobiiliac repair of AAA. **(B)** Iliac disruption repaired by coiling right hypogastric artery and deploying a tapered iliac limb (16 mm proximal to 12 mm distal) to bridge the disruption.

prolonged period may seal the perforation if it is small. For larger ruptures, a covered stent of appropriate size can be chosen and deployed to allow completion of the case without open surgical conversion. Often, a series of rapid exchanges for a more proximal occlusion balloon followed by a stent graft can be accomplished if bleeding is not massive. Alternatively, contralateral balloon control can be used while endovascular repair is undertaken. An example of proximal coil embolization and stent graft into the external iliac artery to bridge the gap is depicted in Figure 30–5. Again, passage of any sheath through the newly deployed covered stent should be done under fluoroscopic guidance to prevent the stent from being dislodged.

Iliac disruption may be suspected when significant force is required to insert or remove the large sheath and there is a sudden "give," which may correspond to avulsion of the external iliac artery, usually just distal to the hypogastric artery origin. The injury may cause immediate hypotension or may not manifest with overt hemodynamic changes until the sheath is withdrawn. A sudden release of tension may be felt during removal of the large sheath associated with the "iliac-on-a-stick" (Figure 30–6) phenomenon where a portion of avulsed external iliac artery is wrapped around the delivery catheter or sheath. This is almost always associated with rapid and profound hypotension. If iliac avulsion is suspected, an aortic occlusion balloon can be inserted through the contralateral iliac artery, but prompt laparotomy or retroperitoneal cutdown is usually indicated. A rapid determination of avulsion will help forego potentially futile endovascular repair and result in

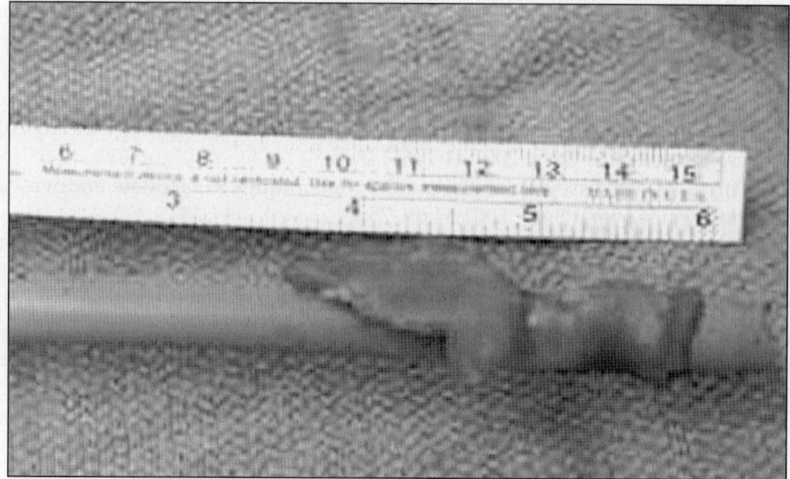

Figure 30-6. "Iliac-on-a-stick" or avulsed external iliac artery adherent to large-diameter sheath.

proceeding sooner to open repair. Retroperitoneal exposure and ligation of the hypogastric artery may be required to stop persistent backbleeding. Open repair will also be necessary if no appropriate covered stent is available. A soft-jawed clamp may be used safely on the endograft limb for proximal control, and an iliofemoral bypass performed to complete the repair.

CONCLUSIONS

Preoperative imaging and planning can reduce the risk of iliac complications by liberally using conduits or other alternative access techniques. Intraoperative techniques can successfully address some access challenges and result in earlier diagnosis of these inevitable complications. As EVAR and TEVAR technology advances and other large profile device treatments evolve to treat a wider spectrum of patients, the ability to deal with challenging iliac anatomy will become increasingly important.

REFERENCES

1. Makaroun MS, Dillavou ED, Kee ST, et al. Endovascular treatment of thoracic aortic aneurysms: results of the phase II multicenter trial of the GORE TAG thoracic endoprosthesis. *J Vasc Surg.* 2005;41:1–9.
2. Fairman RM et al SVS Oral Presentation: "Pivotal Results of the Medtronic Vascular Talent Thoracic Stent Graft System for Patients with Thoracic Aortic Disease. The VALOR Trial." June 2007.
3. Matsumura JS et al SVS Oral Presentation: "Early Results of an Internation Controlled Trial of TEVAR. The STARZ-TX2 clinical trial" June 2007.
4. Parmer SS and Carpenter JP. Techniques for large sheath insertion during endovascular thoracic aortic aneurysm repair. *J Vasc Surg.* 2006;43 supplement:62A–68A.
5. Queral LA, Criado FJ, Patten P. Retrograde iliofemoral endarterectomy facilitated by balloon angioplasty. *J Vasc Surg.* 1995;22:742–748.

6. von Segesser LK, Marty B, Tozzi PG, et al. In situ introducer sheath dilatation for complex aortic access. *Eur J Cardio Thor Surg*. 2002;22:316–318.

7. Abu-Ghaida, AM, Clair DG, Greenberg RK, et al. Broadening the applicability of endovascular aneurysm repair: The use of iliac conduits. *J Vasc Surg*. 2002;36:111–117.

8. Eidt JF and Ali AT. Iliac Conduit for Deploying Aortic Endografts: An All-Autogenous Option. *Vasc Endovascular Surg*. 2007 41:146–148.

9. Yano OJ, Faries PL, Morissey N, et al. Ancillary techniques to facilitate endovascular repair of aortic aneurysms. *J Vasc Surg*. 2001;34:69–75.

10. Wain RA, Lyon RT, Veith FJ, et al. Alternative techniques for management of distal anastomoses of aortofemoral and iliofemoral endovascular grafts. *J Vasc Surg*. 2000;32:307–314.

11. Lee WA, O'Dorisio J, Wolf YG et al. Outcome oafter unilateral hypogastric artery occlusion during endovascular aneurysm repair. *J Vasc Surg*. 2001; 33:921–926.

12. Heidenreich, MJ, Neschis DG, Costanza MJ, et al. Endovascular repair of a penetrating thoracic aortic ulcer by way of the carotid artery. *J Vasc Surg*. 2003;38:1407–1410.

13. Carpenter JP. Delivery of endovascular grafts by direct sheath placement into the aorta or iliac arteries. *Ann Vasc Surg*. 2002;16:787–790.

31

Management of Ischemic Complications Following Endovascular Graft Repair

Daniel Clair, M.D.

Endovascular aneurysm repair was first described by Parodi, et al[1] in 1991. Since that time, the technique has gained widespread acceptance. Over the time since the introduction of this technique, there have been significant strides made in the technology of the devices used in these repairs. Combined with improved experience in the performance of this procedure, most would now view this as the procedure of choice in those with favorable anatomy presenting with aneurismal disease of the infrarenal aorta.

While the nature of the treatment of aortic aneurysm has been undergoing change, the nature of the complications one deals with in these patients has changed as well. Complications that were formerly associated with the performance of open aneurysm repair are different from those seen with endovascular repair. The skilled vascular surgeon needs to understand these complications and their causes in order to avoid them, if possible, and to recognize them and treat them when they do occur. Although there has been much written regarding the recognized complications of open aneurysm repair, there is still much to be learned about the problems of this procedure. In addition, as the devices change, the problems associated with these repairs change and the issues one needs to be aware of in terms of planning and sizing endografts can change dramatically.

Complications of endovascular aneurysm repair, like those of open repair, can be divided into systemic complications such as cardiac, pulmonary, and renal complications, and those local complications such as arterial injury, bleeding, and vessel thrombosis. There are, in addition, a number of complications that are viewed as local complications, but are directly related to the device or the device performance such as endoleak, migration, device integrity failure, and graft limb thrombosis. Many of these latter complications will prove to be directly related to the device utilized in the repair; however, some will clearly be related to the interaction of a particular endograft with a specific patientís anatomic situation. These complications are somewhat unique for surgeons in that they are an assessment of the effect of the technology rather than an evaluation of the ability of the surgeon to perform the procedure safely. In this light, it is important that those using endografts understand the limitations of the devices they use and the situations where one technology may be specifically prone to failure. One such example would be the use of tube endograft devices to repair abdominal aortic aneurysm. With the understanding that these devices have resulted in a much higher incidence of migration and distal type I endoleak, the use of these types of devices is essentially nonexistent at this point. The critical point here is that an understanding of the type of complication and its association with a specific type of graft has led to a change in practice, which benefits patients and physicians alike.

MORTALITY

An evaluation of the risk of mortality of endovascular repair is not quite as simple as one might initially believe. In assessing the risks of open repair, the evaluation of numerous case series and statewide and national databases allow an assessment of the mortality risk of those patients undergoing aneurysm repair. In the setting of open repair being the only option available for patients, the risk of the open repair was easily identifiable; however, the introduction of an alternative technique challenges the concept that one can easily report risks associated with either procedure. Biases in choice of patients may make one procedure appear preferable over another. In addition, operator experience with one technique or another may also skew the data in favor of one type of procedure. Initial reports of endovascular repair contained widely disparate mortality rates varying from 0%–28%. However, these studies reported the risk associated with a new technology utilized in high-risk patients who were felt to be poor candidates for open repair. Many authors initially concluded, as did Woodburn et al.,[2] that the mortality risk of this new technique was similar to what one might expect with open surgical repair. With the approval of devices by the FDA in 1999, the ensuing dissemination of the technology has led to more widespread use, and the application of the technology in those who are otherwise healthy and might be considered good candidates for open repair as well. This approval was based on studies evaluating the outcome of endovascular repair and comparing it with the outcomes in concurrent controls undergoing open repair. In evaluating these outcomes (Table 31–1),[3-7] the perioperative mortality results of endovascular repair are clearly comparable with those of open repair, and from this table, one can see that each of these differing devices are fairly similar in mortality outcomes as well. In none of the studies noted in this table was a significant difference between the mortality of open repair and endovascular repair noted.

In addition to these studies, evaluation of the procedure with more widespread distribution reveals an apparent lower mortality in patients undergoing endovascular

TABLE 31-1. REPORTED MORTALITY FOR OPEN AND ENDOVASCULAR ANEURYSM REPAIR

Author	Device	Endo Mortality	Open Mortality
Zarins[3]	AneuRx	3%	0%
Moore[4]	EVT (phase I)	0%	N/A
Moore[5]	EVT (bifurcated)	1.7%	2.7%
Matsumura[6]	Gore Excluder	1%	0%
Greenberg[7]	Cook Zenith	0.5%	2.5%

repair.[8] In an analysis of aneurysm repair in New York state following approval of endografts for commercial use, these authors looked at the incidence of endovascular repair and the associated in-hospital mortality and length of stay for patients undergoing standard open repair versus those having endovascular repair. Despite the fact that the patients undergoing endovascular repair had increased preoperative risk factors, they had significantly lower mortality and shorter hospital length of stay.

More recently, two trials have compared the results of open and endovascular repair in a randomized trial format. The Dutch Randomized Endovascular Aneurysm Management (Dream) trial[9] was a multicentered, randomized trial comparing the two types of repair directly in nearly 350 patients in need of aneurysm repair who were felt to be good candidates for both types of repair. The trialists recorded a perioperative mortality rate of 4.6% in the open repair group versus 1.2% in the endovascular with a trend to statistical significance of this finding ($p = 0.10$). The second of these trials, the EVAR 1 trial, has only recently had its initial findings published as well.[10] In this trial, over 1,000 patients were randomized to receive either open or endovascular repair for their aneurysms, in patients judged fit for either type of repair. Operative mortality at 30 days in the two groups was 1.6% (endovascular) versus 4.6% (open), revealing a statistically significant difference between the two groups ($p = 0.007$). The results of these trials reveal that the perioperative mortality associated with endovascular repair is lower than that achieved with open repair in the same patient populations. It is expected that the results of the U.S.-based Open versus Endovascular Repair (OVER) study will be completed soon and will allow further assessment of the mortality risks of endovascular aneurysm repair compared with open repair in similar patient populations.

Given this body of evidence, one can state that early mortality is lower for patients undergoing endovascular repair of their aneurysms. It is likely that as the technology continues to improve, these differences may become more substantial. Decreased mortality in these patients may alter the risk-benefit profile for recommendations regarding repair of aneurysms.

SYSTEMIC COMPLICATIONS

Systemic complications of endovascular aneurysm repair have been documented in device trials looking to assess the outcomes of endovascular repair with a particular device versus the outcomes of open repair in a concurrent control population. These complications included cardiac, respiratory, and renal complications, along with other occurrences that have been noted in this patient group, as well as in those patients having undergone repair of an abdominal aortic aneurysm with standard repair. A grading system for these complications allows the standardized reporting of the severity of these complications and has been agreed on by the Society for Vascular Surgery and the American Association for Vascular Surgery.[11] A good assessment of the occurrence of these complications can be found in the reports of the FDA-approved trials evaluating these devices prior to market approval.

A list of the systemic complications noted in these reports[3-7] and others[12-15] is given in Table 31–2. A number of other complications that can occur locally and are related to the devices themselves will be addressed later in this chapter. Specifically, it should be noted that the majority of these complications has been reported in patients

TABLE 31-2. SYSTEMIC COMPLICATIONS OF ENDOVASCULAR AORTIC ANEURYSM REPAIR

Cardiac complications	Pulmonary complications
Myocardial infarction	Prolonged intubation
Cardiac dysrhythmia	Respiratory failure
Congestive heart failure	
Vascular complications	Renal dysfunction
Embolus	Renal failure
Thrombosis	Elevated creatinine
Neurologic complications	Bowel complications
Stroke	Intestinal ischemia
Paraparesis	Ileus
Genitourinary complications	Hepatic failure
Urinary tract infection	
Post-implantation syndrome	Bleeding
Multisystem organ failure	

undergoing open repair of abdominal aortic aneurysms. Additionally, these systemic complications are noted in fewer patients when assessed in concurrent trials comparing the techniques[3-7,16] and also in randomized trials that have compared these techniques.[9,10] Of particular note regarding these complications is the so-called ìpost-implantation syndrome,î[17] which can be seen in patients undergoing endovascular aneurysm repair. Velazquez et al.[17] after first describing this phenomenon, did not relate any evidence of infection to their findings. In fact, they note as well that other authors had previously reported febrile responses in patients undergoing endovascular aneurysm repair[12] while similarly not determining any evidence of infectious cause. A number of investigators have further studied the inflammatory response to endograft placement in comparison to open surgery.[18-23] These authors have noted decreases in a number of inflammatory markers including interleukins, c-reactive protein, and in some studies, tumor necrosis factor-α, although this is not consistent. Additionally, it appears the immune suppression one has following aneurysm repair appears to be attenuated following endovascular repair, compared with open aneurysm repair.[23] While the final implications of these alterations have not been completely clarified, it does appear there are beneficial effects regarding the immune and inflammatory response following endovascular aneurysm repair as compared with open aneurysm repair. The explanation for these differences remains to be shown.

Other systemic complications are similar to those seen after open aneurysm repair and are dealt with in similar fashion. In the majority of instances, this mandates dealing with the organ system separately from the surgical procedure. However, with endovascular surgery as with open surgery, the best results in limiting complications are obtained when the postoperative problems can be avoided by assessing the risk preoperatively. So, for those patients with known coronary disease, preoperative beta blockade and close monitoring of cardiac status should be carried out. In addition, for those patients with evidence of stenosis of the superior mesenteric artery, this issue should be addressed prior to exclusion of the aneurysm and subsequent occlusion of the in-flow to the inferior mesenteric artery. In some instances, anatomic considerations should lead to the performance of open aneurysm repair in preference to endovascular repair; such a choice might be made in treating a patient with severe aortoiliac occlusive disease that may predispose to limb ischemia following endograft placement. The occurrence of bilateral common iliac aneurysms may also be an indication for open aneurysm repair. In most instances, a thorough evaluation of the risks associated with performance of an endovascular aneurysm repair will help to better prevent systemic complications.

LOCAL COMPLICATIONS

Femoral and Iliac Artery Damage

Complications related to the vasculature during performance of the procedure, along with those problems related to the endografts itself, comprise the list of local complications one can encounter during endovascular aneurysm repair. A list of potential local complications is given in Table 31–3. This list is compiled from previously cited reports of endovascular aneurysm repair.[3-7,9,10,12-16] With this list at hand, a review of the differing problems can be undertaken.

Damage to the iliac artery can occur at any point during the delivery, deployment, or completion of the endograft procedure. Its occurrence varies from 0%–10% in reported series[3–7,12,24] and appears to be decreasing in incidence as newer, lower-profile devices and improved delivery systems assist in making insertion of the device easier, and as physicians become more experienced with the performance of this procedure. This is evident from a comparison of the Ancure device trials[4,5] showing decreased iliac artery injuries with the later device and also with the more recent devices trials (Gore Excluder, Cook Zenith)[6,7] showing no incidence of iliac artery damage in their early assessments. It is of benefit to have adequate imaging of the iliac arteries prior to graft placement to assess the difficulty one might encounter with delivery of these devices. This may also alert the clinician to the need of placing an iliac conduit to deliver the device, as has been described previously.[25] Placing conduits in a planned fashion leads to a decrease in the perioperative blood loss, as well as the postoperative length of stay for patients, and can be critical in avoiding more significant systemic complications that may arise as a result of catastrophic bleeding from a damaged iliac artery.

TABLE 31-3. LOCAL AND DEVICE-RELATED COMPLICATIONS OF ENDOVASCULAR ANEURYSM REPAIR

Iliac artery damage	Aortic damage
Perforation	Aneurysm perforation
Dissection	Thrombus embolization
Avulsion	
Femoral artery damage	Endoleak
Perforation	Type I
Dissection	Type II
	Type III
	Type IV
Graft limb thrombosis	Graft migration
Branch artery occlusion	Conversion
Internal iliac artery	
Renal artery	

Less significant damage to an iliac or femoral artery such as dissection limiting flow or local damage can often be repaired with either a direct surgical repair in the case of the femoral artery, or endoluminal stenting. In the case of the femoral artery, this may entail simple suture tacking of the plaque or formal endarterectomy, while some may require more extensive open repair.[4]

Conversion

Conversion to open repair was reported in each of the first three concurrent trials comparing new devices to open surgery.[3-5] However, both of the more recent trials have revealed a decreasing incidence of this complication without the need for emergent conversion.[6,7] There was one patient in the study reported by Greenberg et al.[7] that did not undergo endovascular repair, as the device could not be introduced through heavily calcified arteries.

While traditionally, conversion has been viewed as a complication, in some instances, abandonment of a technically challenging procedure in favor of one that can be performed with less intraoperative difficulty could potentially be seen as the educated decision of an experienced surgeon. Understanding the aspects that will potentially complicate the performance of the procedure makes it possible to address the issues proactively, or alternatively to allow an early decision to desist with attempts that may compromise a successful outcome.

Endoleak

The term ìendoleakî has been used to describe a persistence of flow to within the aneurysm sac, external to a placed endograft.[26] The reported incidence of endoleak varies considerably, in many instances related to the time point at which the leak is identified. At one year assessment, endoleak rates vary from 6%–17% in each of the FDA-approved device trials.[3-7] However, in series assessing device specific results, there do appear to be differences among the devices.[27,28] It also appears from the Eurostar data[29] that there is significant drop-off of endoleaks over the first month alone, with the incidence decreasing from 16% at the time of graft implantation to 10% at one month.

In order to understand endoleaks, it has been helpful to have a classification scheme for the differing types of leaks that can occur.[30] The classification set forth by White et al. has been utilized to define endoleaks and to identify risks associated with differing types of leaks. Type I endoleak refers to those leaks occurring at either the proximal or distal attachment site of the graft (Figure 31–1). With inadequate seal achieved at either of these sites, arterial flow from within the aorta or the iliac artery can directly perfuse the aneurysm sac. Type II endoleak refers to retrograde filling of an aortic branch via collaterals that can lead to branch perfusion of the aneurysm sac and pressurization of the sac (Figure 31–2). Type II endoleaks usually occur via the inferior mesenteric artery, lumbar arteries (fed from the internal iliac artery), or accessory renal arteries. Type III endoleak is one that occurs from a defect within the graft itself. This type of leak can occur at the junction of components as when components separate, or from the interaction of graft materials as can happen from wearing of the fabric by the wire struts of the stent-graft. Type IV endoleak occurs from increased graft porosity and is usually only noted during heparinization that is utilized during graft implantation. Type V endoleak has been used to describe the situation in which there is aneurysm sac enlargement without a detectable endoleak. Further subclassification of these endoleaks has been described as outlined by Veith et al.[31] It is unclear whether this further stratification has any bearing on outcomes for patients; however,

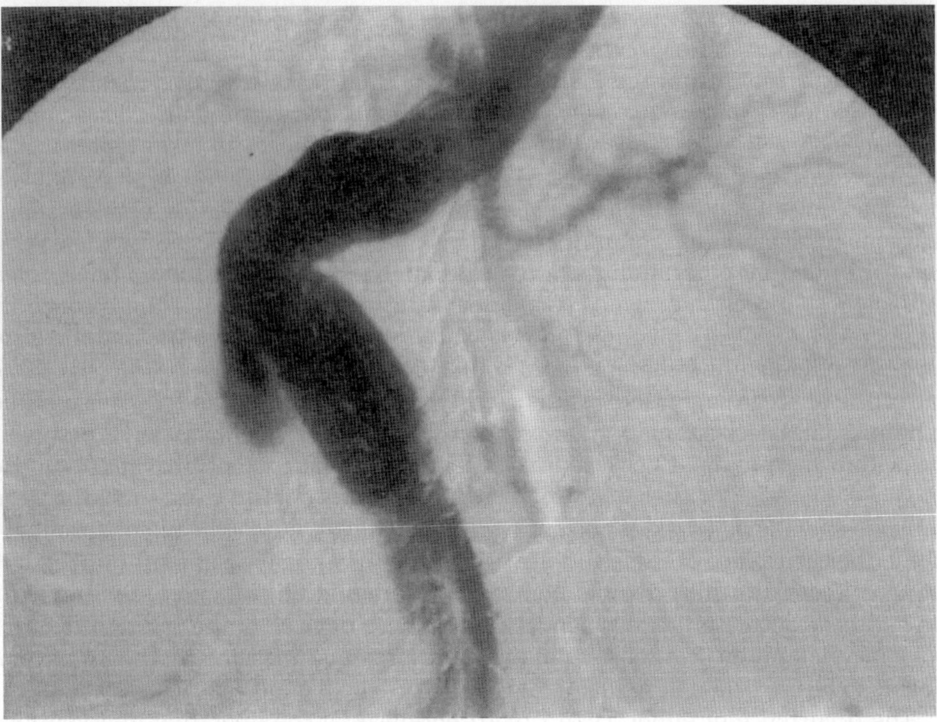

Figure 31-1. Proximal Type I endoleak (arrow) occurring in patient with significant proximal neck angulation.

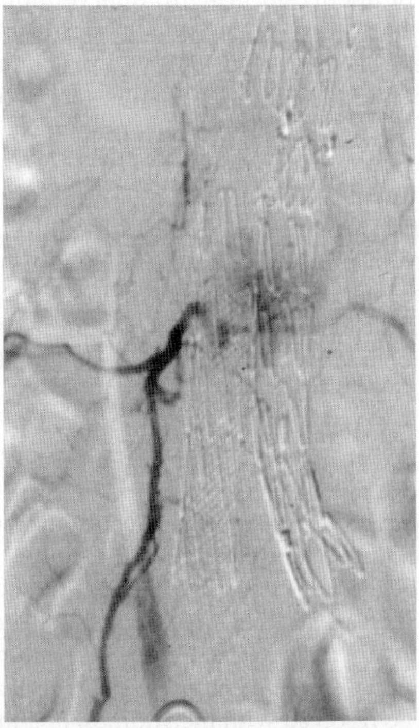

Figure 31-2a. Type II lumbar endoleak filling aneurysm sac.

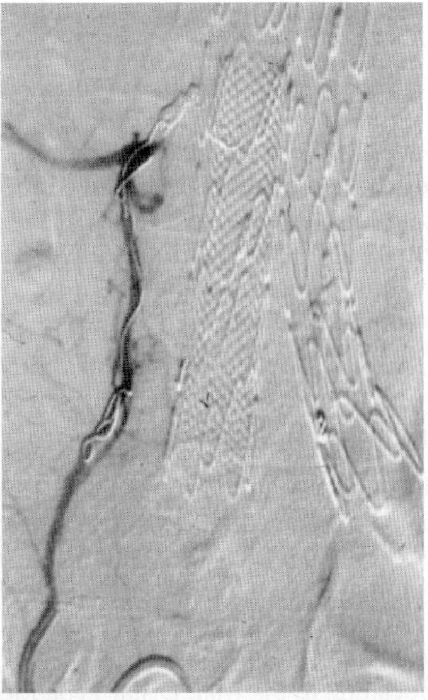

Figure 31-2b. Type II lumber endoleak treated with coil embolization.

it does allow further categorization of these leaks to allow similar comparisons to be made in differing clinical circumstances.

It is clear, again from the EUROSTAR data, that there is a relationship between types of endoleaks and outcomes of endovascular aneurysm repair.[32] These authors noted an increased risk of aneurysm rupture and conversion to open repair in those patients with Type I and III endoleaks as compared with those with Type II endoleaks. They concluded Type II endoleaks need only be treated in the setting of aneurysm sac enlargement. This finding of an increased risk associated with Type I endoleaks has been confirmed by other authors.[33,34] Additionally, these same authors have noted a relationship between aneurysm morphology and the occurrence of these concerning postoperative events. Evaluation by these authors and others have stressed the importance of understanding the anatomic configuration and patient-specific risk factors that can lead to an increased incidence of worrisome endoleaks.[35-37] These authors found proximal neck angulation, proximal neck and aneurysm diameter, and calcification within the proximal neck, led to an increased incidence of proximal type I endoleak. Avoidance of these complicated aneurysms should help to reduce these problems and alleviate risk of postendograft leak and rupture. One other issue that relates to the occurrence of these endoleaks appears to be the type of graft utilized in the setting of these difficult proximal necks. It appears that utilization of suprarenal fixation can help decrease this problem.[38] Use of these devices in the setting of complex proximal anatomy makes sense to allow more proximal placement of the device and appears to be important in reducing the risk of proximal endoleak as well.

The occurrence of either Type I or III endoleak at the operative intervention or early thereafter should be considered an indication to intervene to correct the problem. Type II endoleak, on the other hand, mandates continued follow-up with assessment of the aneurysm sac for growth. In the setting of aneurysm growth, intervention to treat this problem is probably also warranted. Type IV and V endoleak remain somewhat controversial. It is unusual to consider an endoleak beyond 30 days a problem of graft porosity, and one, therefore, should not need to address this as an issue beyond the time in the operating room. The definition of Type V endoleak is clear, however, at conversion; many of these aneurysms have had an alternative explanation for their expansion. For this reason, Type V endoleak is probably best considered a leak of undetermined source that is slow and poorly enhances on the studies performed. In this situation, an extensive evaluation for the source of endoleak should be sought and with continued expansion, conversion may be necessary. Note has been made of an increased incidence of aneurysm expansion without a clear endoleak with the initial version of the Gore Excluder device.[39] It appears this incidence may have been alleviated with a change in the fabric of the graft.

Endoleak Treatment

Most of the need to repair endoleaks relates to Types I and III endoleak. Determining the source can sometimes be difficult, but early recognition makes treatment at the time of repair easier. At initial implantation, extensions, and extended compliant balloon inflations can often resolve the issue. If the problem persists, increased radial force against the aortic wall can be generated by the use of a large, noncompliant balloon sized to the aortic lumen or alternatively, a balloon expandable stent placed at the site of stent graft seal to increase apposition to the wall. Distal Type I leak can often be resolved with the addition of a limb extension. Once out of the operating room and in follow-up, determining the source of the endoleak can continue to be difficult. Often, angiography will be necessary in conjunction with CT scan; however, newer scan technology allowing three-dimensional reconstruction can aid greatly in the determination of the source of an endoleak.[40] Later defined Type I and III endoleaks can often be repaired with the use of extension cuffs, relining of the graft, coil embolization, or conversion, in addition to the application of techniques outlined for use at the time of graft placement.[41] Conversion may involve complete excision of the graft or suturing the area of the endoleak to resolve the issue. Often, this technique will require the potential application of an aortic clamp above the renal arteries because of the proximity of these grafts to the renal ostia. This need for higher aortic cross-clamping, along with the often impaired state of these patients, make this a challenging procedure.

The management of Type II endoleaks varies somewhat with some groups advocating intervention early for all of these, and others recommending a more conservative view. It appears from review of the EUROSTAR data[32] that these types of endoleaks have a much lower association with aneurysm sac enlargement and the need for secondary intervention or conversion. For this reason, observation of these endoleaks with evaluation for increase in sac measurements is the approach most physicians take regarding this problem.[31]

When a Type II endoleak does demand intervention, there are three basic approaches that have been performed.[41-44] For differing problems, each of these approaches has proven useful, and the addition of glue to the armamentarium available to treat these lesions has allowed a continued improvement in the outcomes with endovascular therapies. All of these methods take significant skill and time to ensure a successful result; however, in certain circumstances, this approach will not be successful and conversion will be necessary.

Branch Artery Occlusion

It is important to remember that nearly every infrarenal aortic aneurysm exclusion involves the occlusion of the inferior mesenteric artery. This is an important fact to recall as the internal iliac arteries and the inferior mesenteric artery have significant communication and provide important collaterals for each other. Unplanned occlusion of branch arteries while performing aneurysm exclusion most often involves the internal iliac artery,[45,46] but may involve occlusion of the renal arteries as well.[47-49] In many instances, the occlusion of the internal iliac arteries poses little risk,[46,50] and may occur from either malposition of the endograft or dissection or embolization of the internal iliac artery origin during graft insertion and deployment. In the setting of a contralateral patent iliac artery, it is usually safe to cover an internal iliac artery as either a planned part of the aneurysm exclusion (as might be performed for aneurismal disease of the iliac arteries) or as an unplanned event. In most instances, the coverage does not generate problems for the patient, although rarely, significant consequences can occur.[46] When partial coverage of an internal iliac artery occurs, or if the endograft does not extend a significant length beyond the internal iliac artery orifice, the graft can be displaced proximally by ìpushingî on the iliac limb from below, using the delivery sheath either catching on the end of the graft limb, or advancing it to within the graft limb and pushing within the limb itself.

If there is inadvertent occlusion of both internal iliac arteries, or if this occurs in the setting of contralateral internal iliac artery occlusion, an attempt should be made to revascularize one hypogastric artery, if feasible, as these patients are at higher risk for colonic ischemia and the resultant morbidity this can entail.[51,52] This can be attempted by endovascular means when origin occlusion occurs from dissection or embolization;

however, in many instances, this may require an open surgical approach for surgical reconstruction of the flow through this vessel.[53]

Occlusion of the renal arteries is often more concerning to the clinician because of the risk of renal loss imposed by this event and the time limitation during which re-establishment of blood flow to the kidney must be achieved. It is unclear at this point that the nature of the graft type used has any relationship to the occurrence of this complication,[48] although some authors have implicated endografts with suprarenal extension as a predisposing factor to this problem.[49] The authors implicating graft type in causing this problem have had a very high incidence of partial and complete coverage of the renal arteries in their experience, and it is likely that this may, in fact, account for the differences more than the type of endograft used. In the setting of inadvertent coverage of a small accessory renal artery, little risk is encountered and the patients can merely be followed; however, in the setting of obstruction of flow to the main renal artery, action must be taken. Several authors have described techniques of dealing with this via an endovascular approach,[54-56] and use of these techniques, if effective, is likely the most expeditious method or restoring flow to the kidney. The most commonly described technique involves the placement of a guidewire across the graft bifurcation with downward traction applied from both groin access sites simultaneously. In many instances, this can achieve a caudal displacement of the graft to allow for renal artery stenting to protect the renal artery orifice. In some instances, a brachial approach can afford easier endoluminal access to the renal artery for this purpose. If, however, the endovascular methods fail, the patient should be left anticoagulated and an expeditious surgical reconstruction should be carried out. This is most often performed with an extra-anatomic reconstruction to avoid operation involving the aorta.

Graft Limb Thrombosis

Graft limb thrombosis can occur following placement of a stent-graft for the treatment of abdominal aortic aneurysm.[57-59] These problems can arise either early or late, and may in some instances be predictable and related to the aneurysm morphology, the endograft utilized, or a combination of the two. Assessment of the occurrence in FDA-approved device trials reveals an incidence of 0%–3% in the perioperative period, with the highest rate occurring in the Ancure device.[3,5,6,7] In an assessment of the causes of this problem, Caroccio et al.[57] noted small graft limb diameters extension to the external iliac artery, and while they did not notice an increased incidence of this problem in those with unsupported graft limbs, others have noted this as an additional risk factor,[60] leading to the recommendation by these authors to place stents in all patients undergoing aneurysm treatment with an endograft that does not have stent supported limbs. Patients undergoing endograft placement should have completion angiography performed to assess the status of the iliac arteries following placement of the endograft. In the setting of iliac artery injury, treatment of the pathology noted should be carried out to ensure the optimal outflow for the graft limb. In addition, any abnormalities noted within the graft limb such as kinking or twisting should be treated with balloon angioplasty of the limb or if necessary, stenting within the limb to ensure adequate flow. Once again, as with most complications of surgical procedures, avoidance of the problem by attending to intraoperative abnormalities that are noted can avert problems and risk for the patient.

While some have had uniformly successful outcomes from this problem, critical limb ischemia can result and emergent revascularization should be accomplished.

Limb loss can result from this problem, even when addressed aggressively, and has been noted in >15% of these patients.[61] A number of methods to reestablish flow has been described,[61-63] with endovascular and open surgical approaches. In at least one series, the endovascular solution has offered better long-term patency.[61] The endovascular approaches utilized include mechanical thrombectomy and thrombolysis, along with angioplasty and stent placement. If a surgical approach is preferred or required, cross-femoral grafting offers acceptable results in this setting.

Migration

Migration refers to the movement of the graft in relationship to the arterial implantation site, and has been reported with every FDA-approved endograft system placed to date.[3-7] The occurrence of this problem is concerning because of the potential to develop a Type I endoleak as a result of the graft migration. Graft migration occurs more commonly from the distal motion of the proximal graft and may be related to a number of factors. An early assessment of the EUROSTAR database[64] reveals the occurrence of this to be 3.4% with a smaller number (3.0%) being clinically relevant migrations. These authors also evaluated the demographic, anatomic, and graft-related features of migration, finding that hypertension, aneurysm morphology, and endograft size were all related to endograft migration. Other issues that have been shown by some to have influence on the incidence of graft migration include the absence of suprarenal stent fixation,[65] proximal endograft fixation length,[66] aneurysm neck en-largement,[67] aneurysm diameter,[68] and neck angulation.[69] Of all these factors, the more commonly noted issues relate to aneurysm morphology and include proximal neck length, angulation, and dilatation. In order to ensure adequate fixation of the endograft, the surgeon must assure that the proximal fixation region does not present all of these problems at the same time, and as well, that not one of them is severe enough to lead to this problem as catastrophic consequences can occur.[64] One also needs to recognize that while migration more commonly occurs from the proximal end of an endograft with inadequate fixation in the iliac artery landing zone, proximal migration of the distal end of a stent graft can occur,[7] leading to similarly catastrophic problems.

The treatment for this problem most often is achieved with extension of the endograft; however, in the setting of proximal neck dilation, graft excision and late conversion may be necessary. Aortic banding to treat problematic proximal infrarenal aortic neck anatomy has been described,[70] but experience with this is limited and the long-term results of this approach have yet to be determined. In any instance in which there is concern that the endoluminal approach may not provide adequate long-term fixation again, open repair should be undertaken.

CONCLUSION

Stent-graft repair of the infrarenal aorta is a significant advance in the field of vascular surgery, and provides patients and physicians with an additional method for repairing a complex, life-threatening problem. The technique remains early in its development and will continue to improve through technological advances and improved attention to the performance of the procedure. Each new device and method of treating aneurysm pathology carries with it new risks that must be identified and studied to assess the causes and solutions so that these problems may be treated if they do occur, but more importantly, so that they may be avoided. Physicians treating patients with aneurismal disease using endografts owe it to their patients to thoroughly assess the devices, their positive and negative attributes, and the potential problems that can be encountered both short- and long-term from the use of these devices. Hopefully, reviewing the complications of endovascular aneurysm repair can help in the avoidance of these problems.

Patients undergoing placement of stent-grafts need significant follow-up to ensure the devices are performing as they should and the treatment of the aneurysm has been successful. Endovascular exclusion of an abdominal aortic aneurysm thus becomes part of an agreement between the patient and the treating physician to maintain a long-term relationship to assess the aneurysm, the stent graft, and the success of the procedure.

REFERENCES

1. Parodi JC, Palmaz JC, Barone HD. Transfemoral intraluminal graft implantation for abdominal aortic aneurysms. *Ann Vasc Surg.* 1991;5:491–499.
2. Woodburn KR, May J, White GH. Endoluminal abdominal aortic aneurysm surgery. *Brit J Surg.* 1998;85:435–443.
3. Zarins CK, White RA, Schwarten D, et al., for the investigators of the Medtronic AneuRx Multicenter Clinical Trial. AneuRx stent graft versus open surgical repair of abdominal aortic aneurysms: Multicenter prosective clinical trial. *J Vasc Surg.* 1999;29:292–308.
4. Moore WS, Rutherford RB. Transfemoral endovascular repair of abdominal aortic aneurysm: results of the North American EVT phase 1 trial. EVT Investigators. *J Vasc Surg.* 1996;23:543–553.
5. Moore WS, Matsumura JS, Makaroun MS, et al., for the EVT/Guidant Investigators. Five-year interim comparison of the Guidant bifurcated endografts with open repair of abdominal aortic aneurysm. *J Vasc Surg.* 2003;38:46–55.
6. Matsumura JS, Brewster DC, Makaroun MS, Naftel DC, for the Excluder Bifurcated Endoprosthesis Investigators. A multicenter controlled clilnical trial of open versus endovascular treatment of abdominal aortic aneurysm. *J Vasc Surg.* 2003;37:262–271.
7. Greenberg RK, Chuter TAM, Sternbergh C, Fearnot NE, for the Zenith Investigators. Zenith AAA endovascular graft: Intermediate-term results of the US multicenter trial. *J Vasc Surg.* 2004;39:1209–1218.
8. Anderson PL, Arons Rr, Moskowitz AJ, et al. A statewide experience with endovascular abdominal aortic aneurysm repair: rapid diffusion with excellent early results. *J Vasc Surg.* 2004;39:10–19.
9. Prinssen M, Verhoeven ELG, Buth J, et al., for the Dutch Randomized Endovascular Aneurysm Management (DREAM) Trial Group. A randomized trial comparing conventional and endovascular repair of abdominal aortic aneurysms. *NEJM.* 2004;351:1607–1618.
10. Greenhalgh RM, Brown LC, Kwong GP, et al., for the EVAR trial participants. Comparison of endovascular aneurysm repair with open repair in patients with abdominal aortic aneurysm (EVAR trial 1), 30-day operative mortality results: randomized controlled trial. *Lancet.* 2004;364 (9437);843–848.
11. Chaikof EL, Blankensteijn JK, Harris PL, et al., for the Ad Hoc Committee for Standardized Reporting Practices in Vascular Surgery of The Society for Vascular Surgery/American Association for Vascular Surgery. Reporting standards for endovascular aortic aneurysm repair. *J Vasc Surg.* 2002;35:1048–60.
12. Blum U, Voshage G, Lammer J, et al. Endoluminal stent-grafts for infrarenal abdominal aortic aneurysms. *NEJM.* 1997;336:13–20.
13. Parodi JC. Endovascular repair of abdominal aortic aneurysms and other arterial lesions. *J Vasc Surg.* 1995; 21:549–555.

14. Balm R, Eikelboom BC, May J, et al. Early experience with transfemoral endovascular aneurysm management (TEAM) in the treatment of aortic aneurysms. *Eur J Vasc Endovasc Surg.* 1996;11:214–220.

15. Lawrence-Brown M, Sleunarine K, Hartley D, et al. The Perth HLB bifurcated endoluminal graft: A review of the experience and intermediate results. *Cardiovasc Surg.* 1998;6:220–225.

16. May J, White GH, Waugh R, et al. Improved survival after endoluminal repair with second-generation prostheses compared with open repair in the treatment of abdominal aortic aneurysms: A 5-year concurrent comparison using life table method. *J Vasc Surg.* 2001;33: S21–26.

17. Velazquez OC, Carpenter JP, Baum RA, et al. Perigraft air, fever and leukocytosis after endovascular repair of abdominal aortic aneurysms. *Am J Surg.* 1999;178:185–189.

18. Bolke E, Jehle PM, Storck M, et al. Endovascular stent-graft placement versus conventional open surgery in infrarenal aortic aneurysm: a prospective study on acute phase response and clinical outcome. *Clinica Chimica Acta.* 2001;314:203–207.

19. Galle C, De Maertelaer V, Motte S, et al. Early inflammatory response after elective abdominal aortic aneurysm repair: a comparison between endovascular procedure and conventional surgery. *J Vasc Surg.* 2000;32:234–246.

20. Storck M, Scharrer-Pamler R, Kapfer X, et al. Does a postimplantation syndrome following endovascular treatment of aortic aneurysms exist? *Vasc Surg.* 2001;35:23–29.

21. Swartbol P, Norgren L, Albrechtsson U, et al. Biological responses differ considerably between endovascular and conventional aortic aneurysm surgery. *Eur J Vasc Endovasc Surg.* 1996;12:18–25

22. Odegard A, Lundbom J, Myhre HO, et al. The inflammatory response following treatment of abdominal aortic aneurysms: a comparison between open surgery and endovascular repair. *Eur J Vasc Endovasc Surg.* 2000;19:536–544.

23. Sweeney KJ, Evy D, Sultan S, et al. Enodvascular approach to abdominal aortic aneurysms limits the postoperative systemic immune response. *Eur J Vasc Endovasc Surg.* 2002;23: 303–308.

24. Aljabri B, Obrand DI, Montreuil B, et al. Early vascular complications after endovascular repair of aortoiliac aneurysms. *Ann Vasc Surg.* 2001;15:608–614.

25. Abu-Ghaida AM, Clair DG, Greenberg RK, et al. Broadening the applicability of endovascular aneurysm repair: the use of iliac conduits. *J Vasc Surg.* 2002;36:111–117.

26. White GH, Yu W, May J. ëEndoleakí - a proposed new terminology to describe incomplete aneurysm exclusion by an endoluminal graft. *J Endovasc Surg.* 1996;3:124–125.

27. Ouriel K, Clair DG, Greenberg RK, et al. Endovascular repair of abdominal aortic aneurysms: Device-specific outcome. *J Vasc Surg.* 2003;37:991–998.

28. Torella F, on behalf of the EUROSTAR Collaborators. Effect of improved endograft design on outcome of endovascular aneurysm repair. *J Vasc Surg.* 2004;40:216–221.

29. Buth J, Laheij RJF, on behalf of the EUROSTAR Collaborators. Early complications and endoleaks after endovascular abdominal aortic aneurysm repair: Report of a multicenter study. *J Vasc Surg.* 2000;31:134–146.

30. White GH, Yu W, May J, et al. Endoleak as a complication of endoluminal grafting of abdominal aortic aneurysms: classification, incidence, diagnosis, and management. *J Endovasc Surg.* 1997;4:152–168.

31. Veith FJ, Baum RA, Ohki T, et al. Nature and significance of endoleaks and endotension: Summary of opinions expressed at an international conference. *J Vasc Surg.* 2002;35: 1029–1035.

32. van Marrewijk C, Buth J, Harris PL, et al. Significance of endoleaks after endovascular repair of abdominal aortic aneurysms: The EUROSTAR experience. *J Vasc Surg.* 2002; 35:461–473.

33. Bernhard VM, Mitchell RS, Matsumura JS, et al. Ruptured abdominal aortic aneurysm after endovascular repair. *J Vasc Surg.* 2002;35:1155–1162.

34. Wain RA, Marin ML, Ohki T, et al. Endoleaks after endovascular graft treatment of aortic aneurysms: Classification, risk factors, and outcome. *J Vasc Surg.* 1998;27:69–80.

35. Sternbergh WC, Carter G, York JW, et al. Aortic neck angulation predicts adverse outcomes with endovascular abdominal aortic aneurysm repair. *J Vasc Surg.* 2002;35:482–486.

36. Sampaio SM, Panneton JM, Mozes GI, et al. Proximal type I endoleak after endovascular abdominal aortic aneurysm repair: predictive factors. *Ann Vasc Surg.* 2004;18:621–628.

37. Albertini J, Kalliafas S, Travis S, et al. Anatomical risk factors for proximal perigraft endoleak and graft migration following endovascular repair of abdominal aortic aneurysms. *Eur J Vasc Endovasc Surg.* 2000;19:308–312.

38. Robbins M, Kritpracha B, Beebe HG, et al. Suprarenal endograft fixation avoids adverse outcomes associated with aortic neck angulation. *Ann Vasc Surg.* 2005;19:172–177.

39. Kibbe MR, Matsumura JS, for the Excluder Investigators. The Gore Excluder US multi-center trial: analysis of adverse events at 2 years. *Semin Vasc Surg.* 2003;16:144–150.

40. Stavropoulos SW, Clark TW, Carpenter JP, et al. Use of CT angiography to classify endoleaks after endovascular repair of abdominal aortic aneurysms. *J Vasc Intervent Radiol.* 2005;16:663–667.

41. Faries PL, Cadot H, Agarwal G, Kent KC, Hollier LH, Marin ML. Management of endoleak after endovascular aneurysm repair: cuffs, coils, and conversion. *J Vasc Surg.* 2003;37:1155–61.

42. Haulon S, Tyazi A, Willoteaux S, et al. Embolization of type II endoleaks after aortic stent-graft implantation: technique and immediate results. *J Vasc Surg.* 2001;34:600–605.

43. Baum RA, Carpenter JP, Golden MA, et al. Treatment of type 2 endoleaks after endovascular repair of abdominal aortic aneurysms: camparison of transarterial and translumbar techniques. *J Vasc Surg.* 2002;35:23–29.

44. Richardson WS, Sternbergh WC 3rd, Money SR. Laparoscopic inferior mesenteric artery ligation: an alternative for the treatment of type II endoleaks. *J Laparoendosc Adv Surg Tech.* 2003;13:355–358.

45. Kasirajan K, Matteson B, Marek JM, Langsfeld M. Technique and results of transfemoral superselective coil embolization of type II lumbar endoleak. *J Vasc Surg.* 2003;38:61-66

46. Kalliafas S, Albertini JN, Macierewicz J, et al. Incidence and treatment of intraoperative technical problems during endovascular repair of complex abdominal aortic andeurysms. *J Vasc Surg.* 2000; 31:1175–1192.

47. Karch LA, Hodgson KJ, Mattos MA, et al. Adverse consequences of internal iliac artery occlusion during endovascular repair of abdominal aortic aneurysms. *J Vasc Surg.* 2000;32:676–683.

48. Bockler D, Krauss M, Mansmann U, et al. Incidence of renal infarctions after endovascular AAA repair: relationship to infrarenal versus suprarenal fixation. *J Endovasc Ther.* 2003;10:1054–1060.

49. Lau LL, Hakaim AG, Oldenburg WA, et al. Effect of suprarenal versus infrarenal aortic endograft fixation on renal function and renal artery patency: a comparative study with intermediate follow-up. *J Vasc Surg.* 2003;37:1162–1168.

50. Kramer Sc, Seifarth H, Pamler R, et al. Renal infarction following endovascular aortic aneurysm repair: incidence and clinical consequences. *J Endovasc Ther.* 2002;9:98–102.

51. Rhee RY, Muluk SC, Tzeng E, et al. Can the internal iliac artery be safely covered during endovascular repair of abdominal aortic and iliac artery aneurysms? *Ann Vasc Surg.* 2002;16:29–36.

52. Connolly JE, Ingegno M, Wilson SE. Preservation of the pelvic circulation during infrarenal aortic surgery. *Cardiovasc Surg.* 1996;4:65–70.

53. Yusuf SW, Whitaker SC, Chuter TAM, et al. Early results of endovascular sortic aneurysm surgery with aortouniiliac graft, contralateral iliac occlusion, and femorofemoral bypass. *J Vasc Surg.* 1997;25:165–72.

54. Faries PL, Morrissey N, Burks JA, et al. Internal iliac artery revascularization as an adjunct to endovascular repair of aortoiliac aneurysms. *J Vasc Surg.* 2001;34:892–899.

55. Lin PH, Bush RL, Lumsden AB. Endovascular rescue of a maldeployed aortic stent-graft causing renal artery occlusion: technical considerations. *Vasc Endovasc Surg.* 2004;38:69–73.

56. Ruckert RI, Romaniuk P, Rogalla P, et al. A method for adjusting a malpositioned bifurcated aortic endograft. *J Endovasc Surg.* 1998;5:261–265.

57. Gorich J, Kramer S, Rilinger N, et al. Malpositioned or dislocated aortic endoprostheses: repositioning using percutaneous pull-down maneuvers. *J Endovasc Ther*. 2000;7:123–131.
58. Carroccio A, Faries PL, Morrissey NJ, et al. Predicting iliac limb occlusion after bifurcated aortic stent grafting: anatomic and device-related causes. *J Vasc Surg*. 2002;36:679–684.
59. Amesur NB, Zajko AB, Orons PD, Makaroun MS. Endovascular treatment of iliac limb stenosis or occlusions in 31 patients treated with the Ancure endograft. *J Vasc Intervent Radiol*. 2000;11:421–428.
60. Bohannon WT, Hodgson KJ, Parra JR, et al. Endovascular management of iliac limb occlusion of bifurcated aortic endograft. *J Vasc Surg*. 2002;3:584–588.
61. Carpenter JP, Neschis DG, Fairman RM, et al. Failure of endovascular abdominal aortic aneurysm graft limbs. *J Vasc Surg*. 2001;33:296–302.
62. Erzurum VZ, Sampram ES, Sarac TP, et al. Initial management and outcome of aortic endograft limb occlusion. *J Vasc Surg*. 2004;40:419–423.
63. Krajcer Z, Gilbert JH, Jougherty K, et al. Successful treatment of aortic endograft throbosis with rheolytic thrombectomy. *J Endovasc Ther*. 2002;9:756–764.
64. Parent FN 3rd, Godziachvili V, Meier GH 3rd, et al. Endograft limb occlusion and stenosis after ACCURE endovascular abdominal aneurysm repair. *J Vasc Surg* 2002;35:686–690.
65. Mohan IV, Harris PL, van Marrewijk CJ, et al. Factors and forces influencing stent-graft migration after endovascular aortic aneurysm repair. *J Endovasc Ther*. 2002;9:748–755.
66. Kalliafas S, Albertini JN, Macierewicz J, et al. Stent-graft migration after endovascular repair of abdominal aortic aneurysm. *J Endovasc Ther*. 2002;9:743–747.
67. Zarins CK, Bloch DA, Crabtree T, et al. Stent graft migration after endovascular aneurysm repair: importance of proximal fixation. *J Vasc Surg*. 2003;38:1264–1272.
68. Resch T, Ivancev K, Brunkwall J, et al. Distal migration of stent-grafts after endovascular repair of abdominal aortic aneurysms. *J Vasc Intervent Radiol*. 1999;10:257-264.
69. Cao P, Verzini F, Zannetti S, et al. Device migration after endoluminal abdominal aortic aneurysm repair: analysis of 113 cases with a minimum follow-up period of 2 years. *J Vasc Surg*. 2002;35:229–235.
70. Albertini J, Kalliafas S, Travis S, et al. Anatomical risk factors for proximal perigraft endoleak and graft migration following endovascular repair of abdominal aortic aneurysms. *Eur J Vasc Endovasc Surg*. 2000;19:308–312.
71. Utikal P, Kocher M, Bachleda P, et al. Banding in aortic stent-graft fixation in evar. *Biomedical Papers* 2004;148:1175–178.

32

Gastrointestinal Complications: Serious but Under-appreciated Sequelae of Aortic Surgery

R. James Valentine, M.D.

The development of a gastrointestinal complication (GIC) after cardiovascular surgery is associated with serious morbidity. Affected patients often require additional operations, have prolonged hospitalization, and have an increased mortality rate.[1-3] The mere presence of cardiovascular disease appears to be a risk factor for GICs because these complications develop in patients who undergo cardiovascular operations remote from the abdominal cavity. For example, GICs occur in 2% of patients undergoing coronary artery bypass, in 20% after cardiac transplantation, and in 50% after orthotopic lung transplantation.[1-3] GICs are associated with poor outcome in these circumstances. In addition to prolonged hospitalization, more than 50% of patients with postoperative GICs require abdominal operations, and up to 67% die.[1-3] A common etiology remains unproven, but visceral hypoperfusion appears to be the pathologic mechanism in many cases.[3]

If GICs occur after cardiovascular operations remote from the abdominal cavity, then it follows that GICs should be more prevalent in transabdominal operations for vascular disease, particularly aortic surgery. Some of the risk can be related to direct errors in technique such as inadvertent bowel entry or retractor injury. However, patients with vascular disease may be more prone to GICs because they have a higher prevalence of mesenteric artery disease.[4] Open aortic surgery can be associated with large fluid shifts due to rapid blood loss or prolonged operations. The risk of visceral hypoperfusion due to volume depletion and shock is compounded by the prevalence of mesenteric artery disease in many patients.

The following discussion will examine the scope of the problem and consider specific GICs that occur after aortic surgery. While many of these problems appear to be unavoidable, it is incumbent on the vascular surgeon to recognize and treat patients with GICs to reduce the risk of catastrophic outcome.

THE PREVALENCE OF GIC AFTER AORTIC SURGERY

Each GIC is individually rare, but the aggregation of complications is serious. We prospectively collected data on a group of 120 patients undergoing aortic surgery for aneurysmal (n = 58) or occlusive (n = 62) disease.[5] A secondary analysis was performed on these data to determine the risk factors, associated events, and outcomes for patients who developed GICs. A total of 29 GICs developed in 25 (21%) patients within 30 days of aortic surgery (Table 32–1). The most common complication was paralytic ileus, defined as the requirement for nasogastric tube reinsertion due to gastric distention and vomiting. Other complications included, in descending order: gastrointestinal bleeding, infection, mechanical obstruction, ascites, and colon ischemia. GICs developed in nine patients (16%) with aneurysms, which was not significantly different compared to five patients (8%) with occlusive disease who developed GICs.

Comparing the 25 patients who developed GICs to the 95 patients who did not develop GICs, there were no significant differences in demographics, operative indications, atherosclerotic risk factors, prevalence of mesenteric artery stenoses, perioperative fluid volumes, or operative times. However, mean estimated blood loss was higher for patients who had GICs compared to those who did not (P = .02) (Table 32–2). Seven patients with GICs (28%) and seven patients without GICs (7%) had intraoperative complications (P = .004). Intraoperative complications included hypotension (systolic BP < 90 mm Hg for more than five minutes) in four (16%) patients with GICs and three (3%) without GICs (P = .02); cardiac arrhythmias in three (12%) patients with GIC and three (3%) patients without GICs (NS); and bronchospasm in one patient without GICs (NS). Compared to patients without GICs, those with GICs had a longer duration of mechanical ventilation, length of ICU stay, and duration of hospitalization. Four (3.3%) of the 120 patients in this study died of multisystem organ failure: three (12%) had GICs compared to one (1%) without GICs (P = .007).These data show that GICs are prevalent after transperitoneal aortic surgery and are associated with severe

TABLE 32-1. GASTROINTESTINAL COMPLICATIONS FOLLOWING AORTIC SURGERY IN 120 PATIENTS.

Complication	No. patients (%)	Laparotomy required	Death
Adynamic ileus	12 (10)*		1
Gastrointestinal hemorrhage			
Gastritis	2 (2)		
Duodenal ulcer	2 (2)		
Gastric ulcer	1 (1)		
C. Difficile Enterocolitis	5 (4)†	1	
Acute calculous cholecytitis	2 (2)	2	1
Mechanical bowel obstruction	2 (2)	2	1
Ascites	2 (2)	1	
Colon ischemia	1 (1)	1	
Total	29	7	3

*Three patients had other GICs
†One patient had other GICs
Adapted from Valentine RJ, Hagino RT, Jackson MR, et al. Gastrointestinal complications after aortic surgery. *J Vasc Surg* 1998; 28: 404-412.

TABLE 32-2. COMPARISON OF 25 PATIENTS WHO DEVELOPED GASTROINTESTINAL COMPLICATIONS AFTER AORTIC SURGERY WITH 95 WHO DID NOT.

	GIC	No GIC	P value
Fluid administration (L)			
Preoperative	2.2 ± 1.2	1.7 ± 1.1	NS
Intraoperative	6.0 ± 2.3	5.7 ± 2.3	NS
Postoperative	5.4 ± 2.4	4.3 ± 1.7	.008
Operative time (min)	245 ± 93	243 ± 77	NS
Intraoperative complications	7 (28%)	7 (7%)	.004
Estimated blood loss (L)	1.6 ± 1.7	1.0 ± 1.0	.02
Duration of mechanical ventilation (h)	71 ± 226	7 ± 11	.006
Length of stay (days)			
ICU	16 ± 15	5 ± 2	< .001
Total postoperative	24 ± 20	10 ± 6	< .001
Death	3 (12%)	1 (1%)	.007

Adapted from Valentine RJ, Hagino RT, Jackson MR, et al. Gastrointestinal complications after aortic surgery. *J Vasc Surg* 1998; 28: 404-412.

morbidity rates, increased hospital stay, and increased mortality. However, none of the variables in the study were predictive of GICs. Therefore, these complications may serve as markers of poor outcome but they currently cannot be prevented.

Others have reported the prevalence of GICs following transperitoneal aortic surgery. In a retrospective review, Crowson and colleagues reported acute GICs in 31 (6.6%) of 472 patients undergoing open aortic aneurysm repair.[6] The most common complication was intestinal ischemia (n = 9), followed in descending order by mechanical or paralytic ileus (n = 8), GI bleeding (n = 5), and fistula (n = 2). The associated mortality was high: 21 (68%) of the 31 patients with GICs died. In another retrospective series, Alpagut and associates reported a similar distribution of GICs in 65 (8.6%) of 750 patients undergoing transperitoneal aortic surgery at the University of Istanbul.[7] The patients with GICs had a longer duration of ICU and total hospital stay, but the authors could not identify any risk factors for development of GICs. Data from these two retrospective studies corroborate our findings that GICs are prevalent after transperitoneal aortic surgery and are associated with a worse outcome. Comparing these studies to ours, the difference in overall prevalence of GICs is likely due to the definition of paralytic ileus, which was more liberal in our study. Although paralytic ileus per se appears to be a relatively benign complication, it is nevertheless associated with increased overall costs due to prolonged hospital stay.

REDUCING THE RISK OF GICS IN AORTIC SURGERY

One highly touted advantage of the retroperitoneal incision for abdominal aortic surgery is an overall reduction in GICs, mostly intestinal ileus. In a prospective randomized trial comparing the transabdominal versus retropertineal incisions for aortic operations, Sicard and colleagues reported a higher incidence of prolonged ileus (i.e., nasogastric suction > 72 hours) in patients randomized to transperitoneal compared with retroperitoneal operations (11% versus none, P = .005).[8] In addition, four patients undergoing transperitoneal operations developed mechanical small bowel obstructions, but none undergoing retroperitoneal operations developed obstructions (P = .05). There were no reported instances of GI bleeding, infection, or ischemia in either group. The opposite findings were reported in a prospective randomized study by Cambria and associates.[9] The authors found no overall difference in the recovery of gastrointestinal function after the transperitoneal versus the retroperitoneal approach. It should be pointed out that the decision to discontinue nasogastric suction is often subjective and based on an individual surgeon's personal practice. There were no comparisons of patients who required replacement of nasogastric tubes in these studies, nor were there any reports of other gastrointestinal complications such as infections or ischemia. Thus, the overall benefit of retroperitoneal operations in terms of reducing GICs remains uncertain.

The risk of GICs may also be reduced in patients undergoing endoluminal aortic reconstruction. However, judging by the cardiac and lung transplant experience described above, these patients are not immune to GICs just because the peritoneal cavity is not entered. The prevalence of GICs has not been evaluated per se, but there have been no instances of GI bleeding or intestinal ileus mentioned in large series of patients undergoing aortic stent grafts. On the other hand, overt colon ischemia remains a significant problem after endoluminal aneurysm repair (see below), with a similar incidence to open repair.[10] Colon necrosis has also been reported after thrombin embolization of the inferior mesenteric artery to treat a type II endoleak.[11]

SPECIFIC GASTROINTESTINAL COMPLICATIONS

Intestinal Ileus

Regardless of the definition used, ileus remains problematic in approximately 10% of patients undergoing open aortic surgery (Figure 32–1).[5,8] Nasogastric decompression

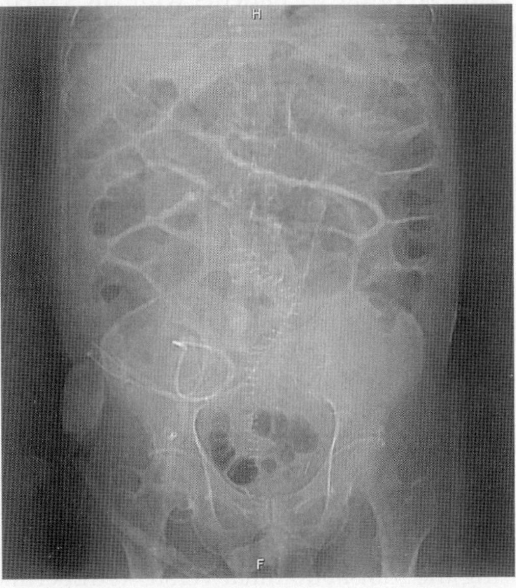

Figure 32-1. Postoperative ileus may be expected to occur in 10–15% of patients undergoing open aortic repair.

after aortic operations is routine in many centers. The optimum duration of nasogastric decompression is unknown, and it remains controversial. In a prospective study of 80 patients undergoing aortic operations, Friedman and associates randomized 40 subjects to immediate removal of the NG tube at tracheal extubation and 40 subjects to retention of the NG tube until passage of flatus.[12] The pathways had similar outcomes: the length of hospital stay was similar between the two groups, and three patients in each group (7.5%) required reinsertion of the NG tube for development of ileus. These data suggest that prolonged nasogastric decompression is not necessary in most patients undergoing open aortic surgery. In another study evaluating a clinical pathway for 50 patients undergoing elective aortic surgery, Podore and Throop placed nasogastric tubes only if gastric distention was directly observed in the operating room.[13] Only two patients (4%) required postoperative nasogastric decompression, and the NG tube was removed in both patients on the first postoperative day. All 50 patients were started on a clear liquid diet on postoperative day one, and 80% were tolerating a regular diet by postoperative day three. There were no instances of paralytic ileus in this series. The authors noted that all 50 subjects were empirically administered 10 mg of metaclopramide every six hours for the first 24 hours to promote gastric emptying.

Why is there such a wide variation in the prevalence of ileus after aortic surgery in these studies? The prevalence rates probably reflect differences in the respective patient populations. Several variables may influence postoperative gastric emptying in these patients. Following uncomplicated elective aortic surgery, gastric emptying returns to normal in approximately eighteen hours.[14] Gastric emptying is significantly delayed by opiates, especially when given via the intrathecal route.[15] Many patients in our study received intrathecal narcotics, while none of the patients received intrathecal opiates in the study by Podore and Throop. Gastric emptying is also delayed in critically ill patients, especially in those requiring prolonged mechanical ventilation.[16] In our study, GICs were significantly associated with prolonged ventilation and increased duration of ICU stay. In contrast, none of the patients in the study by Podore and Throop required prolonged ventilation or long ICU stay. It should also be pointed out that GICs were associated with intraoperative complications possibly leading to visceral hypoperfusion; there were no intraoperative complications reported by Podore and Throop. These data suggest that ileus may be a marker for critical illness in these patients. Intraoperative complications that lead to visceral hypoperfusion represent a common scenario. While the use of opiates probably plays an important role, opiates have not been evaluated as the cause of ileus after aortic surgery. Similarly, the routine use of metaclopramide to prevent ileus has not been evaluated. Based on the foregoing, the following observations can be made: nasogastric decompression is not required in the majority of patients undergoing elective aortic surgery. However, nasogastric tubes should not be removed in patients with intraoperative gastric dilation and in those who have intraoperative complications, require prolonged mechanical ventilation, or have prolonged ICU stays. Although routine metaclopramide use has not been evaluated, intravenous administration may be indicated for patients who do not require mechanical ventilation but have significant gastric residuals after aortic surgery.

Gastrointestinal Bleeding

The widespread use of stress prophylaxis has reduced the incidence of clinically significant gastrointestinal bleeding in critically ill patients. It should not be surprising that the prevalence of GI bleeding after aortic surgery is also low. Five patients (4%) in our series had bleeding episodes; two had a history of duodenal ulcer disease. All five patients had blood in the nasogastric aspirate, and all suffered some degree of hemodynamic instability. However, none required a gastric operation to correct the underlying cause, and all five remained stable without further bleeding after discharge. The incidence in our study was slightly higher compared with 1% in the study by Alpagut et al and 2.5% in the study by Crowson et al.[6,7] In these series as well as in our own, most cases were due to peptic ulceration or gastritis. Aortoduodenal fistulas do not develop in the early postoperative period. The low prevalence of GI bleeding after aortic surgery precludes analysis of associated risk factors or outcome. In large studies of critically ill patients in the intensive care unit, the following have been identified as risk factors for GI bleeding: advanced age, respiratory failure, aneurysm repair, coagulopathy, and sepsis.[17,18] The risk of developing a GI bleed in patients with a history of duodenal ulcer disease does not appear to be increased.[6] Regardless of the etiology, GI bleeding in critically ill patients is associated with increased morbidity and mortality.[19] In general, prophylaxis against gastric stress ulcers is indicated in all patients undergoing aortic surgery. Stress prophylaxis can be discontinued when the patient has resumed a regular diet.

Enterocolitis

C. difficile enterocolitis has been attributed to the use of antibiotics, especially first-generation cephalosporins such as cephazolin. Because prophylactic antibiotics are used routinely in aortic surgery, it should not be surprising that enterocolitis is a relatively common complication. Five patients (4%) in our series developed *C. difficile* colitis, with severe abdominal pain, fevers, and profuse watery diarrhea. All five patients suffered significant morbidity, with two developing paralytic ileus and gastrointestinal hemorrhage, and one requiring a right hemicolectomy for cecal perforation. The diagnosis was made on flexible sigmoidoscopy showing typical pseudomembranes and confirmed with positive stool tests for *C. difficile* toxins. Patients required seven to 10 days of therapy before symptoms resolved, resulting in prolonged hospitalization. These data are in keeping with those of Bulstrode et al who reported an 8.4% prevalence of *C. difficile* enterocolitis after aortic surgery.[20] There was significant associated morbidity, and two patients died of multiple organ failure that resulted directly from the enterocolitis. Although Bulstrode notes that colitis frequently follows prolonged administration of cephalosporins, our patients had a mean of three days of cefazolin therapy. While none would argue with limiting antibiotic usage to one or two doses in the postoperative period, little else can be done to prevent this complication. A high index of suspicion is necessary to limit complications of enterocolitis. Empiric treatment may be indicated in affected patients awaiting the results of stool tests for *C. difficile* toxins. Symptoms may be hard to distinguish from ischemic colitis and flexible sigmoidoscopy may be indicated as an initial test in many patients.

Cholecystitis

The reported incidence of acute calculous cholecytitis developing after open aneurysm repair ranges from 0.3 to 18%.[21] The incidence of postoperative cholecystitis appears to be much lower after endovascular repair.[21] In general, staged laparoscopic cholecystectomy several weeks before open aneurysm repair is preferable to simultaneous

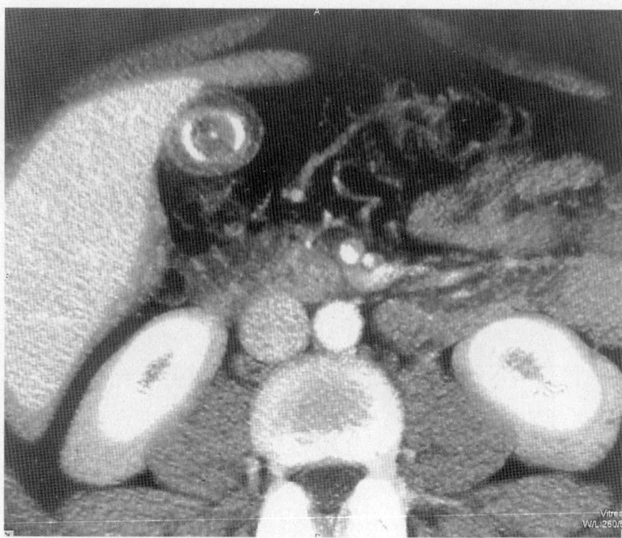

Figure 32-2. Computed tomography scan of a patient with aortic occlusive disease and a large, calcified gallstone.

operations. Much debate has focused on the management of cholelithiasis found incidentally during open aortic operations (Figure 32–2). Although some surgeons do not hesitate to perform simultaneous procedures, many surgeons do not perform cholecystectomy unless the gallbladder appears acutely inflamed at the time of surgery. In the latter circumstance, it may be preferable to delay the aneurym repair in order to reduce the theoretical risk of graft infection.

Acute acalculous cholecystitis is a more common complication after aortic surgery. We reported acalculous cholecystitis in seven of 996 patients who underwent aortic reconstruction at our institution during a 10-year period.[22] Six of the patients had intraoperative hypotension and multiple blood transfusions, and all patients developed multiorgan dysfunction. Other risk factors include prolonged mechanical ventilation and total parenteral nutrition. All seven patients developed fever, leukocytosis, and elevated liver function tests a mean of 32 days after aortic surgery. Five patients underwent cholecystectomy, and two had placement of cholecystostomy tubes. The overall mortality was 71%. These data show that acute acalculous cholecystitis after aortic surgery, while rare, is a highly morbid complication that developed in critically ill patients. Unlike calculous cholecystitis, no preoperative markers are associated with an increased risk of acalculous cholecystitis after aortic surgery. Difficulties in diagnosis may delay definitive care. Therefore, surgeons should maintain a high index of suspicion in patients who are critically ill after aortic surgery, especially in those requiring multiple blood transfusions.

Colon Ischemia

This dreaded complication occurs in 1–2% of patients after elective abdominal aortic aneurysm repair (Figure 32–3). The incidence is much higher after ruptured aneurysm repair, especially in the setting of hypotension. Regardless of the clinical setting, mortality of colon ischemia is 60–100%. Much attention has been focused on the patency and collateral circulation of the inferior mesenteric artery (IMA). While some

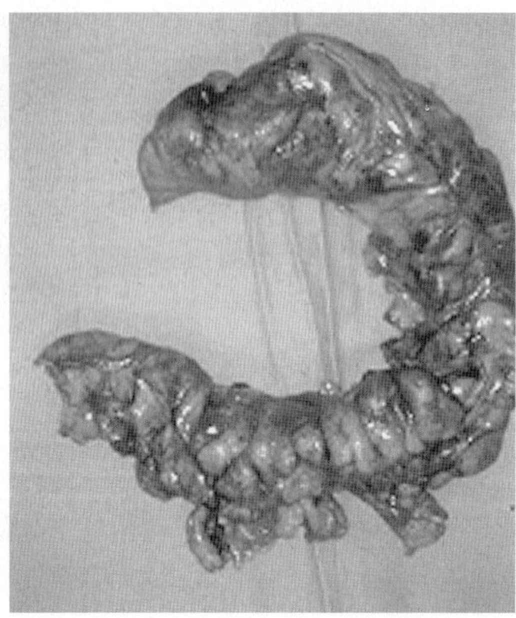

Figure 32-3. Necrotic left colon specimen from a patient who developed colon ischemia two days after emergent repair of a ruptured abdominal aortic aneurysm.

investigators recommend routine IMA reimplantation at the time of open aneurysm repair, most perform this selectively, using a number of different techniques to assess colon viability. However, IMA reimplantation does not ensure colon viability. We reported 10 patients who developed colon ischemia after aortic surgery, five of whom had successful IMA reimplantation at the time of aneurysm repair.[23] All six patients with transmural ischemia had suffered some degree of intraoperative hypotension (systolic blood pressure < 90 mm Hg for greater than five minutes). One patient who had IMA reimplantation had pathologic evidence of microembolization leading to colon necrosis. Survival rates were higher in patients with symptoms manifest in the early postoperative period (24–48 hours) compared to those whose symptoms occurred weeks after the aortic operation. Although transmural necrosis is a highly morbid complication, timely colectomy may lead to survival in some patients.

Intestinal Obstruction

Mechanical small bowel obstruction developed in two patients (1.7%) in our series.[5] Intestinal ileus was initially suspected: both patients required replacement of nasogastric tubes because of vomiting. One patient underwent exploratory laparotomy for peritonitis on postoperative day eight, and the other had the diagnosis made by contrast radiography on postoperative day 10. Intestinal adhesions caused internal hernias associated with segmental bowel infarction in both cases. Our experience is similar to that of Siporin et al who reported small bowel obstruction in 2.9% of their patients undergoing aortic aneurysm repair; 41% of the patients required adhesiolysis.[24] The authors note that surgery for early postoperative small bowel obstruction is associated with significant morbidity including fistulas, sepsis, and recurrent obstruction. Therefore, a one- to two-week period of conservative therapy is appropriate in these patients. However, persistent obstruction lasting more than two weeks almost always requires operative intervention to relieve the obstruction.

Duodenal obstruction after aortic surgery is very rare with a total of 19 cases reported in the English literature. In a review of this literature, Tessier and Brophy report that symptoms of duodenal obstruction begin six to 60 days after aortic surgery with a mean of 13 days.[25] Symptoms typically include increased nsaogastric tube output, bilious vomiting, and pain. Reported causes include hematoma encasing the duodenum, adhesions, sac seroma, and superior mesenteric artery compression. Nearly all cases have been diagnosed with contrast-enhanced studies. Conservative management with nasogastric decompression has been successful in nearly half of the cases, but the mean time to resolution is more than three weeks. Surgical therapy is based on the particular problem identified and has been curative in those who failed conservative management. The combined operative mortality is 10%.

Other Complications

A number of relatively rare GICs have been reported after aortic surgery. The proximity of the aorta to the pancreas and cysterna chili risks damage to these structures during aortic dissection. We reported acute postoperative pancreatitis in 1.8% of our patients who underwent aortic surgery during a six-year period.[26] One likely etiology is pancreatic injury from mobilization or retractors; however, it should be pointed out that pancreatitis also occurs in 0.8–4% patients undergoing cardiovascular operations remote from the abdominal cavity. Therefore, other variables such as decreased perfusion may play a more important role in the development of pancreatic inflammation. Although acute pancreatitis is costly and inconvenient, the complication is usually self-limited and rarely serious.

Clinically apparent chylous ascites is also rare after open aortic surgery. Abdominal distention is the most common presenting symptom and is usually recognized more than two weeks after surgery.[27] Diagnosis is confirmed by paracentesis revealing sterile lipemic fluid. Therapeutic paracentesis combined with a medium chain triglyceride diet or total parenteral nutrition may be expected to resolve chylous ascites in more than half of affected patients. Peritoneovenous shunts may be required in the patients who do not respond to conservative therapy.

SUMMARY AND PERSPECTIVES

The characteristics, risk factors, and outcome of GICs are summarized in Table 32–3. As a group, GICs represent a relatively common problem after open aortic surgery. While no specific etiologies have been identified, common risk factors include visceral hypoperfusion from any cause (hypotension, mesenteric artery occlusion, embolization) and markers of critical illness (prolonged ventilation, multiple blood transfusions, sepsis). These data suggest that many GICs (ileus, acalculous cholecystitis, gastritis, colon ischemia) represent an end-organ response to a systemic complication such as shock or sepsis. Others are due to mechanical complications (bowel obstruction, chylous ascites) or impaired immunity (*C. difficile* enterocolitis). Regardless of the etiology, all GICs are associated with prolonged hospitalization and most are associated with increased mortality. As a group, GICs account for a significant amount of morbidity after aortic surgery.

TABLE 32-3. CHARACTERISTICS AND OUTCOME OF GASTROINTESTINAL COMPLICATIONS AFTER AORTIC SURGERY. DATA COMPILED FROM NUMEROUS STUDIES.

Complication	Incidence	Presentation	Complications	Risk factors
Ileus	10%	Persistent NG output	↑ LOS	Opiates Visceral hypoperfusion Electrolyte imbalance Sepsis
UGI bleeding	2-5%	Blood in NG aspirate	Hypotension ↑ morbidity ↑ mortality	Advanced age Respiratory failure Coagulopathy Sepsis
Enterocolitis	4-8%	Fever Abdominal pain Profuse watery diarrhea	↑ LOS Cecal perforation	Antibiotics
Acalculous cholecystitis	1%	Fever Leukocytosis ↑ LFTs	↑ LOS ↑ Mortality (70%)	Intraoperative ↓ BP Multiple blood transfusions
Colon ischemia	1-2%	Bloody diarrhea	↑ LOS ↑ Mortality (60-100%)	Inadequate IMA flow Ruptured AAA ↓ BP
Intestinal obstruction	1-3%	Prolonged (> 10 days) NG output	↑ LOS ↑ Morbidity	Unknown
Pancreatitis	1-2%	Prolonged ileus Epigastic pain Hyperamylasemia	↑ LOS	↓ BP Visceral hypoperfusion Use of retractors
Chylous ascites	Rare	Abdominal distention Lipemic fluid	↑ LOS	Cysterna injury

NG = nasogastric tube
LOS = length of hospital stay
UGI = upper gastrointestinal
LFTs = liver function tests
BP = blood pressure
IMA = inferior mesenteric artery

REFERENCES

1. Mercado PD, Farid H, O'Connell TX, et al. Gastrointestinal complications associated with cardiopulmonary bypass operations. *Ann Surg*. 1994;60:789–792.
2. Lubetkin EI, Lipson DA, Palevsky HI, et al. GI complications after orthotopic lung transplantation. *Am J Gastroenterol*. 1996;91:2383–2390.
3. Christenson JT, Schmuziger M, Maurice J, et al. Postoperative visceral hypoperfusion: the common cause for gastrointestinal complications after cardiac surgery. *Thorac Cardiovasc Surg*. 1994;42:152–157.
4. Valentine RJ, Martin JD, Myers SI, et al. Asymptomatic celiac and superior mesenteric artery stenoses are more prevalent among patients with unsuspected renal artery stenoses. *J Vasc Surg*. 1991;14:195–199.
5. Valentine RJ, Hagino RT, Jackson MR, et al. Gastrointestinal complications after aortic surgery. *J Vasc Surg*. 1998; 28:404–412.
6. Crowson M, Fielding JW, Black J, et al. Acute gastrointestinal complications of aortic aneurysm repair. *Br J Surg*. 1984;71:825–828.
7. Alagut U, Kalko Y, Dayioglu E. Gastrointestinal complications after transperitoneal abdominal aortic surgery. *Asian Cardiovasc Thorac Ann*. 2003;11:3–6.

8. Sicard GA, Reilly Jm, Rubin BG, et al. Transabdominal versus retroperitoneal incision for abdominal aortic surgery: Report of a prospective randomized trial. *J Vasc Surg*. 1995;21: 174–183.

9. Cambria RP, Brewster DC, Abbott WM, et al. Transperitoneal versus retroperitoneal approach for aortic reconstruction: a randomized prospective study. *J Vasc Surg*. 1990;12: 505–506.

10. Dadian N, Ohki T, Veith FJ, et al. Overt colon ischemia after endovascular aneurysm repair: the importance of microembolization as an etiology. *J Vasc Surg*. 2001;34:986–996.

11. Bush RL, Lin PH, Ronson RS, et al. Colonic necrosis subsequent to catheter-directed thrombin embolization of the inferior mesenteric artery via the superior mesenteric artery: a complication of the management of a type II endoleak. *J Vasc Surg*. 2001;34:1119–1122.

12. Friedman SG, Sowerby SA, Del Pin CA, et al. A prospective randomized study of abdominal aortic surgery without postoperative nasogastric decompression. *Cardiovasc Surg*. 1996;4:492–494.

13. Podore PC, Throop EB. Infrarenal aortic surgery with a 3-day hospital stay: A report on success with a clinical pathway. *J Vasc Surg*. 1999;29:787–792.

14. Avrahami R, Cohen JD, Haddad M, et al. Gastric emptying after elective abdominal aortic aneurysm surgery: the case for early postoperative enteral feeding. *Eur J Vasc Endovasc Surg*. 1999;17:241–244.

15. Lydon AM, Cook T, Duggan F, et al. Delayed postoperative gastric emptying following intrathecal morphine and intrathecal bupivacaine. *Can J Anesth*. 1999;46:544–549.

16. Heyland DK, Tougas G, King D, et al. Impaired gastric emptying in critically ill, mechanically ventilated patients. *Intensive Care Med*. 1996;22:1339–1344.

17. Pimental M, Roberts DE, Bernstein CN, et al. Clinically significant gastrointestinal bleeding in critically ill patients in an era of prophylaxis. *Am J Gastroenterol*. 2000;95:2801–2806.

18. Cook DJ, Fuller HD, Guyatt GH, et al. Risk factors for gastrointestinal bleeding in critically ill patients. *N Engl J Med*. 1994;330:377–381.

19. Cook DJ, Griffith LE, Walter SD, et al. The attributable mortality and length of intensive care unit stay of clinically important gastrointestinal bleeding in critically ill patients. *Crit Care*. 2001;5:368–375.

20. Bulstrode NW, Bradbury AW, Barrett S, et al. Clostridium difficile colitis after aortic surgery. *Eur J Vasc Endovasc Surg*. 1997;14:217–220.

21. Cadot H, Addis MD, Faries PL, et al. Abdominal aortic aneurysmorrhaphy and cholelithiasis in the era of endovascular surgery. *Am Surg*. 2002;68:839–843.

22. Hagino RT, Valentine RJ, Clagett GP. Acalculous cholecystitis after aortic surgery. *J Amer Coll Surg*. 1997; 184: 245–248.

23. Mitchell KM, Valentine RJ. Inferior mesenteric artery reimplantation does not guarantee colon viability in aortic surgery. *J Am Coll Surg*. 2002;194:151–155.

24. Siporin K, Hiatt JR, Treiman RL. Small bowel obstruction after abdominal aortic surgery. *Am Surg*. 1993;59:846–849.

25. Tessier DJ, Brophy CM. Causes, diagnosis, and management of duodenal obstruction after aortic surgery. *J Vasc Surg*. 2003;38:186–189.

26. Burkey SH, Valentine RJ, Jackson MR, et al. Acute pancreatitis after abdominal vascular surgery. *J AmColl Surg*. 2000;191:373–380.

27. Pabst TS 3rd, McIntyre KE Jr, Schilling JD, et al. Management of chyloperitoneum after abdominal aortic surgery. *Am J Surg*. 1993;166:194–198.

33

Management of Endoleaks: Techniques and Results

Patrick J. Geraghty, M.D.
and Gregorio A. Sicard, M.D.

Endoluminal repair of abdominal aortic aneurysm (EVAR) is an acceptable alternative to open repair, especially in high-risk patients.[1-3] National and statewide databases show that at least 50% of elective abdominal aortic aneurysm (AAA) repair is being performed by endovascular techniques.[4,5] Referral centers may treat as high as 60–80% of AAAs by endovascular techniques. Early and midterm outcome of EVAR registries data have been very favorable with very low aneurysm related deaths.[6,7] Risk factors associated with EVAR failure and the need for secondary interventions have been well described.[8,9] Endoleaks, device migration, modular separation, structural failure, aneurysmal sac growth without endoleak, and post-EVAR aneurysm rupture are complications that have been reported, and demand close surveillance following implant of commercially available devices.

Endoleaks represent the most frequent failure mechanism after EVAR. Although Type I and III can be a prelude to post-EVAR aneurysm rupture, their incidence is relatively low. Their finding requires urgent intervention and correction. On the other hand, Type II endoleaks are frequent and reported in 5–25% of patients early after EVAR.[6,8-12] Late appearing Type II endoleaks can occur, which further underlines the importance of long-term surveillance in patients with EVAR.

Vascular surgeons agree that treatment of Type I and III endoleaks is mandatory in order to avoid aneurysm rupture. On the other hand, the treatment of Type II endoleaks has not been as clearly defined. Over 50% of Type II endoleaks seal spontaneously, others persist while the aneurysmal sac size shrinks, and many persist with no change in the aneurysm sac size. Aggressive treatments of Type II endoleaks that persist for six months or longer have been proposed by some authors.[13,14] Most investigators recommend treatment of Type II endoleaks only if associated with growth of the aneurysmal sac of (5 mm.[10-12,14,15] Others recommend the routine measurement of the size of the endoleak nidus since a diameter of 15 mm or greater is associated with an increased risk of aneurysm enlargement.[16] Further verification of the relationship between nidus size and aneurysm sac size change is needed to precisely identify those patients with persistent Type II endoleaks who can benefit from earlier intervention. Most authors agree that endovascular techniques are very effective in treating Type II endoleaks and should be the primary approach when needed. Others have described successful endoscopic ligation of lumbar and inferior mesenteric arteries responsible for persistent Type II endoleaks.[17]

DEFINITION AND DIAGNOSIS

White and collaborators proposed the accepted classification of endoleaks in 1998.[18]

Type I endoleak is the result of an incomplete seal of the endoluminal device at the proximal and/or distal attachment site (Figure 33–1). Factors such as incorrect sizing or deployment site, aortic neck or iliac artery angulation, or oversizing that results in folds that allow perigraft flow into the aneurysmal sac, contribute to the development of Type I endoleaks.

Type II endoleak is the result of retrograde flow from patent lumbars or inferior mesenteric arteries (Figures 33–2 and 33–3). This is the most common form of endoleak and may be detected early (from the time of implantation) or may be late appearing. Most Type II endoleaks will seal spontaneously, but others can persist for many years. The optimal management of persistent (6 months or longer) Type II endoleaks still remains a source of debate.

Type III endoleak occurs through a defect at the junction site of modular components or from a tear in the fabric of the endograft (Figure 33–4). The former can occur late as a result of shrinkage of the aneurysm sac. Alteration of aneurysm sac morphology and associated forces may lead to separation of the modular components of the device.

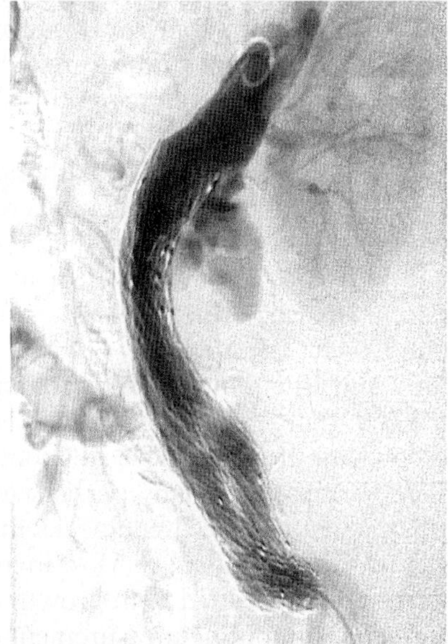

Figure 33-1. Acute Type I endoleak secondary to migration of endograft.

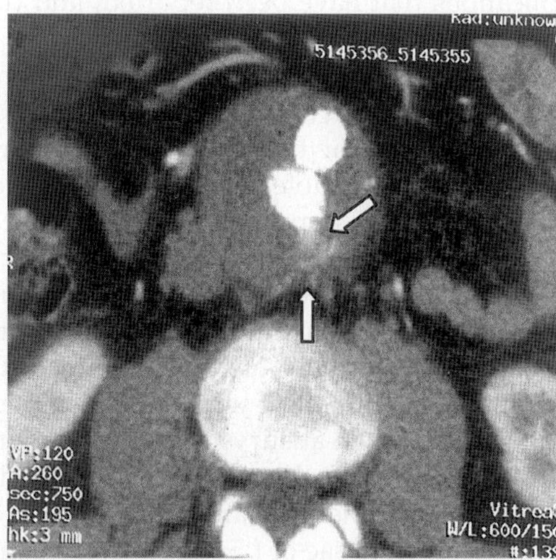

Figure 33-2. Thin-cut contrast CT scan demonstrating Type II endoleak from paired lumbar arteries.

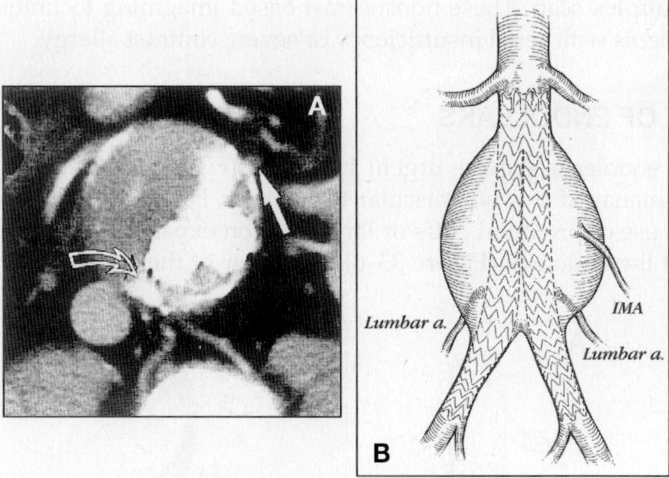

Figure 33-3. Contrast CT scan demonstrating Type II endoleak from paired lumbar (clear arrow) and inferior mesenteric artery (solid arrow).

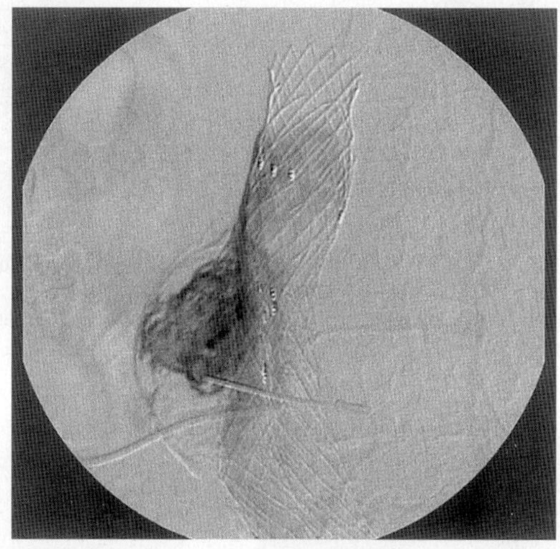

Figure 33-4. Type III endoleak from a hole in the fabric of the endograft.

Type IV endoleak is not considered a device failure, but rather a transient contrast transudation through the graft wall. This type of endoleak tends to disappear early after endograft implantation.

Type V endoleak (endotension) is a persistent growth of the aneurysm sac without demonstrable endoleak. The etiology of this type of "endoleak" is not well understood and although rare, can lead to open surgical conversion.

Detection of endoleaks is best done by thin cut (1–3 mm), contrast spiral computed tomography. Although Type I, II, and III endoleaks are commonly detected with this modality, angiographic verification is important in some cases where the site of the endoleak is in doubt. When endotension is diagnosed, angiographic verification of no demonstrable endoleak is recommended. Endoleaks can also be detected by MRA and/or aortic duplex scan. These noncontrast based imagining techniques are recommended in patients with renal insufficiency or severe contrast allergy.

TREATMENT OF ENDOLEAKS

Type I and III endoleaks require urgent treatment (Figure 33–5). Most Type I and III endoleaks are managed by endovascular techniques. For proximal Type I or Type III endoleaks, the use of proximal cuffs or large balloon expandable transrenal stents can frequently seal the endoleak (Figure 33–6). If neither of these maneuvers is successful

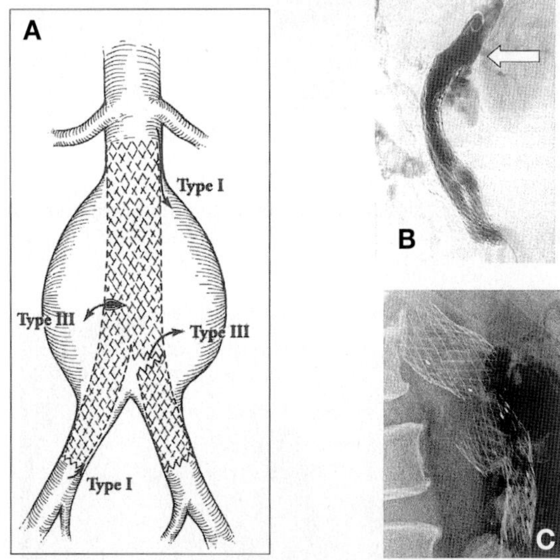

Figure 33-5. Site of Type I and III endoleaks **A**, proximal acute Type I endoleak **B**, and Type III endoleak from migration of main body from proximal cuff **C**.

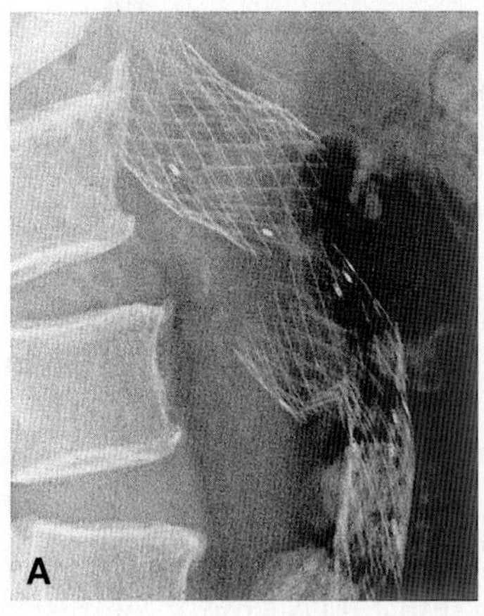

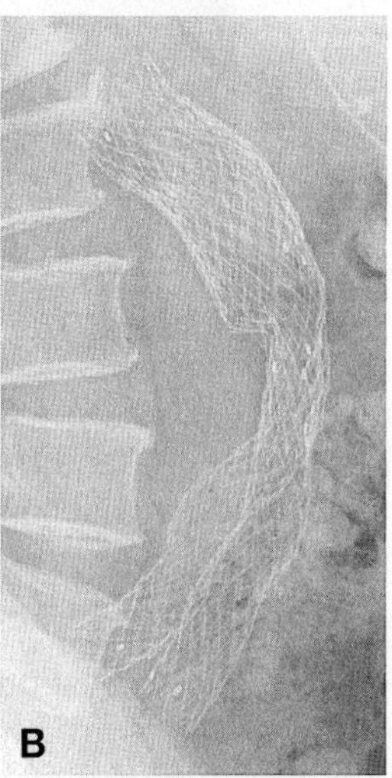

Figure 33-6. Type III endoleak from migration of main body from proximal cuff **A**. Endoluminal repair by placement of new aortic cuff **B**.

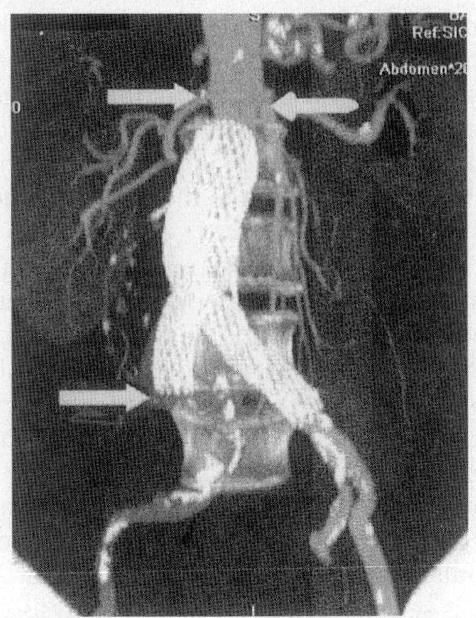

Figure 33-7. Right distal attachment Type I endoleak two years post-EVAR. Notice short right limb inside aneurysm (arrow).

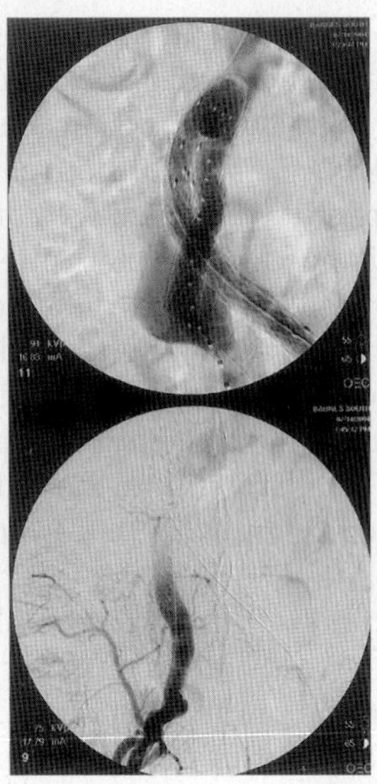

Figure 33-8. Intraoperative arteriogram confirms right limb inside aneurysm sac (a). Repair of Type I endoleak with limb extension into distal right common iliac artery.

in sealing the leak, open conversion is required. The development of fenestrated technology may resolve those proximal Type I endoleaks currently unsolved by endoluminal technique and requiring open conversion. Distal Type I endoleaks can usually be treated by cuff placement or graft extension into the external iliac arteries (Figures 33–7 and 33–8). Type III endoleaks result from modular disconnection of either proximal cuffs or the contralateral limb, and can usually be managed by deployment of another limb from the overlap zone to the ipsilateral iliac system or the disconnected limb. Type IV endoleaks are self-limiting and rarely seen after the completion arteriogram in the operating room. Type V endoleak or endotension with aneurysmal sac growth usually requires open conversion after angiographic verification that there is no detectable perigraft flow.

The management of persistent Type II endoleaks from lumbar and inferior mesenteric artery origin remains a source of debate in the field of endovascular treatment of AAA. Type II endoleaks are a frequent finding in early postoperatively surveillance imaging. Most authors agree that since a large number of these spontaneously seal, initial follow-up in 3–6 months is the indicated approach. The controversy arises in the treatment of persistent ($\geq$ 6 month) Type II endoleaks. The vast majority of experienced vascular surgeons involved in aortic endografting accepts the position of follow-up of persistent Type II endoleaks if the aneurysm sac remains stable or decreases in size. On the other hand, if there is growth of the aneurysm sac ($\geq$ 5 mm), sealing or ligation of the source of the Type II endoleak is indicated, preferably by endoluminal technique.

LUMBAR ARTERIES—TYPE II ENDOLEAK

Type II endoleaks frequently arise from distal aortic paired lumbars or a patent IMA. If the spiral CT scan clearly identifies the lumbar artery as the source of the endoleak, then embolization of the nidus and/or the lumbar arteries is an excellent approach. Preoperative lumbar artery coil embolization or intraoperative filling of the aneurysmal sac with thrombogenic material has not proven efficacious in avoiding delayed endoleaks.[19,20] Prior to the treatment of the presumed Type II endoleak, transfemoral arteriography with selective contrast injection of hypogastrics and superior mesenteric arteries is needed to determine the precise anatomic contribution to the endoleak and to rule out a Type I and/or Type III endoleak.

Persistent Type II endoleak from the inferior mesenteric artery with aneurysmal sac enlargement is best treated by embolization of the IMA at its origin. This is performed by the transfemoral approach with selective cannulation of the SMA. A microcatheter is advanced to the IMA and coil embolization of the origin of the vessel is performed (Figure 33–9). Care must be taken to avoid embolization beyond the branch point of the IMA into the left colic or superior hemorrhoidal arteries to minimize the risk of colon ischemia. Glue embolization of a patent IMA should be avoided.

Access of the aneurysm sac is performed through a translumbar approach with the patient in the prone position on an angiography table. Intravenous sedation and preprocedural antibiotics for coverage against skin contaminants should be administered. A suitable site for puncture of the aneurysmal sac is selected based on careful analysis of the most recent spiral CT scan. The goal is to enter the nidus of the endoleak close to the largest area of active flow. Either the left or right side can be used depending on the position of the endoleak nidus within the sac. An 18-gauge, 15 cm long trocar needle is directed from the flank toward the endograft using C-arm fluoroscopic guidance. Free aspiration of arterial blood or pulsatile flow from the needle confirms proper location of the needle tip. The pressure inside the endoleak nidus should be measured to confirm the similarity of the sac pressure to the mean arterial pressure. Contrast angiography of the aneurysmal sac is performed in order to delineate the sac anatomy and flow lumen (Figure 33–10). Particular attention is paid to any possible communication with the anterior spinal artery. In one patient of our series, visualization of the anterior spinal artery by arteriography led to direct coiling of the lumbar branches rather than using glue.

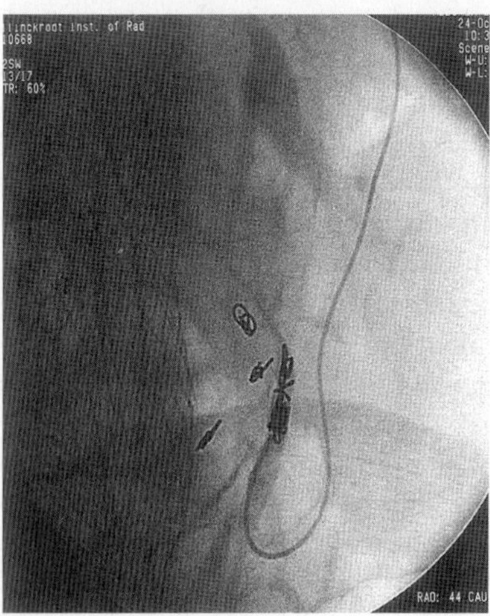

Figure 33-9. Patient with AAA enlargement secondary to persistent Type II endoleak from patient IMA. Transarterial approach via the SMA allowed for coil embolization of the proximal IMA.

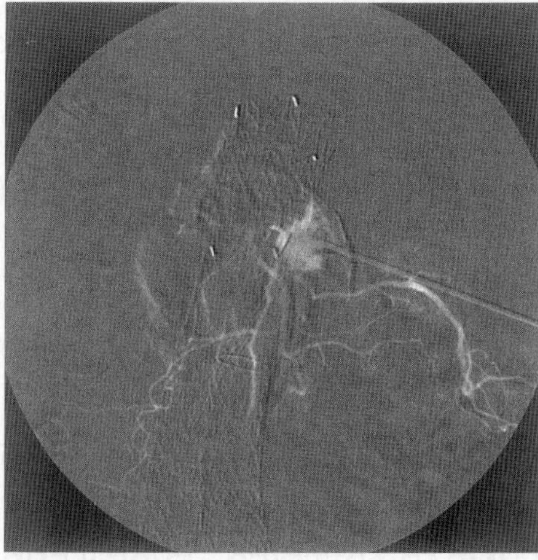

Figure 33-10. Translumbar injection of the nidus of a persistent Type II endoleak demonstrates communication with patient lumbar arteries.

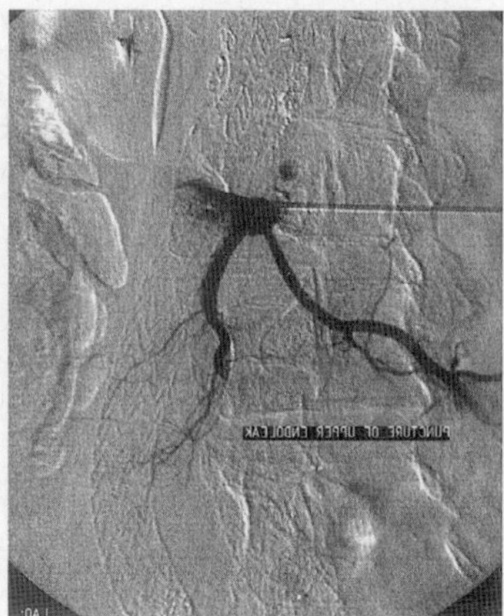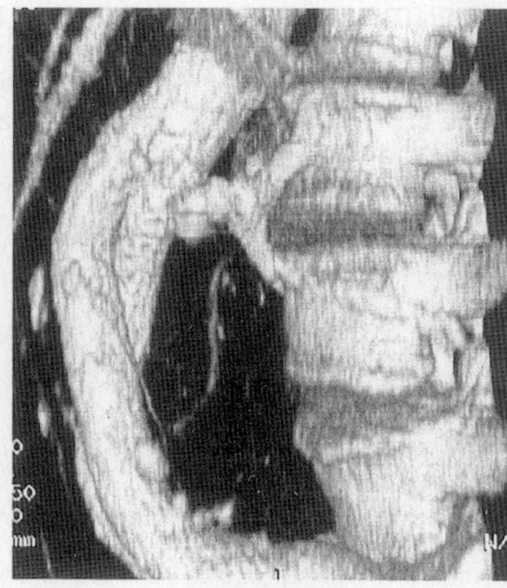

Figure 33-11. Translumbar puncture for treatment of Type II endoleak using glue embolization. CT angiogram is shown at right.

The volume of contrast necessary to fill the flowing portion of the aneurysm sac, with reflux into the feeding lumbar arteries, is then estimated. NBCA glue (Trufill, Cordis Endovascular, Miami Lakes, FL) is prepared according to the manufacturers' instructions, typically in a mixture of 1 cc of N-butyl cyanoacrylate and 2 cc of Ethiodol. The needle must be cleared with dextrose solution to prevent polymerization of the glue. The syringe containing the glue is directly attached to the needle and the glue injected (Figure 33–11). Commonly, after the glue polymerizes, there is absence of pulsatile flow of the nidus. The needle is then removed and the patient observed for signs of neurologic change and bleeding. Most patients can be discharged the same day of the procedure.

RESULTS

Since April 1, 1996 through June 30, 2004, 657 consecutive patients underwent endoluminal repair of AAA (EVAR) at our institution. One hundred forty-three patients (22%) underwent EVAR as part of an FDA approved trial. Patients' data were entered prospectively into a database developed at our institution with preoperative, intraoperative, and postoperative data sets. Postdischarge information was obtained primarily from clinic physician office notes. Devices used in our series are shown in Table 33–1.

TABLE 33-1. INCIDENCE OF TRANSIENT AND PERSISTENT TYPE II ENDOLEAKS FOLLOWING EVAR AT WASHINGTON UNIVERSITY MEDICAL SCHOOL, 1996–2004.

Device	Number of Patients	Number (%) with any Type II Endoleaks	Number with Persistent Type II Endoleaks
AneuRX	397	67 (17%)	18 (4.5%)
Zenith	82	18 (22%)	2 (2.4%)
Ancure	75	21 (28%)	7 (9.3%)
Excluder	74	15 (20%)	10 (13.5%)
Talent	25	2 (3%)	0 (0%)
Endologix	4	2 (50%)	2 (50%)
Total	657	125 (19%)	39 (5.9%)

TABLE 33-2. PATIENTS WITH PERSISTENT TYPE II ENDOLEAK AND GROWTH OF ANEURYSMAL SAC

Patients	Type of device	Preop. AAA size (cm)	Increase in AAA size (cm)	Origin of Type II endoleak	Procedure	Post-embolization f-u
1	AnuRX	5.4	0.8	L	TL glue	30
2	Excluder	5.8	0.7	L	TL glue	40
3	AneuRX	4.4	1.3	L	TL coils	32
4	AneuRX	5.8	1.5	IMA	TA coils	39
5	AneuRX	6.5	0.7	L	TL glue	10
6	AneuRX	5.4	0.9	L	TL glue	2
7	AneuRX	4.7	1.2	L	TL glue	3

TL = Translumbar; TA= Transarterial

Details of the seven patients with persistent Type II endoleak and AAA sac growth who required intervention. Follow-up in months is shown at far right. No patient has required further intervention.

Follow-up thin-cut spiral CT scans were obtained at a minimum of 1, 6, and 12 months, and yearly thereafter. Patients who demonstrated persistent Type II endoleaks for six months or longer underwent spiral CT at six-month intervals to assess the persistence of the endoleak and the aneurysm sac size. The maximal diameter of the aneurysm was measured with electronic calipers and compared to a similar level sac size in the previous CT scan. Patients with renal insufficiency were evaluated by noncontrast CT scan and Duplex ultrasound scans at the same time intervals.

In patients with a persistent Type II endoleak clearly defined by spiral CT scan, preparations were made for translumbar puncture of the endoleak nidus and either glue or coil embolization. In patients with clearly defined IMA fed Type II endoleaks, a transfemoral approach with cannulation and coiling of the IMA was preferred. In situations in which the source of the endoleak was unknown by spiral CT, transfemoral arteriography was performed with selective injection of the hypogastric arteries and the superior mesenteric artery to evaluate which vessel(s) contributes to the endoleak and to rule out a Type I or Type III endoleak.

Of 657 EVARS implanted at our institution, seven (1.1%) have been successfully treated for persistent Type II endoleaks associated with aneurysmal sac growth of (5 mm (Table 33–2). The follow-up ranges from two to 40 months. In all patients, the Type II endoleak was successfully treated either by translumbar glue (N = 5), translumbar coils (N = 1) or transarterial IMA embolization (N = 1). In all patients, nearly systemic pressure was found in the endoleak nidus and the pressure obliterated by the embolization procedure. No patients have required conversion after successful treatment of Type II endoleak.

SUMMARY

Endoluminal repair of AAAs has been established as a viable alternative to traditional open surgical repair. Despite the low morbidity of EVAR and excellent rates of initial success in aneurysm exclusion, the early and late occurrence of endoleaks and other device-related complications necessitates long-term clinical follow-up with serial aneurysm imaging.

Thin-cut spiral CT scanning is the most commonly employed imaging modality for assessment of aneurysm sac size and the presence of endoleak. In the presence of renal insufficiency, magnetic resonance angiography and abdominal duplex scanning may supplement or replace the role of spiral CT scans. Transfemoral and translumbar angiographic approaches are employed to clearly define the origin of subtle endoleaks, as well as to treat endoleaks by cuff/extension deployment, stent placement, and glue/coil embolization.

Type I and III endoleaks expose the aneurysm sac to systemic pressure from antegrade aortic flow, and mandate prompt intervention by the vascular surgeon to prevent aneurysm rupture. Fortunately, the majority of Type I and III endoleaks can be successfully addressed by an endoluminal approach. The ongoing development of branched and fenestrated stent-graft components promises to further expand the vascular surgeon's armamentarium for dealing with complex Type I endoleak anatomy. For those patients not amenable to endoluminal repair of Type I or III endoleak, conversion to open repair is recommended.

Type IV endoleaks appear to be a transient phenomenon, infrequently seen at operative completion angiography, and rarely thereafter. Type V endoleak (endotension) is generally addressed by conversion to open repair after angiographic attempts to demonstrate perigraft flow have been exhausted.

Much debate currently centers on the appropriate management of persistent (>six months duration) Type II endoleaks. In the presence of a stable or shrinking aneurysm sac, most experienced vascular surgeons will manage this issue conservatively with serial clinic examinations and aneurysm sac imaging. Our institution has demonstrated excellent outcomes using this approach in a large series of EVAR patients.[14] However, intriguing research is being conducted to define subsets of patients with persistent Type II endoleak who may benefit from a more aggressive policy of intervention, using the size of the endoleak cavity (nidus) as a guide for therapeutic recommendations.[16] When treatment of persistent Type II endoleak is required, embolization with polymerizing glue or coils is the most frequently employed means of repair.

In summary, EVAR has become firmly established in the treatment of AAA. Long-term freedom from aneurysm rupture is dependent on the vascular surgeon's facility with endoluminal techniques paired with vigilant surveillance, detection, and appropriate treatment of device-related complications.

REFERENCES

1. Parodi JC, Palmaz JC, Barone HD. Transfemoral intraluminal graft implantation of abdominal aortic aneurysms. *Ann Vasc Surg*. 1991;5:491–499.
2. Sicard GA, Rubin BG, Sanchez LA, et al. Endoluminal graft repair for abdominal aortic aneurysms in high-risk patients and octogenarians. *Ann Surg*. 2001;234:427–437.
3. May J, White GH, Waugh R, et al. Improved survival after endoluminal repair with second-generation prostheses compared with open repair in the treatment of abdominal aortic aneurysms: A 5-year concurrent comparison using life-table methods. *J Vasc Surg*. 2001;33:521–526.
4. Anderson PL, Arons RR, Moskourtz AJ, et al. A statewide experience with endovascular abdominal aneurysm repair: Rapid diffusions with excellent early results. *J Vasc Surg*. 2004;39:10–19.
5. Lee WA, Carter JW, Upchurch G, et al. Perioperative outcomes after open and endovascular repair of intact abdominal aortic aneurysms in the United States during 2001. *J Vasc Surg*. 2004;224:739–767.

6. Lifeline Registry of Endovascular Aneurysm Repair (EVAR): 6-year results. Presented at the SVS Plenary Session, June 2004 (submitted to *J Vasc Surg*).

7. Buth J, Laheis RLF. Early complications and endoleaks after endovascular abdominal aortic aneurysm repair: Report of a multicenter study. *J Vasc Surg*. 2000;31:134–140.

8. Harris PF, Rao Vallabhaneni S, Desgranges P et al. Incidence and risk factors of late rupture, conversion, and death after endovascular repair of infrarenal aortic aneurysms: the EUROSTAR experience. European Collaborators on Stent/graft techniques for aortic aneurysm repair. *J Vasc Surg*. 2000;32(4):739–749.

9. Ouriel K, Clair DG, Greenberg RK, et al. Endovascular repair of abdominal aortic aneurysms: Device-specific outcome. *J Vasc Surg*. 2003;37(5):991–998.

10. Veith FJ, Baum RA, Ohki T, et al. Nature and significance of endoleaks and endotension: summary of opinions expressed at an international conference. *J Vasc Surg*. 2002;35(5): 1029–1035.

11. Parent FN, Meier GH, Godziachvili V, et al. The incidence and natural history of Type I and II endoleak: A 5-year follow-up assessment with color duplex ultrasound scan. *J Vasc Surg*. 2002; 35(3):474–481.

12. van Marrewijk C, Buth J, Harris PL, et al. Significance of endoleaks after endovascular repair of abdominal aortic aneurysms: The EUROSTAR experience. *J Vasc Surg*. 2002;35(3): 461–473.

13. Baum RA, Carpenter JP, Cope C, et al. Aneurysm sac pressure measurements after endovascular repair of abdominal aortic aneurysms. *J Vasc Surg*. 2001;33(1):32–41.

14. Steinmetz E, Rubin BG, Sanchez LA, et al. Type II endoleak after endovascular abdominal aortic aneurysm repair: A conservative approach with selective interventions is safe and cost-effective. *J Vasc Surg*. 2004; 39:306–313.

15. Tuerff SN, Rockman CB, Lamparello PJ, et al. Are type II (branch vessel) endoleaks really benign? *Ann Vasc Surg*. 2002;16(1):50–54.

16. Timaran CH, Ohki T, Rhee SF, et al. Predicting aneurysm enlargement in patients with persistent Type II endoleaks. *J Vasc Surg*. 2004;39:1157–1162.

17. Wisselink W, Cuesta MA, Berends FJ, et al. Retroperitoneal endoscopic ligation of lumbar and inferior mesenteric arteries as a treatment of persistent endoleak after endoluminal aortic aneurysm repair. *J Vasc Surg*. 2000;31(6):1240–1244.

18. White GH, May J, Waugh RC, el al. Type I and II endoleaks: A more useful classification for reporting results of endoluminal AAA repair. *J Endovasc Surg*. 1998;5:189–191.

19. Gould DA, et al. Aortic side branch embolization before endovascular aneurysm repair: incidence of type II endoleak. *J Vasc Interv Radiol*. 2001;12(3):337–341.

20. Walter SR, Macierewicz J, and Hopkinson BR. Endovascular AAA repair: prevention of side branch endoleaks with thrombogenic sponge. *J Endovasc Surg*. 1999;6(4):350–353.

34

Translumbar Approaches to Type II Endoleaks

Lindsay Machan, M.D.

Persistent or recurrent flow into an aneurysm around a stent graft is called an endoleak. They generally are divided into four categories depending on the source of inflow.[1] A Type I endoleaks result from failure of the stent graft to make an effective seal with the native vessel at the proximal or distal attachment sites. Blood flows around the stent graft resulting in filling of the aneurysm sac. There is no controversy about the fact that these virtually always require immediate treatment by creating a tighter seal at the attachment site by balloon dilatation, additional stenting, or most often stent graft extension or surgical conversion.

Type II endoleaks are more complex, both in their structure and the algorithms for indications and methods of treatment. They occur when blood flow enters the aneurysm sac via retrograde flow in branch vessels (usually lumbar arteries or inferior mesenteric artery, less commonly internal iliac arteries), transmitting arterial pressure into the aneurysm sac. Type III endoleaks are caused by fabric tears, graft disconnection, or disintegration of the stent graft and generally have the same implications at Type I endoleaks. Flow through the endograft associated with porosity of the graft material is categorized as a type IV leak. Type IV endoleaks virtually all resolve spontaneously. Types I and II endoleaks represent the majority of endoleaks encountered in stent graft patients.[2]

Type II endoleaks, which occur in up to 43.9% of patients at discharge and 29.8% at one month after endovascular stent grafting,[3] transmit systemic blood pressure to the aneurysm sac, can be associated with continued aneurysm expansion, and have been implicated in delayed aneurysm rupture.[4,5] The literature as to whether type II endoleaks require treatment varies considerably. Occlusion of all type II endoleaks has been advocated by some since the pressure within the sac may measure systemic levels and, therefore, promote sac rupture.[6] Others[7] have recommended that in the absence of an expanding aneurysmal sac, observation is sufficient since many small type II endoleaks will seal spontaneously.

If one decides to intervene, the goal of treatment is the elimination of flow through the branch vessels perfusing the aneurysm sac in order to protect the aneurysm from systemic pressure. Both surgical and endovascular treatments have been described.

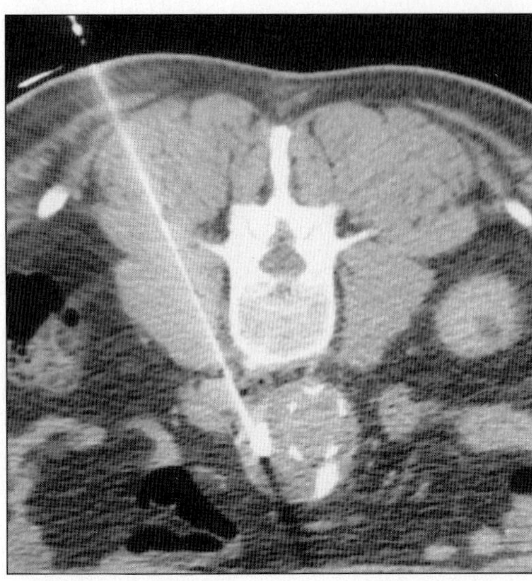

Figure 34-1. Axial CT scan demonstrating CT guided translumbar needle placement into endoleak sac. A slurry of thrombin and gelfoam was injected under fluoroscopic guidance.

Surgical treatments for type II endoleaks include open surgical graft explantation, and open or endoscopic retroperitoneal ligation of collateral feeding vessels.[8,9] These invasive methods require hospital admission and carry with them the accompanying morbidity of surgery. The earliest reports of endovascular type II endoleak treatment involved retrograde catheterization of the endoleak sac via feeding vessels and coil embolization.[10,11] This method is possible in the majority of cases, particularly if the feeding vessel is of large calibre. However, traversal of feeding vessels is technically challenging and time-consuming. While coils can result in angiographic success, there is concern that they may not be effective in reducing intrasac pressure.[12] In addition, recanalization of blood flow within the interstices of coils, coil compaction, and difficulty in directly occluding all inflow and outflow vessels with coils potentially limit the effectiveness and durability of coil repair of type II endoleaks.

Direct translumbar puncture may allow more rapid and reliable access of the endoleak sac (Figure 34–1). Intra-aneurysmal pressure can be measured, which can help confirm the effectiveness of leak embolization. Reported embolic materials used in conjunction with translumbar access include coils, cyanoacrylate, thrombin, thrombin/gelfoam slurry, tetradecyl sulphate, or Onyx. Virtually every combination of the above listed agents appears to have been tried.

TECHNIQUE OF TRANSLUMBAR ACCESS OF THE ENDOLEAK SAC

The patient is placed prone on the fluoroscopy table. We provide sedation with intravenous midazolam and fentanyl at the commencement of the procedure. All patients will have preexisting CT images demonstrating the endoleak, and from these we estimate the location of the endoleak. Usually, this is done by determining from CT the most accessible area of the endoleak and assessing its position in relation to the stent graft flow divider from the scout images. A fluoroscopically guided puncture of the aneurysm sac is performed, initially with a 21 gauge needle. Once the endoleak sac is accessed, a Fr translumbar arteriography puncture kit (Cook Inc, Bloomington, IN) is inserted using the parallel needle puncture technique. The needle/sheath combination is advanced just beyond the estimated endoleak site, the needle removed, and the sheath slowly withdrawn until pulsatile blood flows from the sheath. A left-sided approach is used most commonly; however, if necessary, a transcaval right-sided approach is used. Angiography is performed through the translumbar sheath or coaxial catheter and pressures recorded. Depending on the anatomy of the endoleak sac, position of the puncture, and choice of embolic agent, the embolization may be performed just through the sheath where it is, or a coaxial microcatheter may be advanced through the sac into the origins of feeding and draining vessels, and selective embolization performed. Pressure measurements and angiogram are performed at the completion of embolization. After the translumbar sheath is removed, the patient is positioned supine to apply pressure from his or her own weight to the puncture site. Most patients undergoing translumbar puncture are discharged home after six hours of observation.

LIQUID EMBOLIC AGENTS

The principal advantage of using a liquid embolic agent in the treatment of type II endoleaks relates to the ability of a liquid to fill the endoleak sac completely, including all inflow and outflow vessels, without selective catheterization of each patent vessel. As a single patent vessel leading to the aneurysm sac could conceivably result in transmission of systemic blood pressure, occlusion of all vessels involved in a type II leak would ideally be achieved to ensure that the leak does not continue to pressurize the aneurysm sac.

Thrombin has been described in endoleak treatment, although because of its very liquid nature, recurrences and nontarget embolization have been reported.[13] The author prefers its use in a slurry with gelfoam.

Cyanoacrylate is another commercially available liquid embolic agent that possesses sufficient radio opacity and controlled delivery to be used for endoleak development. Its use in endoleak management has been described.[14,15] Catheter occlusion after cyanoacrylate injection occurs even with small injection volumes, necessitating repeated catheter introduction.

The liquid embolic agent Onyx (Micro Therapeutics Inc. [MTI], Irvine CA) has been used successfully to seal endoleaks in animal models and humans.[16,17] Onyx is a biocompatible liquid embolic agent consisting of ethylene-vinyl-alcohol copolymer (EVOH) dissolved in dimethyl sulfoxide (DMSO). Micronized tantalum powder is added to the polymer/solvent as a contrast agent for visualization under fluoroscopy. Although somewhat tricky to use, in our experience, Onyx filled the origins of nearly all patent vessels when used in embolization of endoleaks. The solid cast formed by Onyx results in a noncompressible structure suggesting that Onyx may provide a more durable and reliable repair compared to that provided by coils. Onyx can be infused in a slower more controlled manner than cyanoacrylate, and essentially unlimited volumes can be injected through a single catheter (although there are theoretical but as yet undefined limitations of the injectable amount due to the possibility of DMSO toxicity).

When using Onyx, translumbar access is achieved in the usual manner. Pressure within the endoleak sac was measured and angiography performed through the translumbar sheath. A 3 Fr DMSO compatible microcatheter (Rebar-14 or Rebar-27,

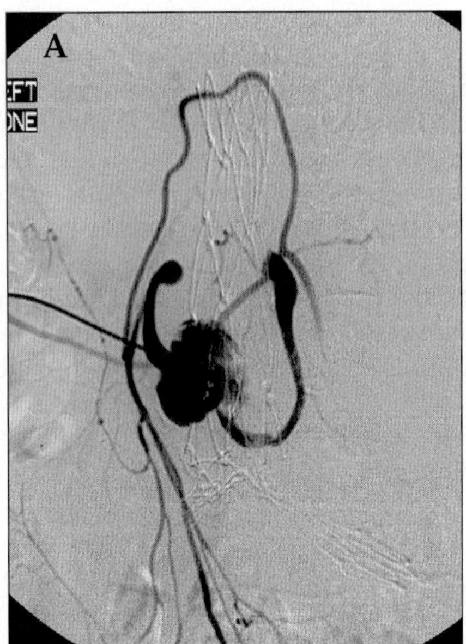

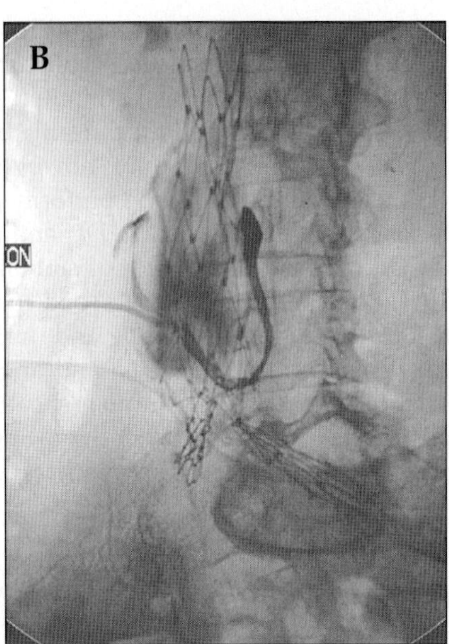

Figure 34-2. (A) Prone angiogram via translumbar sheath demonstrating the endoleak sac, IMA, and a lumbar artery. **(B)** Onyx cast opacified by tantalum filling the endoleak sac.

MTI, Irvine, CA) is passed coaxially through the translumbar sheath into the endoleak sac. If inferior mesenteric artery (IMA) filling was present, the IMA is selectively catheterized. The dead space of the microcatheter is flushed with DMSO to prevent precipitation of Onyx within the catheter. A small quantity of Onyx is then injected, forming a small plug of embolic material at the tip of the catheter. In cases where the IMA is selected, this results in immediate vessel occlusion. Onyx is then injected while the delivery catheter is gradually withdrawn. The endoleak sac fills with Onyx, as do feeding and outflow vessels, resulting in formation of a cast of the endoleak (Figure 34–2). We have not needed to selectively catheterize patent lumbar arteries when using Onyx, but have achieved occlusion by reflux.

SUMMARY

The debate as to whether to treat type II endoleaks persists; however, when intervention is required, treatment via direct translumbar needle/catheter insertion offers several advantages including ease, decreased fluoro time, durability, and the ability to measure sac pressure before and after embolization. The choice of embolic agent is a matter of physician preference, although it would appear that liquid embolic agents without embolic coils are more efficacious than coils alone.

REFERENCES

1. White GH, Yu W, May J, Chaufour X, Stephen MS. Endoleak as a complication of endoluminal grafting of abdominal aortic aneurysm: classification, incidence, diagnosis and management. *J Endovasc Surg*. 1997;4:152–168.

2. Hiatt, M. and Rubin, G. Surveillance for endoleaks: how to detect all of them. *Semin Vasc Surg*. 2004;17(4):268–278.
3. Katzen BT. The Guidant/EVT Ancure Device. *JVIR* Suppl 2000;11:62–66.
4. Hinnen JW, Koning OH, van Bockel JH, Hamming JF. Aneurysm sac pressure after EVAR: the role of endoleak. *Eur J Vasc Endovasc Surg*. 2007 Oct;34(4):432–441.
5. Politz JK, Newman VS, Stewart MT. Late abdominal aortic aneurysm rupture after AneuRx repair: A report of three cases. *J Vasc Surg*. 2000;31:599–606.
6. Gorich J, Rilinger N, Sokiranski R, et al. Treatment of leaks after endovascular repair of aortic aneurysms. *Radiology*. 2000; 215:414–420
7. Tolia A, Landis R, Lamparello P, et al. Type II Endoleaks after Endovascular Repair of Abdominal Aortic Aneurysms: *Natural History. Radiology*. 2005;235:683–686.
8. Wisselink W, Cuesta MA, Berends FJ, van den Berg FG, Rauwerda JA. Retroperitoneal endoscopic ligation of lumbar and inferior mesenteric arteries as a treatment of persistent endoleak after endoluminal aortic aneurysm repair. *J Vasc Surg*. 2000;31:1240–1244
9. Faries PL, Cadot H, Agarwal G, et al. Management of endoleak after endovascular aneurysm repair: cuffs, coils, and conversion. *J Vasc Surg*. 2003 37:1155–1161.
10. Dorffner R, Thurnher S, Polterauer P, Kretschmer G, Lammer J. Treatment of Abdominal Aneurysms with Transfemoral Placement of Stent Grafts: Complications and Secondary Radiologic Intervention. *Radiology*. 1997;204:79–86.
11. LaBerge JM, Sawhney R, Wall SD, et al. Retrograde Catheterization of the Inferior Mesenteric Artery to Treat Endoleaks: Anatomic and Technical Considerations. *JVIR*. 2000;11:55–59.
12. Marty B, Sanchez L, Ohki T, et al. Endoleak after endovascular repair of experimental aortic aneurysms: Does coil embolization with angiographic "seal" lower intraaneurysmal pressure? *J Vasc Surg*. 1998;27:454–462
13. Kasthuri RS, Stivaros SM, Gavan D. Percutaneous ultrasound-guided thrombin injection for endoleaks: an alternative. *Cardiovasc Intervent Radiol*. 2005;28:110–112.
14. Yamaguchi T, Maeda M, Abe H, et al. Embolization of Perigraft Leaks after Endovascular Stent-Graft Treatment of Distal Arch Anastomotic Pseudoaneurysm with Coil and n-Butyl 2-Cyanoacrylate. *JVIR*. 1998;9:61–64.
15. Chao CP, Paz-Fumagalli R, Walser EM, et al.Percutaneous protective coil occlusion of the proximal inferior mesenteric artery before N-butyl cyanoacrylate embolization of type II endoleaks after endovascular repair of abdominal aortic aneurysms. *JVIR*. 2006 (11 Pt 1):1827–1833.
16. Martin ML, Dolmatch BL, Fry PD, Machan LS. Treatment of Type II endoleaks with Onyx. *JVIR* 2001;12:629–632.
17. Maffra R, Dong Y, Brennecke L, Davros W, Dolmatch B. Sealing of Endoleaks with Onyx. *JVIR*. Suppl 2000;11:174.

35

Complications of EVAR and Cases to Avoid

Heron E. Rodriguez, M.D.
and Hung Chu, M.D.

Since its introduction in 1991,[1] endovascular aortic aneurysm repair (EVAR) has rapidly evolved and gained wide acceptance. When compared to open abdominal aortic aneurysm repair, EVAR offers the advantages of decreased perioperative morbidity and mortality, and decreased length of hospitalization. Because of its minimally invasive nature, it is often perceived as a more attractive option by many patients. Over a decade of data are now available regarding the outcome of EVAR. In this chapter, we discuss the nature and management principles of some of the complications unique to EVAR. Also, we describe specific situations in which the use of this minimally invasive technique for the treatment of abdominal aortic aneurysms may not be the best available option.

EARLY COMPLICATIONS OF EVAR

Intraoperative Endoleak

An endoleak is defined as flow outside the lumen of the endograft but within the aneurismal sac. Endoleaks are classified according to the origination of flow into the aneurismal sac.[2] Accurate intraoperative diagnosis of endoleaks can be accomplished with a high-flow power-injected completion arteriogram with imaging continuing through the venous phase. Early recognition of type I and III endoleaks should prompt intervention at the time of implantation. The EUROSTAR data documented that device related leaks (type I or III) are associated with a higher rate of later rupture (3.37%) compared to type II endoleaks (0.52%) and no endoleak (0.25%).[3] A proximal type I endoleak can often be fixed with repeat balloon expansion of the proximal attachment zone. When that fails to correct the endoleak and there is space between the origin of the lowest renal artery and the most proximal covered portion of the

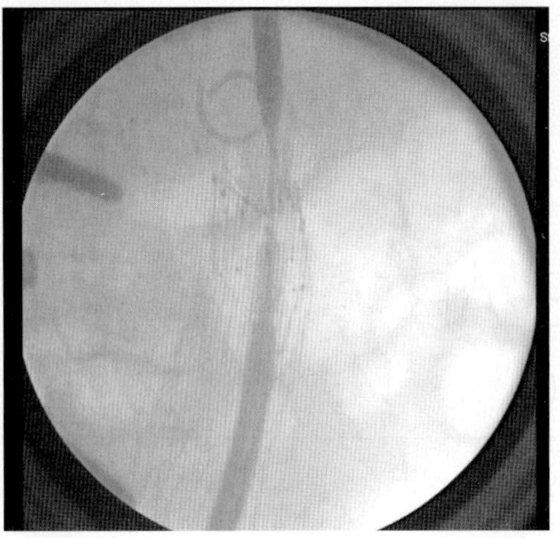

Figure 35-1. An aortic extension is being deployed (partially deployed cuff with the first of the two stents in the extension already deployed) for the treatment of a type IA endoleak. A pigtail catheter was inserted via the left brachial approach to allow for continuous injection of contrast.

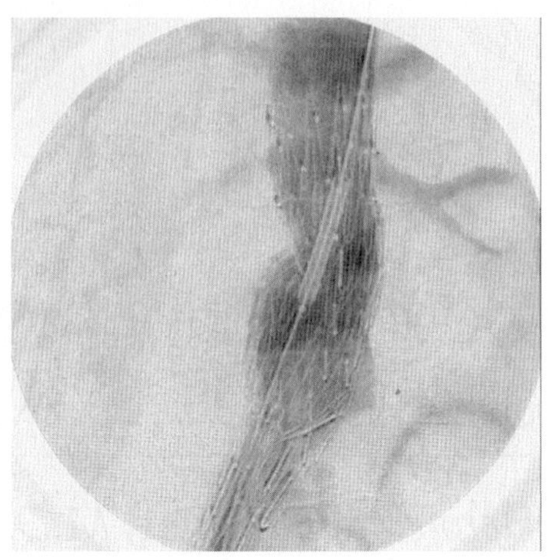

Figure 35-2. A type IA endoleak persists after balloon remolding. A "Giant Palmaz" stent (P3010, Palmaz XL, Cordis Endovascular) is positioned across a kink in the attachment zone. After deployment, the endoleak was no longer present.

endograft, an aortic extension can be used (Figure 35–1). If extending the graft will compromise flow into renal arteries, a balloon-expandable uncovered stent can increase endograft-to-wall apposition (Figure 35–2). Typically, this "giant" stent is deployed across the orifices of the renal arteries without adverse effects to these vessels.

A similar approach is followed to treat distal type I endoleaks. Balloon reinflation, the use of iliac extensions into the distal common iliac or the external iliac artery, and the use of uncovered stents usually are successful maneuvers to correct the radiographic abnormality. Preserving flow into at least one of the hypogastric arteries is a principle that we strictly adhere to in our practice.

The management of type III endoleaks also includes remolding with repeat balloon inflations or the use of "bridging" extensions to seal the defect within the components of the graft.

Inability to Deploy or Complete the Case

Successful implantation of an endograft depends on the ability to reach the aneurysm through the available access channels and to deploy the device in its intended location. Careful anatomic selection and accurate planning are determinant factors in achieving successful deployment and adequate aneurysm exclusion. In order to overcome some adverse anatomic factors, we have a low threshold to use preimplantation iliac artery angioplasty, to expose the retroperitoneal iliac artery, and to use conduits. Once again, adequate planning and the use of the many adjunctive maneuvers described elsewhere are crucial to avoiding tedious bond potentially dangerous intraoperative complications. Nevertheless, when technical misadventures occur, the case can often be completed by converting the repair into an aortouni-iliac configuration and with the aid of a femoro-femoral crossover bypass (Figure 35–3). Some graft designs (i.e., Zenith. Cook Inc., Bloomington, Indiana) include additional components specifically

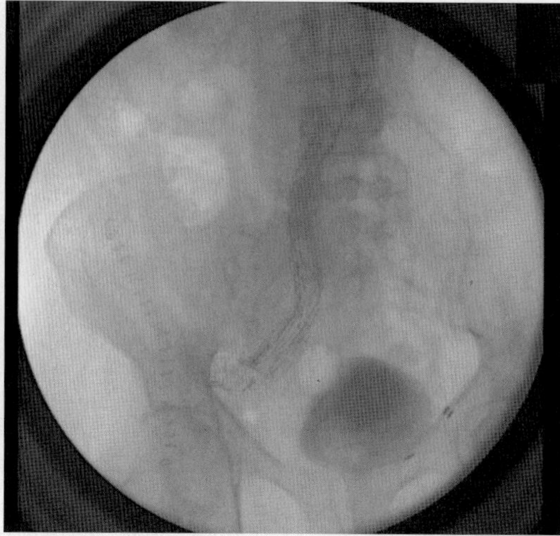

Figure 35-3. A complex aneurysm was excluded by deploying an aortouni-iliac device through a right retroperitoneal exposure of the iliac vessels and with the use of a conduit. A femoro-femoro crossover bypass was used to perfuse the left leg.

designed to convert a modular bifurcated graft into an aortouni-iliac configuration. Other bifurcated grafts can be converted into such configuration by inserting a separate bifurcated graft and deploying both limbs into the iliac limb to remain patent. This effectively excludes the contralateral limb of the original graft, and by using an uncovered stent in the distal portion of the graft limb to remain patent, the desired configuration is achieved.

When all other measures fail, open conversion should be considered. Improved graft designs and operator experience has led to a general decreasing trend in primary conversion rate. In an intent-to-treat analysis, the conversion rate at the time of implantation in the EVAR 1 and DREAM randomized, prospective clinical trials was 0.8% and 1.7%, respectively.[4,5] Of the patients enrolled in the EUROSTAR Registry, the early (less than 30 days) conversion rate was 0.7% in patients enrolled between 1999 and 2002 vs. 2.5% between 1996 and 1998.[6]

Visceral Artery Occlusion

This complication occurs more frequently as a result of attempting to exclude aneurysms with adverse anatomic features (i.e., short aortic necks) than as a technical complication due to poor imaging or lack of attention to detail during deployment. In the event of occlusion, expeditious restoration of flow likely impacts renal function recovery, and endovascular rescue techniques have been described to salvage these situations. One maneuver is to attempt to cannulate the orifice of the occluded artery (Figures 35–4A and 35–4B). Approaching the renal artery from the brachial route often facilitates this. Once a wire is advanced through the partially occluded artery, an arteriogram is done to exclude the possibility of intra-arterial thromboembolism that should be promptly treated with suction embolectomy. A balloon-expandable stent is then deployed across the ostium of the affected artery making sure that at least 0.5 to 1 cm of the stent protrudes into the aortic lumen past the endograft.

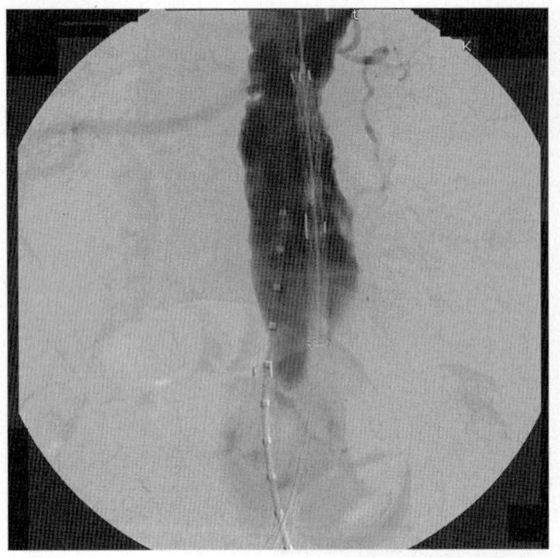

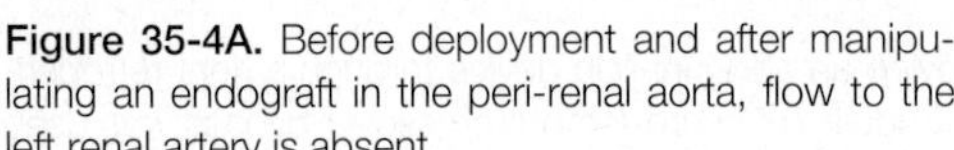

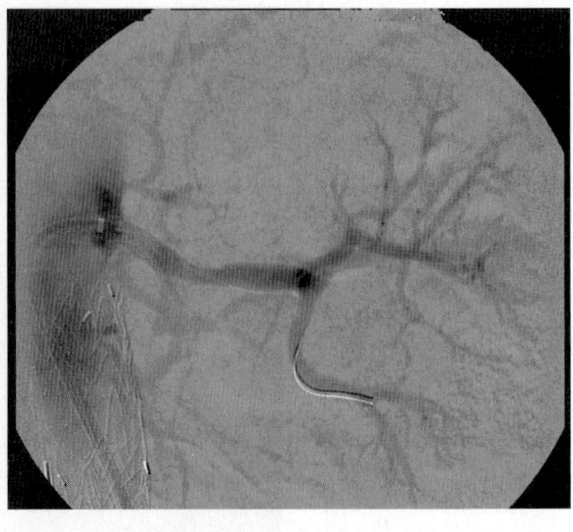

Figure 35-4B. The renal artery occlusion was treated by deploying a balloon-expandable stent through its origin.

Figure 35-4A. Before deployment and after manipulating an endograft in the peri-renal aorta, flow to the left renal artery is absent.

Device Kinking and/or Limb Obstruction

The presence of an endograft kink is significantly associated with endoleaks (type I and III), endograft migration, endograft stenosis, and limb thrombosis and conversion to open repair.[7] We have a low threshold to use balloon-expandable stents to correct any evident abnormality observed during the completion arteriogram. If a limb is completely thrombosed, suction or Fogarty balloon embolectomy is performed prior to attempting to correct any underlying abnormality. If this abnormality is not corrected by the use of intraluminal stents, conversion to an aortouni-iliac device with a femoro-femoral bypass should be considered.

LATE COMPLICATIONS OF EVAR

Randomized, prospective data from the EVAR 1 and DREAM trials showed 30-d mortality rate of 1.2% to 1.7%.[4,5] At 30 days, the conversion rate was 1.7% to 1.9%. The overall conversion rate of the EUROSTAR Registry data was 2% of patients with about two-thirds of these occurring within the first month. Events leading to conversion include endoleak, device migration, device stenosis or thrombosis, aneurysm expansion, or rupture.[6] Significant complications associated with late conversion were proximal type I endoleak ($P =$. 001), midgraft (type III) endoleak ($P =$.001), type II endoleak ($P =$. 003), graft migration ($P =$.001), graft kinking ($P =$.001), and distal type I endoleak ($P =$.001).[8] The short term advantage of EVAR is not in doubt; however, data regarding durability and late complications continue to delineate the role of EVAR as a standard of care. Two-year data from the DREAM trial showed no difference in the rate of complication-free survival and aneurysm-related survival,[9] while four-year data from the EVAR 1 showed improved aneurysm-related survival at the expense of higher cost and higher reintervention rate.[10] The decrease in perioperative morbidity and mortality with EVAR must be balanced with the need for intensive surveillance to identify late complications that are unique to this modality and may be indicative of increased risk of graft failure.

Endoleak

Late endoleaks can be detected indirectly by continued expansion of an aneurysm sac on subsequent imaging studies. Duplex represents an alternative modality to identifying sources of endoleaks that is comparable in specificity but less sensitive than CT scans.[11] Two-thirds of endoleaks identified early (prior to discharge) will resolve without specific treatment within one month. The rational for treating endoleaks is to prevent rupture. The cumulative rate of rupture after EVAR is 1% per year.[8] Significant risk factors for rupture were proximal type I endoleak (P =.001), midgraft (type III) endoleak (P =.001), graft migration (P =.001), and postoperative kinking of the endograft (P =.001).[8] Despite the associations, predicting rupture after EVAR is difficult. From the EUROSTAR Registry database, 39% out of 34 ruptures had no identified complications prior to being diagnosed with rupture.[12]

Though type I and III endoleak should be addressed at the initial operation, not all device-related endoleaks are readily apparent at the time of implantation. The EUROSTAR data showed that of the 488 patients with endoleaks identified at any time during the postoperative period, 297 patients had a type I or III endoleak or multiple endoleaks with a combination of different types.[3]

The clinical significance of type II endoleaks is a subject of debate. It is our practice to treat only those type II endoleaks that are associated with aneurismal sac expansion. Our approach is as follows. If the endoleak can be traced to a lumbar branch originating from the hypogastric vessels, coil embolization is performed (Figure 35–5). We make all efforts to embolize the involved vessels as close to the aneurismal sac as possible. If the endoleak persists, translumbar or transabdominal sac embolization is performed (Figure 35–6). In case the endoleak persists after these interventions and the sac continues to enlarge, we consider open conversion. When sac expansion occurs in the absence of a visible endoleak, relining the endograft with a new device is considered.

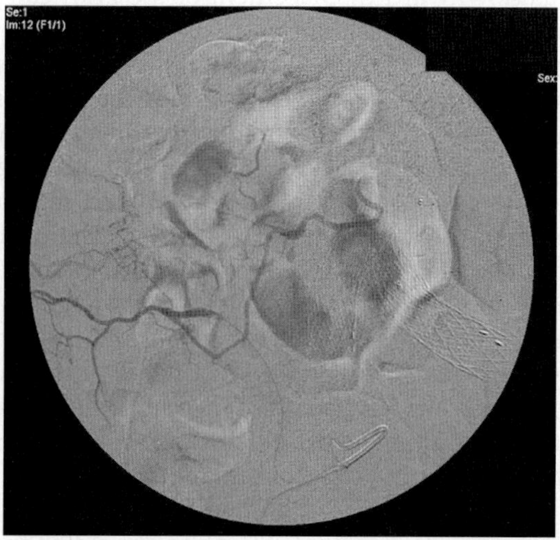

Figure 35-5. Superselective cannulation in preparation for percutaneous transluminal coil embolization of a lumbar branch associated with a late type II endoleak and sac enlargement.

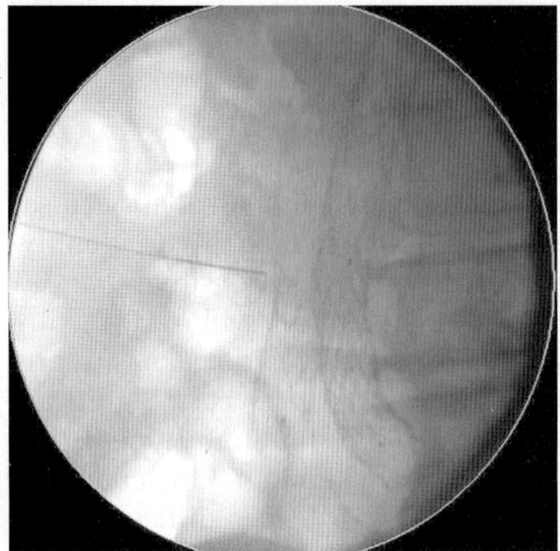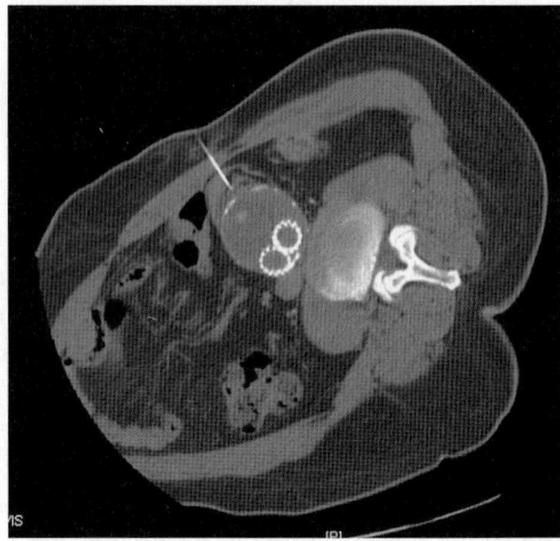

Figure 35-6. A Translumbar cannulation in preparation for sac embolization under fluoroscopic guidance for the treatment of a type II endoleak and sac enlargement. **B** Alternatively, the sac can be approached under CT guidance via the transabdominal approach.

Device Migration

Aortic stent-graft migration is the longitudinal movement of all or part of the stent graft. Stent-graft migration has been reported with nearly all types of endovascular designs.[13-16] Many hemodynamic and biomechanical forces interact between the endograft, its attachment systems, and the aortic wall.[17] Migration is not an innocent event. It can be associated with proximal seal failure, device kinking, occlusion, and disconnection.[18] It has also been associated with post EVAR rupture.[8] Several studies have reported the need for late conversion to open repair,[8,14-15] laparoscopic removal of the stent graft,[19] renal artery stenting,[20] or reinterventions for type I endoleaks using additional aortic cuff placement.[15] The occurrence of endoleaks and the association with rupture is intuitive, as downward displacement of the graft can result in sealing failure and repressurization of the aneurysm sac.

Several recommendations can be given for prevention of stent migration. The avoidance of short (<15mm), wide (>30mm), conical or flared necks ($\geq$ 3mm aortic neck enlargement that measured 15mm caudal to the lowest renal artery ostium) with significant angulation, calcification, or thrombus is strongly suggested. Devices that include hooks or barbs, providing suprarenal fixation and higher radial force, appear to have a protective benefit from migration. Proper oversizing to 10% to 20% of the original size is also desired since excessive or insufficient oversizing may contribute to dilation and migration, and are, therefore, not recommended. Lastly but not less important, atherosclerotic risk factor control, especially tight blood pressure control, is advised as there is evidence suggesting their influence over migration rates.

Routine serial, lifelong imaging surveillance after endografting is mandatory. Routine measurement and comparison of the distance between the most proximal portion of the endograft and stable anatomic landmarks (i.e., renal artery, superior mesenteric artery) must be included in every study performed.

As a general rule, it is our feeling that migration should be treated when the actual overlap between the endograft and aortic neck is <5–10 mm[21] or when evidence of proximal seal zone failure associated with clinically significant events such as type I endoleak or aneurysm expansion occur. Failure to treat migration could lead to repressurization and subsequent rupture of the aneurysm. Traditionally, this has been accomplished either through proximal extension, placement of a new endograft, or conversion to an open procedure. The secondary durability of aortic cuff extensions is unknown. If caudal migration continues, component separation may occur. Therefore, very careful observation is warranted after this type of therapy. Very recently, a novel appliance (Zenith Renu AAA Ancillary Graft; Cook Inc.) was developed for the treatment of migration.[21] Main body extensions and one-piece converters of various sizes are available, preloaded into 18 and 20 French sheaths, to proximally extend different previously implanted endovascular devices. Anchoring barbs are placed incrementally on the suprarenal stent to provide additional suprarenal fixation, reduce the risk of further migration, and improve sealing. The clinical use of this device has yet to be reported in the United States, although it has already been utilized elsewhere.[22]

Less invasive alternatives for both the prevention and management of stent graft migration are being tested. Kolvenbach et al.[23] described the application of laparoscopy to accomplish further fixation of the endograft to the aortic neck.

Endograft Infection

Infection of an aortic endoprosthesis is a rare occurrence. The DREAM trial reported one death from an infected endograft out of 169 patients assigned to endovascular repair.[9] Data are limited to case reports. Management of an infected endograft is governed by the same principles applied to infected aortic prostheses implanted in traditional open aneurysm repair. Usually, it involves removing all prosthetic material and infected tissue and providing distal flow by means of extra-anatomic reconstruction, the use of a homograft, or by harvesting a femoropopliteal vein for autogenous reconstruction (Figure 35–7).

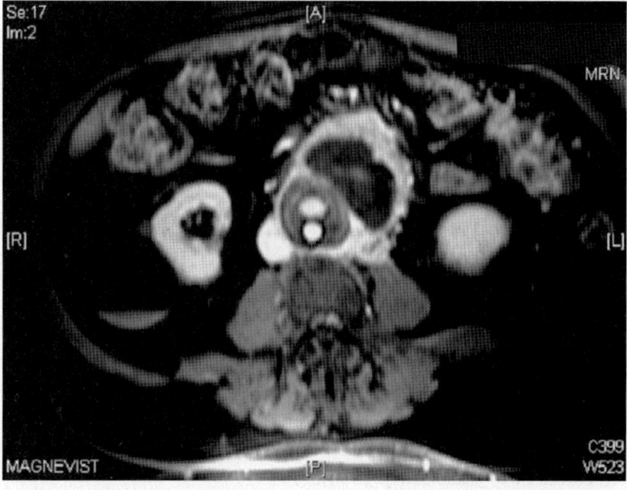

Figure 35-7. MRI of a patient with fever, leukocytosis, and abdominal pain two months after EVAR. A large periaortic fluid collection is seen. The patient underwent explantation of an infected endograft and reconstruction via an axillofemoral bypass.

EVAR: CASES TO AVOID

The Patient with Difficult Anatomy

The best way to avoid most of the early complications of EVAR is by strictly adhering to the anatomic criteria specified for each endograft system. This is particularly critical with regard to the anatomic characteristics of the proximal neck. Attempting to exclude aneurysms with short (<15 mm), angulated (>45°), calcified, thrombus-lined, or irregular infrarenal necks significantly increases the possibilities of proximal attachment zone failure (i.e., type I endoleak, migration).[24,25] Although more often than not, it is possible to complete such cases with acceptable morbidity and reasonable immediate technical results, the durability and long-term results in these circumstances are at least, questionable, and for many reasons, this practice should be discouraged.

On the other hand, adverse anatomic features in the iliac arteries can almost always be solved with the use of retroperitoneal iliac exposure, conduits, hypogastric bypasses, and configurations like aortouni-iliac devices and femoro-femoro bypasses.

The Young Patient with No Comorbidities and Ideal Anatomy

The durability of EVAR is still questionable. The possibility of aneurysm rupture after successful endovascular exclusion is not negligible and has been estimated to be around 1% per year.[8] On the other hand, the long-term results of open aneurysm repair have been well defined and are excellent. For these reasons, it is our strong opinion that young patients with overall good health who can tolerate open surgery should undergo the most durable form of aneurysm management; that is, open repair.

The Small Aneurysm

Multicenter, randomized, prospective clinical trials have established the safety of nonoperative treatment for aneurysms smaller than 5.5 cm.[26,27] The availability of a less invasive treatment modality does not justify—in our opinion—treating aneurysms of small sizes. Any complication occurring after a procedure of questionable indication is a complication that should have not occurred.

CONCLUSIONS

More than a decade of experience regarding EVAR is now available. Most complications related to this procedure can be avoided by proper anatomic selection. When complications occur, many maneuvers have proven effective to overcome the unique problems related to EVAR.

REFERENCES

1. Parodi JA, Palmaz JC, Barone HD. Transfemoral intraluminal graft implantation for abdominal aortic aneurysms. *Ann Vasc Surg*. 1991;5:491–499
2. White GH, Yu W, May J, et al. Endoleak as a complication of endoluminal grafting of abdominal aortic aneurysms: classification, incidence, diagnosis and management. *J Endovasc Surg*. 1997;4:152–168.

3. van Marrewijk C, Buth J, Harris PL, et al. Significance of endoleaks after endovascular repair of abdominal aortic aneurysms: The EUROSTAR experience. *J Vasc Surg.* 2002;35(3):461–473.

4. Prinssen M, Verhoeven EL, Buth J, et al. A randomized trial comparing conventional and endovascular repair of abdominal aortic aneurysms. *N Engl J Med.* 2004;351(16):1607–1618.

5. Greenhalgh RM, Brown LC, Kwong GP, et al. Comparison of endovascular aneurysm repair with open repair in patients with abdominal aortic aneurysm (EVAR trial 1), 30-day operative mortality results: randomised controlled trial. *Lancet.* 2004;364(9437):843–848.

6. Van Marrewijk CJ, Fransen G, Laheij RJF, et al. EUROSTAR Collaborators: Is type II endoleak after EVAR a harbinger of risk? Causes and outcome of open conversion and aneurysm rupture during follow-up. *Eur J Vasc Endovasc Surg.* 2004;27(2):128–137.

7. Fransen GA, Desgranges P, Laheij RJ, et al. Frequency, predictive factors, and consequences of stent-graft kink following endovascular AAA repair. *J Endovasc Ther.* 2003;10(5):913–918.

8. Harris PL, Vallabhaneni SR, Desgranges P, et al. Incidence and risk factors of late rupture, conversion, and death after endovascular repair of infrarenal aortic aneurysms: the EUROSTAR experience. *J Vasc Surg.* 2000;32(4):739–749.

9. Blankensteijn JD, de Jong SE, Prinssen M, et al. Two-year outcomes after conventional or endovascular repair of abdominal aortic aneurysms. *N Engl J Med.* 2005; 352(23): 2398–2405.

10. EVAR trial participants. Endovascular Aneurysm Repair Versus Open Repair in Patients With Abdominal Aortic Aneurysm (EVAR Trial 1): Randomized Controlled Trial. *Perspect Vasc Surg Endovasc Ther.* 2006;18(1):74

11. Raman KG, Missig-Carroll N, Richardson T, et al. Color-flow duplex ultrasound scan versus computed tomographic scan in the surveillance of endovascular aneurysm repair. *J Vasc Surg.* 2003;38(4):645–651.

12. Fransen GA, Vallabhaneni SR Sr, van Marrewijk CJ, et al. Rupture of infra-renal aortic aneurysm after endovascular repair: a series from EUROSTAR registry. *Eur J Vasc Endovasc Surg.* 2003;26(5):487–493.

13. ZarinsCK, White RA, Schwarten D, et al. AneurRx stent graft versus open surgical repair of abdominal aortic aneurysms: multicenter prospective clinical trial. *J Vasc Surg.* 199;29: 292–305

14. Beebe HG, Cronenwett JL, Katzen BT, et al. Results of an aortic endograft trial: impact of device failure beyond 12 months.*J Vasc Surg.* 2001;33(2 Suppl):S55–63.

15. Greenberg RK, Lawrence-Brown M, Bhandari G, et al. An update of the Zenith endovascular graft for abdominal aortic aneurysms: initial implantation and mid-term follow-up data. *J Vasc Surg.* 2001;33(2 Suppl):S157–164.

16. Cao P, Verzini F, Zannetti S, et al. Device migration after endoluminal abdominal aortic aneurysm repair: analysis of 113 cases with a minimum follow-up period of 2 years. *J Vasc Surg.* 2002;35(2):229–235.

17. Leon L, Rodriguez HE. Aortic Endograft Migration. *Perspect Vasc Surg Endovasc Ther.* 2005;17(4):363–373. Review.

18. Sampaio SM, Panneotn JM, Mozes G, et al. AneuRx device migration: incidence, risk factors and consequences. *Ann Vasc Surg.* 2005;19:1–8.

19. Lin JC, Kolvenbach R, Wassiljew S, et al. Totally laparoscopic explantation of migrated stent graft after endovascular aneurysm repair: a report of two cases. *J Vasc Surg.* 2005;41(5): 885–888.

20. Reed AB, Mozes G, Carmo M, et al. Renal artery coverage during endovascular aortic aneurysm repair: proximal migration or misplacement of the stent graft? *Pers Vasc Surg Endovasc Ther.* 2004;16:135–140.

21. Conners MS 3rd, Sternbergh WC 3rd, Carter G, et al. Endograft migration one to four years after endovascular abdominal aortic aneurysm repair with the AneuRx device: a cautionary note. *J Vasc Surg.* 2002; 36(3):476–484.

22. http://www.zenithstentgraft.com/physicians/US/aRenu.php

23. Kolvenbach R, Pinter L, Raghunandan M, et al. Laparoscopic remodeling of abdominal aortic aneurysms after endovascular exclusion: a technical description. *J Vasc Surg*. 2002;36: 1267–1270.

24. Albertini J, Kalliafas S, Travis S, et al. Anatomical risk factors for proximal perigraft endoleak and graft migration following endovascular repair of abdominal aortic aneurysms. *Eur J Vasc Endovasc Surg*. 2000;19(3):308–312.

25. Peppelenbosch N, Buth J, Harris PL, et al. Diameter of abdominal aortic aneurysm and outcome of endovascular aneurysm repair: does size matter? A report from EUROSTAR. *J Vasc Surg*. 2004;39(2):288–297.

26. Mortality results for randomised controlled trial of early elective surgery or ultrasonographic surveillance for small abdominal aortic aneurysms. The UK Small Aneurysm Trial Participants. *Lancet*. 1998;352(9141):1649–55.

27. Aneurysm Detection and Management Veterans Affairs Cooperative Study Group. Immediate repair compared with surveillance of small abdominal aortic aneurysms. *N Engl J Med*. 2002;346(19):1437–1444.

36

Surgical Conversion after Endovascular Aortic Aneurysm Repair

Douglas P. MacMillan, Jr., M.D. and
Elliot L. Chaikof, M.D., Ph.D.

Endovascular repair has become an increasingly accepted treatment option for aneurysmal disease since the initial report of endograft placement in patients with abdominal aortic aneurysm (AAA) more than a decade ago.[1] To date, four endovascular devices, including the AneuRx (Medtronic), Ancure (Guidant), Zenith (Cook), and Excluder (Gore) endografts have been approved by the U.S. Food and Drug Administration (FDA) for clinical use. While the Ancure device is no longer in the clinical marketplace, a number of other devices are at various stages of FDA review. All told, extensive investigations of endovascular AAA repair have been associated with encouraging midterm results.[2-4] Indeed, there is little doubt that endovascular repair of AAA is equivalent to open repair in the short term with enthusiasm for this minimally invasive treatment driven by shorter hospital stays, decreased anesthetic risk, and a rapid postoperative convalescence.[5,6] However, along with numerous positive short-term and midterm reports of AAA endovascular repair, a growing number of studies have also revealed limitations of this evolving technology. Problems with device integrity, component separation, migration, infection, iliac limb occlusion, and aneurysm sac expansion with and without the presence of endoleak have been described.[7]

Although endovascular solutions can, at times, be provided for a failing endograft, many of the aforementioned problems require device explantation and repair of the aneurysm with an open surgical approach. Explantation of an endovascular graft has been termed a *primary* conversion if device removal is performed at the time of the initial procedure, and as a *secondary* conversion if removal is performed at a later date.[8] During the first decade of AAA endovascular repair, the rate of primary conversion has been significantly reduced with improved device design, patient selection, and increasing operator experience.[9,10] Primary conversions have become increasingly rare events with at least two recent multicenter trials reporting 100% primary technical success rates. Several recent investigations, including a report from our center, confirm that secondary operative conversion continues to be a necessary intervention for at least a small cohort of patients treated with endografts. In this chapter, we review our experience and that reported by other centers for patients with late clinical failure in whom secondary conversion was required. In addition, the indications, operative strategies, and technical maneuvers that may facilitate endograft explantation are detailed.

INCIDENCE

The durability and long-term effectiveness of endovascular AAA repair remains under close scrutiny. Conversion-related data, including associated mortality among clinical series reported between 1997 and 2004, are summarized in Table 36–1. Mean follow-up in these 11 studies was 30 months, with mean time to secondary conversion of 20 months. Incidence of secondary conversion ranges between 0.6–4.5% (average 1.9%). Mean perioperative mortality related to secondary conversion is 23%. In a recent review of our experience at Emory,[11] endografts were deployed but subsequently removed in 20 patients (6.3%) and a midline transperitoneal repair was performed. Of these, 11 patients (3.4%) underwent primary conversion and nine patients (2.8%) underwent secondary conversion to open surgical repair after endovascular repair. Time from the original endograft procedure to secondary conversion was 24 ± 13 months (range, two to 48 months). Two grafts were explanted as an urgent procedure, and seven as elective procedures. There were no intraoperative deaths, but one perioperative death occurred 21 days after operation, secondary to bacterial endocarditis and

TABLE 36-1. REPORTED RESULTS OF CONVERSION AND MORTALITY AFTER ENDOVASCULAR REPAIR

Author	Year	Mean follow-up months	Primary conversion %	Primary conversion n	secondary conversion %	secondary conversion n	Mortality with secondary conversion %	Mortality with secondary conversion n	Time to explanation months
May et al.[22]	1997		11.5	13/113	4.4	5/113	20	1/5	
Jacobowitz et al.[23]	1999	40	3	19/669	4	27/669	7	2/27	
Cuypers et al.[24]	2000	6	2	38/1871	0.6	11/1871	27	3/11	8
Harris et al.[18]	2000	12	1.3	34/2464	2.1	53/2464	32	17/53	18
Greenberg et al.[23]	2001	14			0.6	3/528	0	0/3	13
Dattilo et al.[14]	2002	18	1.4	5/362	2.2	8/362			22
Lyden et al.[12]	2002	21	2.7	3/110	4.5	5/110	20	1/5	33
Bockler et al.[9]	2002	23	3.2	17/520	3.8	20/520			12
Chaikof et al.[26]	2002	17	3.8	9/236	1.3	3/236	0	0/3	19
Lipsitz, et al.[21]	2003	46	1	3/386	2.8	11/386	18	2/11	30
Medtronic report[27]	2004	60	1.3	15/1193	3.8	45/1193	18	8/45	
Becquemin, et al.[28]	2004	28	0	0/250	4.4	11/250	0	0/11	31
Average			1.9	156/8174	2.3	202/8702	19.5	34/174	

sepsis. Postoperative complications included respiratory failure in one patient, a non-Q wave myocardial infarction in one patient, and a urinary tract infection in two patients. Likewise, Lyden et al.[12] evaluated 110 patients who received endovascular AAA treatment, five (4.5%) of whom required secondary conversion. Similarly, Dattilo et al.[13] reported a secondary conversion rate of 2.2% (eight patients) over seven years in 362 AAA endovascular grafts and Ohki et al.[14] in a nine-year experience with 239 endovascular grafts, reported a secondary conversion rate of 2.1% (five patients). Together, these data demonstrate that a small but finite risk of secondary conversion is present for all graft types, and perhaps of greater significance, treatment failures requiring operative intervention may occur at any point following initial graft deployment. The detection of clinical failures years after initial treatment, currently mandates life long surveillance for all patients.

INDICATIONS

In our recent review, eight of the nine patients in whom late graft explantation was necessary were men, with mean age 75 years (range, 63–86 years). Indications for secondary conversion, type of device, presence of initial endoleak, and time to explantation in these nine patients are outlined in Table 36–2. None of the patients in whom secondary conversion was required had inadequate anatomy that predisposed to clinical endograft failure. Endografts were explanted because of device infection (AneuRx, n = 1), endotension or aneurysm sac enlargement without evidence of endoleak (Excluder, n = 1; Ancure, n = 1), type I endoleak with aneurysm sac enlargement (Ancure, n = 1; EVT tube, n = 3), and type II endoleak with aneurysm sac enlargement (Ancure, n = 2). No graft thrombosis or aneurysm rupture was identified. Mean AAA diameter at original device implantation was 5.3±0.4 cm, and at secondary conversion was 6.1±0.8 cm. The aneurysm sac enlarged more than 5 mm in all patients except in one patient with graft infection. Device-specific incidence of explantation was 0.8% for AneuRx, 3.7% for Excluder, 3.1% for Ancure, and 10.7% for the EVT tube graft. To summarize, persistent endoleak was the most common indication for conversion. Four patients had type I endoleak. Two patients had enlarging aneurysms, with type II endoleak that persisted despite attempts at percutaneous coil embolization. In addition, two patients exhibited the characteristic features of endotension with increasing aneurysm sac diameter without documented endoleak at ultrasound scanning, CT, or conventional angiography. All told, in our experience, failures to successfully treat endoleak and endotension have been the primary indications for secondary conversion.

Indeed, management of endoleak is evolving and future refinement in treatment strategies offers an opportunity to further decrease the incidence of late surgical conversion. Currently, endoleaks can often be managed with percutaneous techniques of coil embolization and placement of additional stent components. Additional techniques include translumbar access to the aneurysm sac,[15] endoscopic ligation of feeding vessels,[16] and transperitoneal aneurysm sacotomy with direct ligation of feeding vessels.[17] Percutaneous coil embolization of the feeding vessels was attempted in both patients with type II endoleak in our series. However, in both patients endoleak persisted and endograft removal was performed. Admittedly, controversy remains regarding the clinical significance of type II endoleaks, as well as aneurysm growth in the absence of a demonstrable endoleak. The Eurostar database of 2464 patients suggests that significant risk of rupture exists with proximal type I endoleak, type III

TABLE 36-2. DETAILS AND INDICATIONS FOR SECONDARY CONVERSION

Patient	Device type	Initial endoleak*	Months implanted	Indication for conversion
1	EVT tube	No	30	Endoleak type I, distal attachment
2	EVT tube	No	32	Endoleak type I, distal attachment, back pain
3	EVT tube	No	48	Endoleak type I, distal attachment
4	Ancure	Type II	12	Endoleak type II, prior coil embolization
5	Ancure	Type II	15	Endoleak type I, proximal attachment, acute back pain
6	Ancure	No	.27	Endotension, successful coil embolization, type II endoleak
7	Ancure	No	23	Endoleak type II, multiple coil embolizations attempted
8	AncuRx	No	2	Infection
9	Excluder	No	24	Endotension

EVT, Endovascular Technologies.

*Initial endoleak noted on completion angiogram at endograft deployment.

endoleak, device migration, and limb kinking.[18] However, this data does not demonstrate that patients with type II endoleak and endotension are necessarily risk-free. Type II endoleaks may be a more benign phenomenon, but aneurysm rupture solely attributable to the presence of a type II endoleak has been well documented. Likewise, operative conversion for endotension has, on occasion, demonstrated a fully excluded aneurysm sac filled only with proteinaceous debris. This has been particularly true for the Excluder endograft. Nonetheless, it often remains difficult to completely exclude the presence of an underlying endoleak that was not clearly visualized by CT, Duplex, or angiographic imaging. Thus, as in the case of type II endoleak, endotension may represent a relative rather than an absolute indication for endograft removal.

Device migration necessitating operative conversion has been an infrequent event in our experience. However, aneurysm rupture following device migration has been observed. In this regard, some investigators have noted that large preoperative aneurysm size ($d > 55$mm), postoperative neck dilation ($d >10$mm), and circumferential neck thrombus may be predictors of later device migration.[19] To date, when migration has been observed, endovascular salvage has more often than not been feasible. Nevertheless, conversion may be required. Moreover, it bears emphasis that a finite risk of device failure remains, even with the development of novel systems that incorporate suprarenal fixation. Currently, the only absolute indication for open conversion is documented endograft infection.

TECHNICAL CONSIDERATIONS

The surgical details of the secondary conversion procedures in our series mirror those in other reports and are outlined in Table 36–3. All procedures were performed using a midline transperitoneal approach. Removal of Ancure, EVT tube, and Excluder endografts often necessitated suprarenal or supraceliac aortic control to facilitate circumferential detachment of the proximal endograft hooks and barbs. In three of the four patients, the left renal vein was ligated and divided to facilitate suprarenal aortic exposure (Figure 36–1A). None developed renal failure. Ice-cold saline was also used as an adjunct to reduce outward radial forces exterted by nitinol based devices, such as the AneuRx and Excluder endgrafts, so as to facilitate device extraction.

It bears emphasis that devices with barbs or hooks may be more difficult to remove with downward traction alone. Indeed, in three patients (two with Ancure devices and one with an EVT tube), the new aortic prosthetic graft was anastomosed directly to the proximal segment of the endograft and the surrounding tissue (Figure 36–1B). This strategy has gained popularity as vascular surgeons have appreciated the increased level of difficulty that these cases often present.[20,21] Two of our patients had type II endoleak, and one had distal attachment type I endoleak. Thus, in the absence of proximal type I endoleak or graft infection, it was deemed safe to retain the proximal portion of the device. An infrarenal aortic clamp was used in all three patients in whom a portion of the proximal endograft was incorporated into the proximal anastomosis. We believe this reduces potential damage to the infrarenal aorta and eliminates the need to obtain suprarenal aortic control. With this technique of incorporating the proximal portion of the endograft into the anastomosis, yearly CT is recommended to confirm that there is no aneurysm formation at the proximal anastomosis.

Suprarenal aortic control was required in the instance of an AneuRx device infection to allow adequate debridement of infected aortic tissue and oversewing of the

TABLE 36-3. SURGICAL DETAILS OF SECONDARY CONVERSIONS AND POSTOPERATIVE COMPLICATIONS

Patient	Device type	Clamp location	Bypass	Intraoperative findings	Postoperative complications
1	EVT tube	Supraceliac	Aortobiiliac	Distal attachment hook fracture	None
2	EVT tube	Suprarenal	Aortobiiliac	Distal attachment hook fracture	None
3	EVT tube	Infrarenal	Aortobiiliac*	Distal attachment leak	None
4	Ancure	Infrarenal	Aortobiiliac*	Patent lumbar vessel	None
5	Ancure	Suprarenal	Aortobiiliac	Proximal and distal attachment leaks	Pulmonary failure
6	Ancure	Supraceliac	Aortobiiliac	Patent lumbar vessel	UTI, non-Q MI
7	Ancure	Infrarenal	Aortouniiliac*	Patent lumbar vessel and IMA	None
8	AneuRx	Suprarenal	Axillobifemoral	Nonincorporated device	UTI
9	Excluder	Suprarenal	Aortobiiliac	No endoleak found	Endocarditis, death

UTI, Urinary tract infection; MI, myocardial infarction; IMA, inferior mesenteric artery.

*Endograft transected below proximal stent/hook system, and new aortic prosthetic bypass graft was anastomosed end to end to infrarenal aorta and proximal portion of endograft device.

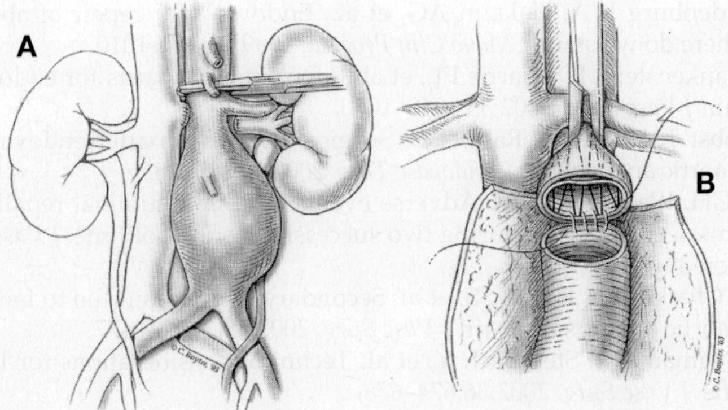

Figure 36-1. A. At the time of operative conversion, the left renal vein may need to be ligated and divided to facilitate suprarenal aortic exposure. **B.** Devices with barbs or hooks may be more difficult to remove with downward traction alone. As an alternative to complete endograft excision, the new aortic prosthetic graft may be anastomosed directly to the proximal segment of the endograft and the surrounding tissue.

aortic stump. With the exception of this case in which an axillobifemoral graft was used to reestablish distal perfusion, direct in-line aortobiiliac reconstruction was the preferred method of operative repair. Mean length of hospital stay was 20±21 days (range, seven to 70 days) and length of ICU stay was 7±8 days. Mean follow-up was 29± 28 months (range, four to 72 months) after surgical conversion. During this period, two patients died from causes unrelated to aortic aneurysmal disease. There were no further aneurysm related morbidity or mortality.

CONCLUSIONS

Despite the overall high technical and clinical success rate of endovascular AAA repair, late failure remains a persistent, albeit infrequent, problem long after initial implantation. Unique challenges are associated with removal of aortic endografts, and preoperative planning requires careful consideration of distinct differences between endograft designs. It is critical to note that secondary conversion is a more difficult operation than primary open AAA repair. However, in most patients, device removal can be safely performed with low morbidity. With tens of thousands of aortic endografts implanted annually in the United States, we estimate that several hundred secondary graft conversions are now performed each year.

REFERENCES

1. Parodi JC, Palmaz JC, Barone HD. Transfemoral intraluminal graft implantation for abdominal aortic aneurysms. *Ann Vasc Surg*. 1991;5:491–499.
2. Carpenter JP, et al. Multicenter trial of the PowerLink bifurcated system for endovascular aortic aneurysm repair. *J Vasc Surg*. 2002;36:1129–1137.
3. Criado FJ, Clark NS, McKendrick C, et al. Update on the Talent LPS AAA Stent Graft: Results with "Enhanced Talent." *Semin Vasc Surg*. 2003;16:158–165.
4. Kibbe MR, Matsumura JS. The Gore Excluder US Multi-Center Trial: Analysis of Adverse Events at 2 Years. *Semin Vasc Surg*. 2003;16:144–150.
5. Moore WS. The Guidant Ancure Bifurcation Endograft: Five year follow up. *Semin Vasc Surg*. 2003;16:139–143.
6. Sternbergh WC 3rd, Money SR, Greenberg RK, Chuter TA. Zenith Investigators. Influence of Endograft oversizing on device migration, endoleak, aneurysm shrinkage, and aortic neck dilation: results from the Zenith Multicenter Trial. *J Vasc Surg*. 2004;39:20–26.

7. Seelig MH, Oldenburg WA, Hakaim AG, et al.. Endovascular repair of abdominal aortic aneurysms: Where do we stand? *Mayo Clin Proceed*. 1999:74;999–1010.

8. Chaikof EL, Blankensteijn JD, Harris PL, et al. Reporting standards for endovascular aortic aneurysm repair. *J Vasc Surg*. 2002;35:1048–1060.

9. Bockler D, Probst T, Weber H, Raithel D. Surgical conversion after endovascular grafting for abdominal aortic aneurysms. *J Endovasc Ther*. 2002;9:111–118.

10. May J, White GH, Waugh R, et al. Adverse events after endoluminal repair of abdominal aortic aneurysms: a comparison during two successive periods of time. *J Vasc Surg*. 1999;29: 32–37. discussion 38-39.

11. Terramani TT, Chaikof EL, Rayan SS, et al. Secondary conversion due to failed endovascular abdominal aortic aneurysm repair. *J Vasc Surg*. 2003;38(3);473–477.

12. Lyden SP, McNamara JM, Sternbach Y, et al. Technical considerations for late removal of aortic endografts. *J Vasc Surg*. 2002;36:674–678.

13. Dattilo JB, Brewster DC, Fan CM, et al. Clinical failures of endovascular abdominal aortic aneurysm repair: incidence, causes, and management. *J Vasc Surg*. 2002;35:1137–1144.

14. Ohki T, Veith FJ, Shaw P, et al. Increasing incidence of midterm and long-term complications after endovascular graft repair of abdominal aortic aneurysms: a note of caution based on a 9-year experience. *Ann Surg*. 2001;234:323–334. discussion 334–335.

15. Baum RA, Carpenter JP, Golden MA, et al. Treatment of type 2 endoleaks after endovascular repair of abdominal aortic aneurysms: comparison of transarterial and translumbar techniques. *J Vasc Surg*. 2002;35:23–29.

16. Wisselink W, Cuesta MA, Berends FJ, et al. Retroperitoneal endoscopic ligation of lumbar and inferior mesenteric arteries as a treatment of persistent endoleak after endoluminal aortic aneurysm repair. *J Vasc Surg*. 2000;31:1240–1244.

17. Hinchliffe RJ, Singh-Ranger R, Whitaker SC, Hopkinson BR. Type II endoleak: transperitoneal sacotomy and ligation of side branch endoleaks responsible for aneurysm sac expansion. *J Endovasc Ther*. 2002;9:539–542.

18. Harris PL, Vallabhaneni SR, Desgranges P, et al. Incidence and risk factors of late rupture, conversion, and death after endovascular repair of infrarenal aortic aneurysms: The EUROSTAR experience. European collaborators on Stent/graft techniques for aortic aneurysm repair. *J Vasc Surg*. 2000;32:739–749.

19. Cao P, Verzini P, Parlani G, et al. Predictive factors and clinical consequences of proximal aortic neck dilatation in 230 patients undergoing abdominal aortic aneurysm repair with self-expandable stent-grafts. *J Vasc Surg*. 2003;37:1200–1205.

20. Milner R, Verhagen HJ, Blankensteijn JD. Salvage of a difficult situation: method for conversion of failed endograft. *J Vasc Surg*. 2003;38:397–400.

21. Lipsitz EZ, Ohki T, Veith FJ, et al. Delayed open conversion following endovascular aortoiliac aneurysm repair: partial (or complete) endograft preservation as a useful adjunct. *J Vasc Surg*. 2003;38:1191–1198.

22. May J, White GH, Yu W, et al. Conversion from endoluminal to open repair of abdominal aortic aneurysms: a hazardous procedure. *Eur J Vasc Endovasc Surg*. 1997;14:4–11.

23. Jacobowitz GR, Lee AM, Riles TS. Immediate and late explantation of endovascular aortic grafts: the endovascular technologies experience. *J Vasc Surg*. 1999;29:309–316.

24. Cuypers PW, Laheij RJ, Buth J. Which factors increase the risk of conversion to open surgery following endovascular abdominal aortic aneurysm repair? The EUROSTAR collaborators. *Eur J Vasc Endovasc Surg*. 2000;20:183–189.

25. Greenberg RK, Lawrence-Brown M, Bhandari G, et al. An update of the Zenith endovascular graft for abdominal aortic aneurysms: initial implantation and mid-term follow-up data. *J Vasc Surg*. 2001;33:S157–164.

26. Chaikof EL, Lin PH, Brinkman WT, et al. Endovascular repair of abdominal aortic aneurysms: risk stratified outcomes. *Ann Surg*. 2002;235:833–841.

27. Medtronic Clinical Update on AneuRx Stent Graft published May 14, 2004.

28. Becquemin JP, Kelley L, Zubilewicz T, et al. Outcomes of secondary interventions after abdominal aortic aneurysm endovascular repair. *J Vasc Surg*. 2004;39:298–305.

New Findings In Thoracic Aortic Endovascular Technology

37

Endovascular Graft for Thoracic Aortic Aneurysms

Heitham T. Hassoun, M.D., Andy C. Chiou, M.D., M.P.H., Kristen L. Biggs, M.D., and Jon S. Matsumura, M.D.

Traditional therapy for descending thoracic aortic aneurysms mandates thoracotomy, aortic clamping, and replacement of the involved segment with a prosthetic graft. Despite significant improvements in surgical techniques and perioperative management, potential for substantial morbidity remains including hemorrhage, visceral ischemia, systemic inflammation, remote organ failure, and paraplegia.[1] Over the past several years, buoyed by the technical success of endovascular repair of infrarenal abdominal aortic aneurysms, several case series reports of endovascular stent-graft placement for descending thoracic aortic aneurysms (DTAs) have been published.[2–6] In addition, results of the first completed U.S. phase II clinical trial have demonstrated short-term safety and efficacy of this treatment modality.[7] While endovascular treatment of a variety of thoracic aortic pathologies have been reported, this chapter will focus on endovascular management of thoracic aortic aneurysms. It will include descriptions of the devices in U.S. trials, general anatomic requirements, technical aspects of the procedure, results and complications with endovascular treatment, and review a compilation of experience of eight world experts.

Thoracic Aortic Aneurysms

Pathology of the thoracic aorta is extensive and includes degenerative aneurysms, dissection, penetrating ulcers, intramural hematoma, fistula, embolizing lesions, coarctation, and traumatic injury. For the most part, device design has been focused on treatment of DTAs, which is the most common pathology treated by thoracic endografts (Table 37–1). The annual incidence of thoracic aortic aneurysms is approximately six cases per 100,000 population,[8] and the five-year survival rate of patients with untreated thoracic aneurysms ranges from 10%–50%.[9–10] Some of these patients have survived acute dissection and developed aneurysmal change in the setting of chronic dissection. This distinction is relevant because

TABLE 37-1. VARIOUS PATHOLOGY TREATED BY ENDOGRAFTS AND PERIPROCEDURAL MORTALITY

Primary aortic pathology	Percent of total cases	30-day Mortality (%)
Degenerative Aneurysm		
Descending thoracic aneurysm	64.2	4.1
Thoracoabdominal aneurysm	1.6	5.0
Posttraumatic		
Acute traumatic disruption	10.0	5.5*
Pseudoaneurysm	3.3	2.7
Dissection		
Acute dissection	7.8	9.9
Intramural hematoma with ulcer	2.2	7.2
Giant penetrating ulcer	1.0	0
Chronic dissection	8.4	3.3
Miscellaneous		
Aortic fistula	0.9	2.6
Embolizing lesion	0.3	0
Stenosis/coarctation	0.1	0

*Often due to concomitant neurologic injury

aneurysms associated with chronic dissection may respond differently to endovascular exclusion if there are numerous untreated reentry points or natural fenestrations that continue to perfuse the aneurysm.

In general, thoracic aortic aneurysms are asymptomatic. When they enlarge, they can produce symptoms by mass effects of surrounding structures or rupture. Typically, the patient may complain of pain in the chest, back, upper abdomen, or flank. Other symptoms include hoarseness, voice changes, stridor, hemoptysis, and shortness of breath from stretch of the recurrent laryngeal nerve or left bronchial compression. In contrast to conventional endoaneurysmorrhaphy, endovascular treatment does not immediately lead to decompression of the aneurysm sac, and symptoms may persist after the endograft is placed.

Diagnostic Imaging

Thoracic aortic aneurysms are usually found incidentally on radiographic studies, and most are small at the time of initial diagnosis. Smaller aneurysms have their size monitored with periodic surveillance, although wall stress is studied as a predictor of rupture risk. When the aneurysm becomes larger, symptomatic imaging objectives become focused on interventional planning. A contrast-enhanced, thin collimation, computed tomography scan of the chest is the primary imaging modality for thoracic aortic lesions. Multiple view digital subtraction angiography with a marker catheter provides complimentary measurement data in regard to lengths, and is routinely used to further evaluate the extent of thoracic aortic and branch vessel lesions in planning open and endovascular intervention. Similar to infrarenal endorepair, anatomic measurements and device selection are critical components to optimize outcomes. Other imaging modalities include magnetic resonance angiography and intravascular ultrasound, which may be particularly useful when assessing the dynamic anatomy of patients with acute dissection. Transesophageal echocardiog-

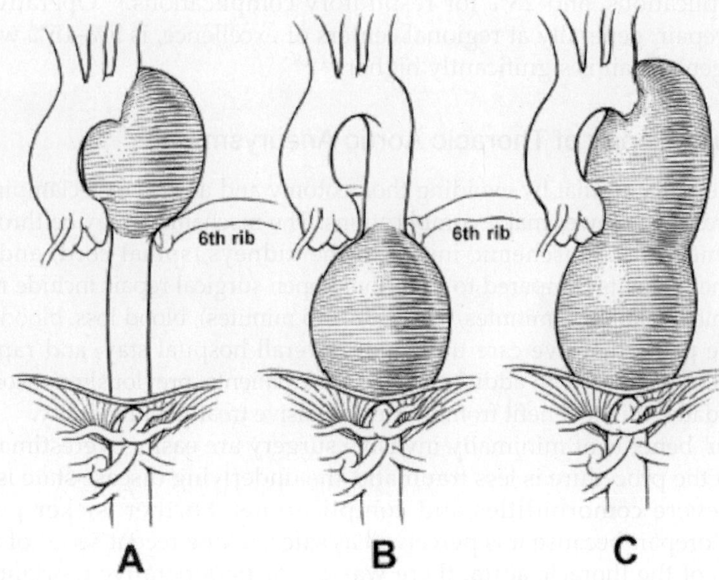

Figure 37-1. Classification of descending thoracic aortic aneurysms. Type **A** aneurysms extend from left subclavian artery to T6. Type **B** aneurysms extend from T6 to the diaphragm. Type **C** aneurysms extend from left subclavian artery to the diaphragm.

raphy with color-flow mapping has also been used to evaluate thoracic disease intraoperatively.[11–12]

Traditional Therapy

Definitive patient selection criteria for repair of DTAs are lacking, and current recommendations for surgical intervention are based on clinical judgement weighing the risk of rupture against the morbidity and mortality associated with operative repair. In general, surgical repair is considered in patients without prohibitive comorbidities when the aneurysm reaches 5–6 cm in diameter or becomes symptomatic.[10,13] DTAs have been classified according to extent (Figure 37–1). This is important since more extensive aneurysms (i.e., extent C) have worse outcomes.[14]

The objectives of surgical repair of descending thoracic aortic aneurysm are to relieve compressive symptoms and prevent rupture of the aorta. Several procedures have been utilized; the most frequent is endoaneurysmorrhaphy with the graft inclusion technique. Open surgical repair usually requires cross-clamping of the aorta and can lead to ischemic (hemodynamic and thromboembolic) complications that are manifest in end-organ failure such as myocardial infarction, stroke, paraplegia, and renal insufficiency. Adjunctive and alternative techniques to reduce aortic clamping or improve distal perfusion are repair with profound hypothermia and total circulatory arrest, left heart bypass and sequential clamping, and partial aortic clamping with multiple bypass grafts. All of these modalities still require thoracotomy, dissection, and aortic anastomosis, and are associated with significant morbidity. In one large series involving 832 patients undergoing open operations using left heart bypass, complication rates were 7% for renal failure, 3% for stroke, 5% for paraplegia, 10% for cardiac complications, and 28% for respiratory complications.[15] Operative mortality for elective repair, generally at regional centers of excellence, is 5%–15% while mortality for emergent repair is significantly higher.[14–18]

Endovascular Repair of Thoracic Aortic Aneurysms

Several studies suggest that by avoiding thoracotomy and aortic cross-clamping, endovascular repair results in fewer major complications. The mechanism may be through less operative trauma and less ischemic injury to the kidneys, spinal cord, and abdominal viscera.[19] Other benefits compared to traditional open surgical repair include reductions in procedure time (mean = 56 minutes, range: 37–215 minutes), blood loss, blood transfusion, postoperative pain, intensive care utilization, overall hospital stay, and rapid return to baseline level of activity.[7,20] In addition, higher risk patients, previously not considered operative candidates, might benefit from this less invasive treatment modality.

However, benefits of minimally invasive surgery are easily overestimated because even though the procedure is less traumatic, the underlying disease state is still associated with severe comorbidities and complications. Further, sicker patients may undergo endorepair because it is perceived as safer. In one recent series of 59 endovascular repairs of the thoracic aorta, there was a 15% perioperative mortality and there were 20% perioperative cardiac events. Of note, the cardiac event rate was 29% for patients who did not receive perioperative beta blockade versus 8% in those who did receive beta blockade. The conclusion was that the mortality associated with endovascular repair of the thoracic aorta remains significant in contrast to some earlier reports.[21]

Initial stent grafts for thoracic endovascular repair were bulky, handmade devices that were difficult to accurately deploy and required large, stiff introducer systems that limited their applicability. Nonetheless, 73% successful repair of thoracic aortic aneurysms was reported with these devices in 1994 with a reintervention rate of 20% and an early mortality rate of 9%.[22] Newer generation stent grafts have improved maneuverability, flexibility, and smaller introducer systems that have led to improved outcomes and the approval of the first endovascular device for treatment of DTAs by the U.S. Food and Drug Administration (FDA).[7]

Current patient anatomical criteria for endovascular devices are variable. There are several relative contraindications for endovascular stenting that include the inability to obtain vascular access, thoracic aortic tortuosity, and poor quality or very short landing zones either proximally or distally. Most devices require iliofemoral access of greater than 8mm to accommodate the introducer systems, aortic arch angulation less than 90° with limited tortuosity, and proximal and distal landing zones that are 20 to 30 mm in length.[7,23-24] Poor iliofemoral access can be bypassed with iliac conduits (Figure 37–2).

Induced hypotension, cardiac asystole, and transvenous balloon occlusion of the right atrium to create partial inflow occlusion have been used to subdue the strong flow dynamics of the proximal thoracic aorta to reduce migration during device deployment.[25] Most physicians now rarely use these techniques with the advent of newer generation devices and improved deployment systems. One group reported that only three of 67 patients required systemic hypotension during stent deployment.[25] Another group completed 73 out of 74 of their thoracic stent grafts under general anesthesia without significantly lowering any heart rates or systolic blood pressures during stent deployment.[20]

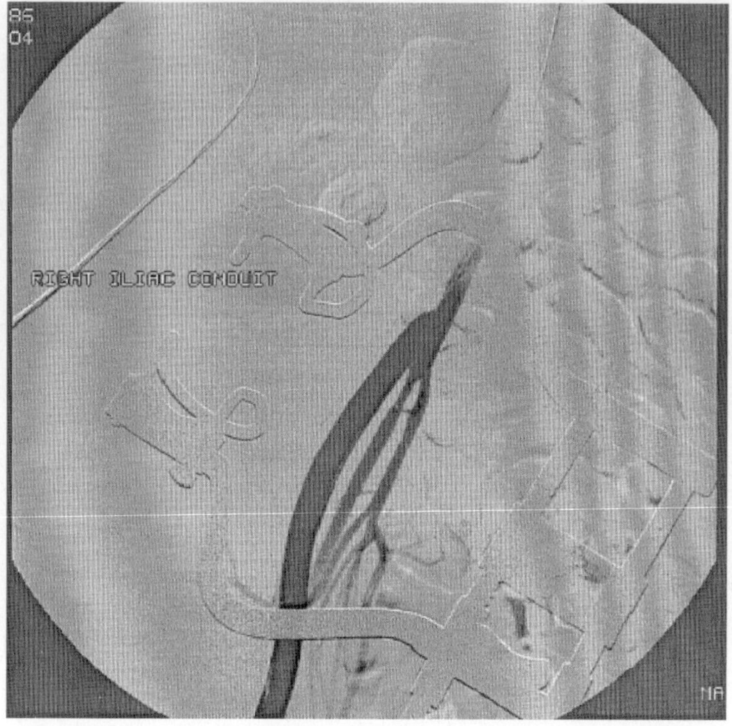

Figure 37-2. Angiogram of a 10 mm PTFE iliac conduit anastamosed to the right common iliac artery enabling advancement of a 24-F sheath into the thoracic aorta.

Thoracic Aortic Zones of the Proximal Neck

Five different anatomic zones of the aortic arch and descending thoracic aorta have been described that are helpful to consider when evalutating patients for thoracic endorepair (Figure 37–3). Thoracic aortic disease that occurs within specific zones may require specific adjunctive procedures to obtain adequate proximal landing areas for sealing and fixation. Zone 0 refers to the ascending aorta, which includes the innominate artery. Zone 1 involves the portion of the aortic arch that provides the takeoff for the left common carotid artery. Zone 2 involves the portion of the aortic arch that includes the left subclavian artery origin. Zone 3 is located distal to the left subclavian artery, within the curved portion of the arch. Zone 4 disease involves the straight portion of the descending thoracic aorta.

The extent of proximal disease correlates with the complexity of the endovascular solution. In cases only involving zone 4, or the straight portion of the descending thoracic aorta, additional surgical procedures are usually not necessary. If disease involves zone 3, an adequate landing zone for proximal fixation of the device may approach or cover the origin to the left subclavian artery. Zone 2 disease, by definition, requires subclavian coverage. Although at times sufficient collateralization may obviate the need for surgery, patients with symptoms of left upper extremity ischemia will need an adjunctive procedure that may be done before or after endovascular coverage. In addition, patients with a dominant left vertebral artery or left internal mammary artery (LIMA) bypass graft will need an adjunctive procedure. Restoration of blood flow to the left subclavian artery can be achieved by a kissing stent, left subclavian transposition, or a left carotid-subclavian bypass. Thoracic endograft placement for

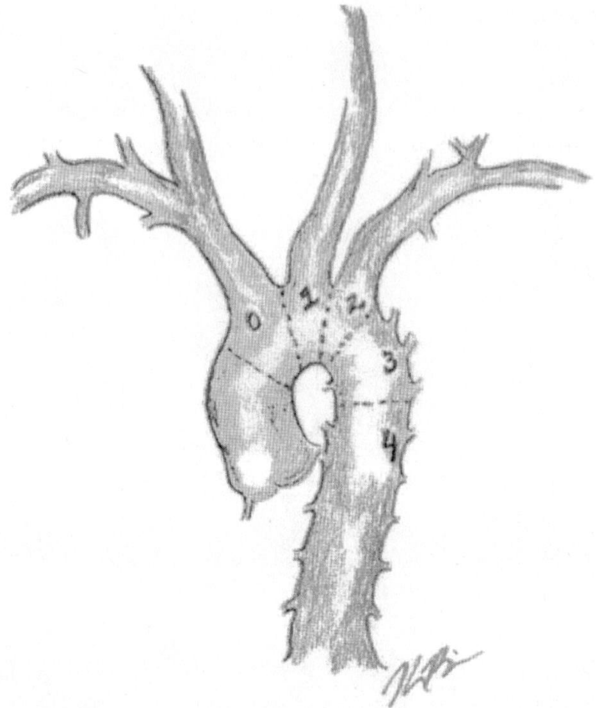

Figure 37-3. Thoracic aorta proximal landing zones.

zone 1 and 0 disease will require coverage of the left common carotid and innominate arteries, respectively. Surgical alternatives for restoring blood flow can involve a variety of creative solutions.

PROBLEMS AND COMPLICATIONS

Complications resulting from thoracic endograft placement include complications common to infrarenal aortic endovascular repair, plus increased concern for specific problems of (1) paraplegia, (2) stroke, (3) ischemia from occlusion of aortic branch vessels, (4) dissection or rupture of access vessel, and (5) device failure, fracture, or migration.

Neurologic Injury

Endovascular exclusion of the thoracic aorta, including coverage of the intercostal arteries, may lead to transient neurologic deficits or permanent paraplegia. Cerebrospinal fluid (CSF) drainage is often used as a protective mechanism during open surgical repair because CSF pressure increases during aortic cross-clamping, and reduction of CSF pressure improves spinal perfusion pressure. A randomized clinical trial showed benefit of drainage to a pressure threshold during open repair, with an 80% reduction in the relative risk of postoperative neurologic deficits.[26] However, CSF drainage can result in complications and its role in patients treated with endoluminal thoracic stent grafts is still unknown. One large series of 103 patients with thoracic aortic aneurysms treated with stent grafts reported only three cases (2.9%) of paraplegia.[27] Recent studies have also found a similarly low incidence of paraplegia.[11,19-20,24] Fattori et al. had no cases of paraplegia arise in their group of 70 patients, despite covering the entire descending thoracic aorta in 21 cases.[11]

Stroke is one complication that may be more frequent in endovascular repair compared to open repair. Coexistent arch/carotid disease, manipulation of stiff wire guides and long leading parts of deployment systems, coverage of arch vessels, and air embolism are potential etiologies of stroke. Better understanding and recognition of these issues should result in modified device design and techniques to reduce stroke rates.

Endoleak

It is interesting that with thoracic endografts, the rate of endoleak seems to be lower when compared with infrarenal endorepair. Endoleak rate may be further reduced by increasing landing zone distance to 20 mm from 10 mm.[20] In general, most groups have reported endoleak rates of 7% to 10%.[7,11,20,24] Late neck dilation and subsequent graft migration is rare, similar to endovascular repair of infrarenal aortic aneurysms. Nevertheless, this is an etiology of late endoleak after endovascular DTA repair and that should be monitored.

Dissection and Arterial Perforation

One major problem with thoracic devices is the larger and often stiff introducer sheath required for their deployment. Iliac artery dissection, perforation, and even avulsion can occur and lead to fatal hemorrhage. More liberal use of conduits, a high index of suspicion, and rapid treatment may reduce the mortality of these events. Another unsuspected late problem with thoracic endovascular repair is the development of aortic dissection or frank perforation of the aorta at the proximal end of the endograft. This has been a catastrophic late complication, but fortunately it appears to be uncommon. Although some investigators suspect this late proximal arterial injury is more frequent with some device features, direct rigorous comparison of rates has not been performed.

Device Failure

The second generation of thoracic stent grafts, although an improvement from earlier "homemade" devices, still have had shortcomings. Stent fracture related to the considerably higher thoracic aortic fatigue forces, migration due to poor proximal, intercomponent, distal fixation, and mechanical device failures such as failure to deploy are some of the problems that have occurred.

In one series of 84 patients receiving thoracic stent grafts under U.S. FDA-approved clinical trials, 11 patients (13%) were found to have stent fracture at a mean of 20 months of follow-up.[23] Nine of these patients did not have an associated endoleak and were being followed with CT scans.

Mortality

In initial reports, mortality rates for endovascular repair of thoracic aortic disease are similar or less than with open repair. The 30-day mortality for electively placed endografts in one study was as low as 2% (one of 42 patients).[19] In this series, the one cause of death was mesenteric ischemia from embolization via the celiac axis. The 30-day mortality for urgent or emergently placed thoracic endografts in the same study was 16% (four of 25 patients).

The causes of death were perioperative myocardial infarction in two patients, on-table aortic rupture in one patient, and rupture of an unrecognized false aneurysm of the distal thoracic aorta in one patient. Other authors report mortality rates between 6% and 10%.[20,23]

Device Durability

The long-term device durability rate of thoracic endografts is unknown. As described above, reports are surfacing regarding stent fracture and material fatigue in the second generation of stent grafts. Most studies have relatively short reported patient follow up from one to 72 months with a mean of about two years.[11,19,24]

CLINICAL TRIALS

There is one FDA-approved device and three thoracic stent grafts currently in clinical trials in the United States. The Gore Thoracic Aortic Graft (TAG) endoprosthesis (W. L. Gore & Associates, Flagstaff, Arizona) is made of a composite of expanded polytetra-fluoroethylene (ePTFE) graft and a self-expanding nitinol support structure that is available in diameters of 26–40 mm (Figure 37–4). A multicenter prospective nonrandomized phase II study enrolled subjects at 17 sites in the United States between September 1999 and May 2001. Initial results of this study in 139 patients who under-went successful implantation of the device were published in January 2005.[7] At a mean follow-up of two years, aneurysm-related and overall survival were 97% and 75%, respectively. It is currently the only commercially available thoracic stent graft approved for treatment of DTAs in the United States.

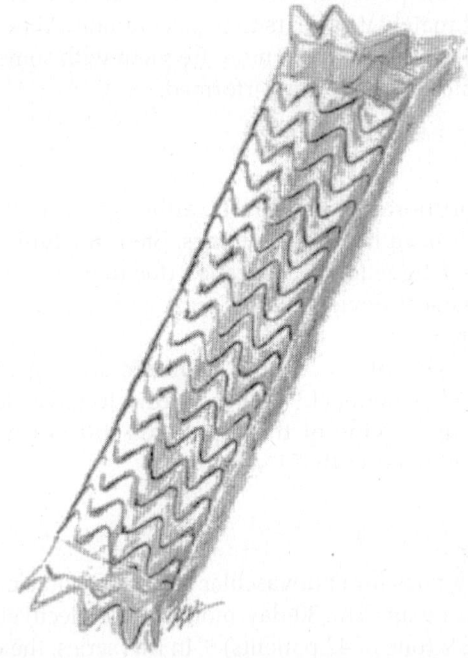

Figure 37-4. Gore TAG endoprosthesis. This version has covered flares and sealing cuffs on the ends, and no longitudinal spines.

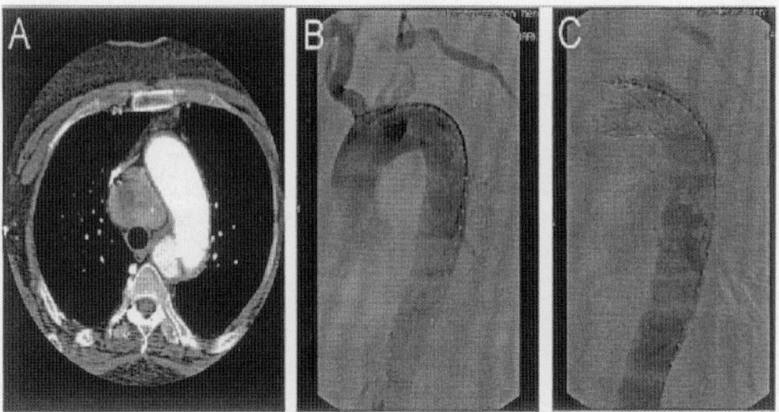

Figure 37-5. A. Axial CT scan image of an extent A DTA with chronic dissection. B. Perioperative angiogram in LAO projection does not reveal the aneurysm but is ideal imaging for graft placement. Note the transposed LSA.

Figure 37–5 depicts the use of a TAG device to treat an aneurysm of the proximal descending thoracic aorta.

The Talent (Medtronic AVE, Santa Rosa, California) thoracic stent graft is a nitinol/polyester endograft (Figure 37–6). This device has been approved for more than five years in Europe and has been implanted in more than 6,000 patients worldwide. The VALOR (Evaluation of the Safety and Efficacy of the Medtronic Vascular Talent Thoracic Stent Graft System for the Treatment of Thoracic Aortic Aneurysms) study began enrolling patients in the United States in November 2003. This trial is being conducted at 35 sites and involves 500 patients. Figure 37–7 depicts pre- and postoperative CT scan images of an extent C DTA in a patient treated with a Talent endograft.

The Zenith TX2 (Cook Incorporated, Bloomington, Indiana) thoracic endovascular graft is also approved for commercial distribution outside the United States (Figure 37–8). This trial compares the outcomes of patients treated with standard operative approach versus endovascular therapy with the Zenith TX2 endograft. The first of these grafts was placed in the trial in March 2004, and the study should complete enrollment

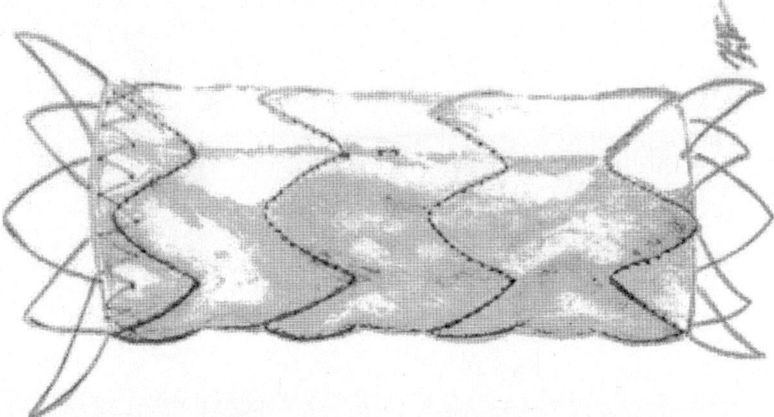

Figure 37-6. Medtronic Talent endograft. There are bare wire flares on the ends.

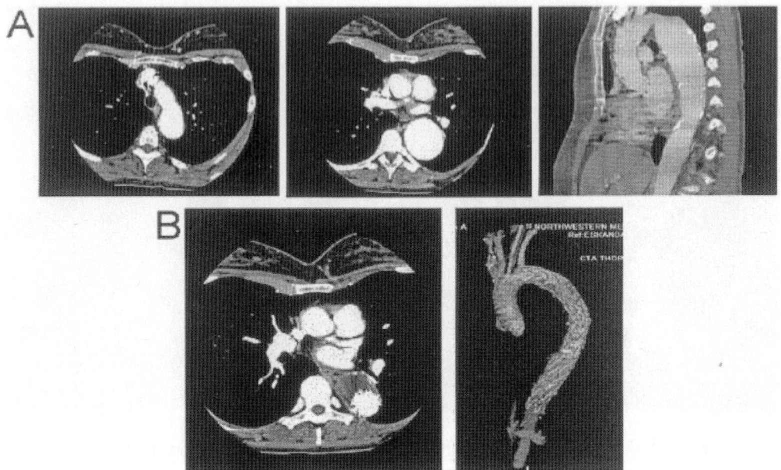

Figure 37-7. A. Axial and sagital CT scan images of an extent C DTA. B. Axial and 3-D-reconstruction images after aneurysm exclusion with a Talent endograft.

of up to 220 patients by the end of 2005. Figure 37–9 depicts pre- and postoperative CT scan images of an extent B DTA treated with a Zenith TX2 endograft.

Worldwide Clinical Review

Peer-reviewed scientific publications are the gold standard of evidence for medical decision making. However, in rapidly emerging technologies, early experiences are dominated by prototype devices, single site small experiences, and initial learning periods. Data from U.S. clinical trials are useful because of the well-defined protocol, regulatory oversight, and generally more diligent follow-up and core lab review. However, practical clinical use often does not match the rigid entry criteria of these studies, and industry-sponsored trials focus on the sponsor's contemporary device version. In order to get a grasp of the general clinical practice in thoracic endografts, a survey was conducted during personal visits with eight physicians from leading thoracic endovascular centers of excellence around the world.[28] Table 37–2 lists the primary investigators who were interviewed and their respec-

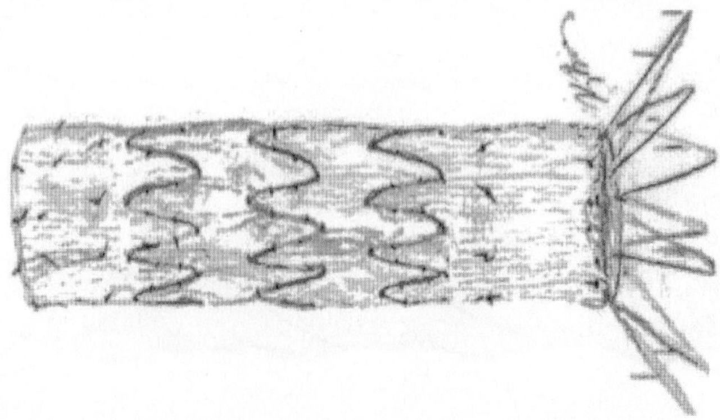

Figure 37-8. Zenith TX2 endovascular graft. A two-piece graft is depicted with large barbs on the ends. The caudal end has a bare stent.

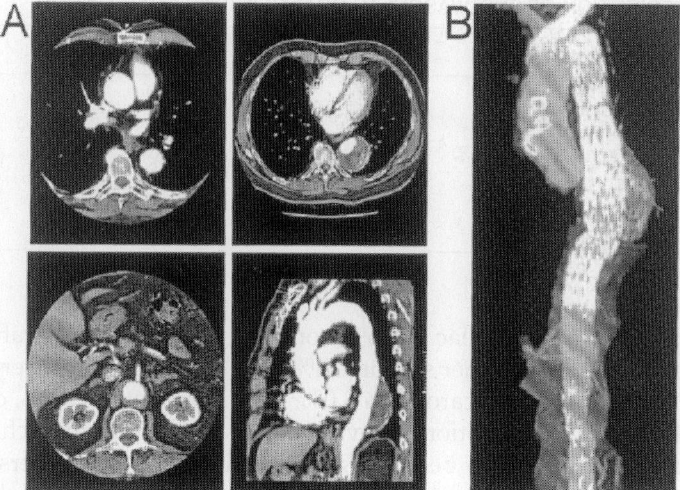

Figure 37-9. A. Axial and sagital CT scan images of an extent B DTA. **B.** 3-D-reconstrction CT scan images after aneurysm exclusion with a Zenith TX2 endograft.

tive medical centers. This pooled data of 1,180 patients provides reflections on a large series of patients from the perspectives of experts in the field. Weaknesses of this compilation are the lack of uniformity in surveillance protocols, definitions, follow-up intervals, and compliance, and overlap with existing publications.

Table 37–1 summarizes the types of thoracic pathology that have been treated and the 30-day mortality in each of these categories. It is the majority impression that endovascular treatment is an equivalent or better therapy compared to conventional treatment in each of these categories except for thoracoabdominal aneurysm, chronic dissection, and stenosis where there was disagreement or it was felt to be unknown. This is conditional on the patient having suitable anatomy for endorepair. The majority of patients (64.2%) have been treated for degenerative descending thoracic aortic aneurysms. A wide variety of endografts have been used for treatment (Table 37–3).

Most patients (70.3%) have been treated in an operating room, and 49.2% used fixed unit fluoroscopy units. Intravascular ultrasound was used in 12%, and transesophageal echocardiography in 38.1%. Primary access was in the femoral artery in

TABLE 37-2. SELECTED PHYSICIANS AND INSTITUTIONS BY REPORTED TOTAL THORACIC ENDOGRAFT VOLUME.

Physician	Location
Shin Ishimaru, M.D.	Tokyo Medical University
Michael Dake, M.D.	Stanford University Medical School
Roy Greenberg, M.D.	Cleveland Clinic
Ludger Sunder-Plassman, M.D.	University of Ulm
Rodney White, M.D.	University of California, Los Angeles-Harbor
Geoffrey White, M.D.	University of Sydney
Takao Ohki, M.D.	Montefiore Medical Center
Michael Laurence-Brown, M.D.	Perth University

TABLE 37-3. DISTRIBUTION OF ENDOVASCULAR GRAFTS IN THIS COMPILATION

Endograft	Frequency
Homemade	53.6
TAG	19.0
Zenith	11.5
Talent	10.8
Other	5.1

84.4% (percutaneous in 1.1%), iliac in 7.5%, conduit or aortofemoral graft limb in 6.5%, infrarenal aorta in 1.1%, and other sites in 0.4%. The left subclavian artery was covered in 29.8%, and the left common carotid in 8.0%, the innominate in 3.7%, celiac artery in 3.1%, and SMA in 0.8%. The option to revascularize these major branches is exercised at different rates, and seems to be undergoing evolution. Most centers revascularize the carotid, innominate, and visceral arteries when they are occasionally covered. In contrast, revascularization is performed before or concurrently with endorepair in only 36.7% of patients who have coverage of the left subclavian artery. Many centers perform selective subclavian revascularization when there is diseased or hypoplastic right vertebral arteries or fistulas/reconstructions based on left subclavian branches. The majority of patients is managed expectantly, and in the infrequent scenario when symptoms develop after left subclavian coverage, delayed revascularization can be performed.

Spinal cord drainage was used routinely in 1.0% and selectively in 6.8% of patients with extensive descending aortic coverage or history of AAA. Adenosine (2.1%) and high-dose beta blocker (0.1%) were used rarely to arrest or slow the heart for deployment. The 30-day morbidity rates are stroke in 2.8%, renal failure in 1.6%, and paraplegia in 2.5%. Of note, 43% of the paraplegia complications were delayed in onset, and some of these patients respond favorably to spinal cord drainage.

Later outcomes are best described by time-dependent estimates, and are not precisely combinable because of unequal or unknown individual lengths of follow-up. Nevertheless, general estimates are useful to gauge the emerging technology. Endoleak was noted in 10.5% of patients, sac expansion in 4.0%, proximal neck dilation or dissection in 2.7%, distal neck dilation in 2.1%, intercomponent migration in 1.7%, proximal migration in 1.3%, distal migration in 0.4%, asymptomatic device failure such as wire fracture in 6.3%, symptomatic device failure in 0.1%, and aneurysm rupture in 0.9%.

CONCLUSION

The treatment of thoracic aortic disease is rapidly evolving. Endovascular repair is now an available alternative to the traditional, open surgical approach, and newer devices are being developed and evaluated in clinical trials. While mortality rates for open surgical repair of the thoracic aorta have decreased with experience, published reports of thoracic aortic endografts demonstrate that endovascular repair is a less invasive option with lower perioperative morbidity and mortality rates. Midterm data from several series are remarkable for promising overall results, but also some rare but striking late failures.

Several engineering advancements are being pursued to address shortcomings in earlier devices for thoracic endorepair. These include endografts that conform to the individual aortic anatomy, more flexible and accurate delivery systems, more robust construction to accommodate higher thoracic aortic forces, and mechanisms to treat pathology close to or involving the aortic arch and visceral sidebranches. As these technologies mature, it is possible that endovascular therapy will become the preferred initial therapy for most thoracic aortic diseases.

REFERENCES

1. Harward TR, Welborn MB 3rd, Martin TD, et al. Visceral ischemia and organ dysfunction after thoracoabdominal aortic aneurysm repair. A clinical and cost analysis. *Ann Surg.* 1996;223:729–734.
2. Najibi S, Terramani TT, Weiss VJ, et al. Endoluminal versus open treatment of descending thoracic aortic aneurysms. *J Vasc Surg.* 2002;36:732–737.
3. Cambria RP, Brewster DC, Lauterbach SR, et al. Evolving experience with thoracic aortic stent graft repair. *J Vasc Surg.* 2002;35:1129–1136.
4. Ellozy SH, Carroccio A, Minor M, et al. Challenges of endovascular tube graft repair of thoracic aortic aneurysm: midterm follow-up and lessons learned. *J Vasc Surg.* 2003;38: 676–683.
5. Grabenwoger M, Hutschala D, Ehrlich MP, et al. Thoracic aortic aneurysms: treatment with endovascular self-expandable stent grafts. *Ann Thorac Surg.* 2000;69:441–445.
6. Taylor PR, Gaines PA, McGuinness CL, et al. Thoracic aortic stent grafts - early experience from two centres using commercially available devices. *Eur J Vasc Endovasc Surg.* 2001;22: 70–76.
7. Makaroun MS, Dillavou ED, Kee ST, et al. Endovascular treatment of thoracic aortic aneurysms: results of the phase II multicenter trial of the GORE TAG thoracic endoprosthesis. *J Vasc Surg.* 2005;41:1–9.
8. Bickerstaff LK, Pairolero PC, Hollier LH et al. Thoracic Aortic Aneurysms: A Population-Based Study. *Surgery* 1982;92:1103.
9. Pate JW, Richardson RL, Eastridge CE. Acute Aortic Dissections. *Am Surg.* 1976;42:395.
10. Clouse WD, Hallett JW, Schaff HV, et al. Improved prognosis of thoracic aortic aneurysms: a population-based study. *JAMA.* 1998;280:1926–1929.
11. Fattori R, Napoli G, Lovato L, et al. Descending Thoracic Aortic Diseases: Stent Graft Repair. *Radiology.* 2003;229:176–183.
12. Criado E, Wall P, Lucas P, et al. Transesophageal Echo Guided Endovascular Exclusion of Thoracic Aortic Mobile Thrombi. *J Vasc Surg.* 2004;39:238–242.
13. Davies RR, Goldstein LJ, Coady MA, et al. Yearly rupture or dissection rates for thoracic aortic aneurysms; simple prediction based on size. *Ann Thorac Surg.* 2002;73:17–28.
14. Estrera AL, Rubenstein FS, Miller CC 3rd, et al. Descending thoracic aortic aneurysm: surgical approach and treatment using the adjuncts cerebrospinal fluid drainage and distal aortic perfusion. *Ann Thorac Surg.* 2001;72:481–486.
15. Svensson LG, Crawford ES, Hess KR, et al. Variables Predictive of Outcome in 832 Patients Undergoing Repairs of the Descending Thoracic Aorta. *Chest.* 1993;104:1248–1253.
16. Crawford ES, Hess KR, Cohen ES, et al. Ruptured aneurysm of the descending thoracic and thoracoabdominal aorta. *Ann Surg.* 1991;213:417–426.
17. Kouchoukos NT, Daily BB, Rokkas CK, et al. Hypothermic bypass and circulatory arrest for operations on the descending thoracic aorta and thoracoabdominal aorta. *Ann Thorac Surg.* 1995;60:67–77.
18. Estrera AL, Miller CC, Huynh TT, et al. Neurologic outcome after thoracic and thoracoabdominal aortic aneurysm repair. *Ann Thorac Surg.* 2001;72:1225–1231

19. Bell RE, Taylor PR, Aukett M, et al. Midterm Results for Second Generation Thoracic Stent Grafts. *Brit J Surgery*. 2003;90:811–817.

20. Orend KH, Scharrer-Pamler R, Kapfer X, et al. Endovascular Treatment in Diseases of the Descending Thoracic Aorta: Six Year Results of a Single Center. *J Vasc Surg*. 2003; 37:91–99.

21. Bui H, Haukoos J, Donayre C, et al. *Ann Vasc Surg*. 2004; 18(1):22–25.

22. Dake MD, Miller DC, Semba CP, et al. Transluminal Placement of Endovascular Stent Grafts for the Treatment of Descending Thoracic Aortic Aneurysms. *N Engl J Med*. 1994; 331:1729–1734.

23. Ellozy SH, Carroccio A, Minor M, et al. Challenges of Endovascular Tube Graft Repair of Thoracic Aortic Aneurysm: Midterm Follow Up and Lessens Learned. *J Vasc Surg*. 2003; 38: 676–683.

24. Criado, FJ, Clark NS, Barnatan MF. Stent graft repair in the aortic arch and descending thoracic aorta: a 4-year experience. *J Vasc Surg*. 2002;36:1121–1128.

25. Marty B, Morales CC, Tozzi P, et al. Partial Inflow Occlusion Facilitates Accurate Deployment of Thoracic Aortic Endografts. *J Endovasc Ther*. 2004;11(2):175–179.

26. Coselli JS, LeMaire SA, Koksoy C, et al. Cerebrospinal fluid drainage reduces paraplegia after thoracoabdominal aortic aneurysm repair: Results of a randomized clinical trial. *J Vasc Surg*. 2002;35:631–639.

27. Mitchell RS, Miller DC, Dake MD, et al. Thoracic aortic aneurysm repair with an endovascular stent graft: the "first generation." *Ann Thorac Surg*. 1999;67:1971–1974.

28. Chiou AC, Biggs KL, Matsumura JS. Update on thoracic aortic endograft. In: Pearce WH, Matsumura JS, Yao JST, eds. *Trends in Vascular Surgery*, Evanston: Greenwood Academic; 2005:325–336.

38

Clinical Trial Review for Thoracic Endovascular Aortic Repair

Jon S. Matsumura, M.D.

Thoracic endovascular aortic repair (TEVAR) has emerged as an alternative to traditional open surgical therapy for descending thoracic aortic aneurysm. Open repair techniques have improved, but require thoracotomy, aortic clamping, and replacement of the involved segment with a prosthetic graft, and there is substantial attendant morbidity, including visceral ischemia and the dreaded risk of paraplegia.[1,2] Data on TEVAR were initially limited to case series reports that demonstrated improving results as iterations of device generations progressed.[3-14] Recently, several multicenter trials have completed enrollment and their results are anxiously awaited.[15-18] This chapter will focus on available updates from these clinical trials and a pooled report of worldwide experience that was published in 2006.[19]

THORACIC AORTIC PATHOLOGY

The thoracic aorta is subject to many diseases including aneurysmal degeneration (DTA), dissection, fistula, embolizing lesions, stenosis, and traumatic injury. Most TEVAR clinical trials are focused on treatment of DTAs, and it is the most common pathology treated with thoracic endografts (Table 38–1). DTA has an annual incidence of about six cases per 100,000 of the population.[20]

PREOPERATIVE IMAGING

Contrast-enhanced, multidetector computed tomography (CT) is the primary imaging modality for thoracic aortic lesions. Digital subtraction angiography with a marker catheter provides complimentary length measurements, evaluation of aortic branch

TABLE 38-1. PATHOLOGY TREATED BY TEVAR AND PERIPROCEDURAL MORTALITY

Primary aortic pathology	Percent of total cases	Perioperative Mortality (%)
Degenerative Aneurysm		
Descending thoracic aneurysm	64.2	4.1
Thoracoabdominal aneurysm	1.6	5.0
Posttraumatic		
Acute traumatic disruption	10.0	5.5
Pseudoaneurysm	3.3	2.7
Dissection		
Acute dissection	7.8	9.9
Intramural hematoma with ulcer	2.2	7.2
Giant penetrating ulcer	1.0	0
Chronic dissection	8.4	3.3
Miscellaneous		
Aortic fistula	0.9	2.6
Embolizing lesion	0.3	0
Stenosis/coarctation	0.1	0

Adapted from: Hassoun HT, Chiou AC, Biggs KL, Matsumura JS. Endovascular graft for thoracic aortic aneurysms. In: Pearce WH, Matsumura JS, Yao JST, (eds). *Trends in Vascular Surgery.* Evanston, IL: Greenwood Academic; 2005:329-342.

vessel anatomy, and more information for access planning. Assessment of collateral pathways of the spinal cord such as the vertebral and hypogastric arteries can be helpful. Similar to infrarenal endovascular repair, neck measurements and device selection are critical components to optimize outcomes. Other imaging modalities include magnetic resonance angiography and intravascular ultrasound, which may be particularly useful when assessing the dynamic anatomy of patients with acute dissection. Transesophageal echocardiography is frequently used to supplement intraoperative fluoroscopic imaging.[19,21-22]

OPEN REPAIR

Centers of excellence in open thoracic aortic repair demonstrate 5% to 15% mortality for elective repair and much higher rates for emergent repair.[23-27] A large series of 832 patients with open repair using left heart bypass showed complication rates of 7% for renal failure, 3% for stroke, 5% for paraplegia, 10% for cardiac complications, and 28% for respiratory problems.[24] Clearly, improvement is possible in this therapy even though tertiary centers have achieved progressively better results.

ENDOVASCULAR REPAIR OF THORACIC AORTIC ANEURYSMS

In last year's book, several publications from single centers were reviewed in detail with focus on techniques for deployment and specific outcome measurements of TEVAR.[28] Improved recovery times, less blood loss, and fewer short-term complications are well documented, although late problems like endoleak, dissection, and device failure are also evident. Many studies have short patient follow-up, and it is clear from trials of infrarenal endovascular repair that undiscovered issues are likely to arise in later years.

U.S. CLINICAL TRIALS

Currently, there is one TEVAR device approved by the U.S. Food and Drug Administration (FDA) for treatment of DTA. This is the Thoracic Aortic Graft (TAG) endoprosthesis (W. L. Gore & Associates, Flagstaff, Arizona), which is made of an expanded polytetrafluoroethylene (ePTFE) graft and a self-expanding nitinol support structure. The graft material contains a layer of high density, low permeability film, and is attached with a sutureless composite attachment process. It is commercially available in diameters of 26 to 40 mm (Figure 38–1) and lengths of up to 20 cm. Larger size TAG grafts are in investigational device evaluation clinical trials.

The FDA approval was based on a pivotal, multicenter, prospective, nonrandomized trial at 17 sites between September 1999 and May 2001, and a later confirmatory trial of a modified device discussed below. Initial results of TEVAR subjects who underwent successful implantation of the device were published in 2005.[15] At a mean follow-up of two years, overall survival was 75%, indicating a fairly ill population, and the need for controlled comparisons. Figure 38–2 depicts the use of a TAG device to treat an aneurysm of the proximal descending thoracic aorta.

Longer-term, controlled data on TAG were presented this year.[16] Ninety-four open surgical controls and 140 TEVAR patients were compared out to four years. Freedom from any major adverse event is 21% in controls and 48% with TEVAR

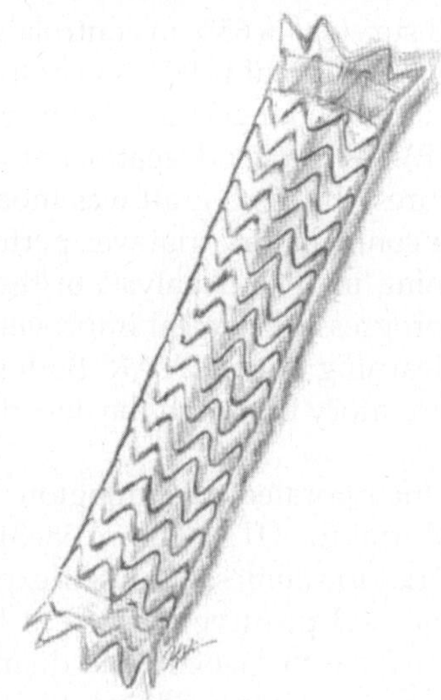

Figure 38-1. TAG endoprosthesis. The current commercial version has covered flares and sealing cuffs on the ends and no longitudinal spines. Reprinted with permission: Hassoun HT, Chiou AC, Biggs KL, Matsumura JS. Endovascular graft for thoracic aortic aneurysms. In: Pearce WH, Matsumura JS, Yao JST, (eds). *Trends in Vascular Surgery*. Evanston, IL: Greenwood Academic; 2005:329-342.

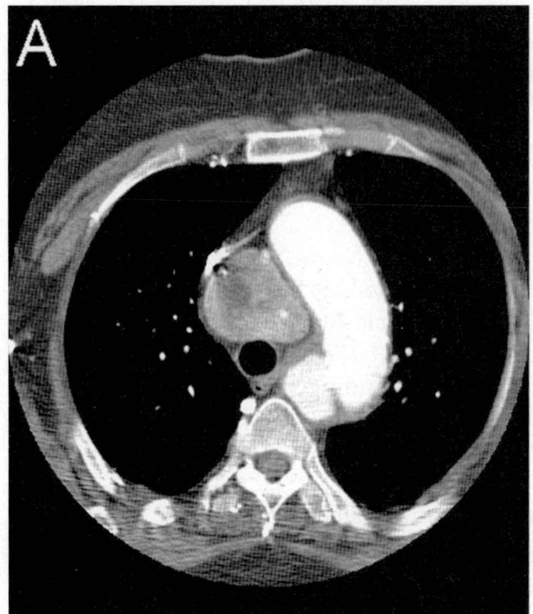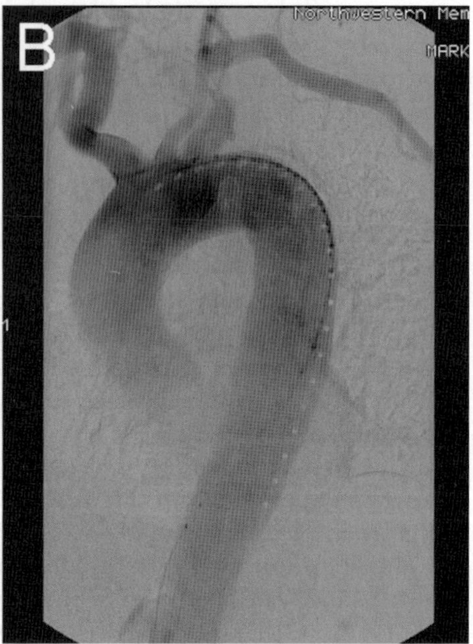

Figure 38-2. (A) Axial CT scan image of an extent A DTA with chronic dissection. **(B)** Perioperative angiogram in left anterior oblique projection is the ideal gantry angle for TAG placement near major side branches. Note the left subclavian-carotid transposition. Reprinted with permission: Hassoun HT, Chiou AC, Biggs KL, Matsumura JS. Endovascular graft for thoracic aortic aneurysms. In: Pearce WH, Matsumura JS, Yao JST, (eds). *Trends in Vascular Surgery*. Evanston, IL: Greenwood Academic; 2005:329-342.

($P<.001$ by logrank). Overall survival is 65% in controls and 70% with TEVAR ($P = .398$ by logrank). Aneurysm-related survival is 90% in controls and 98% with TEVAR ($P = .011$ by logrank). These data are the longest available controlled data from FDA trials, and strongly support that TEVAR is a good treatment for anatomically suitable DTA.

Because of fatigue fractures, the TAG graft was modified to remove the longitudinal deployment spine and a confirmatory trial was performed. Fifty-one patients were enrolled in this trial beginning in 2003. Analysis of these trials with minimal device changes demonstrates the progressive clinical improvement attained by investigators over the first few years of learning with TEVAR. Both safety and efficacy were superior in the more recent confirmatory trial with the new device compared to the original TAG in short-term follow-up.

The Zenith TX2 (Cook Incorporated, Bloomington, Indiana) thoracic endograft is being evaluated in a pivotal trial for DTA (Figure 38–3). It is composed of a standard surgical polyester graft sutured to stainless steel self-expanding stents. This device has a staged deployment system and positive fixation at the proximal and distal ends. Device lengths range from 16.2 cm to 36.4 cm, and diameters range from 28 mm to 42 mm. The trial also is a controlled, nonrandomized design that compares patients treated with standard operative approach versus endovascular therapy with the TX2. The first patient was enrolled in March 2004, and the study has completed enrollment this year and is in the follow-up stages. Figure 38–4 depicts pre- and postdeployment images of an extent B DTA treated with a TX2 endograft.

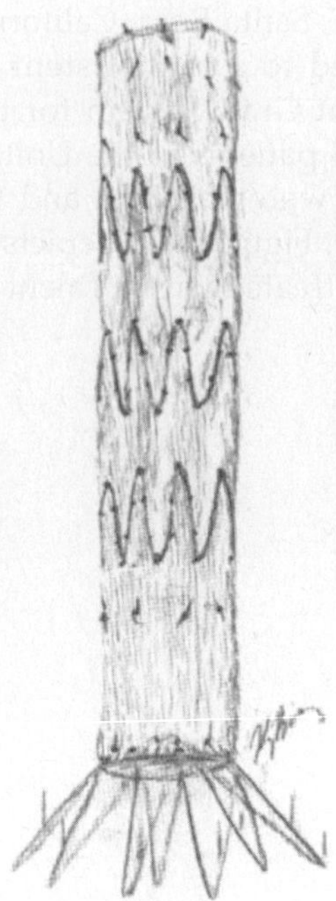

Figure 38-3. Zenith TX2 endovascular graft. A two-piece graft is shown with barbs on the ends, and the caudal end has a bare stent. Reprinted with permission, Hassoun HT, Chiou AC, Biggs KL, Matsumura JS. Endovascular graft for thoracic aortic aneurysms. In: Pearce WH, Matsumura JS, Yao JST, (eds). *Trends in Vascular Surgery*. Evanston, IL: Greenwood Academic; 2005:329-342.

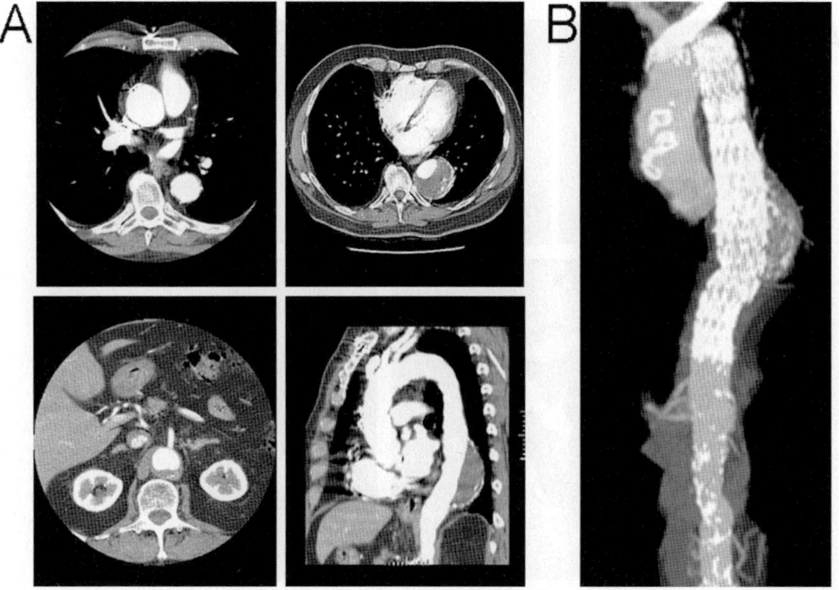

Figure 38-4. (A) Axial and sagital images of an extent B DTA. **(B)** 3-D reconstrction CT scan images after aneurysm exclusion with a TX2. Reprinted with permission: Hassoun HT, Chiou AC, Biggs KL, Matsumura JS. Endovascular graft for thoracic aortic aneurysms. In: Pearce WH, Matsumura JS, Yao JST, (eds). *Trends in Vascular Surgery*. Evanston, IL: Greenwood Academic; 2005:329-342.

The Talent (Medtronic AVE, Santa Rosa, California) thoracic stent graft is made of thin LP polyester graft sutured to a nitinol stent (Figure 38–5). The VALOR trial (Vascular Talent Thoracic Stent Graft System for the Treatment of Thoracic Aortic Aneurysms) study enrolled 394 patients in the United States from November 2003 to June 2005. No control subjects were enrolled, and the TEVAR subjects will be compared to others in the literature. Figure 38–6 depicts pre- and postdeployment images of an extent C DTA in a patient treated with a Talent endograft.

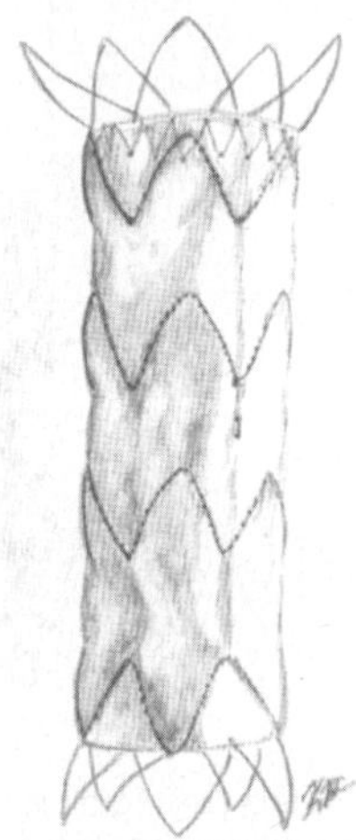

Figure 38-5. Talent endograft with bare nitinol wire flares on the ends. Reprinted with permission: Hassoun HT, Chiou AC, Biggs KL, Matsumura JS. Endovascular graft for thoracic aortic aneurysms. In: Pearce WH, Matsumura JS, Yao JST, (eds). *Trends in Vascular Surgery*. Evanston, IL: Greenwood Academic; 2005:329-342.

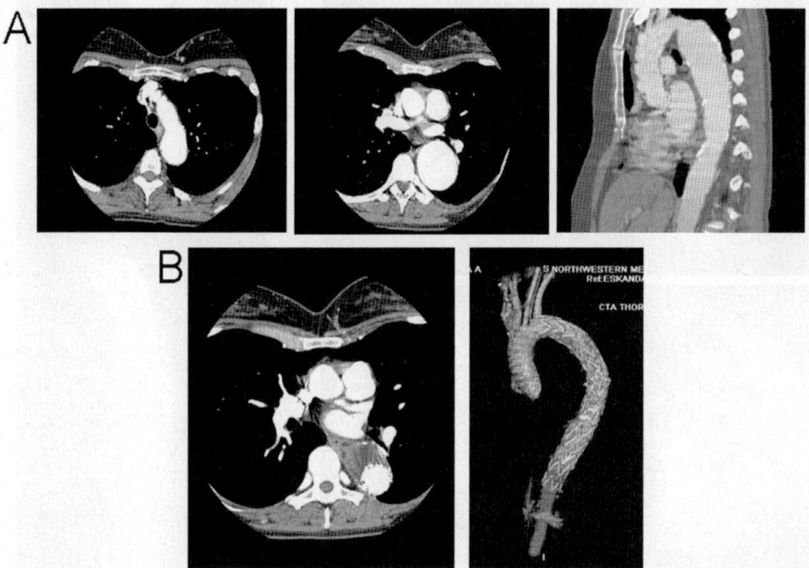

Figure 38-6. (A) Axial and sagital CT scan images of an extent C DTA. **(B)** Axial and 3-D reconstruction images after aneurysm exclusion with a Talent. Reprinted with permission: Hassoun HT, Chiou AC, Biggs KL, Matsumura JS. Endovascular graft for thoracic aortic aneurysms. In: Pearce WH, Matsumura JS, Yao JST, (eds). *Trends in Vascular Surgery*. Evanston, IL: Greenwood Academic; 2005:329-342.

The VALOR trial has multiple arms, and one-year data (the primary safety and efficacy endpoint) on the pivotal standard risk group of 144 patients are not yet available. A high-risk arm of 137 nonsurgical subjects has been presented.[18] Thirty-day mortality was 7.3%, stroke 7%, and paraplegia 1%. With median follow-up of eight months, the actuarial 12-month mortality was 25%. This high-risk cohort outcome is reminiscent of EVAR 2 Trial, and it may be that no intervention is best for the truly "unfit" patient.[29]

The Talent device had short components (12.5 cm), and treatment of longer lesions required either a larger initial sheath or multiple passages by each individual modular piece through the iliofemoral arteries. This shortcoming is addressed, along with other device improvements in the Valiant device, and is being studied in the VALOR 2 trial, which is in the enrollment phase.

Bolton Medical has completed enrollment in a 30-patient feasibility study, and has received conditional FDA approval to begin a phase II trial. This pivotal study will include 120 TEVAR patients and a nonrandomized control group of 60 open repair patients. The Relay device has a nitinol stent structure and polyester graft, and its appearance is similar to the Talent graft. A distinguishing feature is that the device has a three-staged deployment system that may contribute to more precise placement. The device has a modified spiral longitudinal bar, and this endograft also comes in longer lengths.

WORLDWIDE CLINICAL SAMPLE

Pooled data of 1,180 TEVAR patients were gathered during personal visits with eight physicians from leading thoracic endovascular centers.[19] Table 38-1 lists the procedures by thoracic pathology along with 30-day mortality. These experts' assessments are that current technology is equivalent or better compared to conventional treatment in most pathology except for thoracoabdominal aneurysm, chronic dissection, and stenosis. Overall, 30-day morbidity rates are stroke in 2.8%, renal failure in 1.6%, and paraplegia in 2.5%.

The survey includes many types of TEVAR devices (Table 38–2). Debranching or fenestrations for treatment into the arch and thoracoabdominal aorta is common. The left subclavian artery was covered in 30%, the left common carotid artery in 8%, the innominate artery in 4%, celiac artery in 3%, and superior mesenteric artery in 1%. Later outcomes included radiographic findings of endoleak in 10%, sac expansion in 4%,

TABLE 38-2. TYPES OF TEVAR DEVICE USED IN THIS SERIES

Endograft	Frequency
Custom made	54%
TAG	19%
Zenith	11%
Talent	11%
Other	5%

Adapted from: Hassoun HT, Chiou AC, Biggs KL, Matsumura JS. Endovascular graft for thoracic aortic aneurysms. In: Pearce WH, Matsumura JS, Yao JST, (eds). *Trends in Vascular Surgery.* Evanston, IL: Greenwood Academic; 2005:329-342.

proximal neck dilation or dissection in 3%, distal neck dilation in 2%, intercomponent migration in 2%, proximal migration in 1%, distal migration in 0.4%, and device failure such as wire fracture in 6%. Clinically symptomatic device failure is rare at 0.1%, and late aneurysm rupture is 1%.

CONCLUSION

TEVAR is in its infancy, and rapid developments are proceeding as more is learned about the shortcomings of current device designs. It is estimated that 2,892 TEVAR procedures are performed annually compared to 12,212 open DTA repairs in the United States.[30] However, TEVAR rates are doubling every six months. When device maturity and clinical experience is sufficient, randomized clinical trials should be carried out to fully delineate the role of TEVAR. Based on the data now available, it is quite possible that endovascular therapy will become the preferred initial therapy for many thoracic aortic diseases.

REFERENCES

1. Harward TR, Welborn MB 3rd, Martin TD, et al. Visceral ischemia and organ dysfunction after thoracoabdominal aortic aneurysm repair. A clinical and cost analysis. *Ann Surg*. 1996;223:729–734.
2. Coselli JS, LeMaire SA, Koksoy C, et al. Cerebrospinal fluid drainage reduces paraplegia after thoracoabdominal aortic aneurysm repair: Results of a randomized clinical trial. *J Vasc Surg*. 2002;35:631–639.
3. Dake MD, Miller DC, Semba CP, et al. Transluminal Placement of Endovascular Stent Grafts for the Treatment of Descending Thoracic Aortic Aneurysms. *N Engl J Med*. 1994;331:1729–1734.
4. Mitchell RS, Miller DC, Dake MD, et al. Thoracic aortic aneurysm repair with an endovascular stent graft: the "first generation." *Ann Thor Surg*. 1999;67:1971–1974.
5. Grabenwoger M, Hutschala D, Ehrlich MP, et al. Thoracic aortic aneurysms: treatment with endovascular self-expandable stent grafts. *Ann Thorac Surg*. 2000;69:441–445.
6. Taylor PR, Gaines PA, McGuinness CL, et al. Thoracic aortic stent grafts - early experience from two centres using commercially available devices. *Eur J Vasc Endovasc Surg*. 2001; 22:70–6.
7. Cambria RP, Brewster DC, Lauterbach SR, et al. Evolving experience with thoracic aortic stent graft repair. *J Vasc Surg*. 2002;35:1129–1136.
8. Najibi S, Terramani TT, Weiss VJ, et al. Endoluminal versus open treatment of descending thoracic aortic aneurysms. *J Vasc Surg*. 2002;36:732–7.
9. Orend KH, Scharrer-Pamler R, Kapfer X, et al. Endovascular Treatment in Diseases of the Descending Thoracic Aorta: Six Year Results of a Single Center. *J Vasc Surg*. 2003; 37:91–99.
10. Bell RE, Taylor PR, Aukett M, et al. Midterm Results for Second Generation Thoracic Stent Grafts. *Br J Surg*. 2003;90:811–817.
11. Ellozy SH, Carroccio A, Minor M, et al. Challenges of Endovascular Tube Graft Repair of Thoracic Aortic Aneurysm: Midterm Follow Up and Lessens Learned. *J Vasc Surg*. 2003; 38:676–683.
12. Marty B, Morales CC, Tozzi P, et al. Partial Inflow Occlusion Facilitates Accurate Deployment of Thoracic Aortic Endografts. *J Endovasc Ther*. 2004;11(2):175–179.
13. Peterson BG, Longo GM, Matsumura JS, et al. Endovascular repair of thoracic aortic pathology with custom-made devices. *Surgery*. 2005;138(4):598–605.

14. Peterson BG, Matsumura JS, Morasch MD, et al. Percutaneous endovascular repair of blunt thoracic aortic transection. *J Trauma*. 2005;59:1062–1065.
15. Makaroun MS, Dillavou ED, Kee ST, et al. Endovascular treatment of thoracic aortic aneurysms: results of the phase II multicenter trial of the GORE TAG thoracic endoprosthesis. *J Vasc Surg*. 2005;41:1–9.
16. Makaroun MS. Oral Presentation. Society for Vascular Surgery. Philadelphia, PA; June 2006.
17. Hassoun HT, Dake MD, Svensson LG, et al. Multi-institutional pivotal trial of the Zenith TX2 thoracic aortic stent graft for treatment of descending thoracic aortic aneurysms: clinical study design. *Perspect Vasc Endovasc Ther*. 2005;17(3):255–264.
18. Toucek M. Oral Presentation. Midwestern Vascular Surgical Society. Chicago, IL; September, 2005.
19. Matsumura JS. Worldwide survey of thoracic endografts: Practical clinical application. *J Vasc Surg*. 2006;43(2 Suppl):A20–A21.
20. Bickerstaff LK, Pairolero PC, Hollier LH, et al. Thoracic Aortic Aneurysms: A Population-Based Study. *Surgery*. 1982;92:1103–1108.
21. Fattori R, Napoli G, Lovato L, et al. Descending Thoracic Aortic Diseases: Stent Graft Repair. *Radiology*. 2003;229:176–183.
22. Criado E, Wall P, Lucas P. Transesophageal Echo Guided Endovascular Exclusion of Thoracic Aortic Mobile Thrombi. *J Vasc Surg*. 2004; 39:238–242.
23. Estrera AL, Rubenstein FS, Miller CC 3rd, Huynh TT, Letsou GV, Safi HJ. Descending thoracic aortic aneurysm: surgical approach and treatment using the adjuncts cerebrospinal fluid drainage and distal aortic perfusion. *Ann Thorac Surg*. 2001;72:481–486.
24. Svensson LG, Crawford ES, Hess KR, et al. Variables Predictive of Outcome in 832 Patients Undergoing Repairs of the Descending Thoracic Aorta. *Chest*. 1993;104:1248–1253.
25. Crawford ES, Hess KR, Cohen ES, et al. Ruptured aneurysm of the descending thoracic and thoracoabdominal aorta. *Ann Surg*. 1991;213:417–426.
26. Kouchoukos NT, Daily BB, Rokkas CK, et al. Hypothermic bypass and circulatory arrest for operations on the descending thoracic aorta and thoracoabdominal aorta. *Ann Thorac Surg*. 1995;60:67–77.
27. Estrera AL, Miller CC, Huynh TT, et al. Neurologic outcome after thoracic and thoracoabdominal aortic aneurysm repair. *Ann Thorac Surg*. 2001;72:1225–1231.
28. Hassoun HT, Chiou AC, Biggs KL, Matsumura JS. Endovascular graft for thoracic aortic aneurysms. In: Pearce WH, Matsumura JS, Yao JST, (eds). *Trends in Vascular Surgery*. Evanston, IL: Greenwood Academic; 2005:329–342.
29. EVAR Trial Participants. Endovascular aneurysm repair and outcome in patients unfit for open repair of abdominal aortic aneurysm (EVAR trial 2): Randomised controlled trial. *Lancet*. 2005;365:2187–2192.
30. *United States Vascular and Endovascular Monitor*. First quarter, 2006 Report.

39

Population-based Analysis of Endovascular versus Open Repair of Thoracic Aortic Aneurysms

Gilbert R. Upchurch, Jr., M.D., Babak J. Orandi, M.D., Jonathan L. Eliason, M.D., Himanshu J. Patel, M.D., David M. Williams, M.D., John E. Rectenwald, M.D., Enrique Criado, M.D., G. Michael Deeb, M.D.

Aortic diseases, including aortic aneurysms, are the 12th leading cause of death in the United States.[1] While abdominal and ascending aortic aneurysms are more common, descending thoracic aortic aneurysms are not rare.[2] Isolated descending thoracic aortic aneurysm (TAA) repair is associated with significant morbidity and mortality. This chapter will focus on population-based trials examining the treatment of isolated, degenerative descending TAAs by either open or endovascular therapy.

ORIGINS OF OPEN AND ENDOVASCULAR TAA REPAIR

The technical description of open and endovascular TAA repair are beyond the scope of this chapter. However, the goal of therapy is to prevent the attendant excessive mortality associated with aortic rupture. The modern era of thoracic aortic surgery was introduced by Lam and Aram who used an aortic homograft to replace the thoracic aorta,[3] followed two years latter by surgical repair of a TAA with insertion of a synthetic vascular graft.[4] Over the next 30 years, E. Stanley Crawford developed many of the surgical techniques used today.[5] Over the last 50 years, the diagnosis and open surgical treatment of TAAs have become refined with advances in technology, including the use of distal aortic perfusion, spinal drains, improved critical care, and better blood banking, resulting in improved surgical outcomes. However despite these adjuncts, the elective mortality following elective open thoracoabdominal aortic aneurysm (TAAA) repair in the United States is still 22.3%[6] (Figure 39–1).

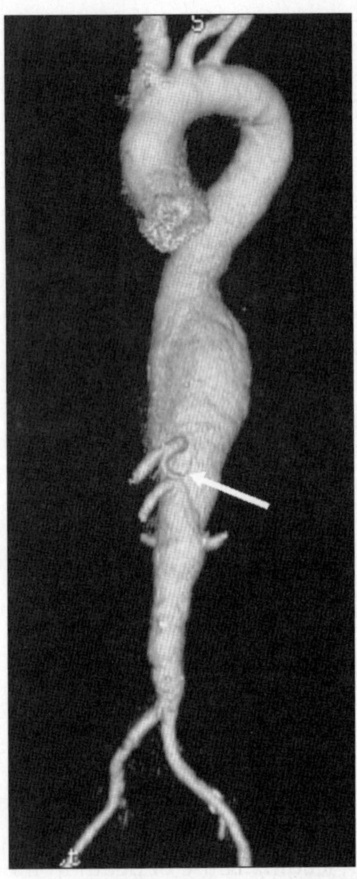

Figure 39-1. Three-dimensional (3-D) CT angiogram documenting a thoracabdominal aortic aneurysm with involvement of the celiac and superior mesenteric arteries (arrow). In the United States today, outside of investigational trials or "homemade" endografts, this patient would not be a candidate for an endovascular approach unless extra-anatomic bypasses were performed first. The patient could then have an endograft placed as the second part of a "hybrid procedure".

An alternative, less invasive technique for the treatment of isolated TAAs in the form of stent-grafting emerged in the 1990s.[7,8] Volodos and colleagues are credited with placement of the first thoracic aortic endograft.[9] The use of stent graft technology has since exploded[10-12] and has been used to treat a number of thoracic aortic pathologies, including elective (Figure 39–2) and ruptured (Figure 39–3) descending thoracic aortic aneurysms. Multiple, single institution studies have documented that endovascular TAA repair (ETAR) is associated with lower physiologic strain, fewer blood transfusions, and fewer hospital and ICU days. Some have suggested a lower in-hospital mortality for ETAR compared with open TAA repair.[13-17] Similar to endovascular abdominal aortic aneurysm (AAA) repair, which was originally used to treat elderly patients with significant cardiac, pulmonary, and renal co-morbidities, an endovascular approach is presently often considered primary therapy for most patients with isolated degenerative TAAs and suitable aortic, brachiocephalic, and iliac arterial anatomy. This will predictably translate into a relative explosion in the number of TAA repairs secondary to the introduction of new "less invasive" technology.

NATURAL HISTORY

As there is no level A or B scientific data determining the timing of operative intervention, size criteria for TAA repair are not as clearly defined as for infrarenal AAAs.[18,19]

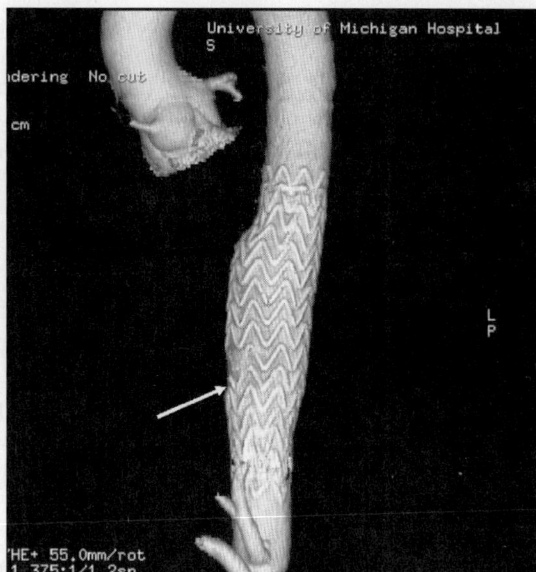

Figure 39-2. 3-D CT angiogram of completed, elective thoracic stent-graft in a patient with a large saccular TAA (arrow). Note the distal stent-graft proximal to a patent celiac artery.

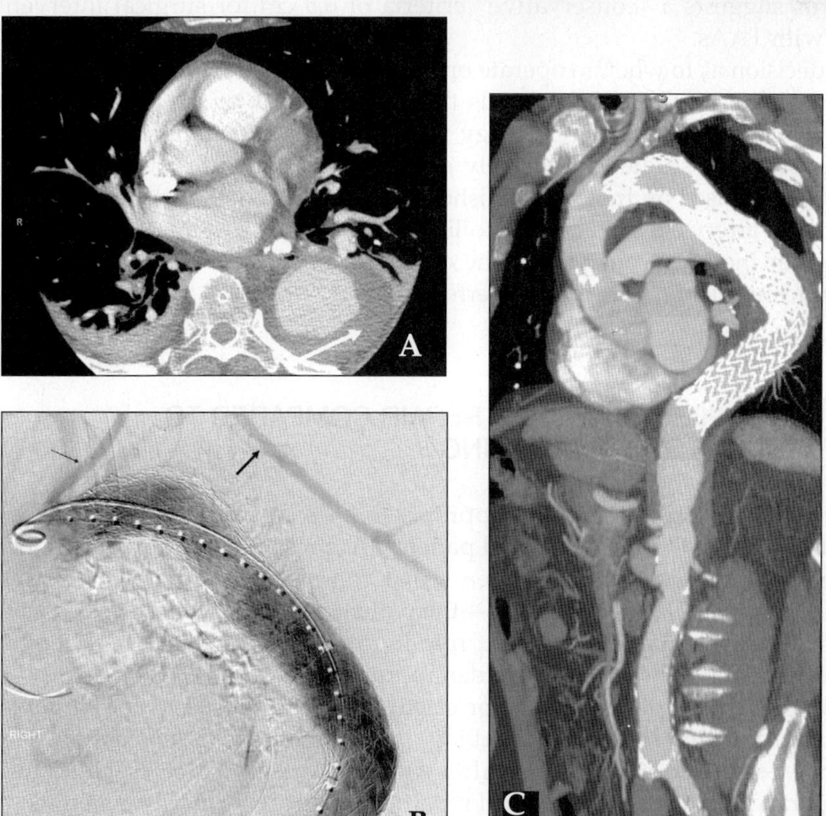

Figure 39-3. (A) Axial CT scan documenting intramural hematoma in a patient with chest pain and a large TAA. Arrow denotes hematoma. **(B)** Completion angiogram documenting patent stent-graft, left common carotid artery (thin arrow), and left subclavian artery (thick arrow) after left common carotid-to-subclavian artery bypass. **(C)** Repeat CT scan six months following placement of thoracic endograft showing resolution of hematoma and exclusion of TAA.

This issue is further complicated by the observation that degenerative TAAs are often not uniform in size and involve aortic segments of varying diameters and morphology (i.e., with or without a dissection component, involves the distal aortic arch, and so on). Based on natural history studies that document an extremely high risk of rupture and death if left untreated, all patients with TAAs should be considered for repair.[4,20-22] The natural history of ruptured TAA repair was first studied extensively by Crawford et al.[23] In a series of more than 100 ruptured TAAs, the authors noted that 80% of ruptures occurred in patients with aneurysms that were less than 10 cm in diameter. Crawford concluded by suggesting that since elective surgery was associated with 92% survival, TAA repair should be considered before rupture when aneurysms are 5 cm or larger in good-risk patients, in patients with symptomatic aneurysms, and in most patients with larger aneurysms. More recently, Elefteiades et al. suggested that the size criteria for surgical intervention for TAAs should be greater than 6.5 cm.[24] These authors also suggested that the threshold for repair should be lowered to 6.0 cm for patients with connective tissue disorders.[24] Coady suggested that in asymptomatic TAA patients who are followed longtitudinally, there are "hinge points" that demarcate highly dangerous aortic thresholds.[25] For the descending thoracic aorta, the hinge point is 7 cm, where a 43% risk of rupture is encountered. This suggests a "conservative" criteria of 6.5 cm for surgical intervention in patients with TAAs.

The decision as to when to operate on a patient with a TAA involves assessment of the likelihood of aortic rupture versus the operative risk of the individual patient.[26] The impact of endovascular technology with its lower attendant morbidity and mortality has not been studied extensively at the population-based level. However, one would predict, based on trends established in the treatment of other disease processes such as renal artery stenosis and aortoiliac occlusive disease, that the introduction of endovascular therapy would lower the diameter threshold for TAA repair, and thus increase the number of TAA repairs performed.[27,28]

TREATMENT SELECTION: OPEN REPAIR COMPARED TO ENDOVASCULAR STENT-GRAFTING

The decision as to which therapy is appropriate for a particular patient is an evolving aspect of the care of these complicated patients. At present, there are no specific guidelines regarding the indication for open repair compared with ETAR performed in a *randomized* fashion. Two major factors—the patient's physiologic reserve as well as the vascular anatomy—play a significant role in determining whether a patient is best suited for open repair or an endovascular approach.[29]

Until recently, surgical therapy for elective TAAs involved major surgery with a significant risk for mortality and morbidity postoperatively. Even centers of reputed excellence report combined mortality and paraplegia rates of close to 10%.[22] Contemporary results of open surgical repair of TAAs are primarily generated at institutions with great expertise in this area. There is little doubt that TAA repair, despite the disease itself being relatively rare, is one of the few operations where surgeon and hospital volume impact mortality.[6,30] Based on 1,898 cases, a mortality rate of 4.8% can be attained following open TAA repair in centers of excellence.[31] This is compared with a national mortality of over 20% from administrative data.[6] In addition, the risk of paralysis and stroke are 3.4 and 2.7%, respectively, following open TAA repair in centers of excellence. Five- and 10-year survival rates are 60 and 38%, respectively.[31]

Examination of a few specific population-based rather than single center studies comparing open and endovascular therapy for TAAs is warranted.

Gore TAG Trial Reports

Bavaria and coauthors documented follow-up on the initial multicenter trial including 140 patients with stent-grafts (Gore TAG Thoracic endograft, Flagstaff, AZ) compared to an open surgical cohort of 94 patients, which included historic and concurrent open controls. Perioperative mortality was significantly lower in the endograft group versus open surgical controls (2.1% for ETAR vs. 11.7% for open repair, P<.001). Perioperative complication rates, ICU, and hospital length of stay were also significantly reduced in the ETAR group. The incidence of endoleaks at two years was 9% in the ETAR group with three inteventions performed in the endograft cohort. At two years, Kaplan-Meier analysis revealed no difference in overall mortality.[32]

Makaroun et al. reported five-year follow-up using the Gore TAG device in degenerative TAAAs with an additional 51 patients added to the trial after the endograft was redesigned in 2003. This study documented no difference in all-cause mortality between endovascular and open TAAA repair at five years (67% vs. 68%).[33] Major adverse events at 5 years were significantly reduced in the ETAR group (57.9% vs. 78.7%, P = .001). Endoleaks in the TAG group decreased from 8.1% at one month to 4.3% at five years. Five TAG patients had undergone major aneurysm-related reinterventions at five years (3.6%), including one arch aneurysm repair for type 1 endoleak and migration, one open conversion, and five endovascular procedures for endoleaks in three patients. For the ETAR patients, sac size at 60 months decreased in 50% and increased in 19% compared to the one-month baseline. Comparison with the modified low-porosity device at 24 months showed sac increase in 12.9% of original versus 2.9% in modified grafts (P = .11). At five years, there have been no ruptures, one migration, no collapse, and 20 instances of stent fracture in 19 patients, all before the redesign of the TAG graft. The authors concluded that while the rates of secondary intervention were much higher in the stent graft group, ETAR was superior to open repair at five years.

TX2 Stent Graft Trial

In this study, 42 international trial sites enrolled a total of 230 subjects with descending thoracic aortic aneurysms. The study compared 160 patients undergoing ETAR treated with the Zenith TX2 Endovascular Graft (William Cook Europe, ApS, Bjaeverskov, Denmark) compared to 70 patients undergoing open TAA repair. The 30-day survival rate was not inferior for the ETAR group compared with the open group (98.1% vs. 94.3%, P < .01). The ETAR group had fewer cardiovascular, pulmonary, and vascular adverse events, although neurologic events were not significantly different. No ruptures or conversions occurred in the first year in the ETAR group and reintervention rates were similar in both groups. At 12 months, aneurysm growth was identified in 7.1% (8/112) of patients (3.9% endoleak rate). Matsumura and coauthors concluded that thoracic endovascular aortic repair with the TX2 is a safe, effective alternative to open surgical repair for the treatment of anatomically suitable descending thoracic aortic aneurysms at one year of follow-up.[34]

VALOR Stent Graft Trial

A recent report summarized the 30-day and 12-month results of endovascular treatment using the Medtronic Vascular Talent Thoracic Stent Graft System (Medtronic Vascular, Santa Rosa, CA) for patients with TAAs, who were also candidates for open repair. Similar to the TAG trial, the study was a prospective, nonrandomized, multicenter trial. ETAR results were compared to a retrospective open surgical cohort from three centers of excellence. In this trial, 195 patients underwent ETAR and 189 underwent open TAA repair. The 30-day ETAR group had a perioperative mortality of 2.1%. Major adverse events occurred in 41% of the stent-graft group, including 1.5% with paraplegia, 7.2% with paraparesis, and 3.6% with stroke. At 12 months, the ETAR group had an all-cause mortality of 16.1% and an aneurysm-related mortality of 3.1%. The Talent Thoracic Stent Graft showed statistically superior performance with respect to acute procedural outcomes (P < .001), 30-day major adverse events (41% vs. 84.4%, P < .001), perioperative mortality (2% vs. 8%, P < .01), and 12-month aneurysm-related mortality (3.1% vs. 11.6%, P < .002) compared to open TAA repair. The authors concluded by suggesting that the Talent Thoracic Stent Graft System is a safe and effective endovascular therapy as an alternative to open surgery in patients with TAAs.[35]

It is important to note that while all of the device-specific trials are prospective in nature, they are not randomized. They also suffer from primary use of historical control patients undergoing open TAA repair. In addition, they were not designed to help us to determine which patient is best served by stent-grafting compared to open repair.

Meta-analysis

A recent meta-analysis reviewing open repair and stent-grafting for thoracic aortic pathology by Walsh et al. included 17 eligible studies totaling 1,109 patients. The meta-analysis included a number of different pathologies, including TAAs, dissections, as well as aortic transections. However, the study demonstrated that stenting was associated with a significant reduction in mortality (pooled odds ratio 0.36, P<.0001) and major neurological injury (pooled odds ratio 0.39, P<.0001), with no difference in major reintervention rate. There was also a reduction in both ICU and hospital length of stay, even though the authors noted bias and heterogeneity with respect to the outcomes. Subgroup analyses documented that ETAR reduced mortality (pooled odds ratio 0.91; 95% CI 0.09-0.66) and neurologic morbidity (pooled odds ratio 0.28; 95% CI 0.13-0.61) following elective TAA repair. The authors concluded by suggesting that ETAR reduces perioperative mortality and neurologic complications in patients undergoing elective TAA repair, while suggesting that there may be less benefit in other thoracic aortic conditions.[36]

Comparison of Open TAA Repair vs. ETAR using National Inpatient Sample Database

A nationally representative database, the Nationwide Inpatient Sample, was used to assess perioperative outcomes after open and endovascular repair of intact thoracic aortic aneurysms from 9/1/05 to 12/31/05.[37] This dataset is a stratified, random sample of 20% of the hospitals in the United States. Using analysis techniques designed for complex sampling, national estimates of outcomes and utilization can be obtained. ICD-9 codes for elective thoracic aortic aneurysm repair without mention of rupture (441.2) were used with appropriate procedure codes to identify all patients in the

TABLE 39-1. DEMOGRAPHIC DATA FOR OPEN VS. ENDOVASCULAR TAA REPAIR

	Open		Endovascular		
	n	(%)	n	(%)	
	500	67.3	243	32.7	P
Age (mean + SD)	67.9 + 9.5			69.6 + 9.8	<.0001
Sex					
Male	345	69.0	180	74.1	
Female	155	31.0	63	25.9	<.1494
Race					
White	318	88.6	112	71.3	
Nonwhite	41	11.4	45	28.7	<.0001
# of comorbidities					
0-1	287	57.4	94	38.6	
2-3	208	41.6	124	50.9	
>4	5	1.0	25	10.5	<.0001

dataset who underwent either open or endovascular TAA repair over the first three months the endovascular code for TAA was available. Patients with an ICD-9 code for both open and endovascular TAA repair and those individuals less than 50 years of age were excluded. Sample survey weights were utilized and statistical comparisons were made using t-test for continuous variables and chi-square for categorical variables with the SAS statistical software package (Linux version 9.13, Cary, NC).

Using the national dataset, 743 patients underwent open or endovascular TAA repair during the three-month study period. Patients undergoing endovascular repair were older, more likely to be nonwhite, and have more comborbidities (Table 39–1). Patient comorbidities were typical for this patient population in that many patients had hypertension and ischemic heart disease (Table 39–2).

ETAR was not associated with a lower in-hospital mortality rate compared to open repair (6.5% for ETAR vs. 6.9% for open repair, P=0.8413). However, patients undergoing ETAR had a significantly shorter hospital length of stay (4.8 days for ETAR vs. 12.4 days for open repair, P<.0001) and were more often dispositioned to home

TABLE 39-2. CARDIOVASCULAR COMORBID CONDITIONS OF PATIENTS UNDERGOING OPEN OR ENDOVASCULAR THORACIC AORTIC ANEURYSM REPAIR.

Comorbid Condition	Open (%)	Endovascular (%)	P value
Diabetes	11.0	8.4	0.2829
Hypertension	61.8	75.8	0.0001
Renal Insufficiency	17.2	15.7	0.6057
COPD	11.4	14.7	0.2062
Ischemic Heart Disease	27.4	37.2	0.0060
CVOD	5.1	16.8	<.0001
PAD	5.1	20.6	<.0001

COPD- chronic obstructive pulmonary disease
CVOD- cerebrovascular occlusive disease
PAD- peripheral arterial occlusive disease.

TABLE 39-3. PREDICTORS OF PATIENT DISCHARGE TO HOME.

Variable	OR	95% CI	P-value
Female gender	1.3	.4 - 4.3	0.6354
0-1 comorbidities (vs. 2-3)	2.2	.8 - 6.0	0.1406
Age<75 years	3.5	1.1 -11.4	0.0360
0-1 comorbidities (vs. >4)	6.2	1.4 - 27.8	0.0171
Endovascular repair	20.8	.6 -57.3	<.0001

OR- odds ratio
CI- confidence interval.

(100% for ETAR vs. 79.3% for open repair, P<.0001). When predictors of discharge to home were examined by multivariate analysis, ETAR was the strongest predictor (Table 39–3). Hospital charges were also significantly higher in the open TAA repair group ($103, 395 for ETAR vs. $141, 913 for open repair, P=.0194). In-hospital complication rates (Figure 39–4) in general were higher for open repair than for ETAR.

These data suggest that while there is no difference in mortality between ETAR and open repair, similar to endovascular AAA repair, patients undergoing ETAR have significantly shorter hospital stays, are more likely discharged to home, and sustain fewer complications compared to open TAA repair. In addition, patients undergoing ETAR have lower hospital charges. These data suggest that given similar mortality rates, ETAR is a favorable alternative to open TAA repair.

Society of Thoracic Surgeons Endovascular Task Force

A recent report from the Society of Thoracic Surgeons (STS) Endovascular Surgery Task Force is useful in trying to determine which patients should undergo open

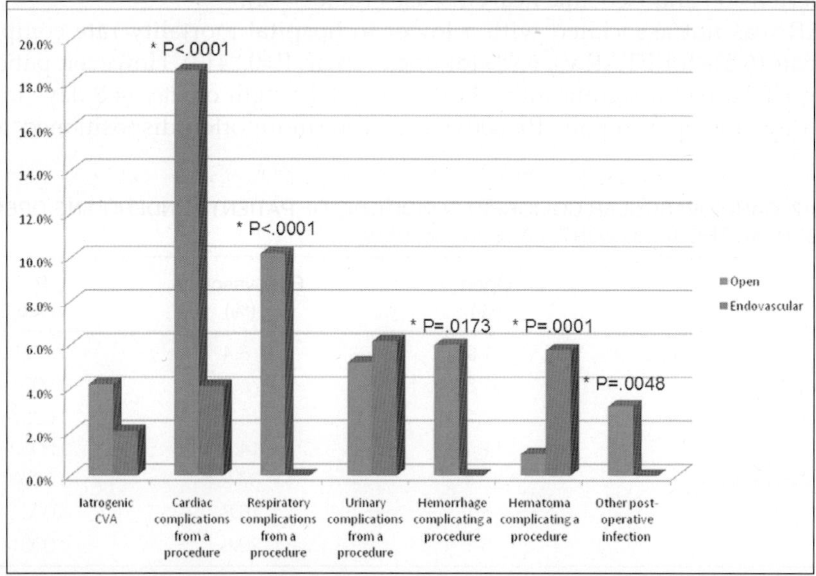

Figure 39-4. Complication rates from the National Inpatient Sample from 9/1/05 to 12/31/05 following open or endovascular repair of TAA in the United States. Data suggest increased complication rates following open repair.

TAAA repair versus endovascular stent-grafting.[31] The expert panel acknowledged that diseases of the thoracic aorta are increasingly being treated by stent-grafts. Yet, no prospective randomized trials, comparing the two types of repair in the same type of pathology, have been performed. At present in the United States, there are three FDA-approved endografts approved for the treatment of type I degenerative TAAAs.[13] First generation stent-grafts suffered a number of graft-related complications (stent fractures, graft collapse, and so forth), as well as complications from the introduction of new technology (increased stroke risk, ascending aortic dissections, and the like). It should be recognized that thoracic stent-grafting is relatively new with little long-term follow-up. In general, while a TAA is a serious disease, it is also relatively indolent. The authors concluded by emphatically stating that identification of small TAAs does not justify the use of endovascular stent-grafting as the rates of rupture, dissection, and death in TAAs less than 5 cm are relatively low.

SUMMARY

Despite the reviewed data suggesting many advantages of ETAR compared to open repair, few would argue for treatment of all TAAs to the exclusion of open repair. Indications for endovascular intervention are not presently defined and instead are based on reports of open TAA repair from institutions with great expertise. Long-term results following endografting are lacking, as the first five-year report of follow-up from the only FDA-approved endograft has only recently become available.[33] Mortality rates following endovascular TAA vary widely between 2 and 26%, depending largely on the nature of the indication for the operation (elective vs. urgent vs. emergent), patient comorbidities, and the experience of the endovascular specialist.[31] Midterm results suggested that moderate term survival (three to eight years) also varied greatly between 25 and 90%. While there should clearly be enthusiasm for the use of endovascular therapies to treat many TAAs, it should be recognized that late complications such as endoleaks, stent fractures, and stent migration, are not uncommon after endovascular TAA repair. The issue of increased downstream cost (multiple CT scans in follow up, secondary procedures, and so on) associated with endografting will also need to be figured into the equation when considering which therapy is correct for a particular patient. Importantly, it also is not clear at present whether a more aggressive endovascular approach will impact long-term survival or freedom from aortic complications compared to open surgical therapy.

There are likely subpopulations of patients best served by endovascular stent-grafting. It is reasonable to conclude that patients older than 75 years of age, if anatomically feasible, should be directed toward stent-grafting.[6] The subset of patients with significant COPD are also likely to benefit from stent-grafting, when possible, in order to avoid the attendant risks incurred from a thoracotomy. Patients presenting with increasing pain or with ruptured TAAs should also be considered for stent-grafting, which often can be performed more expeditiously than open repair, if the anatomy is appropriate for an endovascular approach.

At present, outside of "off label use" of thoracic and abdominal stent-grafts or IDEs, indications for endovascular stent-grafting are only for degenerative Crawford type I TAAs. As with the evolution of many new technologies, the indication for stent-grafting is based on similar to lower short-term operative mortality rate and morbidity compared to open TAA repair or medical therapy, not necessarily long-term outcomes. New, less invasive therapies such as stent-grafting, often need to only document clinical equipoise in order to gain market share. Regardless, the physician caring for the patient with a TAA should consider a constellation of issues including age, comorbidities, symptoms, expected life expectancy, quality of life, aortic diameter, aneurysm morphology and extent, suitability of landing zone for a stent-graft, route of iliac access, compliance with appropriate follow-up, cost of therapies, and operator experience when deciding to commit their patient to any intervention.[31]

ACKNOWLEDGEMENT

The authors would like to acknowledge and thank Mr. Vivek Sharma for his assistance with the analysis of NIS data.

REFERENCES

1. National Center for Health Statistics (NHCS), National Vital Statistics System, WISQARS Query: 20 Leading Causes of Death, United States, 1999–2004, All Races, Both Sexes. Available at: http://webappa.cdc. gov/sasweb/ncipc/leadcaus10.html. Accessed July 25, 2007.
2. Bickerstaff LK, Pairolero PC, Hollier LH, Melton LJ, Van Peenen HJ,et al. Thoracic aortic aneurysms: a population-based study. *Surgery.* 1982;92(6):1103–1108.
3. Lam CR, Aram HH. Resection of the descending thoracic aorta for aneurysm; a report of the use of a homograft in a case and an experimental study. *Ann Surg.* 1951;134(4):743–752.
4. De Bakey ME, Cooley DA. Successful resection of aneurysm of thoracic aorta and replacement by graft. *J Am Med Assoc.* 1953;152(8):673–676.
5. Crawford ES. Thoraco-abdominal and abdominal aortic aneurysms involving renal, superior mesenteric, celiac arteries. *Ann Surg.* 1974;179(5):763–772.
6. Cowan JA, Jr., Dimick JB, Henke PK, Huber TS, Stanley JC, Upchurch GR, Jr. Surgical treatment of intact thoracoabdominal aortic aneurysms in the United States: hospital and surgeon volume-related outcomes. *J Vasc Surg.* 2003;37(6):1169–1174.
7. Dake MD, Miller DC, Semba CP, Mitchell RS, Walker PJ, Liddell RP. Transluminal placement of endovascular stent-grafts for the treatment of descending thoracic aortic aneurysms. *N Engl J Med.* 1994; 331(26):1729–1734.
8. Mitchell RS, Miller DC, Dake MD, Semba CP, Moore KA, Sakai T. Thoracic aortic aneurysm repair with an endovascular stent graft: the "first generation". *Ann Thorac Surg.* 1999;67(6): 1971–1974; discussion 1979–1980.
9. Volodos NL, Karpovich IP, Troyan VI, Kalashnikova Yu V, Shekhanin VE, et al. Clinical experience of the use of self-fixing synthetic prostheses for remote endoprosthetics of the thoracic and the abdominal aorta and iliac arteries through the femoral artery and as intraoperative endoprosthesis for aorta reconstruction. *VASA Suppl.* 1991;33:93–95.
10. Buffolo E, da Fonseca JH, de Souza JA, Alves CM. Revolutionary treatment of aneurysms and dissections of descending aorta: the endovascular approach. *Ann Thorac Surg.* 2002;74(5):S1815–1817; discussion S1825–1832.
11. Dake MD, Miller DC, Mitchell RS, Semba CP, Moore KA, Sakai T. The "first generation" of endovascular stent-grafts for patients with aneurysms of the descending thoracic aorta. *J Thorac Cardiovasc Surg.* 1998;116(5):689–703; discussion 703–684.
12. Greenberg R, Resch T, Nyman U, Lindh M, Brunkwall J, et al. Endovascular repair of descending thoracic aortic aneurysms: an early experience with intermediate-term follow-up. *J Vasc Surg.* 2000;31(1 Pt 1):147–156.

13. Makaroun MS, Dillavou ED, Kee ST, Sicard G, Chaikof E, et al. Endovascular treatment of thoracic aortic aneurysms: results of the phase II multicenter trial of the GORE TAG thoracic endoprosthesis. *J Vasc Surg.* 2005;41(1):1–9.

14. Gawenda M, Brunkwall J. Device-specific outcomes with endografts for thoracic aortic aneurysms. *J Cardiovasc Surg* (Torino). 2005;46(2):113–120.

15. Leurs LJ, Bell R, Degrieck Y, Thomas S, Hobo R, Lundbom J. Endovascular treatment of thoracic aortic diseases: combined experience from the EUROSTAR and United Kingdom Thoracic Endograft registries. *J Vasc Surg.* 2004;40(4):670–679; discussion 679–680.

16. Orend KH, Scharrer-Pamler R, Kapfer X, Kotsis T, Gorich J, Sunder-Plassmann L. Endovascular treatment in diseases of the descending thoracic aorta: 6-year results of a single center. *J Vasc Surg.* 2003;37(1):91–99.

17. Rachel ES, Bergamini TM, Kinney EV, Jung MT, Kaebnick HW, Mitchell RA. Endovascular repair of thoracic aortic aneurysms: a paradigm shift in standard of care. *VASA Endovasc Surg.* 2002;36(2):105–113.

18. The UK Small Aneurysm Trial Participants. Mortality results for randomised controlled trial of early elective surgery or ultrasonographic surveillance for small abdominal aortic aneurysms. *Lancet.* 1998;352(9141):1649–1655.

19. Lederle FA, Wilson SE, Johnson GR, Reinke DB, Littooy FN, et al. Immediate repair compared with surveillance of small abdominal aortic aneurysms. *N Engl J Med.* 2002;346(19):1437–1444.

20. McNamara JJ, Pressler VM. Natural history of arteriosclerotic thoracic aortic aneurysms. *Ann Thorac Surg.* 1978;26(5):468–473.

21. Griepp RB, Ergin MA, Galla JD, Lansman SL, McCullough JN, et al. Natural history of descending thoracic and thoracoabdominal aneurysms. *Ann Thorac Surg.* 1999;67(6):1927–1930; discussion 1953–1928.

22. Coselli JS, LeMaire SA, Miller CC, 3rd, Schmittling ZC, Koksoy C, et al. Mortality and paraplegia after thoracoabdominal aortic aneurysm repair: a risk factor analysis. *Ann Thorac Surg.* 2000;69(2):409–414.

23. Crawford ES, Hess KR, Cohen ES, Coselli JS, Safi HJ. Ruptured aneurysm of the descending thoracic and thoracoabdominal aorta. Analysis according to size and treatment. *Ann Surg.* 1991;213(5):417–425; discussion 425–416.

24. Elefteriades JA. Natural history of thoracic aortic aneurysms: indications for surgery, and surgical versus nonsurgical risks. *Ann Thorac Surg.* 2002;74(5):S1877–1880; discussion S1892–1878.

25. Coady MA, Rizzo JA, Hammond GL, Mandapati D, Darr U, et al. What is the appropriate size criterion for resection of thoracic aortic aneurysms? *J Thorac Cardiovasc Surg.* 1997;113(3):476–491; discussion 489–491.

26. Coady MA, Rizzo JA, Elefteriades JA. Developing surgical intervention criteria for thoracic aortic aneurysms. *Cardiol Clin.* 1999;17(4):827–839.

27. Knipp BS, Dimick JB, Eliason JL, Cowan JA, Henke PK, et al. Diffusion of new technology for the treatment of renovascular hypertension in the United States: surgical revascularization versus catheter-based therapy, 1988–2001. *J Vasc Surg.* 2004;40(4):717–723.

28. Upchurch GR, Dimick JB, Wainess RM, Eliason JL, Henke PK, et al. Diffusion of new technology in health care: the case of aorto-iliac occlusive disease. *Surgery.* 2004;136(4):812–818.

29. Greenberg RK, Clair D, Srivastava S, Bhandari G, Turc A, et al. Should patients with challenging anatomy be offered endovascular aneurysm repair? *J Vasc Surg.* 2003;38(5):990–996.

30. Cowan JA, Jr., Dimick JB, Wainess RM, Henke PK, Stanley JC, Upchurch GR, Jr. Ruptured thoracoabdominal aortic aneurysm treatment in the United States: 1988 to 1998. *J Vasc Surg.* 2003;38(2):319–322.

31. Svensson LG, Kouchoukos NT, Miller DC, Bavaria JE, Coselli JS, Curi MA, et al. Expert consensus document on the treatment of descending thoracic aortic disease using endovascular stent-grafts. *Ann Thorac Surg.* 2008;85(1 Suppl):S1–41.

32. Bavaria JE, Appoo JJ, Makaroun MS, Verter J, Yu Z-F, Mitchell RS. Endovascular stent grafting versus open surgical repair of descending thoracic aortic aneurysms in low-risk patients: a multicenter comparative trial. *J Thorac Cardiovas Surg*. 2007;133(2):369–377.

33. Makaroun MS, Dillavou ED, Wheatley GH, Cambria RP. Five-year results of endovascular treatment with the Gore TAG device compared with open repair of thoracic aortic aneurysms. *J Vasc Surg*. 2008;47(5):912–918.

34. Matsumura JS, Cambria RP, Dake MD, Moore RD, Svensson LG, Snyder S. International controlled clinical trial of thoracic endovascular aneurysm repair with the Zenith TX2 endovascular graft: 1-year results. *J Vasc Surg*. 2008;47(2):247–257; discussion 257.

35. Fairman RM CF, Farber M, Kwolek C, Mehta M, White R, et al. VALOR Investigators. Pivotal results of the Medtronic Vascular Talent Thoracic Stent Graft System: The VALOR Trial. *J Vasc Surg*. 2008;[Epub ahead of print].

36. Walsh SR, Tang TY, Sadat U, Naik J, Gaunt ME,et al. Endovascular stenting versus open surgery for thoracic aortic disease: Systematic review and meta-analysis of perioperative results. *J Vasc Surg*. 2008;47(5):1094–1098.

37. Orandi BJ, Sharma V, Upchurch GR Jr. Perioperative outcomes after open and endovascular repair of intact thoracic aortic aneurysms: Results of the Nationwide Inpatient Sample. Paper presented at: Society for Clinical Vascular Surgery 36th Annual Symposium; March 6, 2008; Las Vegas, NV.

Aortic Dissection

40

Minimally Invasive Endovascular Repair of Acute and Chronic Thoracic Aortic Pathology

Mark D. Morasch, M.D.
Katherine E. Brown, D.O.

The traditional operative approach to the treatment of thoracic disease remains a highly morbid, and often mortal, procedure for elderly patients with pre-existing illnesses. Advances in endovascular technology used in the treatment of abdominal aortic aneurysms have been applied to thoracic aortic pathologies. Thoracic endovascular repair is now a viable alternative to open thoracic aortic reconstruction.[1-4] From the early use of custom-made stent-grafts in 1994 through the development of industry-designed and FDA-approved thoracic aortic endografts, a number of significant advances have been made.[1] Despite this technical revolution, there remains significant risk associated with minimally invasive treatment of the thoracic aorta.

PATIENTS AND METHODS

A retrospective review was conducted of all thoracic endovascular aortic repairs (TEVAR) performed between April 2000 and July 2008. There were a total of 144 TEVAR procedures performed on 140 patients at Northwestern Memorial Hospital

Indications for treatment included asymptomatic degenerative thoracic aneurysms (DTA), aortic dissections with chronic aneurysmal change ≥5.5 cm, or thoracic aneurysm rupture; traumatic aortic disruption; anastomotic pseudoaneurysm; acute complicated dissection; penetrating aortic ulcer; intramural hematoma; and Diverticulum of Kommerell (Table 40–1).

Proximal and distal landing zones of at least 2 cm were required for suitable fixation of the endograft. Arch or mesenteric artery revascularization procedures were performed ahead of time or during the index procedure in 62 cases to allow for adequate proximal or distal fixation when indicated and time permitted.

TABLE 40-1. THORACIC AORTIC PATHOLOGY TREATED AND DEVICES IMPLANTED

Thoracic Aortic Pathology	Thoracic Device (n=101)	Aortic cuff extender (n=22)	Custom (n=17)
Degenerative Aortic Aneurysm			
Elective	55	1	10
Rupture	13	1	1
Aortic dissection, complicated	11	0	1
Traumatic injury	6	17	0
Pseudoaneurysm	11	0	3
Intramural hematoma	1	2	1
Penetrating aortic ulcer	2	1	1
Diverticulum of Kommerell	2	0	0

Procedural Details and Devices.   All procedures were performed in an operating suite equipped with a fixed fluoroscopic unit (Philips V5000, The Netherlands). Prophylactic spinal drains were placed in 26 patients (18%). Devices used included industry designed thoracic aortic endografts (n= 101) [GORE TAG, W.L.Gore & Associates, Flagstaff, AZ (n= 93); COOK TX2, Cook, Inc, Bloomington, IN (n=5); Medtronic Talent, Medtronic/AVE, Santa Rosa, CA (n=3)], endovascular aortic proximal extension cuffs (n=22) [Excluder, W.L. Gore & Associates, Flagstaff, AZ (n= 1; AneuRx, Medtronic/AVE, Santa Rosa, CA (n= 21], or custom made stent grafts (n=17) constructed of 5 cm long stents (Gianturco Z-stents; Cook, Inc., Bloomington, IN) covered with ironed woven polyester fabric (Cooley Veri Soft, Boston Scientific Corp., Oakland, NJ). Aortic arterial access was obtained via percutaneous (n=59; 41%) or cutdown femoral arterial approach (n=64; 44%), direct iliac access (n=4; 3%) or iliac arterial conduit (n=12; 8%), and direct aortic access (n=4; 3%) or via the aortic arch (n=1; 1%).

RESULTS

Patient Demographics.   Thirty-eight percent of the procedures were considered emergent. The average age of the patient cohort was 63.9 years old ($\pm$ 15.9 years, range 20–93 years old). Sixty-eight percent of the patients were male. Of the total patients treated, 85% were ASA class $\geq$ 3 and 13% of the patients were $\geq$ 80 years old.

Subclavian transposition was performed in 33 patients and a carotid-to-subclavian bypass was performed in three patients with prior left internal mammary artery coronary revascularization. The subclavian artery was covered without revascularization in a total of 11 cases. Total arch debranching was performed in six patients and hybrid elephant trunk procedures were utilized in nine patients. Mesenteric arterial revascularization was utilized in 11 patients. Of the mesenteric procedures, three patients underwent celiac bypass alone while eight patients underwent multivisceral revascularization. One patient had celiac artery coverage without prior revascularization.

Early Mortality.   The 30-day mortality rate was 4.8% (n=7) for all primary and secondary endograft procedures. Five of seven deaths followed emergent operations. As such, the 30-day mortality for emergency procedures was 9%.

TABLE 40-2. PROCEDURAL ADVERSE EVENTS

Complication	Total	%
Arterial access site injury	14	9.7
Limbs amputated	3	2.1
Access site infection	2	1.4
Acute myocardial infarction	2	1.4
Cardiac arrhythmias	4	2.8
Acute renal failure	3	2.1
Respiratory failure	8	5.6
Pulmonary embolism	2	1.4
Inadvertent branch vessel coverage	1	0.7
Branch vessel dissection	1	0.7
Visceral infarcts	2	1.4
Pancreatitis	2	1.4
Retroperitoneal hematoma	2	1.4
Access site hematoma	3	2.1
Vocal cord palsy	2	1.4
Device collapse	1	0.7
Late subclavian steal	1	0.7
Death	7	4.9
Stroke	11	7.6
Paraplegia/Paresis	4	2

Early Complications.   Neurological complications, consisting of stroke or spinal cord ischemia, occurred in 10% of the patients treated with both primary and secondary interventions (Table 40–2). Major stroke and paraplegia or paresis rates were 7.6% (n=11) and 2.8% (n=4), respectively.

Arterial access injuries occurred in 14 cases (10%) (cut-down approach [n= 9], percutaneous approach [n= 3], iliac conduit [n= 2]). Eight patients (5.6%) suffered from respiratory failure requiring prolonged intubation or tracheostomy. One young trauma patient experienced device collapse. Three patients experienced acute postoperative renal failure.

Follow-up.   Mean follow-up with imaging of the graft was 21 months (±15 months, range 1–88 months). There were eight patients who were lost to follow-up after their one-month CTA. Five of these were trauma patients treated for acute aortic transection.

Late Mortality.   A total of 22 patients died after the 30-day perioperative period. Causes of death included coronary artery disease or heart failure (n=6), rupture or sepsis from an infected graft (n=5), sepsis from other causes (n=3), respiratory failure (n=3), pneumonia with endocarditis (n=1), perforated duodenal ulcer following ascending arch repair (n=1), rupture awaiting reintervention (n=1), aspiration (n=1), and unknown causes (n=1). The overall delayed infection rate, including one patient who is still alive, was 4.2% (n=6).

Nonfatal Late Complications.   Nine patients developed type I or type III endoleaks (6.3%). Of the nine patients, four were originally treated with custom-made stent-grafts. The average time to appearance of endoleak was 10.2 months. Seven patients underwent repeat operative intervention. Nine additional patients (6.3%) were found to have type II endoleaks on surveillance imaging. None have resulted in sac enlargement and, therefore, have not been treated. Only three (33%) of these patients with type II leaks have persisted beyond one year.

Three additional patients underwent operative intervention for progression of their aortic disease in the absence of an endoleak. One patient underwent an aortic arch repair simultaneous with coronary bypass grafting procedure for aneurysmal degeneration of the ascending arch at seven months. Another patient who was initially treated for a symptomatic subacute type B dissection developed an asymptomatic retrograde type A dissection noted on a six-month surveillance CTA and underwent conversion to a hybrid procedure with an arch replacement. This likely resulted from aortic penetration by the endoprosthesis. A third patient, originally treated for an acute complicated dissection, developed aneurysmal degeneration of the visceral segment with rupture, and underwent emergent open reconstruction and replacement of the aorta from the endograft to the aortic bifurcation.

DISCUSSION

The natural history of untreated major thoracic aortic pathology is a strong impetus for patients to consider operative repair, even if they are severely compromised or elderly. Several large series report significant morbidity following traditional open approaches to thoracic aortic reconstruction, especially when performed under emergent circumstances.[5,6] The use of endovascular devices for the treatment of thoracic aortic aneurysms, and for off-label indications such as traumatic aortic disruptions and dissection, has resulted in decreased rates of mortality, renal failure, and paralysis in both small series and large trials.[2-4,7-9] This new technology has provided higher risk patients, originally denied treatment via conventional operative repair, the opportunity to be treated with satisfactory results. Data from this series would support continued use of TEVAR in a high-risk group; however, our data suggest that the incidence of significant complications remains high in this patient population. Our results are consistent with other reports with similar risk patients noting a combined stroke, death, and paralysis/paresis rate of 15%[2,10,11] and a periprocedural mortality rate of 4.8%.[5,12] The combined rate of stroke, death, and paralysis/paresis for emergent procedures in our series was nearly 20%. In comparison, large series of open repair quote mortality rates as high as 26%.[12,13] Our midterm results with the endovascular treatment of thoracic aortic pathology reflect the relative high risk patient population that we have treated at our institution. The life table analysis indicates that a significant portion of the patients died within one year of their index procedure, the causes of which are not related to their endograft procedure. These results reinforce the severity of illness in patients with thoracic aortic pathology and also brings forth the question of who will reap the most benefit from a minimally invasive method of treatment of aortic disease.

The durability and effectiveness of minimally invasive treatment of the thoracic aorta warrants discussion, and continued imaging surveillance of these devices remains paramount.[8,14,15] In our series, the rate of type I or III endoleaks was significant at 6.3%. Many of the leaks were early type II, none required immediate conversion to open repair, and most followed treatment with custom-made devices. Industry-manufactured devices seem to perform more favorably, provided they are used in the appropriate setting. Excluding devices placed for traumatic aortic injury (which would not be expected to leak), the type I and type III endoleak rate for industry-manufactured devices and custom-made devices in this series was 5.2% and 23.5%, respectively. In midterm reports, endoleak rates as high as 24% have been reported for custom-made grafts.[14-17] The GORE TAG investigators report an incidence of any endoleak at two years to be 9%; of these, only three patients required endovascular revision.[4] The Talent thoracic registry, which included 457 patients treated for various thoracic aortic pathology, reports a persistent primary endoleak rate of 9.6% with type I endoleak being the most common and the most important risk factor for late rupture.[2] Other series of patients treated with industry-designed thoracic stent-grafts have reported rates of endoleaks ranging between 6–20%, type I being the most common.[3,8,9,17,18] Early type I leaks, defined as those identified on completion angiography or on a ≤1 month CT scan, should be expected to resolve spontaneously. As such, a period of observation is not unreasonable. However, early leaks that persist beyond six months should be treated. Type I leaks that develop late (after six months) rarely resolve spontaneously, and should be considered for open or endovascular treatment.

Patients with concomitant ascending arch disease may require even more strict surveillance. Two of our patients developed type I endoleaks, with sac expansion, as a result of progression of arch pathology. Demers et al. did not report graft migration in their series, but instead proposed inadequate fixation as the contributing factor to the development of type I endoleaks.[19] They suggest that continued aortic aneurysmal degeneration changes the morphology of the landing zones, thus making late endoleaks possible. This would appear to be a plausible mechanism for late failure in our series as well. These patients require intervention, usually with open arch reconstruction incorporating the endograft into the distal anastomosis, as these leaks would not be expected to resolve spontaneously and most are adjacent to the great vessels.

In patients with traumatic aortic disruption, the rate of endoleak was 0%. Trauma patients generally have a healthy, normal caliber, aorta with an acute tear, and without aneurysmal pathology. Endoleaks would not be expected to occur in these patients and, therefore, should probably not be included in the context of early or late complications of TEVAR for this subgroup. In fact, all patients treated with aortic extender cuffs for this indication in this series did not experience any device-related complications during follow-up. The primary concern for endograft placement in a healthy but acutely transected aorta is the possibility of device collapse.[20,21] In these young, hyperdynamic patients, when grafts are oversized relative to the aorta, there is a risk for device collapse and distal malperfusion. We did observe this complication in one patient with aortic transection who was treated with a GORE TAG device. Our experience, as well as current literature, reflects the decreased morbidity and mortality with endograft placement for the treatment of polytrauma patients with thoracic aortic injury, and the low rate of repeat intervention for device-related complications. We consider making it a preferred alternative to open surgical repair.[3,22]

Delayed endograft infection and subsequent type I endoleak from presumed aortic wall degeneration was a cause for both early and late aneurysm-related deaths in our series. Patients in our series who developed graft infection within six weeks of device implantation may have had a primary aortic infection that was not recognized at the time of initial presentation. The patients that presented with delayed graft infection likely had seeding of their graft from remote infections that developed after the index procedure. What is evident from our experience is that graft placement in the setting of primary aortic or active remote infection may result in endograft infection, and subsequent rupture and death. Since there are few reports of endografts placed for thoracic aortic infections or fistulas, and fewer reports of delayed thoracic aortic graft infection, the natural history of endovascular repair in the setting of infection is relatively unknown.[23,24] The treatment of a known thoracic aortic infection with an endograft should be undertaken with caution and perhaps should not be performed at all. If active infection is evident at the time of device implantation, lifelong antibiotic coverage should be considered. Similarly, late remote infections need to be promptly diagnosed and treated as late endograft seeding may be more common with thoracic endoprostheses than with sewn in grafts.

The stroke rate of 7.6% in this report is on the higher end of the spectrum compared to other series including those with open surgical repair.[3,18,25] Our stroke rate may be higher due to the large number of patients treated for very proximal disease in this series. Thoracic aortic disease that is adjacent to the great vessels requires manipulation of the arch with wires, catheters, and the device prior to device deployment. Our stroke rate was highest in the earlier part of our series when most patients were treated with custom-made grafts. Other authors have also described a higher incidence of stroke with the use of custom-made devices. This is likely related to the size and stiffness of the delivery system.[14,19] The stroke rate in the second half of our series was reduced to 2% after developing an aggressive policy regarding minimal wire and catheter manipulation in the arch and routine branch vessel revascularization, and after we began to deploy only industry-designed devices.

Posterior circulation strokes occurred alone or in combination with anterior circulation strokes in five patients in our series. Early in our series, we identified two patients with isolated posterior circulation strokes who had endograft coverage of the subclavian artery. As a result, we now routinely perform subclavian artery transposition or carotid-to-subclavian bypass in patients with dominant left vertebral arterial circulation, LIMA coronary bypass grafts, anticipated extensive thoracic intercostal vessels coverage, or when the potential exists for retrograde perfusion of a type B dissection via a patent subclavian artery. We suspect that this aggressive policy of arch branch reconstruction has contributed to an improvement in stroke rate over time and may also contribute to optimal spinal cord perfusion.

Endovascular thoracic aortic repair is associated with a decreased incidence of paraplegia, compared with conventional operative repair. Patients with compromised thoracic intercostal arterial circulation or lack of compensatory lumbar or pelvic circulation due to prior aortic reconstruction are at higher risk for developing paraplegia or paresis.[17,18,26] To prevent spinal ischemia in a high-risk subset of patients, we selectively use spinal drainage when technically feasible and avoid perioperative hypotension.

In conclusion, advances in the endoluminal technology used to treat thoracic aortic pathology have allowed many patients to undergo life-saving treatments with decreased morbidity and mortality. On the other hand, it is clear that the elderly and infirm may not fare well, even with a "minimally invasive" therapy. Furthermore, unlike open surgical repair, the long-term durability of thoracic aortic endograft remains to be seen. Long-term imaging surveillance is required to monitor for endoleaks and repeat interventions may be required if device failure or migration should occur. Overall, TEVAR for thoracic aortic pathology is safe and efficacious, but it is not without significant high risk in the complex patient population who come to endovascular repair.

REFERENCES

1. Dake MD, Miller DC, Semba CP, Mitchell RS, Walker PJ, Liddell RP. Transluminal placement of endovascular stent-grafts for the treatment of descending thoracic aortic aneurysms. *N Engl J Med*. Dec 29 1994;331(26):1729–1734.
2. Fattori R, Nienaber CA, Rousseau H, et al. Results of endovascular repair of the thoracic aorta with the Talent Thoracic stent graft: the Talent Thoracic Retrospective Registry. *J Thorac Cardiovasc Surg*. Aug 2006;132(2):332–339.
3. Leurs LJ, Bell R, Degrieck Y, Thomas S, Hobo R, Lundbom J. Endovascular treatment of thoracic aortic diseases: combined experience from the EUROSTAR and United Kingdom Thoracic Endograft registries. *J Vasc Surg*. Oct 2004;40(4):670–679; discussion 679–680.
4. Makaroun MS, Dillavou ED, Kee ST, et al. Endovascular treatment of thoracic aortic aneurysms: results of the phase II multicenter trial of the GORE TAG thoracic endoprosthesis. *J Vasc Surg*. Jan 2005;41(1):1–9.
5. Coselli JS, Bozinovski J, LeMaire SA. Open surgical repair of 2286 thoracoabdominal aortic aneurysms. *Ann Thorac Surg*. Feb 2007;83(2):S862–864; discussion S890–862.
6. Crawford ES, Hess KR, Cohen ES, Coselli JS, Safi HJ. Ruptured aneurysm of the descending thoracic and thoracoabdominal aorta. Analysis according to size and treatment. *Ann Surg*. May 1991;213(5):417–425; discussion 425–416.
7. Cambria RP, Brewster DC, Lauterbach SR, et al. Evolving experience with thoracic aortic stent graft repair. *J Vasc Surg*. Jun 2002;35(6):1129–1136.
8. Patel HJ, Williams DM, Upchurch GR, Jr., et al. Long-term results from a 12-year experience with endovascular therapy for thoracic aortic disease. *Ann Thorac Surg*. Dec 2006;82(6): 2147–2153.
9. Wheatley GH, 3rd, Gurbuz AT, Rodriguez-Lopez JA, et al. Midterm outcome in 158 consecutive Gore TAG thoracic endoprostheses: single center experience. *Ann Thorac Surg*. May 2006;81(5):1570–1577; discussion 1577.
10. Orend KH, Scharrer-Pamler R, Kapfer X, Kotsis T, Gorich J, Sunder-Plassmann L. Endovascular treatment in diseases of the descending thoracic aorta: 6-year results of a single center. *J Vasc Surg*. Jan 2003;37(1):91–99.
11. Riesenman PJ, Farber MA, Mendes RR, et al. Endovascular repair of lesions involving the descending thoracic aorta. *J Vasc Surg*. Dec 2005;42(6):1063–1074.
12. Conrad MF, Crawford RS, Davison JK, Cambria RP. Thoracoabdominal aneurysm repair: a 20-year perspective. *Ann Thorac Surg*. Feb 2007;83(2):S856–861; discussion S890–852.
13. Girardi LN, Krieger KH, Altorki NK, Mack CA, Lee LY, Isom OW. Ruptured descending and thoracoabdominal aortic aneurysms. *Ann Thorac Surg*. Oct 2002;74(4):1066–1070.
14. Dake MD, Miller DC, Mitchell RS, Semba CP, Moore KA, Sakai T. The "first generation" of endovascular stent-grafts for patients with aneurysms of the descending thoracic aorta. *J Thorac Cardiovasc Surg*. Nov 1998;116(5):689–703; discussion 703–684.
15. Greenberg R, Resch T, Nyman U, et al. Endovascular repair of descending thoracic aortic aneurysms: an early experience with intermediate-term follow-up. *J Vasc Surg*. Jan 2000;31 (1 Pt 1):147–156.
16. Ishida M, Kato N, Hirano T, Cheng SH, Shimono T, Takeda K. Endovascular stent-graft treatment for thoracic aortic aneurysms: short- to midterm results. *J Vasc Interv Radiol*. Apr 2004;15(4):361–367.
17. Stone DH, Brewster DC, Kwolek CJ, et al. Stent-graft versus open-surgical repair of the thoracic aorta: mid-term results. *J Vasc Surg*. Dec 2006;44(6):1188–1197.
18. Bavaria JE, Appoo JJ, Makaroun MS, Verter J, Yu ZF, Mitchell RS. Endovascular stent grafting versus open surgical repair of descending thoracic aortic aneurysms in low-risk patients: a multicenter comparative trial. *J Thorac Cardiovasc Surg*. Feb 2007;133(2):369–377.
19. Demers P, Miller DC, Mitchell RS, et al. Midterm results of endovascular repair of descending thoracic aortic aneurysms with first-generation stent grafts. *J Thorac Cardiovasc Surg*. Mar 2004;127(3):664–673.

20. Muhs BE, Balm R, White GH, Verhagen HJ. Anatomic factors associated with acute endograft collapse after Gore TAG treatment of thoracic aortic dissection or traumatic rupture. *J Vasc Surg*. Apr 2007;45(4):655–661.
21. Neschis DG, Moaine S, Gutta R, et al. Twenty consecutive cases of endograft repair of traumatic aortic disruption: lessons learned. *J Vasc Surg*. Mar 2007;45(3):487–492.
22. Lettinga-van de Poll T, Schurink GW, De Haan MW, Verbruggen JP, Jacobs MJ. Endovascular treatment of traumatic rupture of the thoracic aorta. *Br J Surg*. May 2007;94(5): 525–533.
23. Sayed S, Choke E, Helme S, et al. Endovascular stent graft repair of mycotic aneurysms of the thoracic aorta. *J Cardiovasc Surg* (Torino). Apr 2005;46(2):155–161.
24. Semba CP, Sakai T, Slonim SM, et al. Mycotic aneurysms of the thoracic aorta: repair with use of endovascular stent-grafts. *J Vasc Interv Radiol*. Jan-Feb 1998;9(1 Pt 1):33–40.
25. Khoynezhad A, Donayre CE, Bui H, Kopchok GE, Walot I, White RA. Risk factors of neurologic deficit after thoracic aortic endografting. *Ann Thorac Surg*. Feb 2007;83(2):S882–889; discussion S890–882.
26. Gravereaux EC, Faries PL, Burks JA, et al. Risk of spinal cord ischemia after endograft repair of thoracic aortic aneurysms. *J Vasc Surg*. Dec 2001;34(6):997–1003.

41

Understanding Acute Dissection

Peter S. Liu, M.D.
David M. Williams, M.D.

Understanding aortic dissection is a three-fold problem: understanding what causes aortic dissection, how to diagnose it, and how best to treat it. Astonishingly, the medical community is little closer now to an understanding of the pathogenesis of aortic dissection than it was 250 years ago when King George II of England abruptly died of this condition. Despite our incomplete understanding of the pathogenesis, however, patients with aortic dissection have benefited from recent improvements in diagnosis and treatment, in particular from multidetector CT scans, and from ongoing refinements in endovascular approaches to treating aortic and arterial disease.

Aortic dissection is classically characterized by separation of the vascular intima from the vascular adventitia by blood in the vascular media, often with two resultant parallel flow channels.[1] The disease can have protean clinical manifestations that overlap substantially with other acute cardiopulmonary diseases.[2] Contemporary approaches to the understanding of aortic dissection now utilize the concept of an "acute aortic syndrome", which describes a spectrum of disease that encompasses penetrating atherosclerotic ulcers, intramural hematoma, and classic aortic dissection.[3] Central to the management of aortic dissection is detailed morphologic evaluation of suspected aortic pathology.[4] Advances in modern tomographic imaging techniques now allow fast, reproducible, and accurate imaging of aortic dissection, facilitating appropriate patient triage into medical or surgical therapy.

BACKGROUND

Once thought to be relatively rare, the incidence of aortic dissection has been estimated in well-defined population studies to be approximately three per 100,000 per year.[5] Men are affected more frequently than women, approximately a 2:1 ratio.[6] Commonly recognized risk factors for the development of aortic dissection include long-standing arterial hypertension, bicuspid aortic-valve, pregnancy, connective tissue diseases, and deceleration trauma.[1,4] Additionally, postoperative or iatrogenic etiologies constitute over 20% of cases, particularly in patients less than 40 years of age.[4,6]

In the classical paradigm, the critical inciting event in the pathogenesis of spontaneous aortic dissection involves intimal disruption, often referred to as an entry tear.[3,7] The mechanism of intimal tear is unclear. This tear typically occurs perpendicular to the direction of flow and at a site of high hydraulic stress; in the thorax, this most frequently affects the right lateral wall of the ascending aorta and the proximal segment of the descending aorta.[3] The disruption of the vascular intima allows blood to flow into the vascular wall itself, subsequently separating the vascular media and creating two distinct flow channels—the true lumen and the false lumen—with an interposed flap that results from delaminated vascular media. An abnormal underlying vascular media has been cited as important to the genesis and longitudinal propagation of the dissection flap.[1,7] Physiologically, the flow of blood into the intimal injury/false lumen is often greater than the rate at which blood is able to exit, if at all. Consequently, a tunnel forms parallel to the direction of blood flow. Poor outflow also leads to asymmetric pressurization of the false lumen versus the true lumen, particularly during diastole.[1] This results in progressive enlargement of the false lumen, which can compress or efface the true lumen; end-organ ischemia can result if the organ perfusion is diminished.[1] A dominant re-entry tear may also be present distally, often in the abdominal or iliac arteries.[3]

In an alternative paradigm, the dissection begins as spontaneous hemorrhage of the vasa vasorum into the aortic media.[8] The cause of the hemorrhage is unclear. If the interlamellar attachments of the medial layers are weak, the hematoma may grow in size and propagate within the media. As the hematoma spreads, it can injure small branches such as nearby vasa vasorum or even intercostal arteries, causing them to bleed within the media and amplify the intramedial hemorrhage. In addition, the propagating intramural hemorrhage severs the interlamellar attachments of the inner wall to the adventitia. As larger areas of the inner wall overlie intramedial hemorrhage, radial and longitudinal stretching of the inner wall during systole is unbuttressed by the tough outer adventitial layer, and the inner wall may tear.

CLINICAL EVALUATION

The clinical manifestations of aortic dissection are diverse, and overlap significantly with other acute cardiopulmonary disease processes including myocardial infarction, acute pulmonary embolism, or aortic rupture. Frequently, the patient with acute aortic dissection presents with an abrupt onset of tremendous chest pain; 90% of patients in one series qualified the pain as "worst ever".[6] Traditionally, the pain has been characterized as "tearing" or "ripping", though one population study suggests that this quality is only seen in 50% of patients.[1,2,6] The pain can have an anterior or posterior component, which can be suggestive of the dissection type.[4,6] Only 25% of cases will report radiation of the pain, which is more commonly associated with myocardial infarction. Pain in aortic dissection can be paroxysmal, which further complicates the clinical picture.[1] There may be concomitant branch artery involvement with resultant end-organ ischemic changes; rarely are these ischemic sequelae the sole manifestation of dissection. Extension of the dissection flap into certain anatomic and vascular territories can have catastrophic consequences, resulting in varied clinical presentations, including cardiac tamponade, critical aortic insufficiency, myocardial infarction, or hemispheric stroke. Additionally, 4% of patients with dissection may present with pain predominantly localized to the abdomen.[6] Therefore, a high index of clinical suspicion and appropriate imaging are often required to work up suspected aortic dissection.

Clinical classification of aortic dissection is based on morphologic features. The Stanford system simply classifies dissections on the basis of whether the ascending aorta is involved (Type A) or is not involved (Type B). The DeBakey system utilizes three categories: Type I is characterized by both ascending and descending aortic involvement (accounting for approximately 35% of dissections); Type II is characterized by involvement of the ascending aorta only (15%); and Type III is characterized by involvement of the descending aorta only, distal to the takeoff of the left subclavian artery (50%).[1] Currently, the Stanford system is the more commonly employed classification system in modern clinical practice.

Proper classification of a dissection is critical to proper management and offers important prognostic information. Stanford Type A dissections have a poor natural history with a mortality rate of 1–2% per hour after symptom onset.[4] In the absence of surgical intervention, Type A dissections have a dismal prognosis with a mortality approaching 50–80% at two weeks.[1,4] Because of this, management for Type A dissections is predicated on surgical revision of the ascending aorta utilizing an interposed graft. Even with surgery, in-hospital mortality for repaired Type A dissections remains approximately 20% at two weeks, underscoring the tremendous mortality associated with these types of dissections. In contrast, Stanford Type B dissections are considerably less lethal than Type A dissections with a one-month mortality of approximately 10% due to fewer life-threatening sequelae.[4] Currently, patients with Type B dissections are treated with aggressive medical management including blood pressure control and pain relief. Visceral organ/limb ischemia, progression of dissection, and intractable pain have been considered indications for operative management of Type B dissections.

IMAGING WORKUP

The primary goal of imaging is identification of the cause of chest pain so as to begin proper and timely treatment. Once the presence of aortic dissection is established, a number of anatomical features of the patient's dissection must be established. These include involvement of the ascending aorta; longitudinal extent of the dissection; identification of true and false lumens; source of perfusion to the superior mesenteric, renal, and common iliac arteries; the presence of complications including false lumen rupture, pericardial fluid, and branch artery compromise; location of entry and reentry tears with respect to critical branch arteries; and diameters of the total aorta and aortic true lumen in the aortic arch, at the level of the entry tear(s) and in the mid-descending aorta.

CONVENTIONAL RADIOGRAPHY

Although frequently employed as the first study in the diagnostic algorithm for chest pain, the conventional chest radiograph lacks sufficient diagnostic accuracy for aortic dissection.[9] Features of aortic dissection on chest radiograph include widening of the mediastinum, enlargement of the aortic knob, pleural effusion, and displaced vascular calcifications (Figure 41–1). Unfortunately, interobserver agreement on these

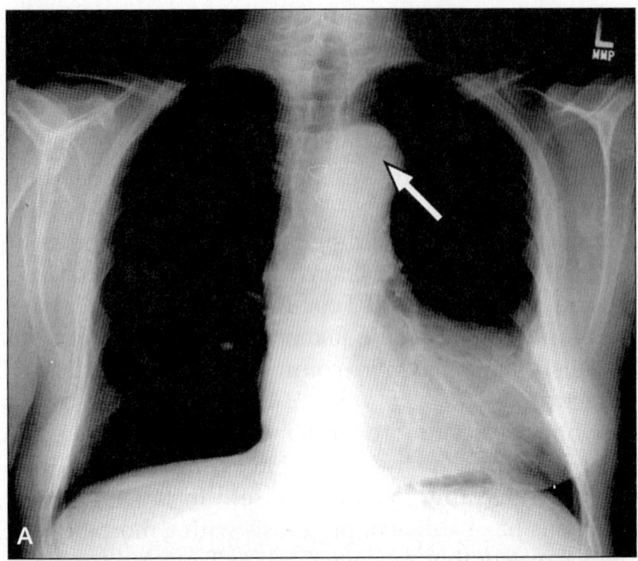

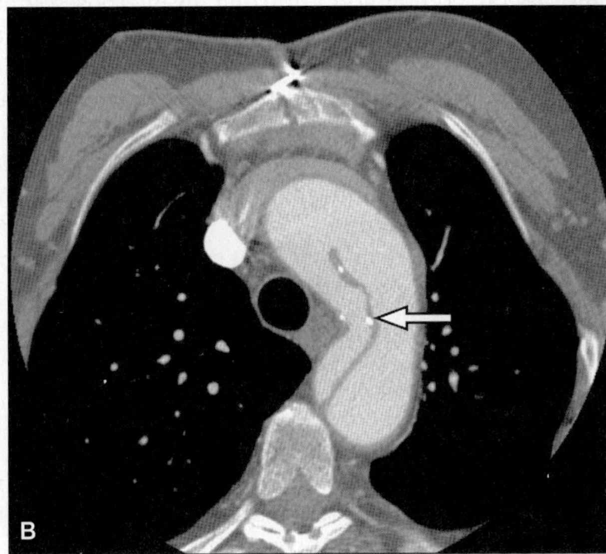

Figure 41-1. A Frontal chest radiograph demonstrates very subtle linear calcification projecting over the aortic knob (arrow). There is apparent displacement from the normal curved surface of the aortic arch. B Axial CT arteriogram image with intravenous contrast demonstrates a dissection flap in the aortic arch with focal flap calcification (arrow) corresponding to the linear density on chest radiograph.

radiographic features has been shown to be poor.[10] Furthermore, several of these radiographic features can be seen in other disease processes, which can decrease specificity. The sensitivity and specificity of radiographs in the diagnosis of aortic dissection have been reported to vary between 64–81% and 86–89%, respectively.[9-10] Thus, the chest radiograph cannot be reliably used to make the diagnosis of aortic dissection.

COMPUTED TOMOGRAPHY

Computed tomography (CT) is a method of generating tomographic images using a rotating X-ray source and detector element combination.[1] The advent of helical scanning, maturation of multidetector technology, and routine use of power injectors has made computed tomography angiography (CTA) a robust tool for modern vascular imaging. CT/CTA has many advantages as an imaging modality. Computed tomography technology is widely available, including in emergency departments, and requires less operator oversight to produce diagnostic and reproducible images than does echocardiography or magnetic resonance imaging.[11] Short scan times facilitate imaging of patients with borderline hemodynamic stability. The CT examination suite can readily accommodate patients who have indwelling medical devices or who require mobile life-support apparatuses without the difficulty encountered by such patients in magnetic resonance imaging suites. The disadvantages of CT/CTA include the use of ionizing radiation and nephrotoxic contrast agents.

The evaluation of suspected acute aortic dissection is best accomplished with CTA.[9] CTA can accurately assess the morphology of the dissection, evaluate for branch artery involvement, and look for other complications of dissection such as hemopericardium (Figures 41–2 and 41–3).[2] Because of the high prevalence of branch artery compromise, the imaging volume should extend from the brachiocephalic arteries to the femoral heads. Sensitivity and specificity of CTA for suspected aortic pathology approaches 95% and 100%, respectively.[12] In addition, CTA can also accurately evaluate the surrounding nonvascular structures to provide an alternative explanation for the patients symptoms.[13] Evaluation usually is accomplished with a multiphase protocol, including precontrast imaging and thin-section postcontrast imaging during the arterial phase of vascular enhancement. Some institutions also acquire a second postcontrast image set during a delayed phase of vascular enhancement. Power injectors allow delivery of a compact bolus of iodinated contrast, which is ideal for arteriographic applications. A bolus tracking technology is frequently used to optimize arterial enhancement. Synchronizing the acquisition of image data to the patient's EKG, via either prospective triggering or retrospective gating, can dramatically reduce apparent motion throughout the thoracic aorta, including near the aortic valve (Figure 41–4).[14]

Diagnosis of aortic dissection on CTA is predicated on demonstration of the intimomedial flap, usually best seen on contrast-enhanced images. The morphology of the

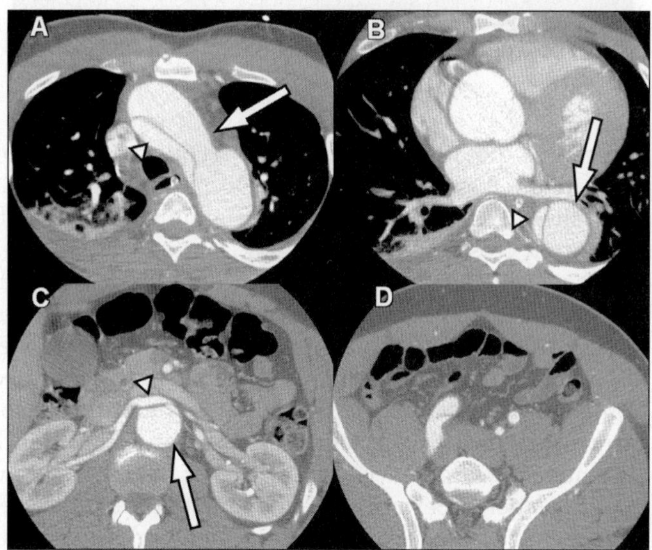

Figure 41-2. Several axial CT arteriogram images with intravenous contrast reveals the typical appearance of aortic dissection **(A)** at various levels from cranial to caudal. There is a Type A dissection that extends from the ascending aorta through to the right iliac artery. Note compression of the true lumen **(B)**, particularly around the level of the renal arteries **(C)**. Re-entry tear is present in the right iliac artery, as depicted in **(D)** Arrow = false lumen; arrowheads = true lumen.

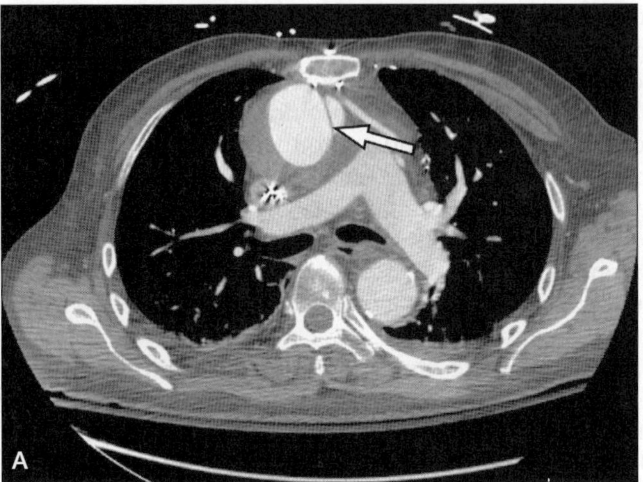

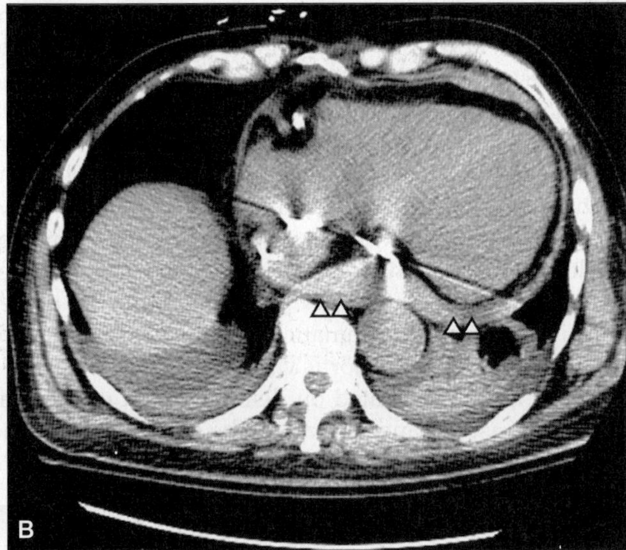

Figure 41-3. A Axial CT arteriogram image with intravenous contrast demonstrates Type A aortic dissection in this patient with chest pain and hypotension (arrow = intimomedial flap). There is increased attenuation in the extravascular space of the mediastinum. B Axial CT arteriogram image without intravenous contrast demonstrates increased attenuation in the pericardial space (arrowheads), measuring 50–60 Hounsfield units, compatible with hemorrhage on noncontrast imaging.

flap can be quite tortuous, and may require data postprocessing on a workstation to generate a reformatted image that accurately depicts the flap geometry and entry/reentry sites.[9] Discrimination of the true lumen from the false lumen is particularly important on cross-sectional imaging, particularly in the era of endovascular repair.[15] This is usually best accomplished for the true lumen by tracing luminal continuity with a nondissected portion of aorta. In contrast, the false lumen often has a larger cross-sectional area than the true lumen, and may demonstrate acute angulation between the dissection flap and the outer vascular wall, the so-called "beak sign" (Figure 41–5).[15] Complete evaluation requires review of the precontrast images as well, particularly if there is diagnostic uncertainty between an intramural hematoma and a thrombosed false lumen; the former is usually higher in attenuation versus background blood pool than the latter.[2,9] Several well-document artifacts can decrease diagnostic certainty on CTA including streak artifact from metal or dense contrast bolus, prominent normal

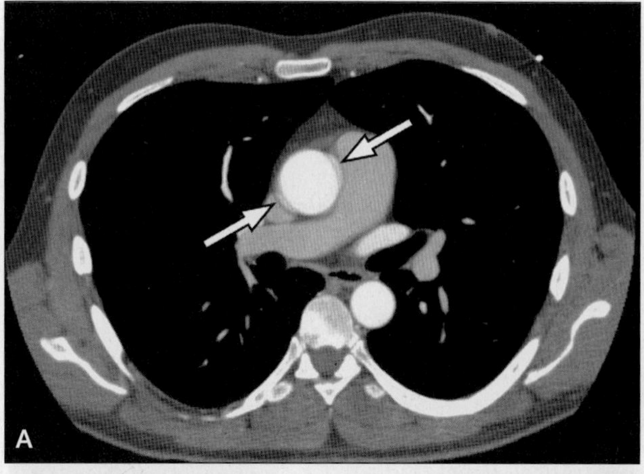

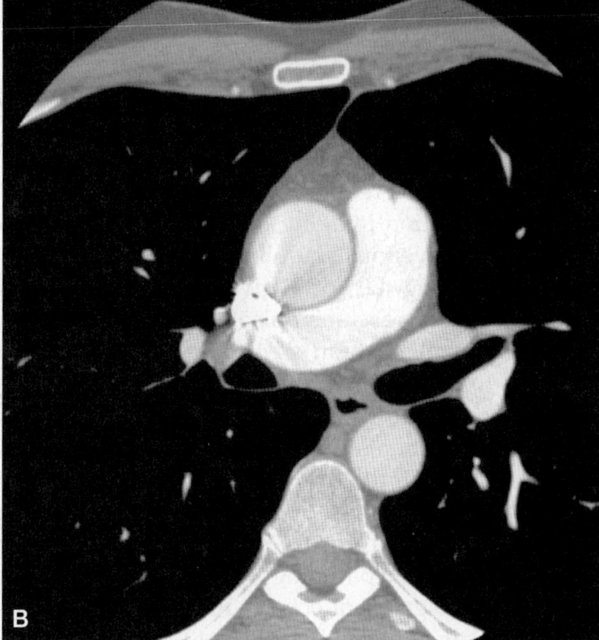

Figure 41-4. A Axial CT arteriogram image with contrast; no ECG gating was performed at the time of scan acquisition, leading to motion artifact at the aortic root that could be confused for aortic dissection. **B** Axial CT arteriogram image with contrast; repeat imaging with ECG gating was performed to evaluate for occult dissection. No dissection is apparent when scan technique accounts for cardiovascular motion.

periaortic structures, or aortic anatomical variants.[1,16] CTA offers a robust method of evaluating suspected aortic dissection with high diagnostic accuracy; a normal CTA in a patient with suspected dissection essentially excludes the diagnosis.[1]

MAGNETIC RESONANCE IMAGING

Magnetic resonance imaging (MRI) generates tomographic images without ionizing radiation utilizing a strong magnetic field and a series of radiofrequency pulses to elicit signals from proton relaxation in the body.[17] Magnetic resonance angiography

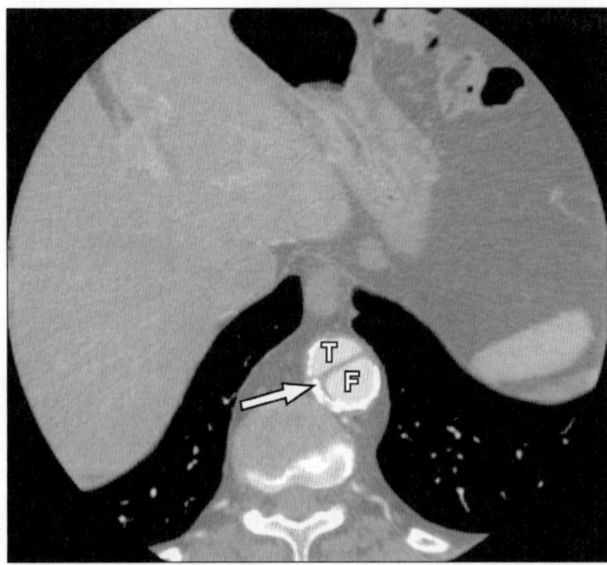

Figure 41-5. Axial CT arteriogram image with contrast demonstrates aortic dissection involving the descending thoracic aorta. The true lumen (T) can frequently be distinguished from the false lumen (F) on axial imaging by looking for the "beak sign" (arrow). This represents a wedge of hematoma that cleaves a space for the propagating false lumen.

(MRA) has numerous benefits, including excellent soft tissue contrast, high sensitivity to subtle flow, and native multiplanar capabilities. Advances in technology now permit high-resolution imaging of the entire aorta in acceptable acquisition times, often relying on intravenous Gadolinium contrast agents. This addresses the inherent challenges of imaging the aorta, given the length of coverage required and speed needed to accommodate vascular pulsatility and respiratory motion. Unfortunately, MRA is less widely available than CTA, takes longer to perform, and requires greater operator oversight to achieve consistent results.[9] Furthermore, the high field strength environment of most clinical scanners requires special life-support apparatuses and precludes evaluation of patients with certain medical devices, including pacemakers and defibrillators. Although often not used in the acute setting, MRA is an excellent option for long-term dissection follow up or evaluation of the hemodynamically stable patient.[1]

Modern MRA protocols often utilize both pre- and postcontrast imaging to evaluate suspected aortic pathology, similar to CTA. The primary method of evaluating the aorta is the 3-D gradient echo sequence with minimally short repetition time, resulting in severe T1-weighting. Injection of Gadolinium contrast shortens the relaxation time of the blood pool, resulting in positive intravascular signal and single-breathhold acquisition times (Figure 41–6).[17] Similar to CTA, power injectors and accurate bolus tracking methods are required to produce optimal arterial phase enhancement and data acquisition. Precontrast images serve two purposes: 1) identify intramural hemorrhage that could be less conspicuous on postcontrast images; and 2) generate a mask for data subtraction during postprocessing. Almost all postprocessing techniques benefit from the decreased background signal intensity inherent to MRA, which can be a common source for artifact during CTA postprocessing (i.e., osseous structures).[18] Although recent news suggests a possible link between intravenous Gadolinium contrast and a skin disorder called nephrogenic systemic fibrosis, noncontrast MRI techniques can also produce angiographic images, a distinct advantage versus CT.[17,19] Traditionally, this has been accomplished with specific sequences that generate high intravascular signal, such as time-of-flight or phase contrast techniques. Newer non-

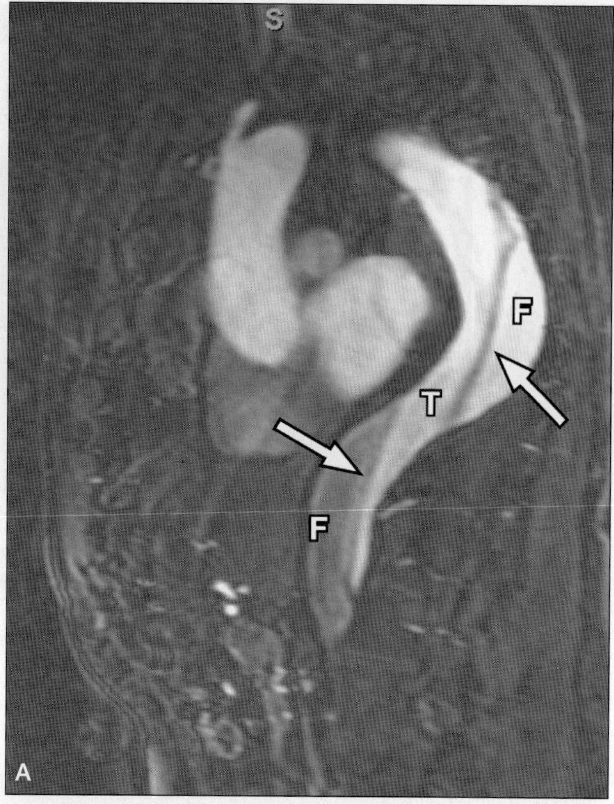

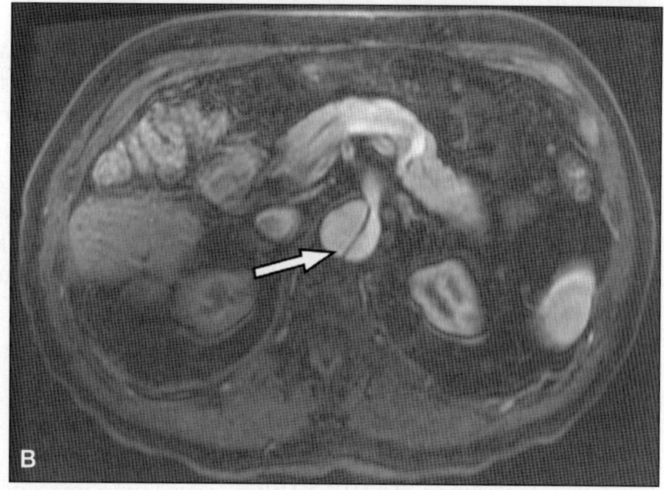

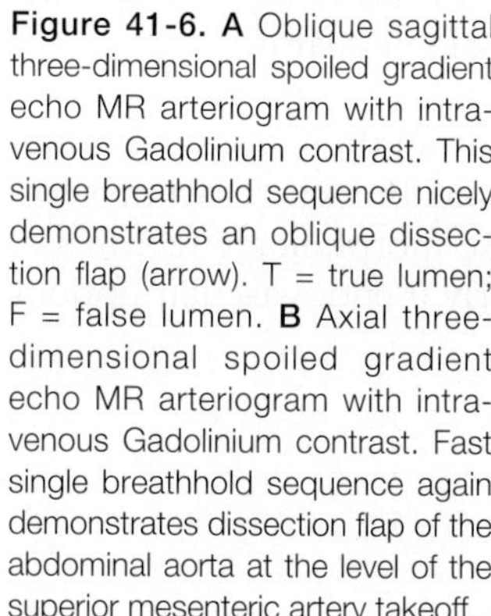

Figure 41-6. A Oblique sagittal three-dimensional spoiled gradient echo MR arteriogram with intravenous Gadolinium contrast. This single breathhold sequence nicely demonstrates an oblique dissection flap (arrow). T = true lumen; F = false lumen. **B** Axial three-dimensional spoiled gradient echo MR arteriogram with intravenous Gadolinium contrast. Fast single breathhold sequence again demonstrates dissection flap of the abdominal aorta at the level of the superior mesenteric artery takeoff.

contrast techniques, such as steady state free precession, produce images with high intravascular signal and excellent background detail, and require substantially shorter imaging times than traditional noncontrast techniques (Figure 41–7).[20] The overall diagnostic accuracy of MRA for the diagnosis of aortic dissection is high, with reported sensitivities and specificities of 95–100% and 94–98%, respectively.[2] Because of the

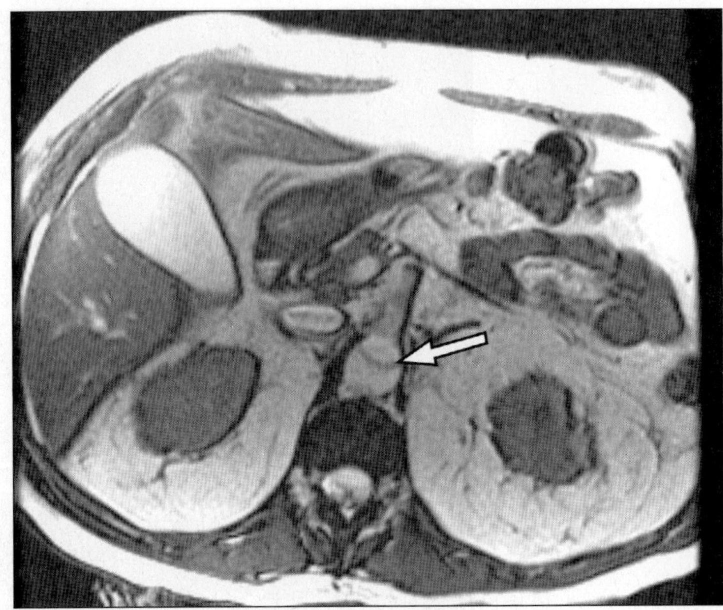

Figure 41-7. Axial steady state-free precession image in the upper abdomen. No intravenous contrast was administered. A dissection flap (arrow) involving the abdominal aorta is well delineated despite lack of intravenous contrast. The sequence was acquired in a single breathhold.

variety of techniques available, MRA offers a valuable alternative to CTA in the evaluation of aortic dissection.

The diagnosis of aortic dissection of MRA is similar to CTA, relying on morphologic identification of the intimomedial flap. This is best accomplished on images with high intravascular signal, usually postcontrast 3-D gradient echo images or specific noncontrast angiographic sequences. Again, certain morphologic features can be applied to differentiate the true lumen from the false lumen, including greater signal intensity in the true lumen on arterial phase imaging and smaller cross-sectional diameter.[18] Similar to CTA, MRA can define the entry-tear site, branch vessel involvement, and the degree of thrombus in the false lumen. These morphologic features of the dissection are important for planning therapy, particularly if endovascular options are entertained.

INTRAVASCULAR ULTRASOUND

Intravascular ultrasound (IVUS) allows real-time imaging of the aorta and is nearly indispensable when performing endovascular treatment of aortic dissection. IVUS of the aorta requires an 8 F sheath, while IVUS of branch arteries can be performed through a 5 F sheath. The 8 F ultrasound catheter is quite stiff and hugs the greater curve of the ascending aorta and aortic arch. In a large diameter aorta, the eccentric lie of the IVUS catheter in the lumen may make it difficult to demonstrate anatomical features on the opposite wall. However, IVUS allows identification of the true and false lumen with nearly absolute certainty, maps the luminal path of the guidewire from puncture site to area of interest, demonstrates the relation of the dissection flap with respect to vessel origins, identifies the mechanism of branch-artery obstruction as dynamic or static, localizes entry and reentry tears, and identifies anatomical changes in the dissection flap in response to endograft placement or fenestration.[21] Moreover, it provides all this information without the use of nephrotoxic contrast.

ANGIOGRAPHY

Angiography has an important role in the endovascular treatment of aortic dissection, but little role otherwise. In our own experience with fenestration and stenting, the workup of suspected malperfusion begins with intravascular ultrasound of the thoracic and abdominal aorta and common iliac arteries, which demonstrates the relation of the dissection flap to vessel origins, and accordingly identifies the vessel(s) at risk of obstruction and suggests the probable mechanism of obstruction. This is followed by dual manometry with simultaneous pressure measurements in the ascending aorta and in each of the branch arteries. Each branch artery pressure measurement is followed by hand-injection of 4–8 cc of contrast, which is sufficient to verify that the location of pressure measurement is reliable and does not need to be repeated at a more distal point such as beyond the termination of a branch artery dissection. These hand injections also identify significant branch artery emboli or localized arteriopathy. Aortography, with standard 2-sec machine injections of contrast material at 15–25 cc/sec is rarely needed or performed. Endograft treatment of aortic dissections also requires careful demonstration of the entry tear with respect to the left common carotid and subclavian arteries. It is not clear whether or under what conditions IVUS provides sufficient anatomical information to allow safe implantation of an endograft in the distal arch.

CONCLUSION

Numerous advances in aortic imaging and endovascular treatment have improved our ability to diagnose and treat aortic dissection. We are hopeful that, in the near future, our knowledge of the pathogenesis of aortic dissection, specifically the sequence of biochemical steps necessary to induce spontaneous hemorrhage of the vasa vasorum and promote propagation of the hematoma, catch up with our technical advances in imaging and treatment, and perhaps contribute to the prevention of this vascular catastrophe.

REFERENCES

1. Kaufman, JA. Thoracic Aorta. In: Kaufman JA, Lee MJ, ed. *Vascular and Interventional Radiology: the Requisites 1st Ed*, Philadelphia: Mosby, 2004:219–245
2. Chughtai A, Kazerooni EA. CT and MRI of acute thoracic cardiovascular emergencies. *Crit Care Clin.* 2007;23(4):835–853, vii.
3. Vilacosta I, Rom·n JA. Acute aortic syndrome. *Heart.* 2001;85(4):365–368.

4. Tsai TT, Nienaber CA, Eagle KA. Acute Aortic Syndromes. *Circulation*. 2005;112;3802–3813
5. Mészáros I, Mórocz J, Szlávi J, et al. Epidemiology and clinicopathology of aortic dissection. *Chest*. 2000;117(5):1271–1278.
6. Hagan PG, Nienaber CA, Isselbacher EM, et al. The International Registry of Acute Aortic Dissection (IRAD): New Insights Into an Old Disease. *JAMA*. 200016;283(7):897–903
7. Macura KJ, Corl FM, Fishman EK, et al. Pathogenesis in acute aortic syndromes: aortic dissection, intramural hematoma, and penetrating atherosclerotic aortic ulcer. *AJR Am J Roentgenol*. 2003;181(2):309–16.
8. Krukenberg E. Beitrage zur Frage des Aneurysma dissecans. *Beitr Pathol Anat Allg Pathol*. 1920;67:329–351
9. De MonyÈ W, Murphy M, Hodgson R, et al. Acute aortic syndromes: pathology and imaging. *Imaging*. 2004;16:230–239
10. Jagannath AS, Sos TA, Lockhart SH, et al. Aortic dissection: a statistical analysis of the usefulness of plain chest radiographic findings. *AJR Am J Roentgenol*. 1986;147(6):1123–1126.
11. Hartnell GG. Imaging of aortic aneurysms and dissection: CT and MRI. *J Thorac Imaging*. 2001;16(1):35–46.
12. Hayter RG, Rhea JT, Small A, et al. Suspected aortic dissection and other aortic disorders: multi-detector row CT in 373 cases in the emergency setting. *Radiology*. 2006;238(3):841–52.
13. Olin JW, Kaufman JA, Bluemke DA, et al. Atherosclerotic Vascular Disease Conference: Writing Group IV: Imaging. *Circulation*. 2004;109(21):2626–2633.
14. Roos JE, Willmann JK, Weishaupt D, et al. Thoracic aorta: motion artifact reduction with retrospective and prospective electrocardiography-assisted multi-detector row CT. *Radiology*. 2002 Jan;222(1):271–7.
15. LePage MA, Quint LE, Sonnad SS, et al. Aortic dissection: CT features that distinguish true lumen from false lumen. *AJR Am J Roentgenol*. 2001;177(1):207–211.
16. Batra P, Bigoni B, Manning J, et al. Pitfalls in the diagnosis of thoracic aortic dissection at CT angiography. *Radiographics*. 2000 Mar-Apr;20(2):309–20.
17. Roberts D, Siegelman ES. Imaging and MR Arteriography of the Aorta. In: Siegelman ES , ed. *Body MRI 1st Ed*, Philadelphia: Elsevier 2005:481–507
18. Liu Q, Lu JP, Wang F, et al. Three-dimensional contrast-enhanced MR angiography of aortic dissection: a pictorial essay. *Radiographics*. 2007 Sep-Oct;27(5):1311–1321.
19. Marckmann P, Skov L, Rossen K, et al. Nephrogenic systemic fibrosis: suspected causative role of gadodiamide used for contrast-enhanced magnetic resonance imaging. *J Am Soc Nephrol*. 2006; 17:2359–2362
20. Mueller-Mang C, Wunderbaldinger P, Janata-Schwatzek K, et al. Acute dissection and contained rupture of a thoracic aortic aneurysm: emergency diagnosis with nonenhanced MR angiography. *Cardiovasc Intervent Radiol*. 2006 Sep-Oct;29(5):930–933.
21. Lee DY, Williams DM, Abrams GD. The dissected aorta: II. Differentiation of the true from the false lumen with intravascular US. *Radiology*. 1997;203:32–36.

42

Endovascular Treatment for Type B Aortic Dissection

David S. Wang, M.D., and Michael D. Dake, M.D.

Aortic dissection occurs when flowing blood enters the aortic wall through a disruption in the intimal lining and cleaves a longitudinal plane within the medial layer. Propagation of the delamination process can progress in variable lengths in a proximal and/or distal direction from the entry tear (with isolated antegrade progression being the more common pattern). As the process extends, a dissection flap or septum consisting of the cleaved lamellar layer of intima and partial thickness of media is created and partitions the original intima-lined lumen ("true" lumen) from a newly formed intramural channel ("false" lumen). This process may lead to additional disruptions in the intimal flap, producing exit or entry sites for flow between the dual lumens. Dissection propagation can also obstruct flow into aortic branch vessels, compromising downstream perfusion and causing distal ischemia (termed malperfusion syndrome). Potentially involving the coronaries to iliac arteries, aortic branch vessel compromise occurs by two mechanisms: static obstruction, where the aortic dissection flap extends directly into an aortic branch, or dynamic obstruction, where the dissection flap prolapses over the ostium of the branch vessel or collapses the true lumen of the aorta above it.[1] The eventual trajectory of flap progression results in a unique morphology for each case; thus, idiosyncratic anatomic relationships are formed between the flap, true lumen, false lumen, and the aortic branch vessels that are involved.

With an incidence of 2.6 to 3.5 per 100,000 person-years,[2-4] aortic dissection is considered the most common aortic catastrophe, occurring two to three times more frequently than AAA rupture.[5-7] It tends to affect males more frequently with a male to female ratio ranging between 2:1 to 5:1.[8-12] Sixty-three is the average age among 464 aortic dissection patients in the International Registry of Acute Aortic Dissection (IRAD).[9] Patients with dissections involving the ascending aorta tend to present at a younger age (50 to 55 years old) than those with dissections of the descending aorta (60 to 70 years old).[6,9,13-14]

The vast majority of aortic dissections originate in one of two locations: the lateral wall of the ascending aorta within a few centimeters of the aortic valve and in the descending aorta just distal to the site of insertion of the ligamentum arteriosum. These regions are presumably subjected to the greatest hemodynamic stress in terms of the first derivative of pressure (dP/dt) and overall pressure.[15] Anatomically, aortic dissections are classified under two systems. Under the DeBakey system, type I begins in the proximal aorta and involves both the ascending and descending thoracic aorta; type II is confined to the ascending aorta; and type III is confined to the descending aorta.[16] Under the Stanford system, type A aortic dissection involves the ascending aorta whereas type B dissection does not.[17] The more simple Stanford system has proven popular as the presence of ascending aortic involvement is associated with well-established prognostic implications and therapeutic considerations. Approximately 60% to 70% of aortic dissections are type A.[5,9] Aortic dissections are also classified according to duration. In general, dissections present less than two weeks are considered acute while those greater than two weeks are chronic. At two weeks, mortality curves of untreated aortic dissections begin to plateau.[11] A review of aortic dissection patients evaluated at the Mayo Clinic found a third to be chronic at diagnosis.[13]

Although the etiology of aortic dissection is not well defined and the precise initiating event remains unclear, several predisposing factors have been identified.[18] As seen with aortic aneurysms, conditions that cause medial degeneration and, in turn, decrease aortic wall integrity and cohesiveness, increase the risk of dissection. Patients with inherited connective tissue disorders, such as Marfan's syndrome and Ehlers-Danlos syndrome, display vascular CMN and are at high risk for aortic dissection. Such patients tend to present at a younger age with dissection of the ascending aorta.[19-21] In an IRAD study, Marfan's syndrome was present in half of those age 40 and under.[22] Necropsy studies have demonstrated, however, that medial degeneration is neither the predominant histological pattern of these lesions nor a prerequisite for dissection formation.[23] Other congenital predispositions to dissection include Turner's syndrome,[24-26] Noonan's syndrome,[27] aortic coarctation,[23,28] and bicuspid aortic valve.[29-30] In the absence of congenital risk factors, systemic hypertension, found in 70% to 80% of all dissection patients, is the most important predisposing factor.[9-13,23,31] The incidence of coexisting hypertension is higher in type B dissections (70% versus 36%).[9,11,23] By placing a greater mechanical strain on the arterial wall, hypertension may accelerate the normal medial degeneration associated with aging. The potential causative role of hypertension is underlined by the near exclusive occurrence of pulmonary artery dissection in the setting of pulmonary hypertension.[32] Other less common acquired risk factors include giant cell aortitis,[33-34] cocaine-use,[35-39] and deceleration and iatrogenic trauma.[40-43] There also exists a controversial association between pregnancy and dissection in young women.[43-47]

The cardinal feature of acute aortic dissection is severe chest and/or back pain that is sharp, ripping, or tearing in nature, and almost always abrupt in onset.[9,48,49] Patients with type A dissections more frequently experience anterior chest pain, whereas patients with type B dissections tend to experience back and abdominal pain.[9] Chronic dissection, in contrast, is usually painless and mostly without symptoms.[13] At least a third of acute aortic dissection patients are complicated by manifestations secondary to aortic branch occlusion, proximal extension to the aortic root, and leakage to surrounding structures.[50-51] Such complications include acute aortic regurgitation, myocardial ischemia/infarction, cardiac tamponade, stroke, syncope, pulse deficits, visceral ischemia, limb ischemia, and renal failure.[9,50]

The natural history of acute aortic dissection is particularly poor for type A dissections; the mortality rate for untreated type A dissection approximates 1% to 2% per hour during the first 24 hours after symptom onset and reaches 80% by two weeks.[7,11,52] Type B dissections, however, are less lethal and associated with a better prognosis.[9,17,53-54] Common causes of death include aortic rupture, severe aortic regurgitation, and end-organ compromise secondary to major branch vessel obstruction.[4,9,11] Chronic aortic dissection is also associated with a high incidence of rupture with a five-year survival of 10% to 15%.[52] Progression to aneurysmal dilatation is common in chronic phase dissections. In DeBakey and associates' 20 year follow-up of operated survivors of aortic dissection, the development of and subsequent rupture of aortic aneurysms was the leading cause of late deaths.[10]

With improvements in diagnostic imaging modalities, two radiologic and pathologic variants of aortic dissection have been recently recognized and diagnosed with increasing frequency: intramural hematoma (IMH) and PAU.[18,55-61] When associated with acute symptoms, these three pathologic entities are often grouped together under the general classification termed "acute aortic syndrome." It is estimated that 5% to 17% of diagnosed aortic dissections may actually be IMH or PAU.[18,62-63] IMH, considered a precursor of classic dissection, is characterized by blood in the aortic wall without an intimal disruption and is thought to originate from rupture of the vaso vasorum.[18,64] PAU is defined by an ulceration of aortic atherosclerotic plaque that penetrates the internal elastic lamina, intima, media, and possibly the adventitia.[56-57,65] Compared to classic aortic dissection, both IMH and PAU tend to be found in older patients with a history of hypertension and are more likely to be located in the descending thoracic aorta (43% in IMH and 90% in PAU).18, [57,66-67] Both entities can progress to frank dissection, rupture, or aneurysm formation.[56,59,65,68-70] IMH tends to behave like classic aortic dissection. Like type A dissection, type A IMH is associated with a greater risk of adverse progression.[71] In contrast, PAU rarely progresses to classic dissection and instead, more frequently forms aneurysms (up to 50%).[57]

CONVENTIONAL TREATMENT

A critical event in the evaluation of patients with suspected aortic dissection is the determination of whether the ascending aorta is involved. Therapeutic strategy hinges on whether type A or B dissection is present. In general, acute type A dissections are considered surgical emergencies while uncomplicated type B dissections are treated medically.[72] Regardless of dissection location, however, all patients in whom there is a strong suspicion of aortic dissection should be immediately placed on antihypertensive therapy to limit dissection progression.[73-74]

Given the associated high risk of sudden death due to aortic rupture, aortic regurgitation, cardiac tamponade, or myocardial infarction, type A dissection mandates expeditious diagnosis and emergent operative intervention.[75-76] Surgical therapy involves excision of the intimal tear, removal of the most diseased segment of aorta, obliteration of the false channel, reconstitution of the aorta directly or with the interposition of a synthetic graft, and, if necessary, restoration of aortic valve competence.[75] In a review of 547 type A dissections in the IRAD, the in-hospital mortality was 27% for patients treated surgically and 56% for those treated medically.[77] The associated survival benefit of surgical intervention remained in patients greater than 70 years old.[78]

There is a small subset of type A dissections where the entry tear is in the descending aorta and propagation occurs up to the ascending aorta in a retrograde manner (retrograde type A). The incidence of this subtype ranges from 10% to 27% among DeBakey type III dissections and from 4% to 20% among Stanford type A dissections.[17,79-82] Emergent surgical treatment is still mandated for this subtype although challenging and controversial.[79-83] Graft replacement of only the ascending aorta retains the primary entry tear and consequently the postoperative risk of rupture. On the other hand, excision of the entry tear and replacement of both the ascending aorta and aortic arch is associated with high mortality and morbidity.[81-82]

Patients with acute type B dissection are at lower risk of early death from complications, and tend to be older and of higher surgical risk. A large retrospective series of uncomplicated type B dissection patients from Duke and Stanford suggested equivalent outcome with medical and surgical treatment.[84] Consequently, the preferred treatment for most patients has, therefore, been medical in the form of aggressive antihypertensive treatment predominantly with beta blockers. Surgical intevention is generally reserved for those who develop complications such as rupture, dissection progression, aneurysmal growth, refractory hypertension, intractable pain, and malperfusion syndromes from aortic branch vessel obstruction.[76,85-86] Underlying connective tissue disease should also prompt consideration for early operative repair.[79,87] An IRAD study of the outcomes of this complication-specific approach revealed in-house mortality rates of 11% and 31% for medical and surgical treatment groups, respectively.[9] Surgical treatment is also associated with significant morbidity, particularly paraplegia (7% to 36%).[88-91] However, it is important to note that because medical therapy alone does not stop blood flow to the false lumen, 20% to 50% of patients who survive the acute phase develop aneurysmal dilatation of the false lumen within one to five years after onset.[15,54,92]

By definition, patients with chronic dissection have survived the acute phase of high mortality. In-hospital survival of such patients have approximated 90%, independent of whether they were managed surgically or medically.[93] Medical therapy, therefore, is recommended for patients with both type A and type B chronic dissection, with surgery reserved for those who develop an aneurysm or rupture.[94-95]

Aortic dissection is complicated by malperfusion syndromes resulting from aortic branch vessel obstruction in 30% to 50% of patients.[96-97] Such cases are associated with a particularly poor prognosis; those complicated by mesenteric and renal ischemia have surgical mortality rates of up to 87% and 70%, respectively.[96-99] In type A dissection, aortic branch vessel obstruction is usually corrected concomitantly with surgical management for dissection.[96] In type B dissection, complication with malperfusion syndrome is an indication for surgical intervention, and treatment options include fenestration of the intimal flap, replacement of the diseased aorta, and establishment of bypasses to the ischemic vessels.[99]

The treatment paradigm for IMH parallels the approach in classical aortic dissection.[66,100] A meta-analysis review of 11 IMH studies found cumulative mortality for type A IMH to be 24% for those treated surgically, 47% for those treated medically, and 34% overall; mortality for type B IMH was 14% overall with little difference between surgical (15%) and medical (13%) treatment groups.[101] At present, no consensus therapeutic strategy for PAU exists although a more aggressive surgical approach, independent of location, is being increasingly considered, especially in symptomatic patients.[56,68,102] The Yale Thoracic Aortic Diseases Group has identified a 40% rupture rate among PAU patients managed medically.[56,68] At a minimum, PAU patients with complications should undergo surgical treatment.[103]

ENDOVASCULAR STENT-GRAFT TREATMENT

Aortic dissection is the second most common investigational application of thoracic stent-graft technology. The concept of endovascular stent-graft repair of aortic dissection is predicated on successful placement of the device over the primary entry tear to obliterate blood flow into the false lumen (Figure 42–1). The intent is to mimic the effect of successful operative repair with isolation of the false lumen from the circulation and redirection of blood flow into the true lumen. As demonstrated in experimental models of dissection, coverage of the primary entry tear is the optimal method of relieving true lumen collapse and concomitantly promotes thrombosis of the false lumen.[104] Interestingly, dissections with naturally thrombosed false lumen are associated with improved prognosis.[80,105-106] False lumen patency, in contrast, contributes to progressive aortic dilatation and is a predictor of late mortality.[107] In the typical type B dissection case, progressive thrombosis proceeds distally, irrespective of the location of the primary intimal disruption.[108] The tempo of false lumen thrombosis is variable and influenced by several factors such as the size of the false lumen and amount of residual false lumen flow via uncovered additional tears. Over time, the false lumen thrombus consolidates and the dissection lumen itself resolves. Besides such gains in aortic remodeling, this endovascular surrogate for open surgery confers additional benefits: reversal of downstream branch vessel ischemia (particularly in patients with dynamic obstruction) and protection against thoracic false lumen aneurysm formation. In acute dissection, reversal of dynamic obstruction occurs expeditiously after stent-graft placement.[109]

Clinical evaluation of stent-grafts for the treatment of patients with complicated and uncomplicated acute type B dissection, a select subset of type A dissection, as well as chronic dissection with false lumen aneurysm formation are currently ongoing at a growing number of institutions around the world. Applications are limited to dissections with entry tears distal to the left subclavian artery. Initial results are encouraging. Unfortunately, as with that of TAA, the literature for aortic dissection often mixes

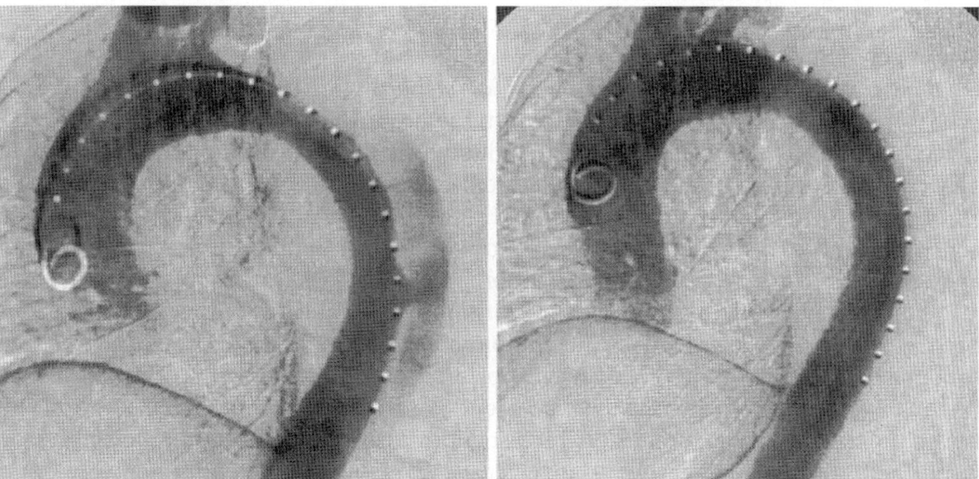

Figure 42-1. Type B aortic dissection in 75-year old woman with acute back pain. Left interior oblique thoracic aortograms performed before and after placement of a Gore TAG endograft over the entry tear in the mid-descending thoracic aorta. The stent-graft has obliterated the communciation between the true and false lumens.

outcomes from applications in different clinical contexts in terms of age of dissection, extent of disease, and presence of complications. Nonetheless, valuable lessons from this early experience have served to fuel progress in our understanding of the disease process as well as its management by less invasive means. Table 42–1[109-124] summarizes the results in published studies on endovascular stent-grafting for aortic dissections. In this section, we will first review clinical experiences within specific categories of acute dissection followed by an overview of aggregate results, trends, and challenges.

Although there is general consensus that acute type B dissection should be managed medically with surgical treatment reserved for cases with complications,[72] the intermediate and long-term outcome resulting from this treatment paradigm remains unsatisfactory. The mortality rate among patients treated medically alone ranges from 11% to 20%;[6,9,86] furthermore, such patients are at continued long-term risk of aneurysm formation and rupture.[15,54,92] Mortality among type B patients treated surgically ranges from 30% to 35% and is significantly worse for those complicated by end-organ ischemia.[79,9,93,96]

Our group recently studied the use of thoracic stent-grafts among 15 complicated acute type B and four retrograde type A dissection patients at Stanford and Mie University School of Medicine in Japan (Figure 42–2).[109] Eleven of these patients exhibited symptomatic branch vessel obstruction. The primary entry tear was sealed in 95% of cases with associated complete and partial thrombosis of the thoracic false lumen in 79% and 21% of patients, respectively. In all cases, true lumen expansion occurred immediately, but no aneurysmal expansion or rupture was found on follow-up. More impressively, follow-up imaging found complete false lumen resolution and no residual evidence of dissection in six cases. Thirty-day mortality was 16% with no additional deaths during mean follow-up of 13 months. Hutschala and associates have also explored the use of stent-grafts in a cohort of acute type B patients who were without indications for surgery and found similar outcomes.[116] In light of these results, the INSTEAD trial (Investigation of STEnt grafts in patients with type B Aortic Dissection), a prospective, multicenter, randomized, controlled clinical study, is underway to compare the one-year outcome of type B aortic dissection treated by stent-graft placement versus conventional antihypertensive therapy.[124]

There remains significant controversy over the proper treatment for patients with acute type A dissection with an entry tear in the descending aorta. Kato and colleagues treated 10 retrograde type A patients without evidence of cardiac tamponade or severe aortic regurgitation using endovascular stent-grafts.[114,125] Entry closure and complete thrombosis of the false lumen of both the ascending and descending aorta was achieved in all patients. During mean follow-up of 20 months, all patients were alive and without rupture or aneurysm formation.

Application of endoluminal stent-grafts in the setting of chronic dissection has been met with skepticism given the anatomic and hemodynamic complexity of such lesions.[126] The thick and fibrotic nature of a chronic dissection flap may limit true lumen expansion following device placement. Additionally, multiple fenestrations between the true and false lumens often exist and may hinder false lumen thrombosis. A number of groups, however, have achieved good results with stent-graft treatment of chronic dissections.[117,120,127-128]

Nienaber et al. prospectively evaluated stent-graft treatment in 12 patients with chronic type B dissection and compared the results with 12 matched surgical controls.[110] Proximal entry closure and complete thrombosis of the false lumen at three

TABLE 42-1. SUMMARY DATA ON STUDIES OF ENDOVASCULAR TREATMENT OF AORTIC DISSECTIONS

Reference	N	Mean Follow-up (months)	Devices	Sealing of Primary Entry Tear	Thrombosis of False Lumen	30-day Mortality	Long-term Survival (time)	Paraplegia
Dake 1999[109]	19: 4 acute retrograde type A, 15 acute type B (11 with symptomatic compromise of branch vessels)	13	Homemade	94.7%	78.9% complete, 21.1%partial	15.8%	84.2% (mean 13 months)	0%
Nienaber 1999[110]	12 chronic type B (12 matched surgical controls)	12	Talent	100%	100% complete	0% stent-graft, 8.7% surgical	100% for endovascular, 66.7% for surgical (12 months)	0%
Czermak 2000[111]	7 type B: 5 acute, 2 chronic	14	Talent, Vanguard	85.7%	85.7%	0%	85.7% (mean 14 months)	0%
Hausegger 2001[112]	5 acute type B uncomplicated	13.4	Talent	100%	100% complete	0%	100% (mean 13.4 months)	0%
Kato 2001[113]	15 chronic: 14 type B, type A	24	Homemade	100%	100% complete	0%	100% (mean 24 months)	0%
Kato 2001[114]	10 type A retrograde (7 acute, 3 chronic)	20	Homemade	100%	100% complete	0%	100% (mean 20 month)	0%
Sailer 2001[115]	7 acute and chronic type B, 4 PAU	8.5	Excluder, Talent, Vanguard	100%	63.6% complete, 27.3% partial	0%	100% (mean 8.5 months)	0%
Hutschala 2002[116]	9 acute type B uncomplicated	3	Excluder, Talent	100%	22.2% complete, 77.8% partial	0%	100% (mean 3 11% months)	0%
Kato 2002[117]	38: 10 acute type A, 14 acute type B, 14 chronic type B	27	Homemade	NA	NA	5.3%	92% acute, 100% chronic (1 year)	3%
Palma 2002[118]	70: 35 acute type B, 23 chronic type B, 6 IMH, 6 PAU	29	Homemade	92.9%	NA	5.7%	91.4% (mean 29 months)	0%
Shim 2002[119]	15 type B	31.5	Homemade	93.3%	66.7% complete	6.7%	86.7% (mean 31.5 months)	NA

(Continued)

TABLE 42-1. SUMMARY DATA ON STUDIES OF ENDOVASCULAR TREATMENT OF AORTIC DISSECTIONS (*Continued*)

Reference	N	Mean Follow-up (months)	Devices	Sealing of Primary Entry Tear	Thrombosis of False Lumen	30-day Mortality	Long-term Survival (time)	Paraplegia
Shimono 2002[120]	37: 16 acute complicated (9 type A retrograde, 7 type B), 8 acute type B uncomplicated, 13 chronic type B	24.5	Homemade	100%	94.4% complete or partial	2.7% overall, 6.3% acute complicated	97.3% overall (actuarial survival 2 years), 93.8% acute complicated, 100% acute uncomplicated, 100% chronic	NA
Lonn 2003[121]	20: 14 acute type B, 4 chronic type B, 2 chronic type A	13	Excluer, Talent, Hemobahn	100%	90%	15%	85% (mean 13 months)	5%
Lopera 2003[122]	10 type B complicated: 4 acute, 6 chronic	20	Homemade	90%	60% complete, 30% partial	0%	90% (mean 20 months)	NA
Bell 2004[123]	115	NA	Commercial	82%	NA	6.9%	NA	0.9%
Nienaber 2004[124]	105: 87 type B, 18 type A	32.4	NA	100%	NA	2.9%	89.5% (mean 32.4 months)	0%

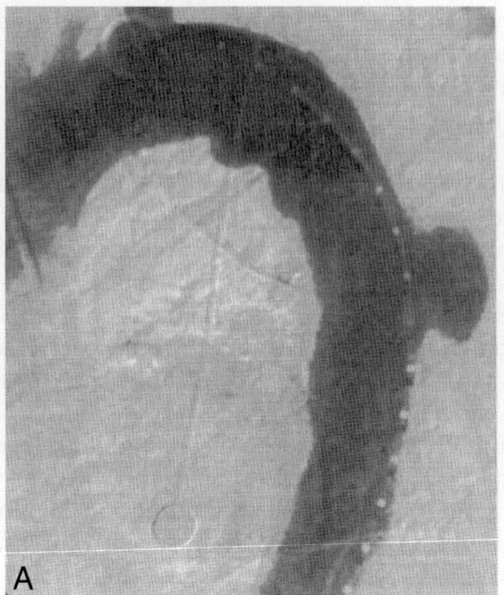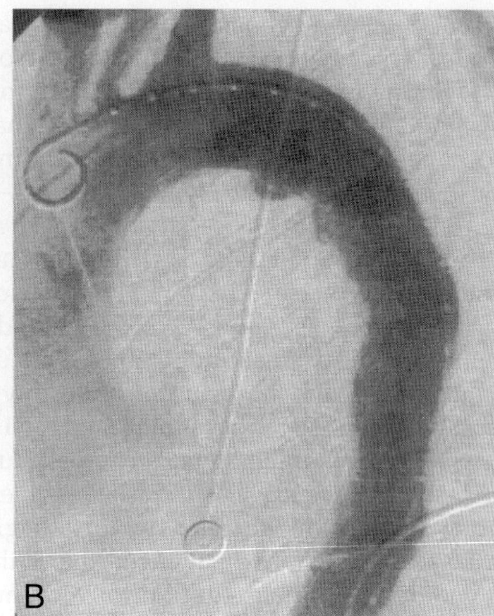

Figure 42-2. 80-year old man complaining of an abrupt onset of severe back pain. **A.** Thoracic aortogram shows a large penetrating aortic ulcer with associated contained rupture of the mid-descending thoracic aortic arch. **B.** After placement of a thoracic endograft in a position bridging the large ulcer, it is no longer evident on a completion aortogram.

months was achieved in all patients. Stent-graft treatment resulted in no mortality or morbidity while surgical treatment resulted in four deaths and five adverse events. At three months, complete thrombosis of the false lumen was achieved in all patients with clear evidence of true lumen expansion and false lumen shrinkage. A similar study by Kato and colleagues also demonstrated favorable aortic remodeling.[113] However, in a second study by the same group that evaluated both chronic and acute dissections, complete false lumen thrombosis was documented in all patients, but complete obliteration of the false lumen was found in only 38.5% of the chronic dissection patients versus 70% of the acute dissection patients (mean follow-up of 27 months).[120]

Endovascular stent-graft treatment of aortic dissections offers the additional benefit of relieving dynamic branch vessel obstruction. In our 1999 study of acute dissection patients,[109] 11 patients presented with symptomatic branch vessel obstruction involving 38 infradiaphragmatic vascular beds. Of these, 22 were obstructed exclusively by a dynamic process, 15 by both dynamic and static mechanisms, and one by static obstruction alone. After stent-graft placement, all 22 of the branch vessels with exclusively dynamic obstruction and six of the 15 arteries with combined dynamic and static involvement were immediately reperfused. Adjunctive endovascular procedures were used to relieve persistent ischemia in the remaining obstructed cases.

Briefly, two endovascular techniques can be used to relieve branch obstruction. Endovascular placement of an uncovered stent in the true lumen of the obstructed branch vessel relieves static obstruction.[129-130] Percutaneous balloon fenestration is used to mitigate dynamic obstructions by creating an artificial tear in the flap to allow communication between the true and false lumens.[131] In this procedure, the intimal flap is usually first punctured using a needle, crossed with a guidewire, and then opened using a balloon. Although the early results of these endovascular treatments appear encouraging,[129-132] the long-term outcomes are unknown.

Efforts to extend application of endovascular stent-graft technology to aortic dissection variants have focused predominantly on PAU.[133-136] Because PAU is usually focal and almost always in the descending aorta, it is an ideal anatomic target for endovascular stent-graft repair (Figure 42–7).[102] To minimize the risk of paraplegia, a short device could be used to locally seal and stabilize the lesion.

In a meta-analysis of 54 patients accumulated from 13 studies, complete sealing of the ulcer was achieved in 94%, neurologic complications occurred in 6%, and in-hospital mortality was 5%.[137] We recently studied a cohort of 26 symptomatic type B PAU patients (half deemed inoperable) treated by endovascular repair.[134] Primary success rate was 92% and perioperative mortality was 12% with no cases of paraplegia. At one and five years, survival estimates were 81% and 65%, respectively.

On review of the literature across multiple subtypes of aortic dissection, it is clear that successful entry closure was possible in 85% to 100% of cases. Since most primary entry tears in the descending aorta begin immediately distal to the left subclavian artery, adequate proximal anchoring of the device may be difficult. In several studies, anatomical selection criterion for minimum distance between entry tear and subclavian artery origin was set at 5 mm.[110,114,117] Intentional coverage of the left subclavian origin with expectant management was commonly used in these studies.[112] Alternatively, a device with a proximal segment consisting of a bare stent can be placed across the left subclavian artery to effectively maximize the length of graft contact with the aortic wall prior to the tear. However, in other settings, where there is a retrograde proximal extension of the dissection from the tear to the subclavian artery, it may be necessary to place the graft over the branch with its leading margin between the left carotid and subclavian arteries. In addition to carefully monitoring the patient postprocedure for ischemic symptoms referable to the covered left subclavian, it is important to carefully image the thoracic aorta to exclude persistent perfusion of the false lumen via retrograde subclavian flow around the device.

In parallel, successful entry tear coverage induced complete or partial thoracic false lumen thrombosis in 85% to 100% of patients, even in the settings of chronic and retrograde type A dissections. Partial thrombosis of the false lumen can still be advantageous and protect the false lumen from enlarging over time since systemic blood pressure is no longer directly transmitted through the primary entry tear. The age of the disease process may play a role in the degree of false lumen thrombosis; it has been found to be most pronounced in those dissections treated within six months of presentation.[108] True lumen expansion and partial or full false lumen resolution was noted in several studies.[109-110,119-120]

Whereas false lumen thrombosis was consistently observed at the level of the implanted stent-graft, thrombosis distal to the device and particularly in abdominal false lumens was less common. It is thought that uncovered portions of a dissection flap oscillate with retrograde flow through distal flap disruptions, preventing false lumen thrombosis. This holds implications regarding device length. Most investigators implant stent-grafts that are clearly longer than the entry tear, usually in the range of 10 to 15 cm long. This added length confers an appearance to the aortic morphology after implantation that is more normal anatomically, especially in the arch, than that observed following placement of a short device focally over the entry tear. In addition, the longer device promotes a more rapid tempo of thrombus formation within the proximal false lumen. Given that aortic rupture is a cause of death after device implantation,[109] acceleration of false lumen thrombosis may also improve mortality outcomes. However, extension of stent-graft coverage into the distal one-third of the descending thoracic aorta increases the risk of spinal cord ischemia. It has thus been suggested that distal extension with bare stents may provide the structural stability needed to promote false lumen thrombosis without sacrificing intercostal flow.

The recent development of endovascular stent-graft technology and its application as an alternative management strategy to medical therapy or open surgical intervention of patients with aortic dissection is an exciting and potentially valuable advance. As conventional treatments for aortic dissection and its attendant complications are often associated with significant failure rates, result in substantial morbidity and mortality, and/or do little to reduce the risk of aneurysm formation as late sequelae, improved treatment options are desired. Here, we have reviewed the current clinical experience with stent-graft placement for treatment of complicated and uncomplicated acute type B dissection, retrograde type A dissection, chronic dissection, and PAU. It is imperative to first appreciate the wide array of clinical, anatomic, and temporal manifestations within the umbrella pathology of aortic dissection. Evaluation of the role of endoluminal stent-graft technology must be performed within the context of each of these subgroups through rigorous, prospective controlled investigations and compared against respective standard treatment. Although this poses a much more significant challenge, the encouraging early results highlighted here underscore the potential for stent-graft therapy to supplant conventional-and often suboptimal-treatment paradigms, and to provide patients with a less invasive therapeutic alternative that may concomitantly achieve gains in survival.

REFERENCES

1. Williams DM, Lee DY, Hamilton BH, et al. The dissected aorta: part III. Anatomy and radiologic diagnosis of branch-vessel compromise. *Radiology.* 1997;203:37–44.
2. Bickerstaff LK, Pairolero PC, Hollier LH, et al. Thoracic aortic aneurysms: a population-based study. *Surgery.* 1982;92:1103–1108.
3. Clouse WD, Hallett JW, Jr., Schaff HV, et al. Acute aortic dissection: population-based incidence compared with degenerative aortic aneurysm rupture. *Mayo Clin Proc.* 2004;79:176–180.
4. Meszaros I, Morocz J, Szlavi J, et al. Epidemiology and clinicopathology of aortic dissection. *Chest.* 2000;117:1271–1278.
5. Sorensen HR, Olsen H. Ruptured and dissecting aneurysms of the aorta. Incidence and prospects of surgery. *Acta Chir Scand.* 1964;128:644–650.
6. Wheat MW, Jr. Acute dissecting aneurysms of the aorta: diagnosis and treatment-1979. *Am Heart J.* 1980;99:373–387.
7. Anagnostopoulos CE, Prabhakar MJ, Kittle CF. Aortic dissections and dissecting aneurysms. *Am J Cardiol.* 1972;30:263–273.
8. Coady MA, Rizzo JA, Goldstein LJ, et al. Natural history, pathogenesis, and etiology of thoracic aortic aneurysms and dissections. *Cardiol Clin.* 1999;17:615–635; vii.
9. Hagan PG, Nienaber CA, Isselbacher EM, et al. The International Registry of Acute Aortic Dissection (IRAD): new insights into an old disease. *Jama.* 2000;283:897–903.
10. DeBakey ME, McCollum CH, Crawford ES, et al. Dissection and dissecting aneurysms of the aorta: twenty-year follow—up of five hundred twenty-seven patients treated surgically. *Surgery.* 1982;92:1118–1134.
11. Hirst AE, Jr., Johns VJ, Jr., Kime SW, Jr. Dissecting aneurysm of the aorta: a review of 505 cases. *Medicine* (Baltimore). 1958;37:217–279.

12. Wilson SK, Hutchins GM. Aortic dissecting aneurysms: causative factors in 204 subjects. *Arch Pathol Lab Med.* 1982;106:175–180.

13. Spittell PC, Spittell JA, Jr., Joyce JW, et al. Clinical features and differential diagnosis of aortic dissection: experience with 236 cases (1980 through 1990). *Mayo Clin Proc.* 1993; 68:642–651.

14. Roberts WC. Aortic dissection: anatomy, consequences, and causes. *Am Heart J.* 1981; 101:195–214.

15. Wheat MW, Jr. Acute dissection of the aorta. *Cardiovasc Clin.* 1987;17:241–262.

16. DeBakey ME, Beall AC, Jr., Cooley DA, et al. Dissecting aneurysms of the aorta. Urg Clin North Am. 1966;46:1045–1055.

17. Daily PO, Trueblood HW, Stinson EB, et al. Management of acute aortic dissections. *Ann Thorac Surg.* 1970;10:237–247.

18. Coady MA, Rizzo JA, Elefteriades JA. Pathologic variants of thoracic aortic dissections. Penetrating atherosclerotic ulcers and intramural hematomas. *Cardiol Clin.* 1999;17:637–657.

19. Roberts WC, Honig HS. The spectrum of cardiovascular disease in the Marfan syndrome: a clinico-morphologic study of 18 necropsy patients and comparison to 151 previously reported necropsy patients. *Am Heart J.* 1982;104:115–135.

20. Smith JA, Fann JI, Miller DC, et al. Surgical management of aortic dissection in patients with the Marfan syndrome. *Circulation.* 1994;90:11235–11242.

21. Stolle CA, Pyeritz RE, Myers JC, et al. Synthesis of an altered type III procollagen in a patient with type IV Ehlers-Danlos syndrome. A structural change in the alpha 1(III) chain which makes the protein more susceptible to proteinases. *J Biol Chem.* 1985;260:1937–1944.

22. Januzzi JL, Isselbacher EM, Fattori R, et al. Characterizing the young patient with aortic dissection: results from the International Registry of Aortic Dissection (IRAD). *J Am Coll Cardiol.* 2004;43:665–669.

23. Larson EW, Edwards WD. Risk factors for aortic dissection: a necropsy study of 161 cases. *Am J Cardiol.* 1984;53:849–855.

24. Birdsall M, Kennedy S. The risk of aortic dissection in women with Turner syndrome. *Hum Reprod.* 1996;11:1587.

25. Clement CI, Brereton J, Clifton-Bligh P. Aortic dissection in Turner syndrome. *Med J Aust.* 2004;180:584.

26. Rubin K. Aortic dissection and rupture in Turner syndrome. *J Pediatr.* 1993;122:670.

27. Shachter N, Perloff JK, Mulder DG. Aortic dissection in Noonan's syndrome (46 XY turner). *Am J Cardiol.* 1984;54:464–465.

28. Moodie DS. Aortic dissection and coarctation. *Curr Opin Cardiol.* 1990;5:649–654.

29. Edwards WD, Leaf DS, Edwards JE. Dissecting aortic aneurysm associated with congenital bicuspid aortic valve. *Circulation.* 1978;57:1022–1025.

30. Roberts CS, Roberts WC. Dissection of the aorta associated with congenital malformation of the aortic valve. *J Am Coll Cardiol.* 1991;17:712–716.

31. Roberts WC. The hypertensive diseases. Evidence that systemic hypertension is a greater risk factor to the development of other cardiovascular diseases than previously suspected. *Am J Med.* 1975;59:523–532.

32. Steurer J, Jenni R, Medici TC, et al. Dissecting aneurysm of the pulmonary artery with pulmonary hypertension. *Am Rev Respir Dis.* 1990;142:1219–1221.

33. Ginsburg R. Aortic aneurysm and dissection in giant cell arteritis. *Ann Intern Med.* 1996;124:615.

34. Liu G, Shupak R, Chiu BK. Aortic dissection in giant-cell arteritis. *Semin Arthritis Rheum.* 1995;25:160–171.

35. Fisher A, Holroyd BR. Cocaine-associated dissection of the thoracic aorta. *J Emerg Med.* 1992;10:723–727.

36. Perron AD, Gibbs M. Thoracic aortic dissection secondary to crack cocaine ingestion. *Am J Emerg Med.* 1997;15:507–509.

37. Hsue PY, Salinas CL, Bolger AF, et al. Acute aortic dissection related to crack cocaine. *Circulation.* 2002; 105:1592–1595.

38. Eagle KA, Isselbacher EM, DeSanctis RW. Cocaine-related aortic dissection in perspective. *Circulation.* 2002;105:1529–1530.
39. Rashid J, Eisenberg MJ, Topol EJ. Cocaine-induced aortic dissection. *Am Heart J.* 1996;132: 1301–1304.
40. Januzzi JL, Sabatine MS, Eagle KA, et al. Iatrogenic aortic dissection. *Am J Cardiol.* 2002;89: 623–626.
41. Rogers FB, Osler TM, Shackford SR. Aortic dissection after trauma: case report and review of the literature. *J Trauma.* 1996;41:906–908.
42. Still RJ, Hilgenberg AD, Akins CW, et al. Intraoperative aortic dissection. *Ann Thorac Surg.* 1992;53:374–379; discussion 380.
43. Nienaber CA, Eagle KA. Aortic dissection: new frontiers in diagnosis and management: Part L from etiology to diagnostic strategies. *Circulation.* 2003;108:628–635.
44. Mandel W, Evans EW, Walford RL. Dissecting aortic aneurysm during pregnancy. *N Engl J Med.* 1954;251:1059–1061.
45. Cavanzo FJ, Taylor HB. Effect of pregnancy on the human aorta and its relationship to dissecting aneurysms. *Am J Obstet Gynecol.* 1969;105:567–568.
46. Schnitker MA, Major MC, Bayer CA. Dissecting aneurysm of the aorta in young individuals, particularly in association with pregnancy: With report of a case. *Ann Intern Med.* 1944;20:486–511.
47. Immer FF, Bansi AG, Immer-Bansi AS, et al. Aortic dissection in pregnancy: analysis of risk factors and outcome. *Ann Thorac Surg.* 2003;76:309–314.
48. Klompas M. Does this patient have an acute thoracic aortic dissection? *Jama.* 2002;287: 2262–2272.
49. von Kodolitsch Y, Schwartz AG, Nienaber CA. Clinical prediction of acute aortic dissection. *Arch Intern Med.* 2000;160:2977–2982.
50. Khan IA, Nair CK. Clinical, diagnostic, and management perspectives of aortic dissection. *Chest.* 2002;122:311–328.
51. Oderich GS, Panneton JM. Acute aortic dissection with side branch vessel occlusion: open surgical options. *Semin Vasc Surg.* 2002;15:89–96.
52. Lindsay J, Jr., Hurst JW. Clinical features and prognosis in dissecting aneurysm of the aorta. A re-appraisal. *Circulation.* 1967;35:880–888.
53. Nienaber CA, Eagle KA. Aortic dissection: new frontiers in diagnosis and management: Part II: therapeutic management and follow-up. *Circulation.* 2003;108:772–778.
54. Doroghazi RM, Slater EE, DeSanctis RW, et al. Long-term survival of patients with treated aortic dissection. *J Am Coll Cardiol.* 1984;3:1026–1034.
55. Dake MD. Aortic intramural haematoma: current therapeutic strategy. *Heart.* 2004;90: 375–378.
56. Coady MA, Rizzo JA, Hammond GL, et al. Penetrating ulcer of the thoracic aorta: what is it? How do we recognize it? How do we manage it? *J Vasc Surg.* 1998;27:1006–1015; discussion 1015–1006.
57. Harris JA, Bis KG, Glover JL, et al. Penetrating atherosclerotic ulcers of the aorta. *J Vasc Surg.* 1994;19:90–98; discussion 98–99.
58. Lui RC, Menkis AH, McKenzie FN. Aortic dissection without intimal rupture: diagnosis and management. *Ann Thorac Surg.* 1992;53:886–888.
59. Nienaber CA, Richartz BM, Rehders T, et al. Aortic intramural haematoma: natural history and predictive factors for complications. *Heart.* 2004;90:372–374.
60. Nienaber CA, Sievers HH. Intramural hematoma in acute aortic syndrome: more than one variant of dissection? *Circulation.* 2002;106:284–285.
61. Song JK, Kim HS, Kang DH, et al. Different clinical features of aortic intramural hematoma versus dissection involving the ascending aorta. *J Am Coll Cardiol.* 2001;37:1604–1610.
62. Bolognesi R, Manca C, Tsialtas D, et al. Aortic intramural hematoma: an increasingly recognized aortic disease. *Cardiology.* 1998;89:178–183.
63. Lansman SL, McCullough JN, Nguyen KH, et al. Subtypes of acute aortic dissection. *Ann Thorac Surg.* 1999;67:1975–1978; discussion 1979–1980.

64. Gore I. Pathogenesis of dissecting aneurysm of the aorta. *AMA Arch Pathol.* 1952;53:142–153.
65. Stanson AW, Kazmier FJ, Hollier LH, et al. Penetrating atherosclerotic ulcers of the thoracic aorta: natural history and clinicopathologic correlations. *Ann Vasc Surg.* 1986;1:15–23.
66. Nienaber CA, von Kodolitsch Y, Petersen B, et al. Intramural hemorrhage of the thoracic aorta. Diagnostic and therapeutic implications. *Circulation.* 1995;92:1465–1472.
67. Maraj R, Rerkpattanapipat P, Jacobs LE, et al. Meta-analysis of 143 reported cases of aortic intramural hematoma. *Am J Cardiol.* 2000;86:664–668.
68. Tittle SL, Lynch RJ, Cole PE, et al. Midterm follow-up of penetrating ulcer and intramural hematoma of the aorta. *J Thorac Cardiovasc Surg.* 2002;123:1051–1059.
69. Ganaha F, Miller DC, Sugimoto K, et al. Prognosis of aortic intramural hematoma with and without penetrating atherosclerotic ulcer: a clinical and radiological analysis. *Circulation.* 2002;106:342–348.
70. Sueyoshi E, Matsuoka Y, Sakamoto I, et al. Fate of intramural hematoma of the aorta: CT evaluation. *J Comput Assist Tomogr.* 1997;21:931–938.
71. von Kodolitsch Y, Csosz SK, Koschyk DH, et al. Intramural hematoma of the aorta: predictors of progression to dissection and rupture. *Circulation.* 2003;107:1158–1163.
72. Erbel R, Alfonso F, Boileau C, Dirsch O, et al. Diagnosis and management of aortic dissection. *Eur Heart J.* 2001;22:1642–1681.
73. Wheat MW, Jr., Palmer RF, Bartley TD, et al. Treatment Of Dissecting Aneurysms Of The Aorta Without Surgery. *J Thorac Cardiovasc Surg.* 1965;50:364–373.
74. Wheat MW, Jr. Current status of medical therapy of acute dissecting aneurysms of the aorta. *World J Surg.* 1980;4:563–569.
75. Miller DC, Stinson EB, Oyer PE, et al. Operative treatment of aortic dissections. Experience with 125 patients over a sixteen-year period. *J Thorac Cardiovasc Surg.* 1979;78:365–382.
76. Masuda Y, Yamada Z, Morooka N, et al. Prognosis of patients with medically treated aortic dissections. *Circulation.* 1991;84:1117–1113.
77. Mehta RH, Suzuki T, Hagan PG, et al. Predicting death in patients with acute type a aortic dissection. *Circulation.* 2002;105:200–206.
78. Mehta RH, O'Gara PT, Bossone E, et al. Acute type A aortic dissection in the elderly: clinical characteristics, management, and outcomes in the current era. *J Am Coll Cardiol.* 2002;40:685–692.
79. Miller DC, Mitchell RS, Oyer PE, et al. Independent determinants of operative mortality for patients with aortic dissections. *Circulation.* 1984;70:I 153–64.
80. Erbel R, Oelert H, Meyer J, et al. Effect of medical and surgical therapy on aortic dissection evaluated by transesophageal echocardiography. Implications for prognosis and therapy. The European Cooperative Study Group on Echocardiography. *Circulation.* 1993;87:1604–1615.
81. Kazui T, Tamiya Y, Tanaka T, et al. Extended aortic replacement for acute type A dissection with the tear in the descending aorta. *J Thorac Cardiovasc Surg.* 1996;112:973–978.
82. Lansman SL, Galla JD, Schor JS, et al. Subtypes of acute aortic dissection. *J Card Surg.* 1994;9:729–733.
83. von Segesser LK, Killer I, Ziswiler M, et al. Dissection of the descending thoracic aorta extending into the ascending aorta. A therapeutic challenge. *J Thorac Cardiovasc Surg.* 1994;108:755–761.
84. Glower DD, Fann JI, Speier RH, et al. Comparison of medical and surgical therapy for uncomplicated descending aortic dissection. *Circulation.* 1990;82:IV 39–46.
85. Fann JI, Miller DC. Aortic dissection. *Ann Vasc Surg.* 1995;9:311–323.
86. Elefteriades JA, Hartleroad J, Gusberg RJ, et al. Long-term experience with descending aortic dissection: the complication-specific approach. *Ann Thorac Surg.* 1992;53:11–20; discussion 20–11.
87. Schor JS, Yerlioglu ME, Galla JD, et al. Selective management of acute type B aortic dissection: long-term follow-up. *Ann Thorac Surg.* 1996;61:1339–1341.
88. Svensson LG, Crawford ES, Hess KR, et al. Variables predictive of outcome in 832 patients undergoing repairs of the descending thoracic aorta. *Chest.* 1993;104:1248–1253.

89. Svensson LG, Crawford ES, Hess KR, et al. Dissection of the aorta and dissecting aortic aneurysms. Improving early and long-term surgical results. *Circulation.* 1990;82:IV 24–38.
90. Miller DC. The continuing dilemma concerning medical versus surgical management of patients with acute type B dissections. *Semin Thorac Cardiovasc Surg.* 1993;5:33–46.
91. Neya K, Omoto R, Kyo S, et al. Outcome of Stanford type B acute aortic dissection. *Circulation.* 1992;86:II1–7.
92. Richter GM, Allenberg JR, Schumacher H, et al. Aortic dissection—when operative treatment, when endoluminal therapy? *Radiologe.* 2001;41:660–667.
93. Crawford ES, Svensson LG, Coselli JS, et al. Aortic dissection and dissecting aortic aneurysms. *Ann Surg.* 1988;208:254–273.
94. Juvonen T, Ergin MA, Galla JD, et al. Risk factors for rupture of chronic type B dissections. *J Thorac Cardiovasc Surg.* 1999;117:776–786.
95. Kato M, Bai H, Sato K, et al. Determining surgical indications for acute type B dissection based on enlargement of aortic diameter during the chronic phase. *Circulation.* 1995;92:II107–112.
96. Cambria RP, Brewster DC, Gertler J, et al. Vascular complications associated with spontaneous aortic dissection. *J Vasc Surg.* 1988;7:199–209.
97. Fann JI, Sarris GE, Mitchell RS, et al. Treatment of patients with aortic dissection presenting with peripheral vascular complications. *Ann Surg.* 1990;212:705–713.
98. Borst HG, Laas J, Heinemann M. Type A aortic dissection: diagnosis and management of malperfusion phenomena. *Semin Thorac Cardiovasc Surg.* 1991;3:238–241.
99. Heinemann MK, Buehner B, Schaefers HJ, et al. Malperfusion of the thoracoabdominal vasculature in aortic dissection. *J Card Surg.* 1994;9:748–755; discussion 755–747.
100. Robbins RC, McManus RP, Mitchell RS, et al. Management of patients with intramural hematoma of the thoracic aorta. *Circulation.* 1993;88:II 1–10.
101. Sawhney NS, DeMaria AN, Blanchard DG. Aortic intramural hematoma: an increasingly recognized and potentially fatal entity. *Chest.* 2001;120:1340–1346.
102. Eggebrecht H, Baumgart D, Herold U, et al. Multiple penetrating atherosclerotic ulcers of the abdominal aorta: treatment by endovascular stent graft placement. *Heart.* 2001;85:526.
103. Braverman AC. Penetrating atherosclerotic ulcers of the aorta. *Curr Opin Cardiol.* 1994;9: 591–597.
104. Chung JW, Elkins C, Sakai T, et al. True-lumen collapse in aortic dissection: part II. Evaluation of treatment methods in phantoms with pulsatile flow. *Radiology.* 2000;214:99-
105. Ergin MA, Phillips RA, Galla JD, et al. Significance of distal false lumen after type A dissection repair. *Ann Thorac Surg.* 1994;57:820–824; discussion 825.
106. Williams DM, Andrews JC, Marx MV, et al. Creation of reentry tears in aortic dissection by means of percutaneous balloon fenestration: gross anatomic and histologic considerations. *J Vasc Interv Radiol.* 1993;4:75–83.
107. Bernard Y, Zimmermann H, Chocron S, et al. False lumen patency as a predictor of late outcome in aortic dissection. *Am J Cardiol.* 2001;87:1378–1382.
108. Kato M, Matsuda T, Kaneko M, et al. Outcomes of stent-graft treatment of false lumen in aortic dissection. *Circulation.* 1998;98:II305–311; discussion II 311–302.
109. Dake MD, Kato N, Mitchell RS, et al. Endovascular stent-graft placement for the treatment of acute aortic dissection. *N Engl J Med.* 1999;340:1546–1552.
110. Nienaber CA, Fattori R, Lund G, et al. Nonsurgical reconstruction of thoracic aortic dissection by stent-graft placement. *N Engl J Med.* 1999;340:1539–1545.
111. Czermak BV, Waldenberger P, Fraedrich G, et al. Treatment of Stanford type B aortic dissection with stent-grafts: preliminary results. *Radiology.* 2000;217:544–550.
112. Hausegger KA, Tiesenhausen K, Schedlbauer P, et al. Treatment of acute aortic type B dissection with stent-grafts. *Cardiovasc Intervent Radiol.* 2001;24:306–312.
113. Kato N, Hirano T, Shimono T, et al. Treatment of chronic aortic dissection by transluminal endovascular stem-graft placement: preliminary results. *J Vasc Interv Radiol.* 2001;12:835–840.
114. Kato N, Shimono T, Hirano T, et al. Transluminal placement of endovascular stem-grafts for the treatment of type A aortic dissection with an entry tear in the descending thoracic aorta. *J Vasc Surg.* 2001;34:1023–1028.

115. Sailer J, Peloschek P, Rand T, et al. Endovascular treatment of aortic type B dissection and penetrating ulcer using commercially available stem-grafts. *Am J Roentgenol.* 2001;177: 1365–1369.

116. Hutschala D, Fleck T, Czerny M, et al. Endoluminal stem-graft placement in patients with acute aortic dissection type B. *Eur J Cardiothorac Surg.* 2002;21:964–969.

117. Kato N, Shimono T, Hirano T, et al. Midterm results of stem-graft repair of acute and chronic aortic dissection with descending tear: the complication-specific approach. *J Thorac Cardiovasc Surg.* 2002;124:306–312.

118. Palma JH, de Souza JA, Rodrigues Alves CM, et al. Self-expandable aortic stem-grafts for treatment of descending aortic dissections. *Ann Thorac Surg.* 2002;73:1138–1141; discussion 1141–1132.

119. Shim WH, Koo BK, Yoon YS, et al. Treatment of thoracic aortic dissection with stem-grafts: midterm results. *J Endovasc Ther.* 2002;9:817–821.

120. Shimono T, Kato N, Yasuda F, et al. Transluminal stent-graft placements for the treatments of acute onset and chronic aortic dissections. *Circulation.* 2002;106:I241–247.

121. Lonn L, Delle M, Falkenberg M, et al. Endovascular treatment of type B thoracic aortic dissections. *J Card Surg.* 2003;18:539–544.

122. Lopera J, Patino JH, Urbina C, et al. Endovascular treatment of complicated type-B aortic dissection with stent-grafts: midterm results. *J Vasc Interv Radiol.* 2003;14:195–203.

123. Bell RE, Buth J, Taylor PR, et al. UK and EUROSTAR thoracic stenting registries: combined experience. *J Endovasc Ther.* 2004;11:I6. Abstract.

124. Nienaber CA, Rehders TK, S., Ince H, et al. Stent-graft intervention for type B aortic dissection: Update of European trail results. *J Endovasc Ther.* 2004;11:I29. Abstract.

125. Shimono T, Kato N, Tokui T, et al. Endovascular stent-graft repair for acute type A aortic dissection with an intimal tear in the descending aorta. *J Thorac Cardiovasc Surg.* 1998; 116:171–173.

126. Fann JI, Miller DC. Endovascular treatment of descending thoracic aortic aneurysms and dissections. *Surg Clin North Am.* 1999;79:551–574.

127. Nienaber CA, Ince H, Petzsch M, et al. Endovascular treatment of acute aortic syndrome. Supplement to Endovascular Today; 2003:12–15.

128. Kato N, Hirano T, Shimono T, et al. Treatment of chronic type B aortic dissection with endovascular stem-graft placement. *Cardiovasc Intervent Radiol.* 2000;23:60–62.

129. Slonim SM, Miller DC, Mitchell RS, et al. Percutaneous balloon fenestration and stenting for life-threatening ischemic complications in patients with acute aortic dissection. *J Thorac Cardiovasc Surg.* 1999;117:118–1126.

130. Slonim SM, Nyman U, Semba CP, et al. Aortic dissection: percutaneous management of ischemic complications with endovascular stems and balloon fenestration. *J Vasc Surg.* 1996; 23:241–251; discussion 251–243.

131. Williams DM, Lee DY, Hamilton BH, et al. The dissected aorta: percutaneous treatment of ischemic complications—principles and results. *J Vasc Interv Radiol.* 1997;8:605–625.

132. Chavan A, Hausmann D, Dresler C, et al. Intravascular ultrasound-guided percutaneous fenestration of the intimal flap in the dissected aorta. *Circulation.* 1997;96:2124–2127.

133. Brittenden J, McBride K, McInnes G, et al. The use of endovascular stents in the treatment of penetrating ulcers of the thoracic aorta. *J Vasc Surg.* 1999;30:946–949.

134. Demers P, Miller DC, Mitchell RS, et al. Stent-graft repair of penetrating atherosclerotic ulcers in the descending thoracic aorta: mid-term results. *Ann Thorac Surg.* 2004;77:81–86.

135. Kos X, Bouchard L, Otal P, et al. Stent-graft treatment of penetrating thoracic aortic ulcers. *J Endovasc Ther.* 2002;9 Suppl 2:1125–1131.

136. Murgo S, Dussaussois L, Golzarian J, et al. Penetrating atherosclerotic ulcer of the descending thoracic aorta: treatment by endovascular stent-graft. *Cardiovasc Intervent Radiol.* 1998; 21:454–458.

137. Eggebrecht H, Baumgart D, Schmermund A, et al. Penetrating atherosclerotic ulcer of the aorta: treatment by endovascular stent-graft placement. *Curr Opin Cardiol.* 2003;18:431–435.

Endovascular Options
for Thoracic Aortic
Dissection

43

*Randy D. Moore, M.D., B.S.C., M.S.C., F.R.C.S.C.,
F.A.C.S., Gary Dobson, M.D., F.R.C.P.C., K. McCune,
M.D., F.R.C.S. (Ed.), and Talal Altuwaijri, M.D.*

Acute aortic dissection is relatively uncommon, affecting five to 30 patients per million per year (compared to 4400/million/year for acute myocardial infarction). It, nevertheless, remains one of the most common acute aortic catastrophes. Mortality for this condition has improved dramatically over the past 20 years with advances in medical armamentarium and surgical techniques for selected populations, early diagnosis and management of branch vessel occlusions, and the development of hybrid surgical and endovascular techniques, but still remains significant. Multiple reports[1] and the large international registry for aortic dissection (IRAD) have confirmed that early (in- hospital) mortality rates approach 30%[2] and can exceed 50% with end-organ ischemia at presentation,[3] and that late mortality due to complications related to the initial dissection continues to accrue even with successful initial medical or surgical treatment. Similar to the observational studies for aortic ruptured aneurysms demonstrating improved survival with endovascular techniques, and based on seminal reports for endovascular repair,[4] further improvements in outcomes for the treatment of aortic dissection will require advanced endovascular or hybrid techniques that are only now emerging, and will require the clinician to have a thorough understanding of the underlying pathophysiology, presentation, and methods of diagnosis and treatment for aortic dissection. This chapter focuses on the emerging importance of endovascular repair for aortic dissection, and discusses endovascular classification, diagnosis, and endovascular strategy, and current outcomes utilizing endovascular technology.

GENERAL CONSIDERATIONS

Primary risk factors for aortic dissection include hypertension and aging. Diffuse weakness of the arterial wall such as that observed in association with bicuspid aortic valve aortopathy, aortic lesions such as intramural hematoma or penetrating ulcer, or more clearly defined connective tissue disorders such as Ehlers-Danlos or Marfan syndromes, or idiopathic cystic medial necrosis have also been implicated, although dissections have also been observed in patients with histologically normal aortas (e.g., cocaine abuse, pregnancy, or anabolic steroid-related hypertension). Irrespective of the associated causes, the initial pathologic event is an intimal tear, leading to pulsatile flow into the aortic wall layers, with primarily subintimal, or intimal-medial extension, antegrade or rarely retrograde, or both, with the development of an aortic false lumen. Typically, the tear is associated with severe pain (85% to 95%), and in contradistinction to classic medical teaching, is often described by patients as sharp (68%) or migratory (19%) rather than tearing or ripping (50%).[1] Abdominal pain may also be observed in 20% to 40% of patients, particularly in the setting of acute mesenteric ischemia. IRAD investigators have identified that patients presenting without the typical back or chest pain have higher in-hospital mortality due to delayed diagnosis, and an increased incidence of coma/altered consciousness, syncope, and hypotension.[5] Other risk factors for in-hospital death included massive (>6cm) widening of the mediastinum on chest radiograph imaging or periaortic hematoma on imaging studies (CT or MRI, respectively). The location of the primary entry tear and the subsequent progression of the intramural hematoma are pivotal to current classification schemes, and relate closely to the natural history of these lesions. Identification of the site of primary entry is, therefore, critical to the current endovascular management of aortic dissection, and modern imaging offers a plethora of complimentary modalities to precisely localize not only the primary entry, but also secondary re-entry tears, branch vessel occlusions, and luminal pressure relationships.

Diagnostic confirmation of clinical suspicion is usually made with a high resolution, fine cut (<3mm), contrast enhanced CT scan (Figure 43–1) given the relatively nonspecific findings of widened aortic profile (60% to 90%) on standard chest radiography.[2] Although digital subtraction aortography has historically been used to diagnose aortic dissection, most contemporary centers treating aortic dissection recognize the limitations of aortography that lead to false negative studies including the inability to identify a false lumen if both lumens fill simultaneously, the inability to identify a thrombosed false lumen or intramural hematoma, or the "artificial" perfusion of dynamically occluded visceral branches due to the pressurized jet of contrast. Cannulation of the friable, freshly dissected aorta during angiography also carries with it the risks of perforation or extension of dissection through the passage of guidewires or catheters. Contemporary centers involved in the management of patients with aortic dissection have eliminated diagnostic aortography, and typically rely on this modality to aid in therapeutic management of malperfusion syndromes or to assist with the completion of endovascular repair. CT scan imaging remains the most commonly utilized modality worldwide in the IRAD registry given the lack of operator dependency, widespread availability, and the high sensitivity (85% to 95%), and the reported specificity of up to 100% for aortic dissection.[6] CT imaging allows for the diagnosis, and the determination of the extent of the dissection, as well as the determination of visceral branch involvement. Our center has coined the term the "dissection battle sign" (Figure 43–2) to describe the typical appearance of the compressed true lumen with

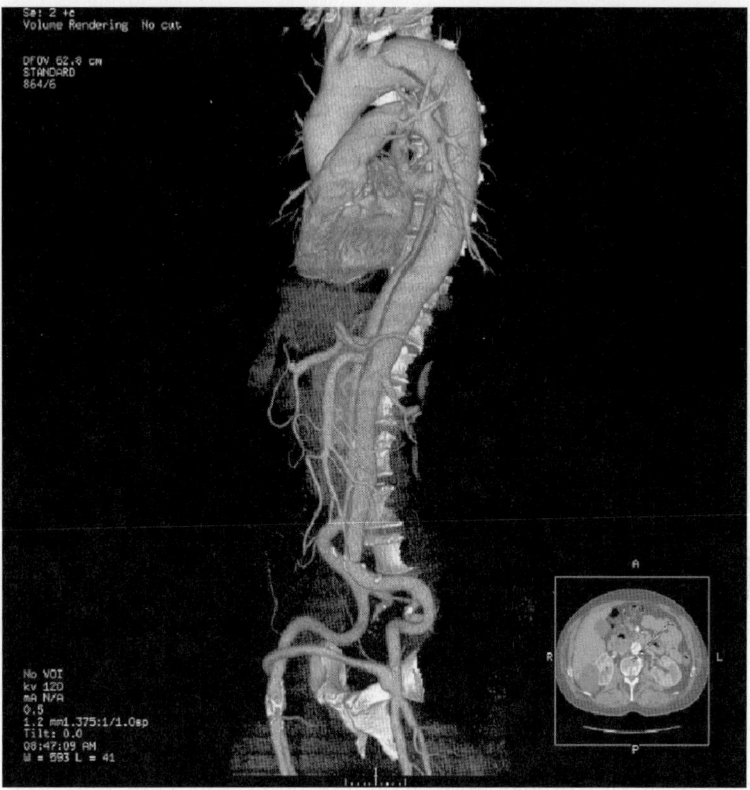

Figure 43-1. Volume-rendered CT diagnosis of aortic dissection. Note easily identifiable longitudinal tear through descending aorta and compressed true lumen on axial view (inset).

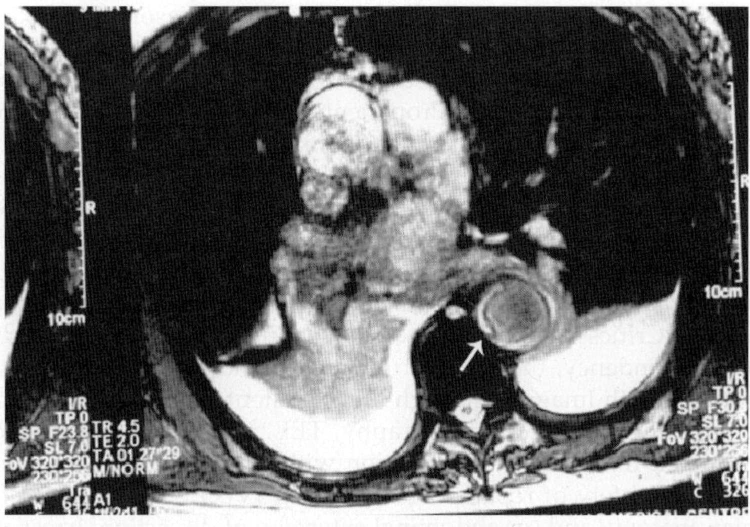

Figure 43-2. Dissection "Battle Sign." MRI image of aortic dissection demonstrates compression of true lumen (arrow) by pressurized false lumen.

acute aortic dissection, and the wall tension disparity that initially exists between the true and false lumens due to the pressure differential. This true lumen compression by the weakened, rapidly expanded and larger false lumen is seen in up to 90% of cases[6] and helps to identify the false lumen on CT scanning, and allows for serial assessment of the relationship between the two channels and any subsequent remodeling.[7] In our experience, the absence of this compression indicates autofenestration, with pressure equalization between the two channels and reduced risk of vascular compromise. Despite the obvious utility of CT analysis for aortic dissection, involvement of the ascending aorta is poorly assessed with CT imaging, even with the maximum intensity projection (MIP), multiplanar reformats (MPR), and volume rendered surface imaging studies obtained with modern 16- or 64-slice CT scanners. Transesophageal echocardiography (TEE) is complementary in this regard, providing highly sensitive imaging of the aortic root and ascending aorta, as well as determining coronary artery involvement, assessing valvular function, and diagnosing pericardial effusion. This notion of complementary diagnostic studies is critical in that IRAD demonstrated that over 65% of patients with acute aortic dissection required at least two imaging modalities.[8]

TEE has the added advantages of easy bedside and intraoperative applicability, with diagnostic sensitivity and specificity rates that approach those for CT scanning.[9] New TEE techniques have reduced the limitations associated with the echocardiographic blind spot in the distal ascending aorta and arch related to the air-filled pulmonary conduits,[9] although TEE imaging beyond the diaphragm is still not reliably obtained. In our center, TEE has been invaluable during aortic endovascular repair in terms of the identification of true lumen cannulation during wire advancement, identification of primary and secondary entry site tears, and arch branch patency. Utilizing new techniques with color flow doppler and echo contrast agents, we, and other investigators,[10] have also been able to reliably demonstrate intraoperative endoseal over both primary entry and secondary re-entry site tears, and subsequent false lumen thrombosis (Figure 43–3) (the "holy grail" of endovascular dissection repair) with good correlation with findings on completion aortography and CT scan imaging. Similar to TEE, Intravascular Ultrasound (IVUS) can easily provide intraoperative imaging support during endovascular repair for experienced users.[11] No large studies have assessed the utility of IVUS for diagnosis, given the invasive nature of this technology. Proponents of IVUS cite the ability to image the entire aorta, including the arch and intra-abdominal segment, and the ability to identify entry sites, confirm guidewire placement in the true lumen, measure the aortic diameters and lengths at the attachment zones, and assess endoseal postdeployment. New "re-entry" devices for peripheral vascular subintimal angioplasty (Pioneer Catheter: MEDTRONIC Inc, Santa Rosa, California) have incorporated IVUS technology for targeting, and may be useful during complex fenestration techniques for visceral occlusions. Critics of IVUS technology remind us of the steep learning curve and operator dependency, the costs of the IVUS catheters, and the occasional difficulties associated with imaging through the endostent fabric and wireforms postdeployment. A recent review of angiography, TEE, and IVUS during endovascular repair determined that TEE, in conjunction with angiography, was advantageous, and improved the safety of repair.[11] Additionally, IVUS was important for patients with complex anatomy and/or abdominal extension of dissection. Irrespective of the combination of imaging modalities utilized, outcome for aortic dissection is dependent on rapid diagnosis and treatment.

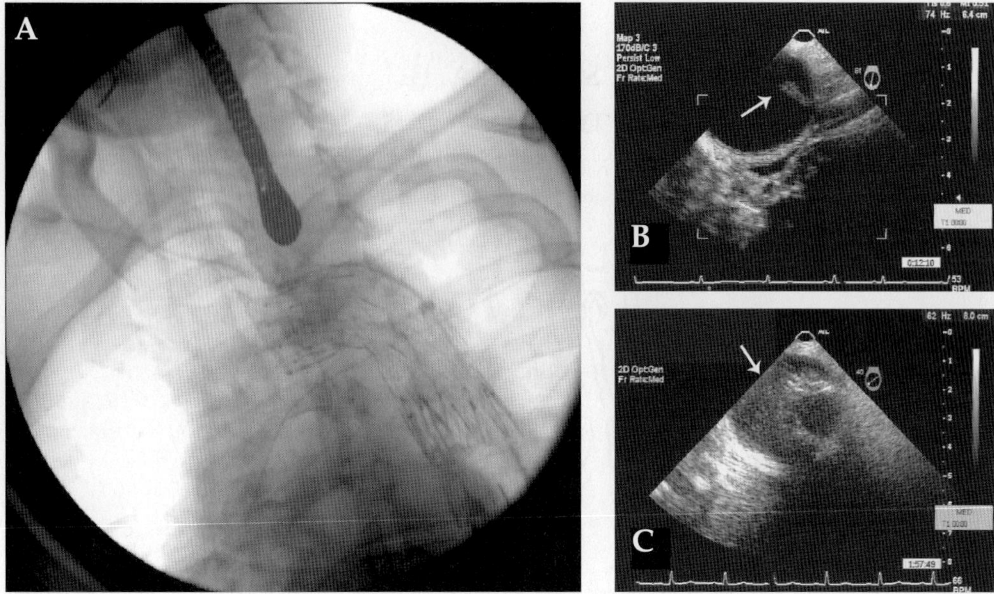

Figure 43-3. Transesophageal TEE echo (top) during proximal thoracic endograft repair for type B dissection. Dissection flap (left arrow) is evident adjacent to left subclavian artery. Echo-dense signal ("smoke") in the false lumen (right arrow) outside the stent, signifies endoseal and false lumen thrombosis.

CLASSIFICATION AND PATHOPHYSIOLOGY

Stanford A (Debakey I and II) dissections (Figure 43–4) involving the aortic arch may progress to aortic root, coronary ostial, aortic valve, and pericardial involvement, and have typically been treated with urgent cardiothoracic bypass and ascending aorta/aortic valve reconstructive procedures. Stanford B (Debakey IIIA and IIIB) dissections (Figure 43–4) have traditionally been treated medically, with management of acute hypertension and monitoring for complications such as acute branch occlusion or aneurysmal degeneration, primarily due to the historic high mortality associated with urgent open reconstruction in the acute phase when tissue integrity may be grossly impaired. Surgical or interventional therapy for Stanford B dissections has been traditionally reserved for acute complications related to the false lumen. This false lumen can be contained and thrombose. Alternatively, aortic flow can re-enter the aortic true lumen through autofenestration with ongoing patency and pressurization. Although acute aneurysm formation and rupture can occur, this is, perhaps, less common with modern medical care, and occurs more frequently with type A proximal dissections. Most of the initial pathology, morbid clinical sequelae, and indications for acute intervention with aortic dissection relate to the behavior of the aortic false lumen relative to the variety of hemodynamic mechanisms by which the pressurized channel produces partial, intermittent (dynamic), or complete (static) occlusions of either the branch vessels or the aorta itself (pseudo-obstruction or pseudocoarctation) (Figure 43–5). These malperfusion syndromes are responsible for the majority of the morbidity and mortality associated with acute aortic dissection, and present some of the most challenging surgical and/or endovascular problems for the clinician involved in the care of these patients. For those patients surviving beyond the acute period (> two

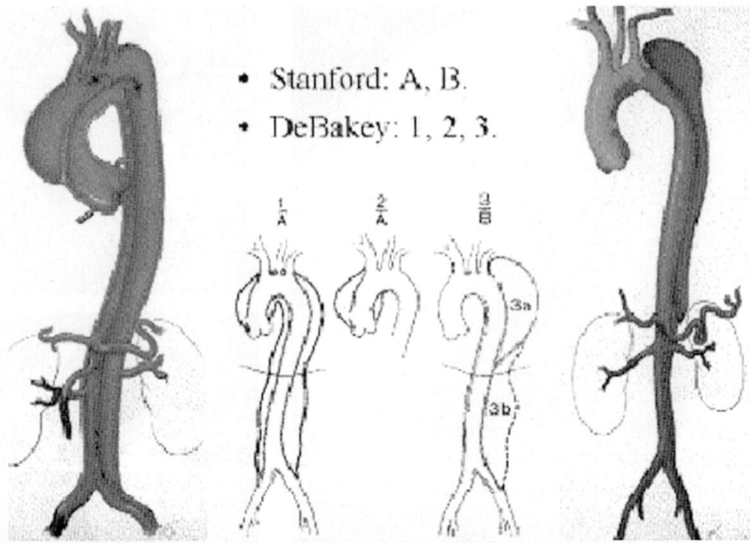

Figure 43-4. Stanford and DeBakey Classification Schemes for Thoracic Aortic Dissection. Reproduced with permission *J Vasc Surg.* 2006;43(supplA):31A.

weeks), ongoing pressurization can lead to aneurysm formation with late complications due to rupture, surgical repair, or late branch vessel occlusions. Data from the IRAD registry has demonstrated that in patients with chronic aortic dissection (> two weeks) treated medically for acute dissection with ongoing false lumen patency, aneurysmal degeneration of the false lumen is seen in up to 25% during the first four years after aortic dissection, with an estimated mortality of 50% at five years related to rupture, ischemic complications, or complications related to surgical repair. For endovascular consideration of aortic dissection, we rely on a classification scheme that more accurately depicts the indications for treatment and the unique therapeutic challenges encountered: acute uncomplicated dissection, Intramural Hematoma (IMH)/Penetrating Atherosclerotic Ulcer (PAU) syndrome, acute complicated dissection, and chronic aortic dissection.

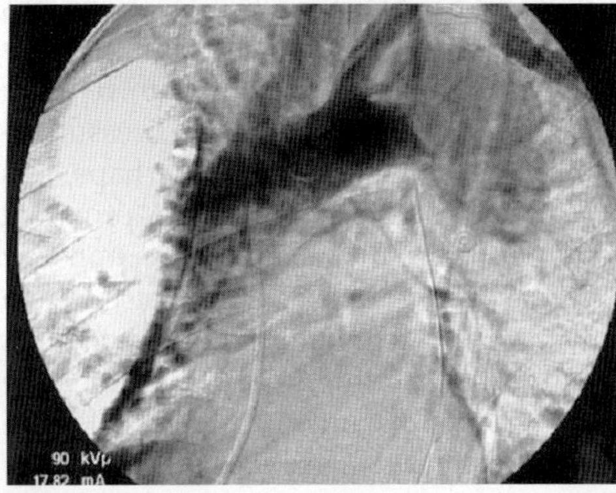
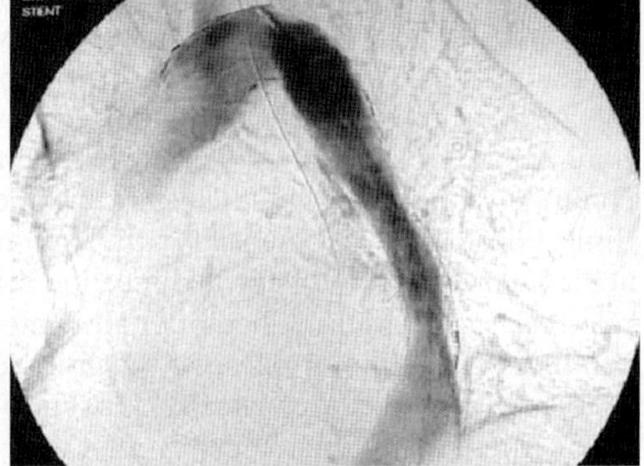

Figure 43-5. Aortic pseudo-obstruction: Occlusion of the aorta just beyond left subclavian artery by pseudoaneurysm after acute dissection. Spinal cord, renal, and hepatic perfusion deficits resolved after urgent placement of endovascular stents (right) to re-expand the thoracic true lumen.

ACUTE UNCOMPLICATED DISSECTION

This is undoubtedly the most controversial of all groups relative to endovascular treatment. Unlike those patients with acute malperfusion syndromes, ongoing bleeding or pain with false lumen expansion, new neurological deficits, or rupture, there are no classic indications for acute intervention. The goal in this patient cohort is to prevent the long-term sequelae of chronic aortic dissection. This is theoretically possible through the coverage of the primary entry site and elimination of false lumen pressurization with false lumen thrombosis, and re-expansion of the true lumen and aortic remodeling (Figure 43–6). The trade-off from a life curve perspective is the finite risk of mortality from early endovascular intervention and from any subsequent reinterventions, a risk that has yet to be clearly defined, although recent IRAD data suggests this may be <5% at one year.[6] Recent studies with nonrandomized patients demonstrated feasibility and an improvement in outcome relative to historical cohorts.[12,13]

Our approach in the past has been to offer repair to patients with acute uncomplicated dissection, excluding those with either early (<two weeks) or spontaneous false

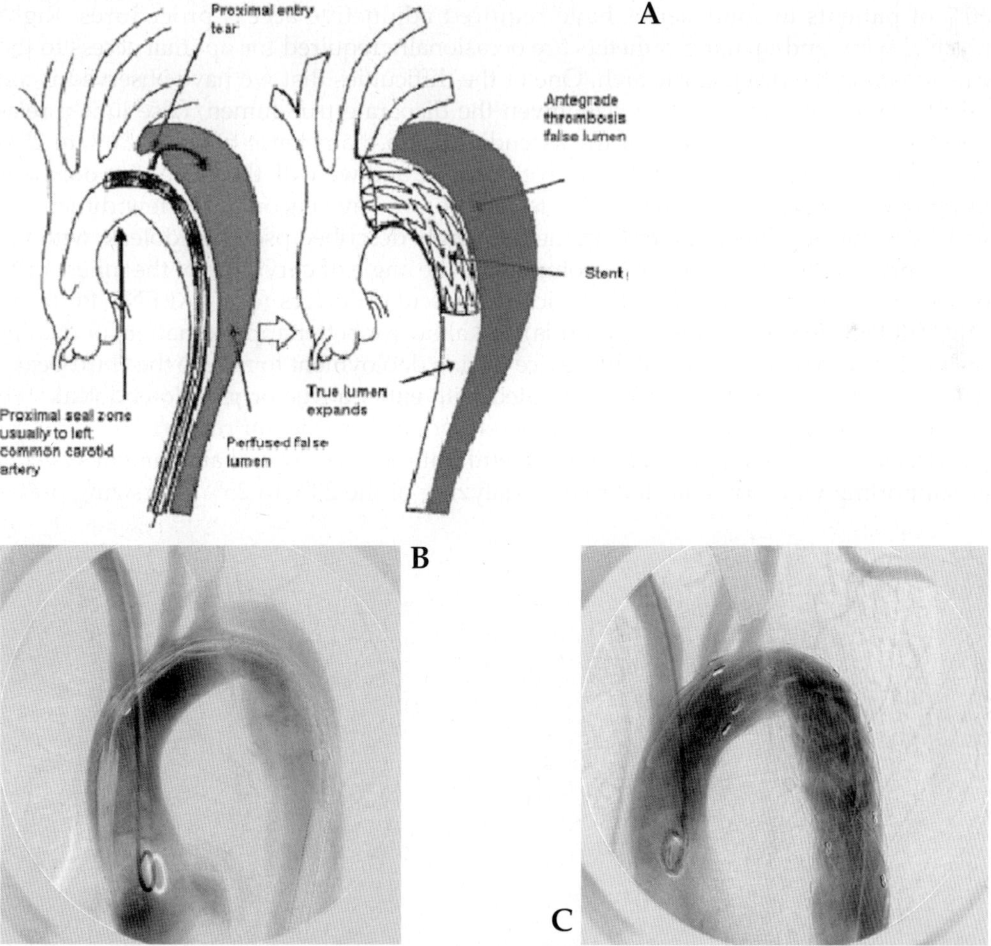

Figure 43-6. Thoracic stent graft deployment across proximal entry site tear resulting in obliteration of false lumen flow and false lumen thrombosis. Re-expansion of true lumen and remodeling of the aorta leads to restoration of aortic wall integrity. Drawing reproduced with permission *J Vasc Surg*. 2006;43(suppl A):38A.

lumen thrombosis, given the improved outcome demonstrated with medical treatment in this cohort of patients. After medical stabilization (elimination of pain, control of hypertension, no further extension of dissection), we use preoperative CT scanning and intraoperative TEE to identify the primary entry site for coverage at the time of stent graft repair, and any other secondary re-entry sites, occasionally stenting all the way to the visceral segment (celiac axis) for type IIIB dissections. We have observed an increased incidence of autofenestration at roughly three weeks after dissection, leading us to offer repair within the first two weeks of the event, which increases the chance that simple primary entry site coverage can be achieved. TEE guidance is also utilized to ensure proper placement of deployment guidewires into the true lumen and to ensure endoseal with the use of echo contrast. For these and all patients requiring endovascular reconstruction of the thoracic aorta, vascular access is a critical issue. Thoracic endovascular devices are larger than abdominal devices, and female patients with their smaller access vessels comprise a larger component of thoracic cohorts, resulting in an increased need for adjunctive procedures during endovascular deployment including trans-iliac or trans-abdominal conduits,[15] or the use of brachial-inominate wires and catheters ("body-floss technique") for extreme tortuosity of the descending thoracic aorta or arch. Up to 30% of patients in some series have required adjunctive access procedures. Right brachial wires and imaging catheters are occasionally required for optimal access to the true lumen in the distal aortic arch. One of the difficulties that we have observed is the calculation of appropriate stent size, given the disparate true lumen/false lumen relationship. We have observed that the ascending aorta diameter is typically 20% to 25% larger than the arch diameter for any given patient, and we will, therefore, size our stent using this measurement. Utilizing this technique, we have encountered few difficulties with proximal attachment other than the frequently described pseudoendoleak, with the inner curve of the stent failing to accommodate the angle of curvature of the inner curve of the arch (Figure 43–7). New thoracic endovascular devices (e.g. TALENT Proform, MEDTRONIC Inc, Santa Rosa, California) will allow for better approximation, or manipulation of the inner curvature of the device during deployment to reduce the "bird-beak" deformity of the stent that can be associated with either a true or pseudo-endoleak. We avoid aggressive ballooning due to risks of retrograde dissection or rupture.[16]

Recently, the development of devices without robust proximal attachment systems or supporting wireforms has led to a reanalyzing of the 20% to 25% oversizing previ-

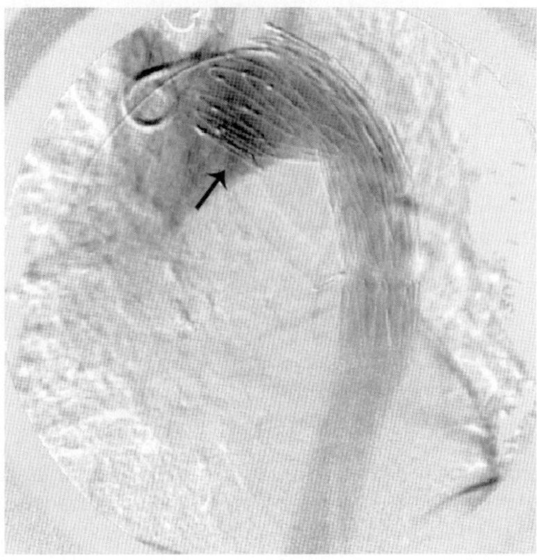

Figure 43-7. Pseudoendoleak. Contrast outside of stent at inner curve of arch (arrow) due to failure of the stent to accommodate the steep angle of curvature.

ously recommended for the endovascular treatment of aortic thoracic pathology. Although some of these thoracic devices can more easily accommodate the angle of curvature at the distal aortic arch, aggressive oversizing of these less robust designs has led to collapse of devices and maldeployments (Figure 43–8). The ideal stent design including the combination of arch trackability, curvature accommodation, and robust attachment has yet to be designed.

The extent of the repair is certainly as controversial as is whether to offer surgical repair at all. Proponents of early repair of the entry tear cite the ability to completely exclude the false lumen flow, eliminate the long-term sequelae of false lumen degeneration, and functionally "cure" the patient. Complete coverage of the entry site tear, and the subsequent depressurization of the false lumen prevents the partial thrombosis that can be observed in medically treated patients - Partial thrombosis is an independent predictor of death (Odds Ratio 2.69)[1] due to the blind loop phenomenon leading to rapid expansion and rupture. In our experience, patients with no further observable false lumen flow after coverage of the entry site tear are at low risk for further dilation, and can be treated with the single covered stent with obliteration of the false lumen due to remodelling (Figure 43–9). For those patients with severe distal true

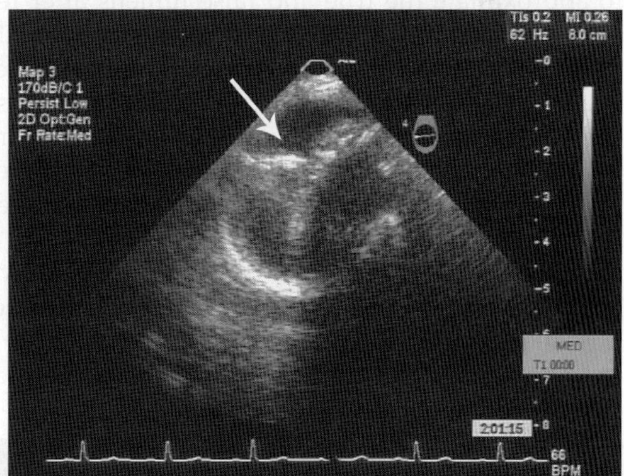

Figure 43-8. Collapse of proximal thoracic aortic stent during endovascular repair for aortic dissection. "Omega sign" as a result of stent folding over on itself.

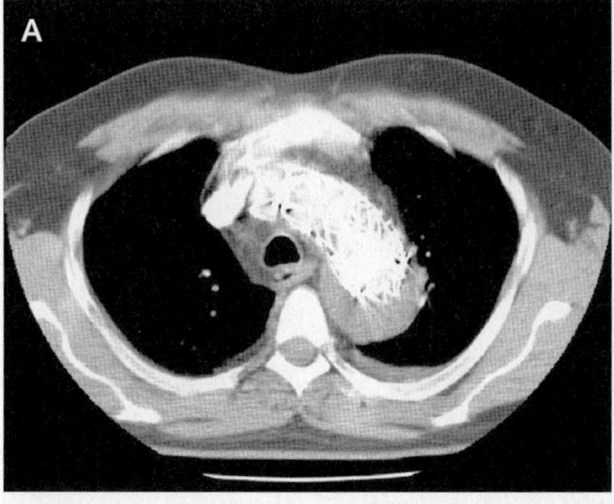
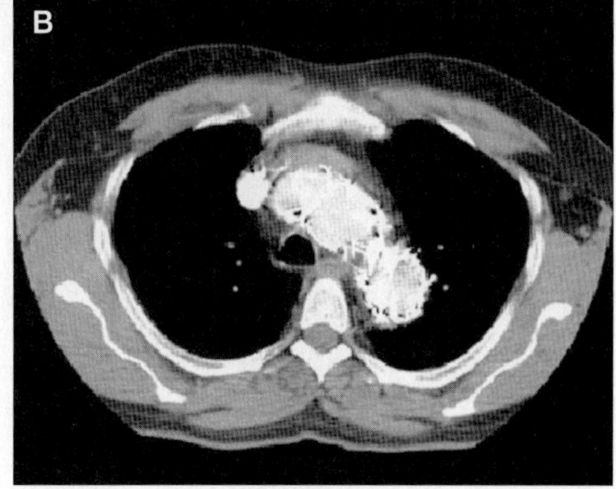

Figure 43-9. Acute thrombosis of false lumen after single stent placement (left) for thoracic dissection. Twenty-four month follow-up CT images (right) demonstrate complete obliteration of thoracic false lumen due to aortic remodeling.

lumen compromise due to compression by the false lumen, we have occasionally utilized uncovered self-expanding stents to enhance aortic remodeling, stabilize the dissection flap, and improve the coaptation of the true and false lumens, which will occur as long as the false lumen has been depressurized. In patients with multiple distal sites of fenestration, which is the typical case for any dissection older than three weeks, we aggressively extend the covered stent to any large fenestration, up to the level of the celiac axis if necessary. The observed rate of paralysis is low, both in the literature[16] and in our own experience (<4%), and may be minimized by the lack of significant inflammatory mediated reperfusion injury observed after open repair. In addition, we use aggressive adjuncts for all patients having distal thoracic coverage including routine CSF drainage and aggressive maintenance of systemic blood pressure to support cord perfusion pressure. The self-expanding stent is typically not ballooned distally due to the extreme friability of the true lumen false lumen interface, and the risks of rupture, or promotion of further perivisceral dilation. If any of the visceral branch vessels are perfused exclusively from the false lumen, or if re-expansion of the true lumen proximally results in impaired visceral perfusion (i.e., conversion to an acute complicated dissection), visceral reperfusion can be achieved through endovascular fenestration techniques[6] just above or at the visceral segment, with use of an uncovered stent to approximate the true and false lumens after fenestrated flow has been achieved. Alternatively, the occluded visceral can be cannulated through the wireforms of the uncovered stent, and stented open with either covered or uncovered devices. This has been eloquently described by other investigators[17] with excellent results reported, even for those patients with complex occlusions or complicated dissections at presentation. Despite extension of the covered or uncovered stent device to the level of the celiac, it is typical to observe retrograde peristent and/or antegrade perivisceral false lumen flow in patients with extensive type B dissection (Figure 43–10). In all dissection cohorts, aneurysmal dilation of this perivisceral or peristent segment could theoretically represent the "Achilles Heal" for endovascular repair for thoracic dissection, particularly given the complex nature of the perivisceral segment, the difficulty in aligning visceral orifices at the true and false lumens (particularly for chronic

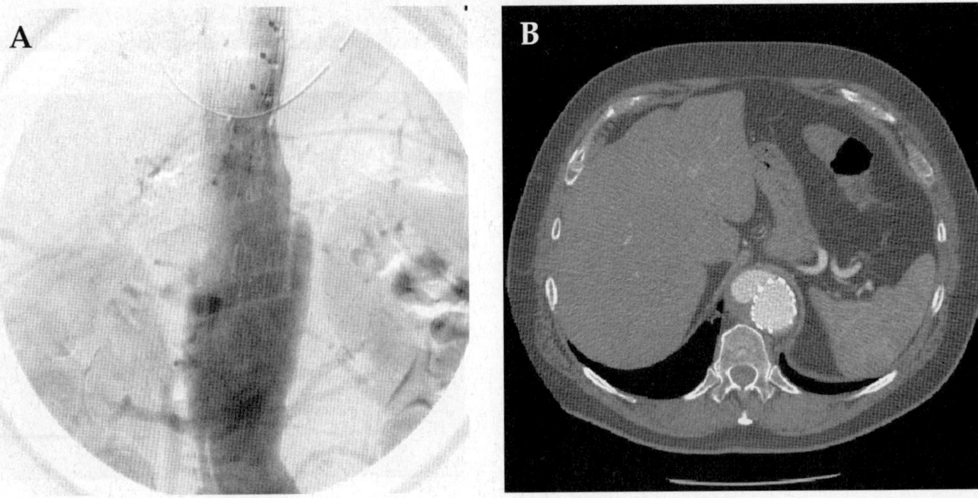

Figure 43-10. Persistent false lumen flow around distal stent through the perivisceral aorta after endovascular stent repair for aortic dissection.

dissections), and the fledgling nature of current branched and perivisceral endovascular technology. Although some patients do go on to develop peri-visceral aneurysmal disease, this is relatively uncommon in the literature, even for patients treated medically,[18] suggesting a resistance to dilation for this segment of the aorta (Figure 43–11). Investigators have reviewed the impact of open surgical fenestration and ongoing false lumen perfusion on the risk of perivisceral dilation, and have also noted a relatively low rate of progression to aneurysm formation.[6] A recent publication reviewed aortic true and false lumen diameters at various levels of the aorta following endovascular repair for aortic dissection, and reported no significant change in the combined aortic true and false lumen diameter at the level of the diaphragm.[7] This was associated with an overall reduction in the false lumen diameter, with an associated increased true lumen diameter, thus demonstrating favorable aortic remodeling after proximal entry site coverage. Even though the reported risk for perivisceral dilation appears to be low, if it does occur, this dilation is easily followed, and may be readily amenable to hybrid open/endovascular procedures, with reduced mortality and morbidity rates compared to total thoracoabdominal repair.

We have observed no deaths, but like other investigators, have observed retrograde dissection requiring conversion to aortic root repair due to a combination of bare proximal wireform interaction with the proximal aortic wall, and possibly overly aggressive balloon dilatation during deployment. In one series, retrograde type A dissection occurred with an incidence of 6.8% and an associated mortality rate of 40%.[19] New aneurysm formation at proximal or distal attachment zones has also been described in the literature,[20] and all of these represent valid criticisms of early repair. We avoid proximal ballooning unless there is obvious evidence of an attachment site leak, and have stopped using devices with bare wire proximal fixation systems.

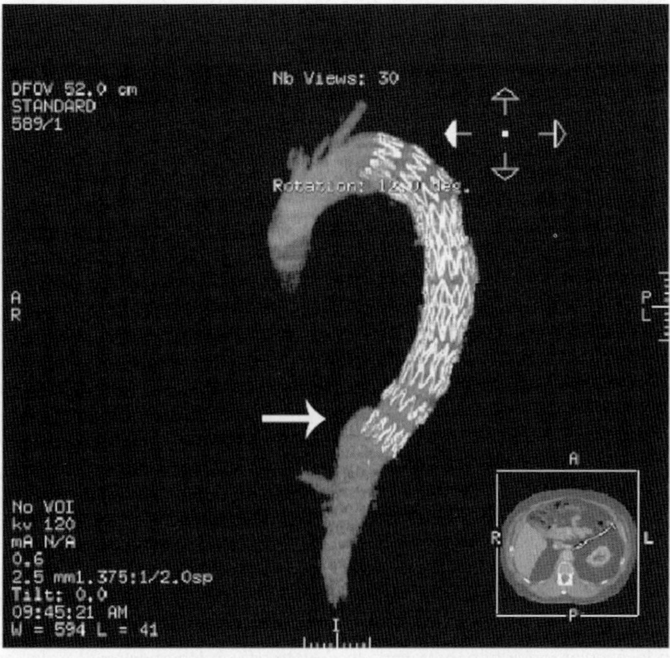

Figure 43-11. Stable (nonenlarging) perivisceral aortic segment in a patient two years after endograft repair for type B dissection despite ongoing peristent perfusion of false aneurysm (arrow).

Nienaber and his group reviewed 80 patients treated with endovascular repair for uncomplicated type B dissection, and compared this series to 80 patients treated medically.[21] His two year outcomes showed a marked improvement in survival in favor of the stented group, and led to the formulation of the randomized prospective INSTEAD trial comparing best medical therapy to best medical therapy plus endovascular repair for 136 patients with chronic (> two weeks, <52 weeks) uncomplicated type B dissection. The preliminary three-month follow-up data are discussed in the chronic aortic dissection segment (below), but have demonstrated a favorable trend toward false lumen thrombosis in the stented cohort. Patients at the highest risk for subsequent complications and death appear to be those with persistent false lumen flow, those patients with partial false lumen thrombosis and blind loop pressurization, and those with initial aortic diameters greater than 40mm.[29] Patients in these categories may be considered for early repair. Given the current lack of prospective data, routine endovascular repair for acute uncomplicated aortic dissection cannot be recommended until further studies to assess outcomes have been completed.

INTRAMURAL HEMATOMA/PENETRATING ATHEROSCLEROTIC ULCER SYNDROME

These clinical/pathological entities have only recently been described, likely representing the spectrum of the same general aortic degenerative illness, and have been documented in 5.7% of acute aortic syndromes in the IRAD database.[6] A penetrating ulcer results in an intramural hematoma, with or without further extension beyond the confines of the true aortic wall, to produce a typical saccular appearance on CT scan or aortography (Figure 43–12A). An intense inflammatory response may limit the disease to a focal area of the aortic wall with subsequent spontaneous resolution, although progression to frank dissection and rupture has been described in the literature in up to 16% of patients,[22-23] and the overall mortality rate for IMH of approximately 20% is only slightly lower than that for typical aortic dissection. High-risk lesions that increase the likelihood for aortic repair include those associated with an initial aortic diameter

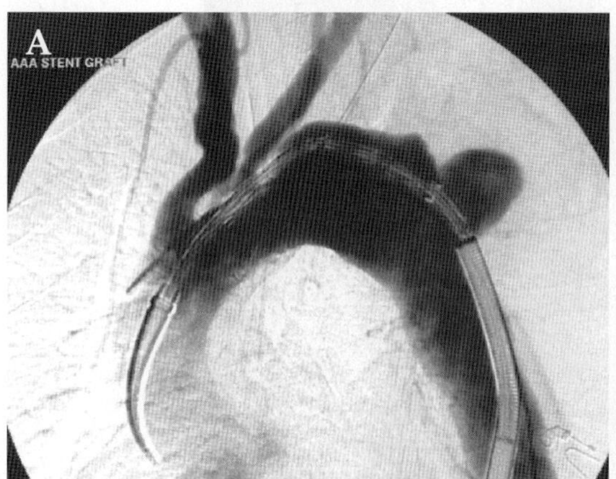

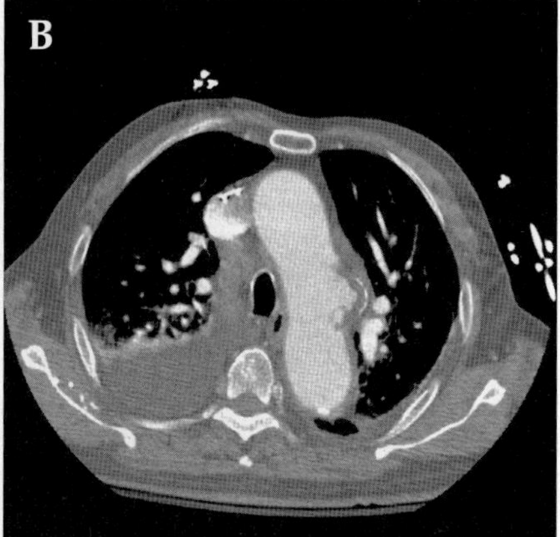

Figure 43-12. (A) Endovascular repair of penetrating ulcer. Note diffuse atherosclerotic irregularity through aortic arch and branch vessels ("shaggy aorta"). **(B)** CT scan of proximal thoracic aortic arch penetrating ulcer. Proximal aortic penetrating ulcers > 1cm deep and >2cm wide demonstrate an increased risk of rupture.

> 40mm, an aortic wall thickness > 10mm, ascending aortic involvement, ulcer depth > 10mm, or ulcer width > 20mm (Figure 43–12B). Endovascular repair of these lesions is tempting, due to the relatively focal appearance of the pathology in imaging studies. However, the absence of a definite intimal flap makes defining the deployment landing zone more difficult, and the disease likely represents diffuse degenerative rather than focal aortopathy that may be quite dynamic on serial imaging. Often, there is associated diffuse atheromatous disease ("shaggy aorta") that increases the likelihood of embolic phenomenon during guidewire, catheter, and sheath manipulation, and degenerative ulceration, aneurysm formation, and rupture of the adjacent unstented segments has been described. Most authors recommend aggressive medical therapy with blood pressure management for all but the high-risk lesions previously discussed, and rely on frequent follow-up imaging to assess resolution or progression of the disease. A mycotic process needs to be excluded for all patients with saccular aneurysm formation.

ACUTE COMPLICATED DISSECTION

Type A Dissection

Type A proximal dissections, which comprise roughly two-thirds of all aortic dissections, are by definition complicated. Endovascular options have traditionally been limited, and open surgical repair has been considered mandatory to avoid the significant early risks of mortality due to retrograde dissection with pericardial tamponade, acute aortic valvular failure, congestive heart failure, myocardial ischemia or infarction, cerebrovascular extension with stroke and/or coma, and mediastinal rupture with shock. IRAD investigators reporting on over 500 cases of type A dissection[24] with an in-hospital mortality of 25.1% have identified high-risk patients presenting with these clinical sequelae, and have demonstrated independent predictive features for operative mortality including hypotension at presentation (odds ratio = 1.95), shock or tamponade (odds ratio = 2.69), history of aortic valve replacement (odds ratio = 3.12), preoperative limb ischemia (odds ratio = 2.10), or migrating chest pain (odds ratio = 2.77). The morbidity of type A repair is increased in the setting of aortic arch replacement, or hemiarch replacement and/or elephant trunk repair, which is considered mandatory in many centers due to the significant risk of arch dilation if aortic root repair alone is utilized, and due to the ability to use the elephant trunk as a proximal landing zone for simultaneous or staged endovascular reconstruction of the dissected descending thoracic aortic segment. In our center, elephant trunk repair is also completed with the addition of suturing a short segment of J-wire to the most distal end of the vascular graft to allow for easy fluoroscopic identification during subsequent endovascular repair of the descending thoracic aortic segment. The J-wire can also be snared and used as a tether to ensure that the graft is not "accordioned" during advancement of the endovascular stent device. On-table retrograde placement of endovascular stent devices through the arch aortotomy has also been described[25] to minimize the risks of further descending thoracic aortic dilation and promote false lumen thrombosis. More recently, investigators have reported a less invasive approach to type A repair[26] involving aortic root repair with simultaneous aortoinominate bypass and ligation of the inominate at its origin. This is followed by staged carotid-carotid bypass and total arch endovascular exclusion. Short-term follow-up has demonstrated complete false lumen thrombosis with no deaths or neurologic complications. Our group has also utilized this total arch exclusion technique after extra-anatomic bypass for chronic dissections and aneurysmal dilation of the aortic arch (Figure 43–13). Other investigators have described the use of branched devices inserted into the arch for elective repair to encompass arch vessel supply, or alternatively, the use of in situ fenestration techniques to improve aortic arch branch endovascular options.[27] In the acute setting, these options are limited by device availability, lack of global expertise, and the need for rapid therapy. Complete proximal endovascular deployment is also limited by the presence of the coronary ostia, the often associated pericardial or valvular involvement, and the excessive length of the nose cone of currently available devices, which may necessitate a high-risk maneuver involving pushing the device through the aortic valve leaflets. Until these technical challenges are overcome, hybrid techniques currently represent the best options for limiting the morbidity associated with open arch reconstructions for type A dissection repair.

ACUTE COMPLICATED DISSECTION

Type B Dissection

Acute complicated type B dissection includes those patients with uncontrollable pain, progression of dissection, mediastinal or pleural hemorrhage due to rupture or direct aortic branch vessel involvement, or branch vessel flow impairment due to proximal true lumen compression by the aortic false lumen (malperfusion syndrome). With modern medical therapy and an increased emphasis on prompt diagnosis and treatment, uncontrolled extension of dissection, hypertension, and rupture rates for dissection have improved dramatically over the past few decades, with only 6% of patients requiring urgent repair for acute rupture in modern series.[6] The majority of patients

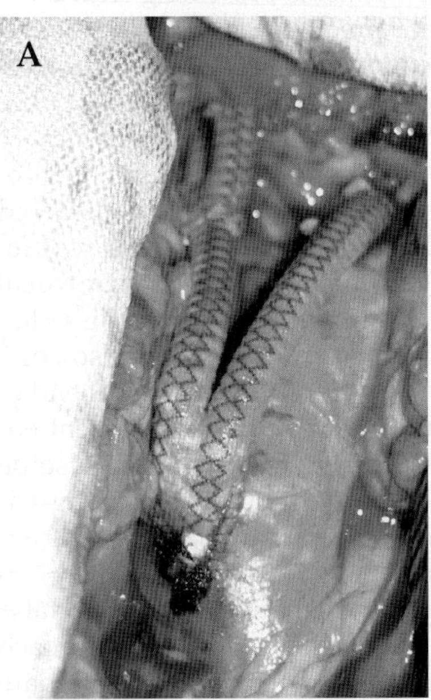
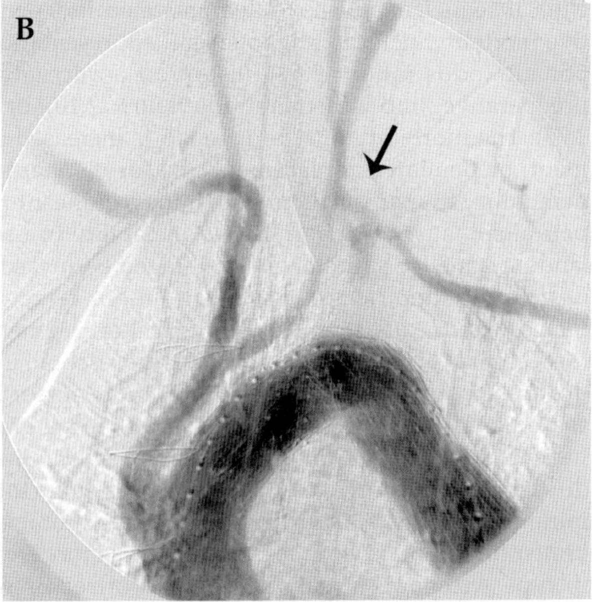

Figure 43-13. Complete aortic arch branch devascularization and extra-anatomic revascularization (left) followed by total thoracic arch stenting. The left carotid-subclavian bypass (arrow) was performed to reperfuse the dominant left vertebral artery.

classified as complicated type B dissection have malperfusion syndrome, with varying levels of branch vessel compromise leading to ischemia in the involved vascular bed, a clinical scenario that occurs in up to 40% of patients.[2] Outcome is related to the vascular bed involved, with the highest mortality observed in those patients with central neurologic (stroke and coma) and mesenteric ischemia. Mesenteric ischemia in particular has emerged as one of the treatment priorities, even in patients with type A dissection, and the strategy of early mesenteric revascularization has contributed to the overall reduction in mortality related to dissection in recent series.[1-3] Interestingly, peripheral ischemia, although a marker for more extensive dissection, does not appear to increase mortality, likely due to its association with a more prompt diagnosis and therapy in patients with dissection. Spinal cord ischemia is a dramatic finding, but relatively rare, seen in only 2% to 3% of all patients.[6] Our understanding of the mechanisms of malperfusion or aortic branch vessel compromise has improved with the advent of endovascular technology. In the majority of cases, either the compressed true lumen results in flow impairment to the branch vessel downstream or the dissection flap prolapses intermittently into the branch vessel origin (Figure 43–14A), resulting in ischemia that can vary in severity depending on hemodynamic factors including the rate at which the aortic pulse wave is generated (dp/dt) and the peripheral vascular resistance, both of which can be manipulated pharmacologically. Stent graft coverage of the primary entry site tear can eliminate this mechanism of obstruction by restoring true lumen flow, and favorably altering the "pressure battle" toward the true lumen side of the equation. Our observation has been that this mechanism is particularly important for those patients with spinal cord ischemic symptoms with excellent results using early primary entry site repair. Dake et al.,[4] in their seminal report on the endovascular treatment for aortic dissection, noted that 80% of perfusion deficits could be overcome by simple primary entry site coverage, leading to the term "dynamic obstruction." A smaller percentage of patients either have dissection flaps that extend directly into the branch origin (Figure 43–14B), or alternatively have flaps that have sheared off the origin of the branch vessel with perfusion from the false lumen (Figure 43–14C). If the dissection flap into the branch vessel results in significant stenosis or thrombosis, or if false lumen thrombosis occurs under those situations where visceral flow is false lumen dependent, then the obstruction is static, with the need for directed revascularization procedures including vessel access and stenting, and/or endovascular fenestration procedures. If required, direct vessel access for stenting should be obtained prior to fenestration techniques due to the risk of misalignment of vessel origins between the true and false lumens after fenestration and subsequent failed cannulation. Multiple endovascular fenestration techniques have been described, but all have in common the strategy of lamellar puncture and passage of a wire from the smaller true lumen to the larger false lumen in order to bridge the two channels, with subsequent use of wires or balloons to create the communicating channel (Figure 43–15). Intraoperative IVUS and/or TEE may be the ideal modalities to assist in this process, particularly since all techniques have a substantive risk of rupture due to the always two-dimensional and often blind nature of the puncture on fluoroscopy. Directional catheters (e.g., Outback Catheter: LuMend Inc, Redwood City, California) can also assist in the passage of wires from true to false lumen during the fenestration procedure. We have utilized the stent graft itself to create a fenestration above the visceral segment by nudging the distal end of the deployed stent with a molding balloon under direct fluoroscopic vision in order to shear the lamellae between the two channels. Mortality rates for patients requiring fenestration of direct endovascular

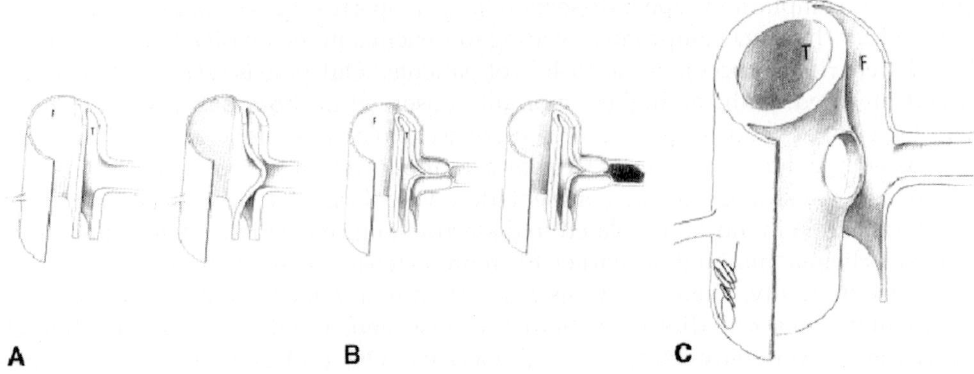

Figure 43-14. Mechanisms of branch vessel malperfusion after aortic dissection. **(A)** Dynamic obstruction of branch flow produced by lamellar compression of lumen during the cardiac cycle. **(B)** Static obstruction produced by dissection into the branch vessel, and subsequent distal thrombosis. **(C)** Commonly, the dissection flap shears off at the orifice of branch vessels leading to perfusion by way of the false lumen. If false lumen flow is obliterated, misalignment of the branch vessel orifice and the branch vessel can result in impaired flow.

revascularization for static obstruction ranges as high as 30%, and are likely related as much to delay in diagnosis and therapy as to the technical procedures themselves. In general, malperfusion syndromes take priority over repair of the entry site tear for type B dissections, although it is important to emphasize that the most effective technique to deal with the majority of malperfusion syndromes is to cover the entry site tear and alter the luminal pressure dynamics. Advanced age, severe mesenteric ischemia, and involvement of multiple vascular beds appear to be the most significant predictors for mortality in patients with malperfusion.[1-3,6] Fenestration techniques theoretically increase the risk for further false lumen dilation, and hence aneurysmal

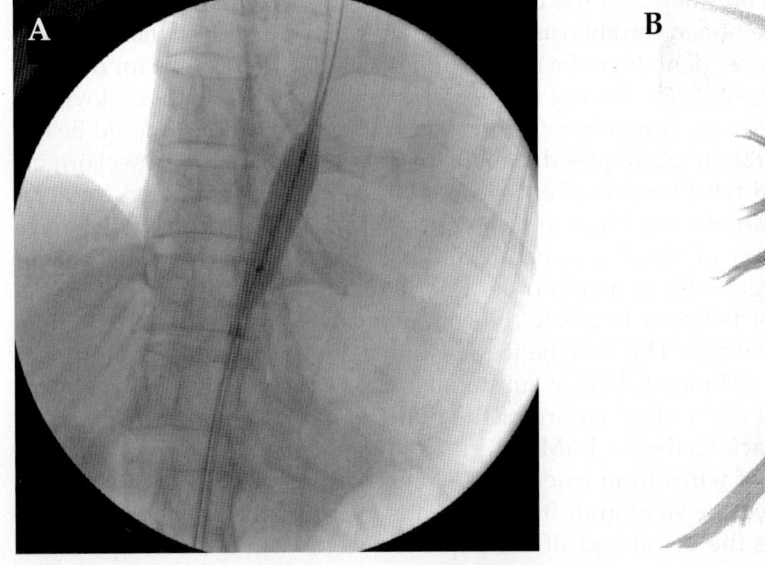

Figure 43-15. Balloon fenestration of the dissection lamella between the true and false lumen to reperfuse the left renal artery. Drawing reproduced with permission *J Vasc Surg*. 2006;43(supplA):41A.

degeneration, although this has not been clearly defined in the literature. We have observed rapid expansion of the false lumen, requiring secondary intervention in those patients having fenestration using the distal end of the stent graft (Figure 43–16), emphasizing the need for early serial imaging in all patients having revascularization procedures for malperfusion.

CHRONIC DISSECTION

In up to 40% of patients with aortic dissection treated with beta-blockade and optimal medical therapy alone, the underlying tissue deficit, associated with the impact of often poorly controlled hypertension and ongoing perfusion of the aortic false lumen, results in aneurysmal degeneration within four years of diagnosis. In addition to uncontrolled hypertension and ongoing false lumen perfusion, patients with a maximal combined true and false aortic diameter > 40 mm are also at increased risk for subsequent aneurysm formation.[6] Although chronic occlusions of branch vessels may occur, aneurysm formation represents the most common indication for intervention in patients beyond the acute phase (two weeks), and up to 20% of patients may experience late rupture of their complex dissection aneurysms with an increased mortality and morbidity rate relative to their degenerative aneurysm counterparts. In fact, 20% to 40% of all extent II thoracoabdominal repairs are completed for patients with aneurysmal degeneration related to aortic dissection.[17] The INSTEAD (**IN**vestigation of **ST**Entgrafts in **A**ortic **D**issection) trial was formulated in response to these significant delayed risks associated with medical treatment for chronic aortic dissection and the 26.5% three-year mortality rate identified by IRAD investigators.[21] Inclusion criteria for the 136 patients recruited included patient older than 18 years, no contraindication to anesthesia with intubation, type B aortic dissection older than 14 days and younger than 52 weeks, diameter of target aortic segment ≤ 6 cm, aortic kinking < 75°, and signed patient informed consent approved by a medical ethics committee. Patients were excluded primarily if they demonstrated early thrombosis of the false lumen, if they had signs of malperfusion syndrome, or if they had significant renal failure or di-

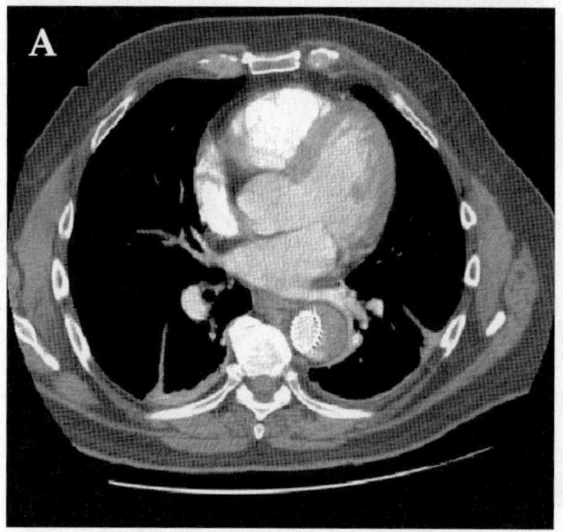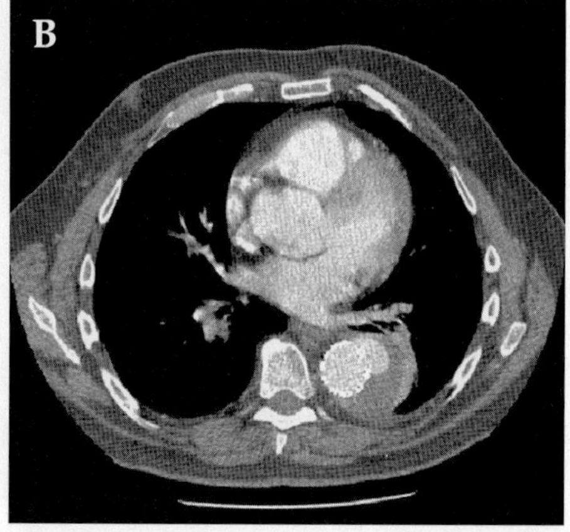

Figure 43-16. Fenestration by balloon dilation of distal end of stent (left) producing rapid (six month) false lumen expansion and aneurysm formation at the distal aspect of the stent (right).

minished life expectancy due to concurrent illness. The primary endpoint was all-cause mortality at one year, with secondary endpoints including thrombosis of the false lumen, degree of aortic expansion, cardiovascular morbidity, quality of life, length of ICU and hospital stay, and crossover between treatment arms. Study inclusion and exclusion criteria, and three-month interim data were presented at the 2006 Charing Cross Symposium (available at www.cxvascular.com), and demonstrated three deaths in the stented treatment arm (vs. 0 deaths in the medical arm), and primary entry site seal in 85% of stented patients at three months, with 52% of patients showing false lumen thrombosis. Only 66% of patients in the stented arm showed no further aortic expansion, with 16% of patients demonstrating further enlargement. These figures for aortic expansion were comparable to those observed in patients in the medically treated arm. One year INSTEAD follow-up data was presented at the ISET 2007 Symposium (http://www.prolibraries.com/iset/?select=session& sessionID=702) and demonstrated a higher (P=NS) all cause mortality in the stented group, with 0% mortality observed in the 11% of patients that required delayed crossover to surgery, leading the authors to conclude that for uncomplicated (chronic) dissection, a period of tailored medical therapy with deferred stent graft therapy for patients failing to respond is the most appropriate option. Criticisms of the study include the inability to achieve proximal entry site seal in 15% of patients, as well as the long mean time to randomization (57 days in the stented group, 83 days in the medically treated arm), both of which, in our experience, predisposes the patient to pressurization and complex fenestrations with increased likelihood of ongoing aortic false lumen perfusion, and death particularly if a single stent is used to cover only the primary entry site tear. Many investigators believe that the complex multiple fenestrations between the true and false lumens (the "Swiss cheese lamellae") that occur in patients with chronic dissection and the fibrous nature of the chronic lamellae, mitigate against successful aortic remodeling and aneurysm resolution after endovascular repair. Using our strategy of complete coverage of the aortic segment with covered endovascular stents from the entry site to celiac axis for this patient population, we have been able to demonstrate successful remodeling with aneurysm resolution (Figure 43–17), even for very old dissections (> one year). Critics of this total thoracic aortic

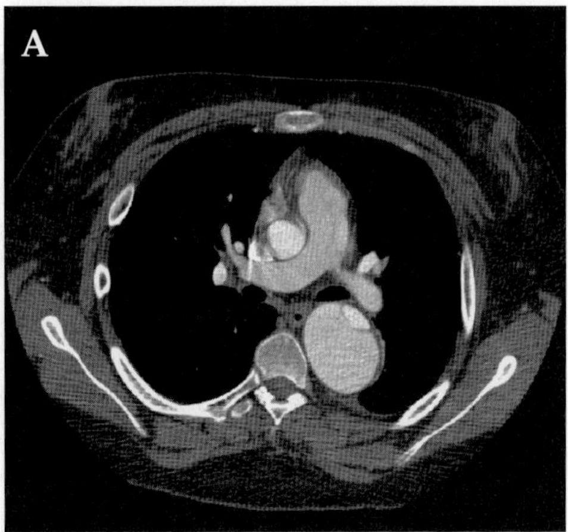
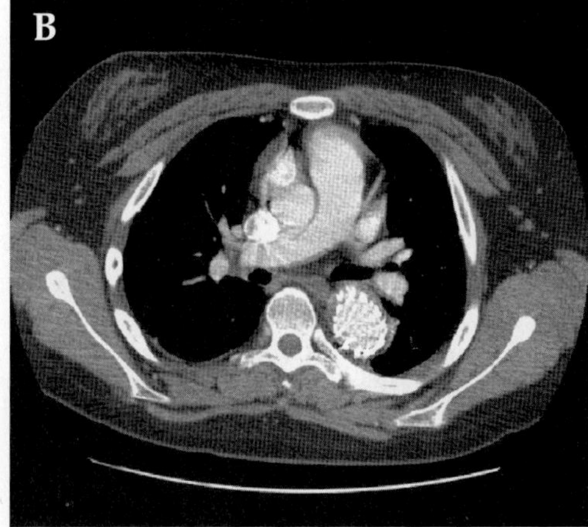

Figure 43-17. Chronic aortic dissection. Note small compressed true lumen due to aneurysmal dilation of false lumen (left). Complete re-expansion of true lumen and obliteration of chronic false lumen (right) 18 months after total thoracic aortic stent graft exclusion of dissection.

coverage strategy cite the ongoing perfusion of the false lumen through the perivisceral segment, although as discussed above, the risk for subsequent aneurysmal degeneration appears to be low, and can be followed with serial imaging. If further aneurysmal degeneration occurs, our approach is to treat the resulting extent IV thoracoabdominal aneurysm with balloon control from a proximal brachial access, with direct anastamosis of the aortic graft to the fabric at the distal end of the endovascular stent. In most cases, this can be completed without thoracotomy or with simple 11th intercostal space extension for exposure, and is associated with a much lower risk than the conventional Extent II thoracoabdominal aneurysm repair that would be required for patients without proximal thoracic endovascular repair. Alternatively, extra-anatomic bypass to all viscerals can be completed with aortic branch origin ligation and without the need for aortic cross-clamping. After devascularization of the perivisceral aorta, endovascular stent graft deployment through the visceral segment can be completed down to the iliac bifurcation if required. As long as left subclavian artery and hypogastric artery flow are preserved, the overall risk of paraplegia with these hybrid extra-anatomic revascularization and transvisceral stenting procedures (Figure 43–18) appears to be comparable to that for complete open reconstruction, without the associated risks of aortic cross-clamp and ischemia/reperfusion.[28] Complete endovascular repair of degenerative thoracoabdominal aneurysms with branched graft technology has become relatively commonly utilized in many large aortic centers, and branched grafts[27] will undoubtedly have a role to play in the treatment of chronic dissection. Limitations of this technology in the chronic dissection patient are related to the misalignment of branch orifices between true and false lumens, and the complex

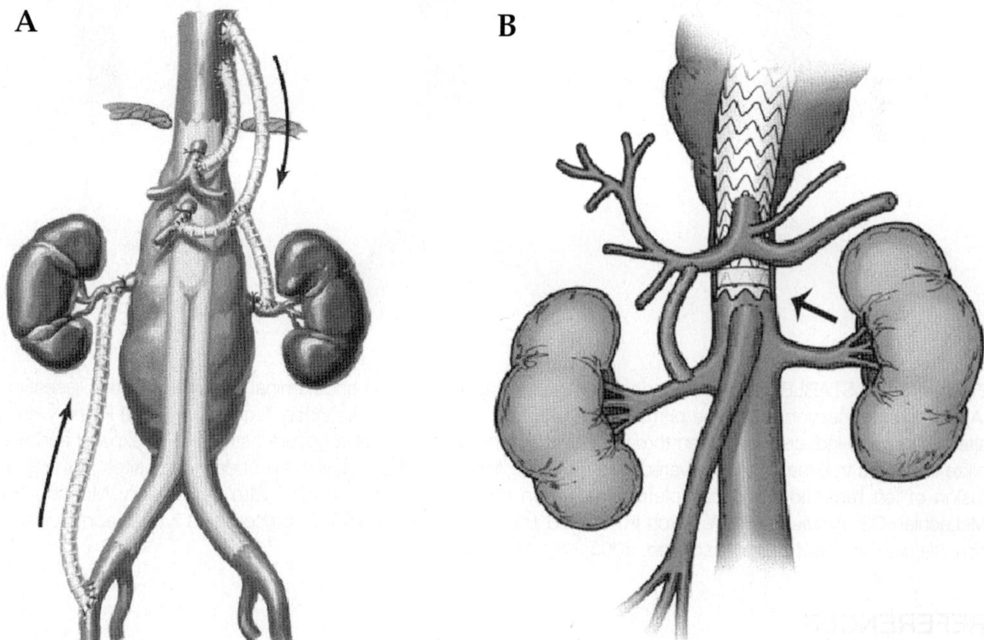

Figure 43-18. Hybrid extra-anatomic visceral bypass techniques associated with endograft repair for the perivisceral aortic segment. The distal end of the thoracic stent graft (right) can also be used as an anastamotic site for open perivisceral aortic repair, eliminating the need for open thoracic aortic reconstruction. Drawings reproduced with permission *J Vasc Surg.* 2006;43(supplA:81A.

visceral flaps that are occasionally present in chronic dissections that can mitigate against successful visceral artery cannulation and stenting. In addition, expertise with these complex devices and access to this technology is limited to a few centers of excellence, and will likely not achieve widespread distribution. Mossop and his colleagues from Australia have successfully developed a strategy for "staged thoracoabdominal and branch vessel endoluminal repair" (the "STABLE" procedure) (Figure 43–19), which entails early covered stent repair of the dissection entry site, with uncovered stent stabilization of the distal thoracic true lumen, followed by direct cannulation and stenting of any malperfused viscerals, with or without coil embolization of communicating fenestrae in order to promote false lumen thrombosis (observed in 85% of patients in their series) and maintain visceral integrity.[17] Similar to the management of complex aortic arch branch disease for type A dissection, these hybrid open and endovascular techniques may represent the future of perivisceral repair for aortic dissection until branched graft technology achieves more widespread acceptance.

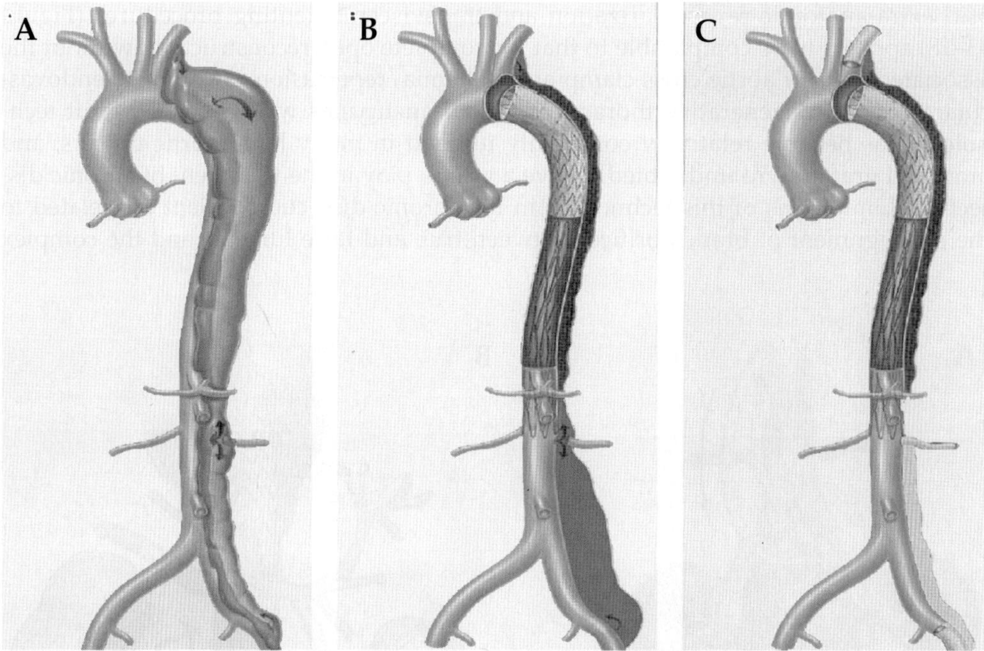

Figure 43-19. STABLE (Staged thoracoabdominal and branch vessel endoluminal repair) for Aortic Dissection. **(A)** Complex dissection with large primary entry site tear and multiple secondary fenestrations. **(B)** Primary entry site coverage to induce false lumen thrombosis and placement of distal uncovered stents to re-expand and stabilize the aortic true lumen. **(C)** Covered stent repair of iliac, and left subclavian secondary entry sites, with reperfusion of left renal flow and complete false lumen thrombosis. Reproduced with permission: Mossop PJ, McLachlan CS, Amukotuwa SA, Nixon IK. Staged endovascular treatment for complicated type B aortic dissection. *Nature Clin Pract Cardiovasc Med.* 2005;2(6):316-321.

REFERENCES

1. Tsai TT, Trimarchi S, Nienaber CA. Acute Aortic Dissection: Perspectives from the International Registry of Acute Aortic Dissection (IRAD). *Eur J Vasc Endovasc Surg.* 2009;37:149–159.

2. Hagan Peter G, Nienaber CA, Isselbacher EM, et al. The International Registry of Acute Aortic Dissection (IRAD) New Insights into an Old Disease. *JAMA*. 2000;283: 897–903.

3. Song T K, Donayre C E, Walot I, et al. Endograft Exclusion of acute and chronic descending thoracic aortic dissections. *J Vasc Surg*. 2006;43(2):247–258.

4. Dake MD, Kato N, Mitchell RS, et al. Endovascular stent-graft placement for the treatment of acute aortic dissection. *N Engl J Med*. 1999;340:1546–1552.

5. Nienaber Christoph A, Eagle, Kim A. Aortic Dissection: New frontiers in Diagnosis and Management Part II: Therapeutic Management and Follow-up. *Circulation*. 2003;108:772–778.

6. Atkins MD Jr, Black J H, Cambria RP. Aortic Dissection: Perspectives in the era of stent-graft repair. *J Vasc Surg*. 2006;43(Suppl A):30A–43A.

7. Gaxotte V, Thony F, Rousseau H, et al. Midterm Results of Aortic Diameter Outcomes After Thoracic Stent-Graft Implantation for Aortic Dissection: A Multicenter Study. *J Endovasc Ther*. 2006;13:127–138.

8. Moore AG, Eagle KA, Bruckman D, et al. Choice of Computed Tomography, Transesophageal Echocardiography, Magnetic Resonance Imaging, and Aortography in Acute Aortic Dissection: International Registry of Acute Aortic Dissection (IRAD). *Am J Cardiol*. 2002;89:1235–1238.

9. Salerno P, Jackson A, Shaw M, et al. Transesophageal echocardiographic imaging of the branches of the aorta: a guide to obtaining these images and their clinical utility. *J Cardiothorac Vasc Anesth* 2009;23:694–701.

10. Rocchi G, Lofiego C, Biagini E, et al. Trans-esophageal echocardiography - guided algorithm for stent-graft implantation in aortic dissection. *J Vasc Surg*. 2004;40:880–885.

11. Koschyk D, Nienaber C, Malgorzata K, et al. How to Guide Stent-Graft Implantation in Type B Aortic Dissection? Comparison of Angiography, Transesophageal Echocardiography, and Intravascular Ultrasound. *Circulation*. 2005;112[suppl I]:I–260–I-264.

12. White RA, Donayre CE, Walot I, et al. Intraprocedural imaging: Thoracic aortography techniques, intravascular ultrasound, and special equipment. *J Vasc Surg*. 2006;43(Suppl A):53A–61A.

13. Dialetto G, Covino FE, Scognamiglio G, et al. Treatment of type B aortic dissection: endoluminal repair or conventional medical therapy? *Eur J Cardiothorac Surg*. 2005;27:826–830.

14. Eggebrecht H, Herold U, Kuhnt O, et al. Endovascular stent-graft treatment of aortic dissection: determinants of post-interventional outcome. *Eur Heart J*. 2005;26:489–497.

15. Moore RD, Villalba L, Petrasek PF, et al. Endovascular treatment for aortic disease: is a surgical environment necessary? *J Vasc Surg*. 2005;42(4):645–649; discussion 649.

16. Pamler RS, Kotsis T, Gorich J, et al. Complications after endovascular repair of type B aortic dissection. *J Endovasc Ther*. 2002;9:822–888

17. Mossop PJ, McLachlan CS, Amukotuwa SA, Nixon IK. Staged endovascular treatment for complicated type B aortic dissection. *Nat Clin Pract Cardiovasc Med*. 2005;2(6):316–321.

18. Sueyoshi Eijun, Sakamoto Ichiro, hayashi Kuniaki, Yamaguchi Tetsuji Imada Tatuya. Growth rate of Aortic Diameter in Patients with Type B aortic Dissection During the Chronic Phase. *Circulation* 2004;110(suppl II):II–256–261.

19. Nuehauser B, Czermak BV, Fish J, Perkmann R, Jaschke W, Chemelli A Fraedrich G. Type A dissection following endovascular thoracic aortic stent-graft repair. *J Endovasc Ther* 2005;12:74–81.

20. Kato Noriyuki, Hirano Tadanori, Kawaguchi Tatsuya, Ishida Masaki, Shimono Takatsugu, et al. Aneurysmal degeneration of the aorta after stent-graft repair of acute aortic dissection. *J Vasc Surg* 2001;34:513–8.

21. Nienaber Christoph, Zannetti Simona, Barbieri Barbara, Kische Stephan, Schareck Wolfgang, Rehders Tim C. Investigation of STEnt grafts in patients with type B Aortic Dissection: Design of the INSTEAD trial - a prospective, multicenter, European randomized trial. *Am Heart J* 2005;149:592–9.

22. Timperley Jonathan, Ferguson John D, Niccoli Giampaulo, Prothero Anthony, Banning Adrian P. Natural History of Intramural Hematoma of the descending Thoracic Aorta. *Am J Cardiol* 2003;91:777–780.

23. Kaji Shuichiro, Akasaka Takashi, Katayama Minako, Yamamuro Atsushi, Yamabe Kenji, et al. Long-Term Prognosis of Patients with Type B Aortic Intramural Hematoma. *Circulation* 2003;108(suppl II):II–307–311.

24. Trimarchi S, Nienaber CA, Rampoldi V, Myrmel T, Suzuki T, Mehta RH, et al. Contemporary results of surgery in acute type A aortic dissection: The International Registry of Acute Aortic Dissection experience. *J Thorac Cardiovasc Surg*; 129:112–22.

25. Yamaki F, Sato W, Yamamoto H, Kouda T, Kouno T. Aortic Arch replacement with covered stent-graft as elephant trunk for a type A acute aortic dissection. *Kyobu Geka* 2002;55:193–7.

26. Bergeron P, de Chaumaray T, Coulon P, Ruiz-Patino M, Mariotti F, Shah A, Gay J. New Approach for Type A Aortic Dissection With Combined Ascending Aortic Repair and Supra-Aortic Vessel Transposition. *J Endovasc Ther* 2006;13(suppl I):I–6.

27. Chuter Timothy AM. Branched and fenestrated stent grafts for endovascular repair of thoracic aortic aneurysms. *J Vasc Surg* 2006; 43(suppl A): 111A–115A.

28. Farber Mark A. Visceral vessel relocation techniques. *J Vasc Surg* 2006;43(suppl A): 81A–84A.

29. Marui A, Mochizuki T, Mitsui N, Koyama T, Kumira F, Horibe M. Toward the Best Treatment for Uncomplicated Patients with Type B Acute Aortic Dissection: A Consideration for Sound Surgical Indication. *Circulation* 1999;100:II-275-II280.

44

Surgical Treatment of Abdominal Aortic Aneurysms Associated with Thoracic Aortic Dissections

James C. Stanley M.D., Gilbert R. Upchurch Jr M.D., G. Michael Deeb M.D., and David M. Williams M.D.

Patients having an abdominal aortic aneurysm (AAA) and thoracic aortic dissection (Figure 44–1) often challenge the diagnostic and therapeutic efforts of clinicians. This scenario will be more common with the aging population, especially in patients with arteriosclerotic cardiovascular disease and systemic hypertension, both of which contribute to aortic aneurysms and dissections. Two factors need better definition for physicians to offer rational advice to patients having these illnesses. The first relates to the true incidence of AAAs and thoracic aortic dissections, as well as the natural history of both these diseases. The second involves the varying therapies available to treat AAAs associated with an acute versus a chronic dissection, especially when the two diseases are juxtaposed anatomically (Figure 44–1), in contrast to their being segregated from each other as isolated diseases within the thoracic and abdominal aorta.

INCIDENCE OF AAAS AND THORACIC AORTIC DISSECTIONS

Information regarding AAAs in the setting of a thoracic aortic dissection has evolved from a small number of clinical reports.[1-13] These two aortic lesions are most likely to occur with Type III dissections, usually in older patients and those having a long-standing history of hypertension. Coexistence of an AAA and an aortic dissection is not rare, with the Massachusetts General Hospital-Yale New Haven Hospital experience documenting AAAs in 18 of 326 patients (5.5%) with aortic dissections,[2] and a NIH autopsy report revealing AAAs in 13 of 182 patients (7%) having thoracic aortic dissections.[9]

A recent University of Michigan experience provides further insight into the relative frequency of these diseases.[10] The series involved 145 patients (95 men, 50 women) encountered from 1992 to 2001 with thoracic aortic dissections, excluding those associ-

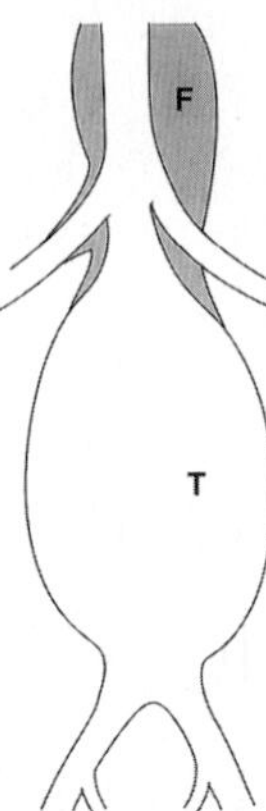

Figure 44-1. Schematic representation of true lumen (**T**) and false lumen (**F**) of a AAA in juxtaposition to the distal extent of the aortic dissection. Reprinted with permission from Anand RJ, Williams DM, Proctor MC, et al. Operative mortality rate for elective abdominal aortic aneurysm repair is not increased by the presence of a previous or concurrent thoracic or thoracoabdominal aortic dissection. *J Vasc Surg* 2002;36:690-695.

ated with trauma, Marfan's syndrome, and those with diffuse degenerative thoracoabdominal aortic aneurysms. Type III dissections affected 59% of these patients and Type I dissections affected the remaining 41%.

Aortic computed tomography (CT) was obtained annually in all of the Michigan series' patients. Five patients (3%) had a history of AAA repair prior to their thoracic aortic dissection diagnosis, three being Type III dissections and two being Type I dissections. Twelve patient's (8%) had a AAA diagnosed at the time of their initial CT study of their thoracic aortic dissection. Type III dissections affected all but one of these patients. Ten additional patients developed AAAs (7%) among the 128 patients having no initial evidence of an AAA. The latter were recognized from one to 48 months (average 16 months) after their thoracic aortic dissection was diagnosed. Type III dissections affected eight of these 10 patients. These 27 patients having AAAs represent 18.6% of a consecutive group of individuals having thoracic aortic dissections.

In the Michigan series, 26% of the AAAs were continuous with the thoracic aortic dissection and 74% occurred independent of the dissection. In the univariate analysis, age (P = .0002), male gender (P = .044), history of smoking (P = .01), chronic obstructive pulmonary disease, COPD, (P<.001), duration of the dissection (P = .05), and presence of Type III dissection (P = .009) were associated with the presence of an AAA In the multivariate analysis, both COPD (OR 5.4, 95% CI, 1.3 to 22.3; p = .02) and age (OR 1.06, 95% CI, 1.02 to 1.11; P = .004) were significant predictors of the development of AAAs.

CLINICAL MANIFESTATIONS

Most patients with an AAA are asymptomatic with a diagnosis usually established by an imaging study for a nonvascular disease. Manifestations of an acutely expanding or ruptured AAA are well established and when classic, the symptoms of a thoracic aortic dissection are well known. However, the latter are not always recognized in an expeditious manner, a fact leading to a relatively high mortality rate in this group of patients. Unfortunately, uncertainty regarding the diagnosis often exists with patients presenting with severe back pain and a known AAA and thoracic aortic dissection.

Any symptoms suggesting aortic expansion in patients having a known thoracoabdominal aortic dissection or an AAA, no matter how mild or uncharacteristic, deserve immediate attention. Unfortunately, patients with preexisting AAAs with superimposed acute dissections may have pain from the dissection that is impossible to distinguish from an expanding AAA or contained AAA rupture. Such patients, if hypertensive but otherwise hemodynamically stable, deserve aggressive blood pressure control and subsequent emergent imaging studies to help determine whether the pain is from expansion of an AAA or the aortic dissection. If the blood pressure elevation becomes well controlled and the patient still has persistent or increasing abdominal pain, one must be most suspicious of an impending dissection-related rupture and consider immediate operative intervention, be it by conventional open surgery or catheter-based endovascular surgery.

The lethal nature of either of these aortic diseases, if symptomatic, was apparent in the NIH autopsy report of 13 patients, in whom the dissection was acute in 10 patients including eight who died from rupture of the dissection's false channel. Among the remaining cases, one died from an AAA rupture, two from attempted AAA repairs, and two from attempted repair of their aortic dissection.[11] The Massachusetts General Hospital experience supports the tenet that the risk of aortic rupture with concomitant AAAs and acute dissections is exceedingly high.[4] Among the 18 patients in the latter series, eight had an aortic dissection that extended into the region of their AAA. Rupture of the AAA affected six of the latter eight patients, occurring in four at the junction of the dissection and aortic aneurysm.

DIAGNOSIS

Urgent aortic imaging will usually confirm the diagnosis of these diseases. Magnetic resonance angiography (MRA) often defines the extent of the thoracic aortic dissection and branch involvement of the AAA (Figure 44–2).[2,3,4,15,16] CT scans with thin cuts are also exceedingly useful in delineating the extent of these two coexistent diseases.[2,5,12,15,16] CT images may at times be inadequate to differentiate irregular thrombus in an aneurysm from hematoma in a dissection's false channel. Conventional catheter-based arteriography may be necessary to precisely define the entry or reentry sites associated with the aortic dissection in the acute setting. Arteriographic examinations not only provide diagnostic information, but also provide access for catheter-based interventions including septum fenestration and stenting of the true lumen in the setting of malperfusion of the splanchnic, renal, or lower extremity vessels as a result of the dissection.[14-16]

OPERATIVE TECHNIQUE

Treatment of Abdominal Aortic Aneurysms

The indications for repairing an AAA in the presence of a thoracic aortic dissection have not been firmly established, but in general parallel those for AAAs unassociated with such dissections. The technique of AAA repair in association with a thoracic dissection is often complex and depends on whether AAA is associated with an acute or a chronic and stable aortic dissection.

In the case of a chronic thoracic aortic dissection that is not in juxtaposition to the infrarenal AAA, a conventional AAA repair in a standard manner is favored. Particular attention is directed to control of the blood pressure with vasodilators to reduce

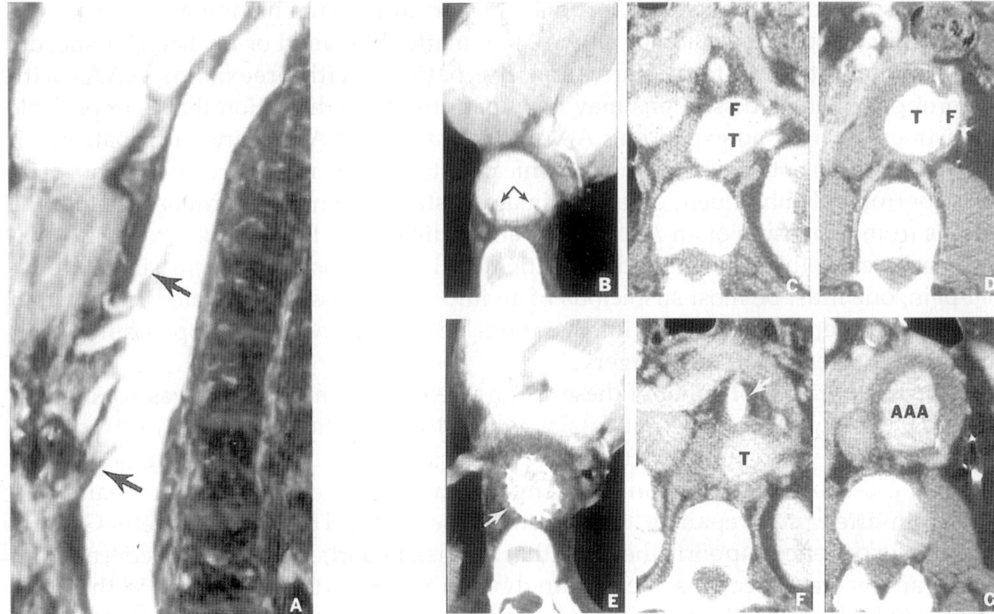

Figure 44-2. Magnetic resonance arteriogram of a thoracic aortic dissection in juxtaposition to an infrarenal **AAA**. **A.** Dissection of the thoracic aorta (arrow) above the celiac artery and the abdominal aorta (arrow) below the superior mesenteric artery. **B.** Origination (arrows) of dissection in the thoracic aorta. **C.** True (**T**) and false (**F**) aortic lumens just above the renal arteries. **D.** Cephalic portion of infrarenal **AAA** and its true lumen (**T**) with diminished false lumen (**F**) size. **E.** Stent endograft (arrow) within the true lumen of the supraceliac abdominal aorta. (**F**) Stent within the superior mesenteric artery (arrow), True (**T**) aortic lumen. **G.** Infrarenal **AAA** that was repaired in a conventional manner 3 months after endograft exclusion of the thoracic dissection.

peripheral arterial resistance and cardiac afterload so as to lessen the likelihood of an acute expansion of the preexisting thoracic aortic dissection. This is important regardless of the type and location of the dissection. Similarly, soft-jaw aortic vascular clamps are preferred over the usual atraumatic serrated metallic clamps for occluding the aorta in these patients because of the potential medial defects that may create a dissection within the abdominal aorta following minimal operative trauma.

In the case of chronic dissections juxtaposed to the AAA, the outer wall of the false channel may be sufficient to anastomose a graft to, with most surgeons favoring its reinforcement with a felt strip. If the false channel is patent and no reentry exists above the graft anastomosis, then either creating a fenestration between it and the true lumen by excising a segment of the intervening septum is recommended.[7] In certain patients with splanchnic or renal branches arising from the false lumen, it is essential to preserve their perfusion. An occasional patient with a preexisting aortic dissection that has been treated may already have undergone a catheter-based fenestration and stenting of the true lumen.[2]

In the case of an acute thoracic aortic dissection, the necessity to treat the AAA is secondary to the management of the dissection. Type I and II dissections are usually treated by expeditious operative intervention. Type III dissections may be treated medically if no organ threatening ischemia exists and the patient's blood pressure and symptoms are easily managed with antihypertensive medications. Treatment of an AAA in the presence of an acute or subacute aortic dissection usually necessitates

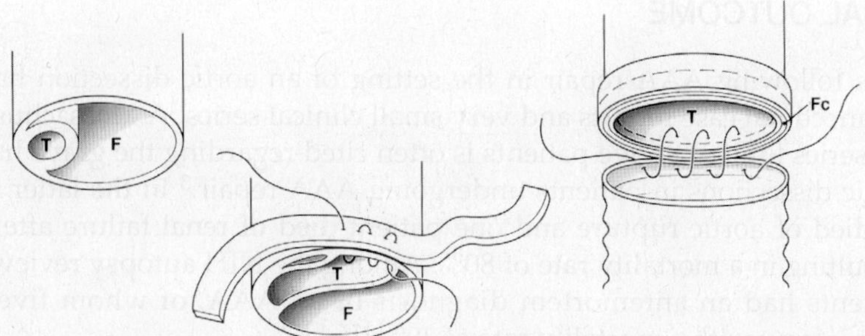

Figure 44-3. Operative technique used in treatment of AAA with associated acute aortic dissection juxtaposed to aneurysm. Wall of true lumen (**T**) is coapted to wall of false lumen (**F**) with external felt strip reinforcing this plication, resulting in collapse of false lumen (**Fc**). Reprinted with permission from Anand RJ, Williams DM, Proctor MC, et al. Operative mortality rate for elective abdominal aortic aneurysm repair is not increased by the presence of a previous or concurrent thoracic or thoracoabdominal aortic dissection. *J Vasc Surg* 2002;36:690-695.

obliteration of the false lumen at the anastomotic site. An externally placed felt pledget may be used to plicate the true and false walls before anastomosing the divided aorta to the graft (Figure 44–3). An end-to-end anastomosis can then be performed with full thickness sutures placed through the felt and plicated aortic walls. Both the proximal and distal anastomoses in this setting are usually performed in this manner. AAAs treated by this means with no proximal reentry point may experience thrombosis of the false channel,[6] although multiple entrance and reentry tears usually exist in these patients.

Treatment of Aortic Dissections

The initiating event in an aortic dissection is a tear or hemorrhage in the aortic wall that results in a separation of the media with potential end organ damage from propagation of the dissection, with occasional collapse of the true lumen and obstruction of the celiac, superior mesenteric, renal, or iliac arteries. When this occurs in a patient with a coexisting AAA, the treatment of the dissection takes priority. Initial therapy directed at end organ ischemia is often focused on less invasive methods such as catheter-directed fenestration of the aortic septum (from the true lumen to the false lumen) and true lumen stenting to relieve the malperfusion that follows collapse of the opposing lumen onto the orifices of the branch vessels. Promising results have been reported with treatment of type III aortic dissections with placement of endovascular stents, and this intervention may prove especially useful in patients who are at particularly high risk for open operative repair.[14-16]

Persistent malperfusion after less invasive catheter-based interventions may necessitate open aortic fenestration or direct surgical revascularization of the affected vessels with their reimplantation or bypass. This is most likely to occur when the dissection enters the aortic branch vessel. Obvious complications of an aortic dissection that necessitate more urgent therapy include contained rupture, continued pain despite intensive medical therapy, or evolving ischemic complications affecting the kidneys, spinal cord, intestines, or legs.

SURGICAL OUTCOME

Outcomes following AAA repair in the setting of an aortic dissection have been defined by anecdotal case reports and very small clinical series. A Massachusetts General Hospital series limited to five patients is often cited regarding the grave hazard of thoracic aortic dissections in patients undergoing AAA repair.[3] In the latter report, three patients died of aortic rupture and one patient died of renal failure after a ruptured AAA, resulting in a mortality rate of 80%. Among the NIH autopsy review of 13 cases, nine patients had an antemortem diagnosis of an AAA, of whom five underwent aneurysmectomy with a mortality rate of 40%.[11]

A slightly larger group of patients with aortic dissections who underwent elective AAA repair at the University of Michigan had a much different outcome with no operative mortality.[2] The latter experience included 11 men and three women with known thoracic or thoracoabdominal aortic dissections. Three patients had acute dissections (less than 14 days) and 11 patients had chronic dissections (14 days or longer). All 14 patients had type III aortic dissections. Stent graft treatment of the aortic dissection was performed in one patient before the AAA repair (Figure 44–2). AAA repair in this series was associated with no 30-day mortality and a one-year mortality rate of 7.1%. Specific preoperative patient characteristics, intraoperative events, or perioperative complications were not predictive of the one late death.

In conclusion, patients with thoracic aortic dissections are clearly at risk to harbor or develop an AAA, and this risk is significantly associated with increasing age and the presence of COPD. It is recommended that yearly CT scans or MRA be undertaken in the follow-up of all patients with known thoracic aortic dissections. This will not only allow recognition of an evolving AAA, but it will also document any aneurysmal expansion of the aortic dissection. AAA repair in the setting of acute or chronic aortic dissection appears to carry a mortality rate similar to that generally attributed to elective AAA repair without an accompanying aortic dissection. However, the conduct of the operation in these cases is often difficult, especially in the setting of an acute aortic dissection, and requires detailed preoperative assessment and deft surgical technique.

REFERENCES

1. Abad C, Ninot S, Guerola M, et al. Aneurysms of the abdominal aorta in patients on a permanent hemodialysis program. *Angiologia*. 1992;44:8–12.
2. Anand RJ, Williams DM, Proctor MC, et al. Operative mortality rate for elective abdominal aortic aneurysm repair is not increased by the presence of a previous or concurrent thoracic or thoracoabdominal aortic dissection. *J Vasc Surg*. 2002;36:690–695.
3. Cambria RP, Brewster DC, Gertler J, et al. Vascular complications associated with spontaneous aortic dissection. *J Vasc Surg*. 1988;7:199–209.
4. Cambria RP, Brewster DC, Moncure AC, et al. Spontaneous aortic dissection in the presence of coexistent or previously repaired atherosclerotic aortic aneurysm. *Ann Surg*. 1988;208: 619–624.
5. Gomes MN, Wallace RB. Present status of abdominal aorta imaging by computed tomography. *J Cardiovasc Surg*. 1985;26:1–6.
6. Gugulakis AG, Matsagas MI, Vasdekis SN, et al. Rupture of an abdominal aortic aneurysm following acute descending thoracic aortic dissection, case report. *J Cardiovasc Surg*. 1998;39:583–585.

7. Jacobs DL, Freischlag JA, Seabrook GR, et al. Acute aortic dissection into a preexisting abdominal aortic aneurysm. *Ann Vasc Surg.* 1984;8:491–495.
8. Kawasaki T, Kambayashi J, Goda K, et al. Dissecting thoracic aorta and fusiform aneurysm of the abdominal aorta. *Cardiovasc Surg.* 1995;3:313–315.
9. Kyosola K, Jarvinen A. Abdominal aortic aneurysm and dissection after blunt trauma. *J Cardiovasc Surg.* 1987;28:737–739.
10. Lee JJ, Dimick JB, Williams DM, et al. Existence of abdominal aortic aneurysms in patients with thoracic aortic dissections. *J Vasc Surg.* 2003;38:671–675.
11. Roberts CS, Roberts WC. Combined thoracic aortic dissection and abdominal aortic fusiform aneurysm. *Ann Thorac Surg.* 2001;52:537–540.
12. Taylor CR, August D, Greenwood L, et al. Aortic dissection with concurrent abdominal aortic aneurysm: computed tomography diagnosis. *J Comput Tomogr.* 1987;11:392–396.
13. Van Schil P, De Vries D, Vanmaele R, et al. Combined type B aortic dissection and fusiform abdominal aortic aneurysm. *Angiology.* 1994;45:655–661.
14. Czermak BV, Waldenberger P, Fraedrich G. Treatment of Stanford type B aortic dissection with stent-grafts: preliminary results. *Radiology.* 2000;217:544–550.
15. Williams DM, Lee DY, Hamilton BH, et al. The dissected aorta: percutaneous treatment of ischemic complications: principles and results. *J Vasc Interv Radiol.* 1997;8:605–625.
16. Williams DM, Lee DY, Hamilton BH, et al. The dissected aorta: part III. Anatomy and radiologic diagnosis of branch-vessel compromise. *Radiology.* 1997;203:37–44.

Renal Artery Revascularization

45

Endovascular Stent-graft Placement for Emergent Traumatic Thoracic Aortic Disruption

Brian G. Peterson, M.D., Mark K. Eskandari, M.D., and Mark D. Morasch, M.D.

If left untreated, thoracic aortic transection in the setting of blunt trauma carries with it an 85% mortality rate.[1] Repair of these injuries has traditionally required left thoracotomy, single lung ventilation, aortic cross-clamping, and interposition grafting. Open repair generally requires full systemic anticoagulation. Complex repairs may require cardiopulmonary bypass or hypothermic circulatory arrest. Previously published studies have shown that mortality rates range from 5% to 28%[2-5] and paraplegia rates after open repair range from 2.3% to 14%.[3,6]

In most settings, disruption of the thoracic aorta in the setting of blunt trauma is not isolated, but rather, due to the complex mechanisms of insult, is associated with concomitant injury. Such injuries can include, but are not limited to, significant closed head trauma, pulmonary contusion, long-bone and pelvic fractures, and solid organ damage, which can make treatment of this patient population quite difficult.[7-8] The presence of associated trauma clearly makes the use of systemic anticoagulation problematic.

Shortly after the first endoluminal stent-grafts were used in the treatment of patients with thoracic aortic aneurysms, Dake et al.[9] applied the same endovascular principles to treat traumatic thoracic aortic transections.[10] There were no specifically designed, commercially-available devices at the time, so custom endografts, created using a meld of metallic stents and standard Dacron grafts, were utilized. Industry-manufactured endoluminal extension cuffs, designed and commercially marketed for use in the infrarenal aorta, have also been used in the thoracic aorta in an off-label fashion to treat traumatic disruption in patients with smaller aortas. This technique has been shown to be feasible in several small series.[11-17] Recently, the Gore TAG device (W.L. Gore & Associates, Flagstaff, AZ) has been approved by the U.S. Food and Drug Administration for treatment of thoracic aortic aneurysms. These devices have also been used off-label to treat traumatic tears.

Theoretical advantages of this "less invasive" treatment modality include the ability to avoid thoracotomy, single lung ventilation, aortic cross-clamping, significant fluid shifts, and perhaps most importantly, systemic heparinization in these patients suffering multiple injuries.

Between February 2001 and June 2005, various pathologies of the thoracic aorta were treated using endovascular stent-grafts in 60 patients at Northwestern Memorial Hospital.[18] Included in this group were 12 (20%) patients who underwent endovascular management of traumatic aortic transections. All patients were involved in high-speed motor vehicle collisions or other rapid deceleration-type events, each suffered multiple injuries, and all underwent endovascular repair for thoracic aortic transection in the acute or subacute setting. Average time from initial injury to endovascular repair was 13 ± 28 days (range 0–94 days), with 75% of repairs occurring within four days of the initial injury.

The average patient age was 41 ± 14 (range 20–73), with eight (67%) males and four (33%) females. Patients suffered multiple injuries that included closed head injury, rib fractures with concomitant pulmonary contusion, extremity or pelvis fractures, and solid organ injury. The mean injury severity score (ISS) of this group of patients was 44 ± 13 (range 25–66). The mechanisms of injury included high-speed motor vehicle collisions (10 patients), a fall from a three-story building (one patient), and a pedestrian versus automobile accident (one patient) (Table 45–1).

Thoracic aortic transection, suggested by CT, was confirmed in all cases with intraoperative aortography (Figure 45–1). Measurements of the proximal and distal neck length and the critical aortic diameters, as well as identification of the location and extent of injury in relation to the origins of the arch vessels, were obtained using the aforementioned imaging modalities.

In four patients, preoperative CT scan showed the area of transection to be in close proximity to the left subclavian artery from which the dominant vertebral artery took origin. In order to ensure an adequate seal proximal to the transection, these patients underwent left subclavian artery to common carotid artery transposition prior to endovascular repair. In all four cases, the origin of the transposed left subclavian artery

TABLE 45-1. PATIENT CHARACTERISTICS, TYPE OF DEVICE AND APPROACH USED, AND POST-OPERATIVE LENGTH OF STAY.

Age	Sex	Mechanism of Injury	ISS	Device	Approach
51	M	MVC	35	Excluder cuff	Cut-down
40	M	MVC	34	Excluder cuff	Percutaneous
40	F	MVC	41	Aneurx cuff	Cut-down
42	M	MVC	66	Excluder cuff	Cut-down
40	F	MVC	66	Excluder cuff	Percutaneous
50	M	MVC	25	Excluder cuff	Cut-down
20	F	MVC	41	Excluder cuff	Percutaneous
73	M	MVC	38	Excluder cuff	Percutaneous
26	M	MVC	38	Excluder cuff	Percutaneous
47	F	30 foot fall	45	Excluder cuff	Percutaneous
43	M	Pedestrian vs. Auto	38	Excluder cuff	Percutaneous
22	M	MVC	66	Thoracic Excluder	Percutaneous

M: male, F: female, MVC: motor vehicle collision, ISS: injury severity score.

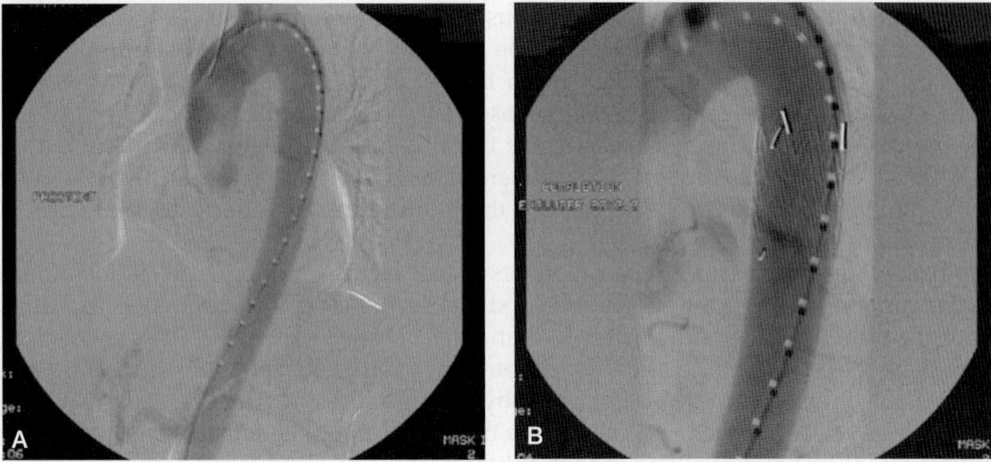

Figure 45-1. A. Angiogram taken at the time of the endovascular intervention demonstrating the thoracic aortic transection along the medial aspect of the descending thoracic aorta. **B.** Completion angiogram demonstrating stent-graft coverage of the aortic tear using an abdominal aortic extension cuff.

was covered with the stent-graft. Two patients who were hemodynamically unstable on admission and required urgent endograft deployment had the origin of the subclavian covered without prior transposition. One of these two patients suffered an ipsilateral cerebellar stroke. In the remaining six cases, the device was deployed distal to the subclavian origin. We recommend transposition or bypass of the left subclavian artery, when time allows, in most patients with an injury where treatment requires coverage of that vessel.

We perform these endograft procedures in an angiography suite in an operating room. The devices we have used to treat transections include commercially available endovascular aortic proximal extension cuffs (AneuRx, Medtronic/AVE, Santa Rosa, CA, and Excluder, W.L. Gore & Associates, Flagstaff, AZ), and more recently, the Gore TAG device. After the induction of local or general anesthesia, access to the aorta is obtained percutaneously via the common femoral artery or by cut-down on the external iliac artery. A floppy tipped J-wire and an angiogram catheter are then passed into the aorta under direct fluoroscopic guidance, and a thoracic aortogram is obtained using steep left anterior oblique projection. In those patients undergoing percutaneous repair, a 10 French Prostar XL suture-mediated arterial closure device (Abbott Laboratories, Abbott Park, IL) can then be deployed using the previously described "preclose" technique.[19] At this point, an 18–24 French sheath is passed proximally over a stiff Amplatz or Lunderquist guidewire. One or more endovascular stent-graft devices are then deployed over a curved-tip stiff wire to cover the area of the transection. Each endoluminal stent-graft is deployed without the use of chemically induced cardiac arrest or hypotension, and without the use of systemic anticoagulation. We usually inflate a compliant flow-through or occluding balloon to seat the device. A completion angiogram is always obtained before leaving the operating room and additional aortic extension cuffs are placed as needed to completely seal the tear. Plain X-rays are obtained prior to discharging the patient from the hospital.

Endovascular repair was technically successful in 11 of 12 patients (92%) as demonstrated by completion angiography at the time of the intervention and plain films prior to discharge. Completion angiograms demonstrated apposition of the stent-grafts to the aortic wall, normal perfusion of the innominate and left carotid vessels, and exclusion of the aortic transection without evidence of extravasation of contrast prior to leaving the operating room in all cases. One patient who was treated with a Gore TAG device developed collapse of the endovascular device after leaving the operating room. The deformity in the metallic nitinol skeleton was identified on plain x-ray films the day following treatment. This patient was successfully treated by reballooning the device and then placing three infrarenal Excluder extension cuffs in the proximal end of the device.

Following endovascular repair, patients underwent CT angiography at one month and at six months, and then were followed yearly thereafter. Mean follow-up of this patient cohort was 21 months (range 3–49 months).

Given the severity and variety of concomitant injuries, it may not be surprising that patient outcome seemed to be determined by the associated injuries present rather than the thoracic aortic transections. There were no procedure-related deaths and no patient suffered paralysis as a result of endograft placement. There was one procedure-related stroke as described above. Follow-up CT scans (Figure 45–2) have demonstrated technically successful endovascular repair of all the traumatic aortic transections. There has been no evidence of endoleak, stent migration, or late pseudoa-neurysm formation throughout follow-up.

DISCUSSION

Mortality rates following traumatic thoracic aortic transection in the setting of blunt trauma are estimated to be 85%.[1] Studies have shown that open repair with graft interposition has mortality rates as high as 28% and paraplegia rates following repair of up to 14%.[3,6] Since Kato et al.[10] first described the endovascular treatment of acute thoracic aortic pathology using stent-grafts, several subsequent case reports have also suggested that this technique is technically feasible.[11-17] We also have been able to demonstrate that acute trau-

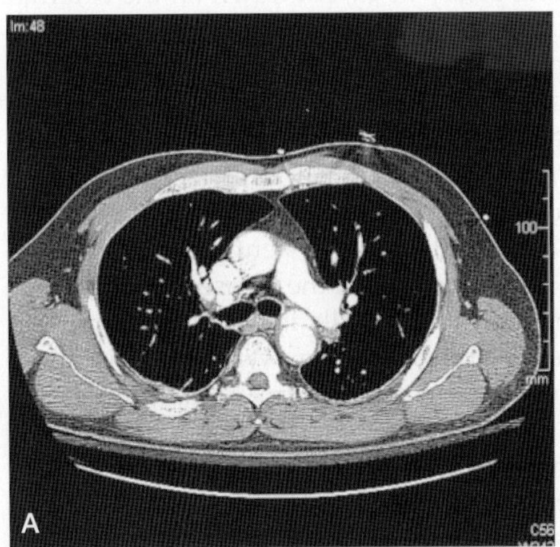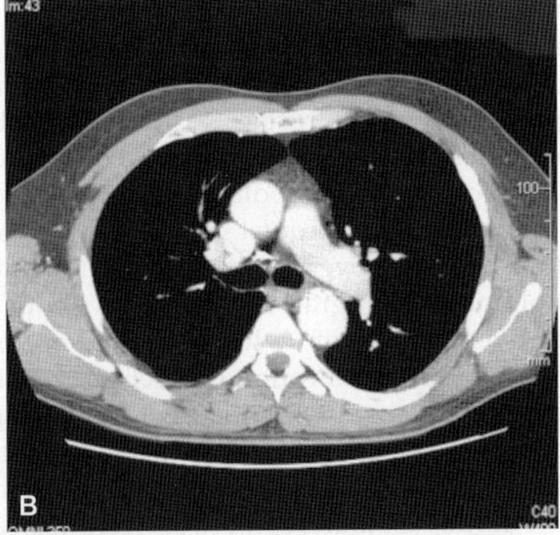

Figure 45-2. A. Admission CT scan depicting thoracic aortic transection. **B.** CT scan obtained at 12-month follow-up demonstrating healing of the tear without evidence of extravasation or pseudoaneurysm formation.

matic aortic transection can safely and effectively be treated using "off-the-shelf," commercially available infrarenal aortic extension cuffs and thoracic endografts.[18]

Thoracic aortic injuries typically occurred in the setting of high-speed motor vehicle collisions and were associated with injuries to multiple organ systems. Endovascular repair, in contrast to traditional open repair, can be performed without the use of systemic heparinization. The ability to avoid the use of systemic heparin in this patient population, especially those suffering multiple injuries that can include long-bone or pelvic fractures and solid organ injury, is an important theoretical advantage to endovascular repair. Additionally, the minimally invasive nature of endovascular repair should significantly reduce blood loss and overall patient length of stay when compared to open surgical reconstruction.

In general, the patients who present with thoracic aortic transection in the setting of blunt trauma are younger than patients who develop aneurysmal degeneration or dissection of the thoracic aorta, and the long-term outcome and durability of these endovascular devices has yet to be proven. As such, follow-up still requires annual CT angiography. With a mean follow-up of nearly two years, our CT scans have demonstrated no evidence of endoleak, stent migration, or late pseudoaneurysm formation. It is possible that since these devices are not required to bridge a fusiform aneurysm and are placed over a short distance within an otherwise normal aorta, the occurrence of late complications like those seen after endovascular repair of abdominal or thoracic aortic aneurysms may be less common.

Our small series demonstrated technical success, safety, and midterm durability of endovascular repair of thoracic aortic transection. Again, the ability to avoid systemic anticoagulation and a thoracotomy in an otherwise multiply injured patient are the main advantages of the endovascular technique. Endovascular repair is possible in the majority of cases. However, while initial results are encouraging, close long-term follow-up is necessary until the durability of these devices can be demonstrated definitively.

REFERENCES

1. Orford VP, Atkinson NR, Thomson K, et al. Blunt traumatic aortic transection: the endovascular experience. *Ann Thorac Surg*. 2003;75:106–112.
2. Lobato AC, Quick RC, Phillips B, et al. Immediate endovascular repair for descending thoracic aortic transection secondary to blunt trauma. *J Endovasc Ther*. 2000;7:16–20.
3. Cowley RA, Turney SZ, Hankins JR, et al. Rupture of thoracic aorta caused by blunt trauma: a fifteen-year experience. *J Thorac Cardiovasc Surg*. 1990;100:652–660.
4. Gott VL. Heparinized shunts for thoracic vascular operations. *Ann Thorac Surg*. 1972;14: 219–220.
5. Verdant A. Traumatic rupture of the thoracic aorta. *Ann Thorac Surg*. 1990;49:686–687.
6. von Oppell UO, Dunne TT, De Groot MK, Zilla P. Traumatic aortic rupture: twenty-year meta-analysis of mortality and risk for paraplegia. *Ann Thorac Surg*. 1994; 58:585–593.
7. Parmley LF, Mattingly TW, Marian WC. Nonpenetrating traumatic injury of the aorta. *Circulation*. 1958;17:1086–1100.
8. Fabian TC, Richardson JD, Croce MA, et al. Prospective study of blunt aortic injury: multicenter trial of the American Association for the Surgery of Trauma. *J Trauma*. 1997;42: 374–383.
9. Dake MD, Miller DC, Semba CP, et al. Transluminal placement of endovascular stent-grafts for the treatment of descending thoracic aortic aneurysms. *N Engl J Med*. 1994;331: 1729–1734.

10. Kato N, Dake MD, Miller DC, et al. Traumatic thoracic aortic aneurysm: treatment with endovascular stent-grafts. *Radiology.* 1997;205:657–662.
11. Sam A II, Kibbe M, Matsumura J, Eskandari MK. Blunt traumatic aortic transection: endoluminal repair with commercially available aortic cuffs. *J Vasc Surg.* 2003;38:1132–1135.
12. Wellons ED, Milner R, Solis M, et al. Stent-graft repair of traumatic thoracic aortic disruptions. *J Vasc Surg.* 2004;40:1095–1100.
13. Dunham MB, Zygun D, Petrasek P, et al. Endovascular stent grafts for acute blunt aortic injury. *J Trauma.* 2004;56:1173–1178.
14. Semba CP, Kato N, Kee ST, et al. Acute rupture of the descending thoracic aorta: repair with use of endovascular stent-grafts. *J Vasc Interv Radiol.* 1997;8:337–342.
15. Ahn SH, Cutry A, Murphy TP, Slaiby JM. Traumatic thoracic aortic rupture: treatment with endovascular graft in the acute setting. *J Trauma* 2001;50:949–951.
16. Doss M, Balzer J, Martens S, et al. Surgical versus endovascular treatment of acute thoracic aortic rupture: a single-center experience. *Ann Thorac Surg.* 2003;76:1465–1470.
17. Orend KH, Pamler R, Kapfer X, et al. Endovascular repair of traumatic descending aortic transection. *J Endovasc Ther.* 2002;9:573–578.
18. Peterson BG, Matsumura JS, Morasch MD, et al. Percutaneous endovascular repair of blunt thoracic aortic transection. *J Trauma.*, in press.
19. Morasch MD, Kibbe MR, Evans ME, et al. Percutaneous repair of abdominal aortic aneurysm. *J Vasc Surg.* 2004;40:12–16.

46

Renal Artery Interventions

Stephen M. Hass, M.D.
Marshall E. Benjamin, M.D.

The treatment of renovascular disease has gone through an evolution over the last 25 years. Surgical revascularization, through the use of bypass or endarterectomy, represents the "gold standard," and has demonstrated excellent long-term durability and clinical results in terms of hypertension management and improvement of renal function.[1-3] However, the morbidity and mortality associated with surgical revascularization are significant, even when performed in centers with extensive experience.[1-3] More recently, endovascular techniques for renal revascularization, including percutaneous transluminal angioplasty with or without endoluminal stenting (PTAS), have emerged as another option for the treatment of occlusive renovascular disease.[4-6] These techniques provide the potential benefits of decreased morbidity, mortality, and recovery times, with the major potential drawback of decreased durability.[7-10] While controversy exists regarding the appropriate application of surgical and endovascular therapy in the treatment of renovascular disease, in today's "endovascular age," PTAS remains the first-line treatment in almost all centers except those specializing in renal surgery. Specialists from several fields (interventional radiology, interventional cardiology, or vascular surgery) all perform PTAS today, but with varying techniques and opinions. This chapter provides an overview of the technical aspects involved in the performance of PTAS from a vascular surgery perspective, as well as a brief review of the current data concerning the technical results and clinical outcomes.

CONTRAST ANGIOGRAPHY OF THE RENAL ARTERIES

Despite recent advances in duplex ultrasound imaging, as well as computed tomographic arteriography (CTA) and magnetic resonance arteriography (MRA)[11,12] (Figure 46–1), the formulation of a surgical or endovascular therapeutic plan continues to depend on visualization of the renal artery anatomy with angiographic techniques. As such, contrast arteriography of the renal arteries should be considered an integral component of the therapeutic armamentarium for clinically significant renal artery lesions.

CONTRAST CONSIDERATIONS

Patients with known renovascular disease typically have a high prevalence of associated medical comorbidities including diabetes mellitus, congestive heart failure, chronic renal insufficiency, and diuretic-induced intravascular volume depletion. Previous investigations have demonstrated that higher volumes of iodinated contrast[13-15] and higher contrast agent osmolarity[13,15] may increase the risk of postprocedure renal function impairment. It is our policy to prepare all patients for aortorenal arteriography with saline hydration (limited in patients with significant heart failure) and periprocedural administration of Acetylcysteine.[16] Furthermore, the use of lower osmolarity iodinated contrast agents should be considered routinely in these patients, and special attention should be paid to limiting the volumes infused. In patients with moderate to severe pre-existing renal insufficiency, carbon dioxide[17-18] also can be used as intra-arterial contrast agents to limit or completely eliminate the use of iodinated contrast (Figure 46–2).

Angiographic Technical Consideratios

Femoral arterial access is still the most versatile and low risk option when possible. Brachial artery access is a useful alternative in patients with downsloping renal arteries or when femoral access is not practicable (Figure 46–3). The left brachial artery is

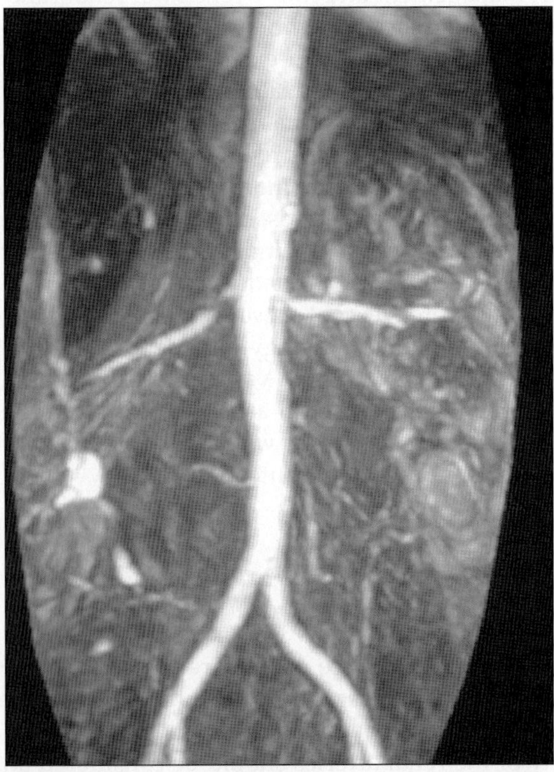

Figure 46-1. Magnetic resonant imaging demonstrating high-grade bilateral renal artery stenosis.

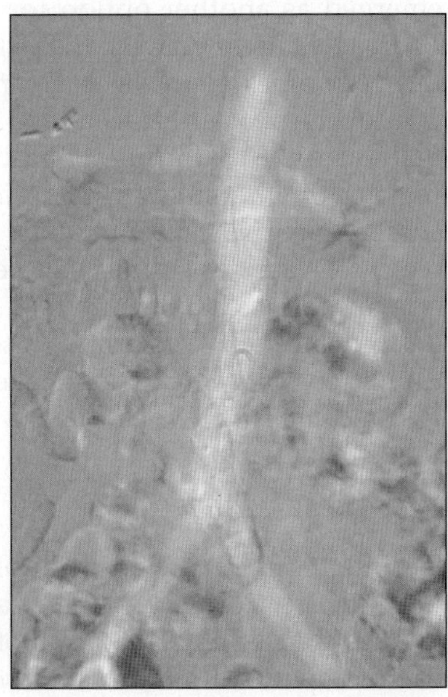

Figure 46-2. Carbon dioxide aortogram demonstrating bilateral renal artery stenosis in a patient with severe renal dysfunction.

preferred as this approach avoids crossing the origin of the left common carotid artery. Brachial artery access may be established using either percutaneous or open techniques. Limitations to percutaneous brachial access include a higher risk of complications[19] and smaller permissible sheath and catheter sizes. It is our practice to perform an open exposure of the brachial artery, with arterial puncture, access, and closure carried out under direct vision.

Aortography and selective renal arteriography, using multiple projections, are necessary to fully examine the renal arteries and juxtarenal aorta. In addition, the inter- and intralobar arteries within the renal parenchyma, as well as the nephrogram

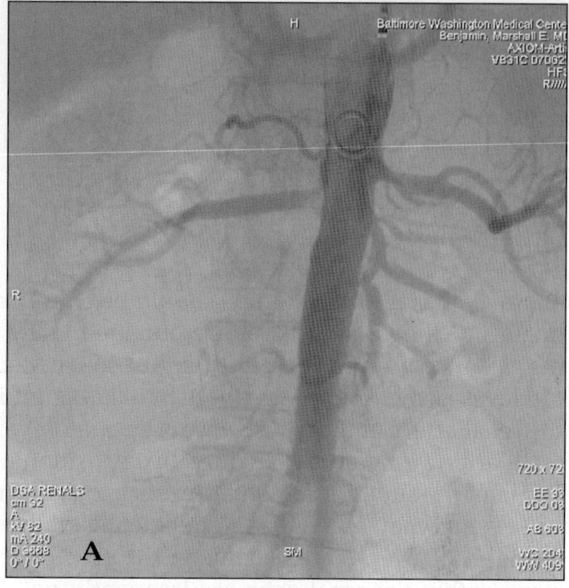

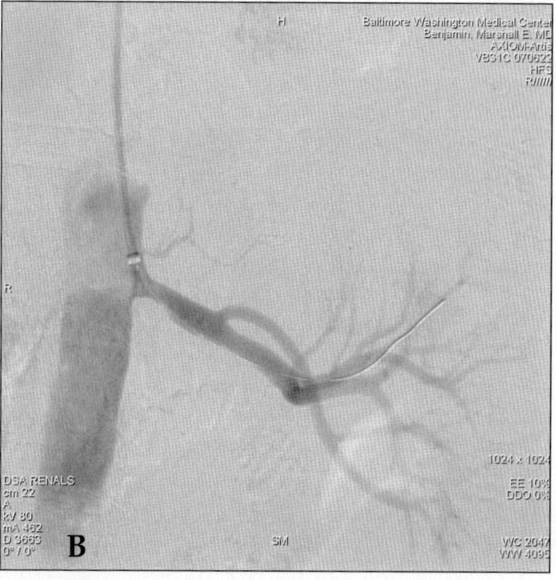

Figure 46-3. (A) Anteroposterior aortogram via a brachial artery access; **(B)** and **(C)** Selective renal arteriograms via a brachial artery access. Note the caudal orientation of the renal arteries. *(Continued)*

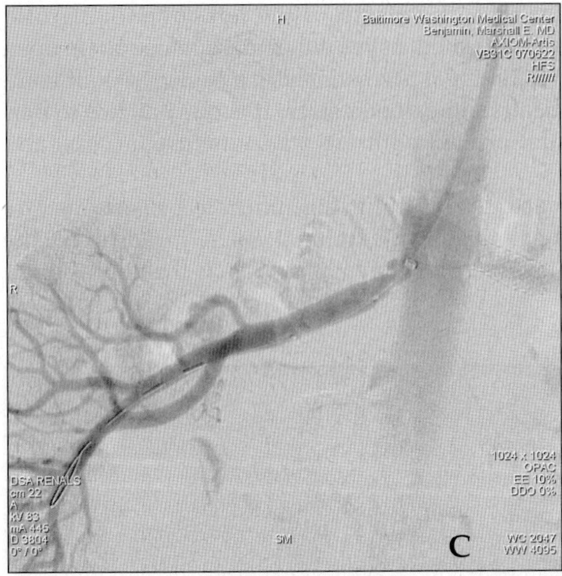

Figure 46-3. *(Continued)*

and overall size of the kidney, should be closely examined. Initial anteroposterior (AP) images of the visceral aorta are obtained using power contrast injections through a multiside holed flush catheter (Figure 46–4) positioned just beneath the diaphragm at the level of the first lumbar vertebra. These initial AP views provide an overview of the renal artery and perivisceral aortic anatomy. All further nonselective images of the renal arteries should be obtained by repositioning the catheter to a location below the origin of the superior mesenteric artery to prevent contrast opacification of the visceral vessels that may obscure anatomic details of the renal arteries (Figure 46–5). The ostia of the renal arteries are usually on the posterolateral aspect of the aorta. Therefore, lesions within the renal ostia are frequently not seen or appear insignificant in an AP projection, due to overlap of the contrast filled aorta. Oblique aortography, or oblique selective renal arteriography, will project these portions of the vessel in profile and

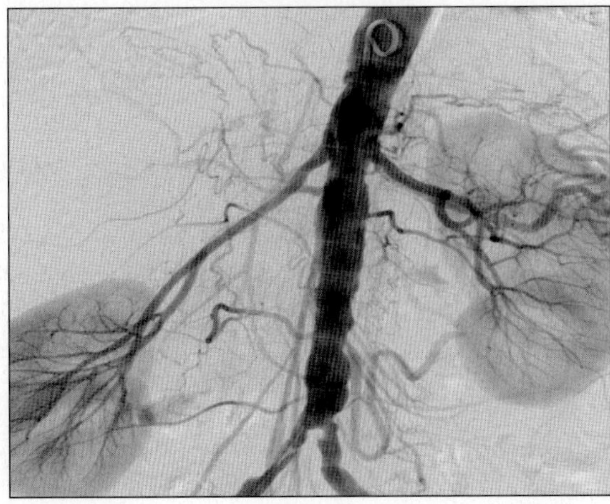

Figure 46-4. Anteroposterior aortogram demonstrating the mesenteric and renal arteries.

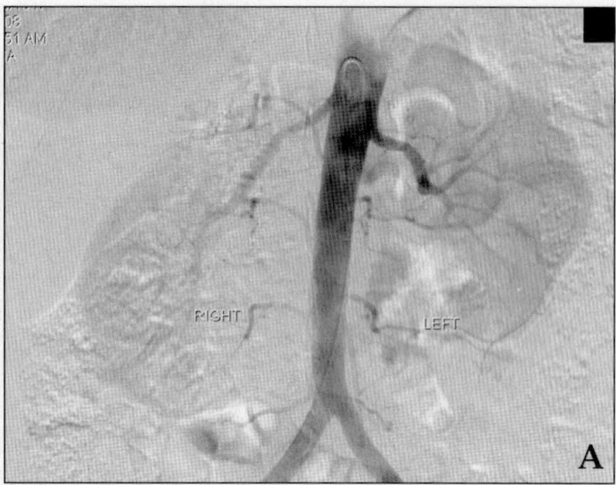

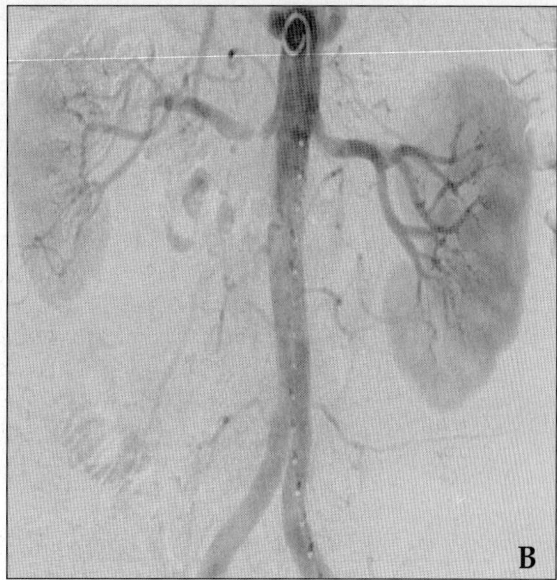

Figure 46-5. (A) and **(B)** Placing the flush catheter below the mesenteric vessels allows for a clearer visualization of the renal arteries.

often better identify lesions, when present. The most useful projections to visualize the renal ostia are usually moderate ipsilateral anterior oblique views (10 to 20°).[20] Recently, rotational angiography has become available (Figure 46–6). Although it requires an increased contrast load, this technique can eliminate the need for multiple oblique images.

Lesions within the mid to distal segments of the renal artery may require selective arteriographic views for full delineation. Selective cannulation is usually performed using an angled catheter such as a cobra, Sos, or renal double curve (RDC) catheter, in combination with a steerable guidewire. There are several catheters of varying shapes offering advantages to particular anatomic situations (Figure 46–7). The Berenstein and JB1 catheters, for example, may be useful in selecting renal arteries that are angled cephalad as they leave the aorta. The more typical down-sloping arteries may be better accessed with the Sos, Simmons, or RDC. Prior to selective renal artery cannulation,

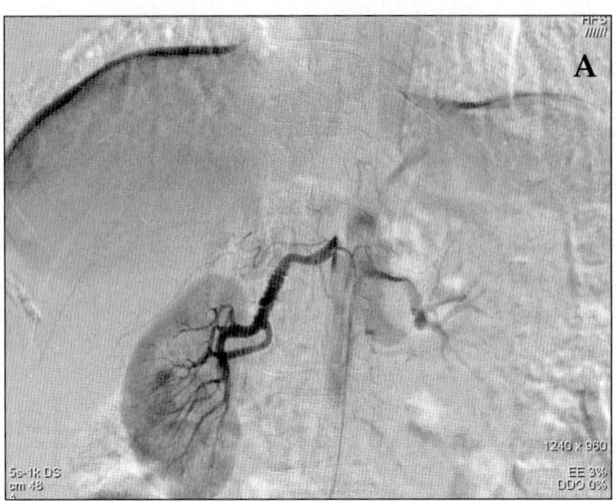

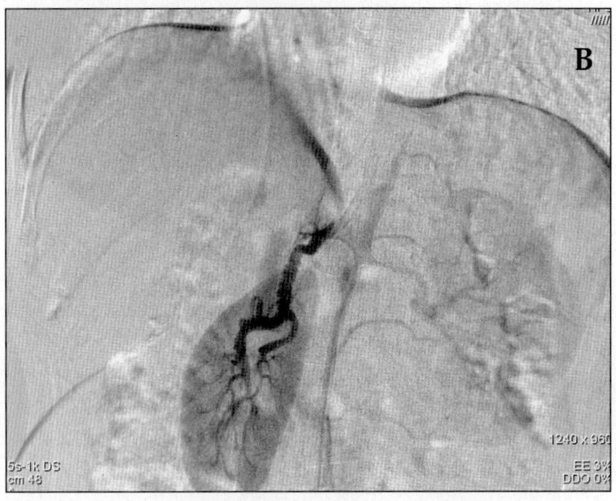

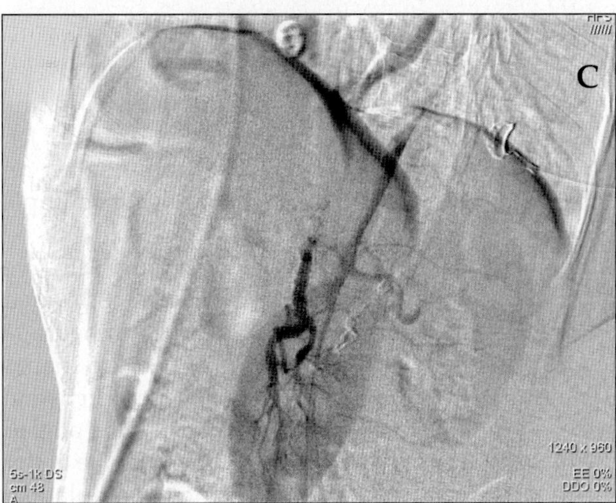

Figure 46-6. Selected images from a right-to-left rotational renal angiography. **(A)** Right lateral projection; **(B)** Right posterolateral projection; **(C)** Posterior projection.

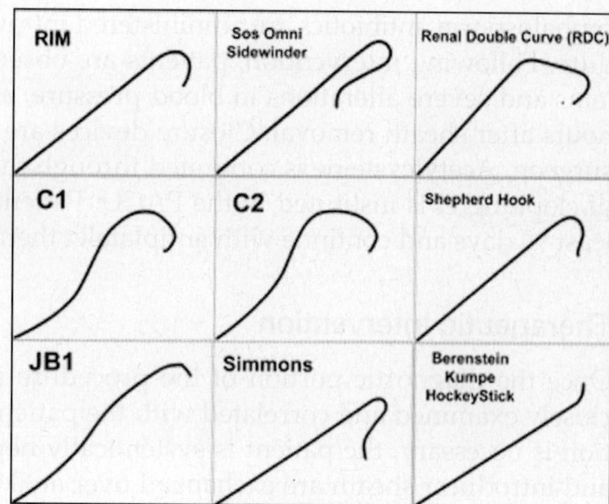

Figure 46-7. Selective catheters commonly used for selective renal cannulation.

intravenous heparin is administered. Once the guidewire and catheter are gently advanced into the renal artery ostia, a hand injection of contrast should be performed to ensure an intraluminal position and the safety of a more vigorous contrast injection. Selective images can then be obtained using low volume power or hand injected images.

ENDOVASCULAR TREATMENT OF RENOVASCULAR DISEASE

Patient Management and Preparation

Patient preparation is similar to that routinely practiced for diagnostic arteriography. Patients are instructed to take no solid food by mouth after midnight the evening before endovascular therapy is planned. If patients are taking Coumadin®, this medication is held for at least four days prior to the procedure. Asprin and or clopidogrel (Plavix®) are not typically stopped. Acetylcysteine is started the evening before the procedure, and continued for 24 hours after the procedure. On arrival in the prep area, an intravenous solution containing bicarbonate is started (Table 46–1). Patients take their routine medications, with the exception of angiotensin converting enzyme inhibitors and angiotensin receptor antagonists, on the morning of the procedure with a sip of water. When renal artery stent placement is anticipated, first generation

TABLE 46-1. PREMEDICATION FOR INTRAVENOUS CONTRAST ADMINISTRATION

Mucomyst (Acetylcysteine)

600 mg orally

Give twice daily on the day before procedure and day of procedure

Sodium Bicarbonate Intravenous Drip

154 mEq/L sodium bicarbonate (1000 mEq/L in 864 cc of dextrose)

3 ml/kg/hr starting one hour prior to procedure

1 ml/kg/hr for six hours postprocedure

cephalosporin antibiotics are administered intravenously 30 minutes prior to the procedure. Following intervention, patients are observed in the PACU for access site problems and severe alterations in blood pressure, and are usually discharged to home six hours after sheath removal. Closure devices are used at the discretion of the operating surgeon. Acetylcysteine is continued through the hospital stay and oral administration of clopidogrel is instituted in the PACU. Patients are maintained on clopidogrel for at least 90 days and continue with antiplatelet therapy (usually aspirin) indefinitely.

˙Therapeutic Intervention

Once the diagnostic portion of the procedure is completed, the images obtained are closely examined and correlated with the patient's clinical presentation. If an intervention is necessary, the patient is systemically heparinized. The 5-Fr diagnostic catheter and introducer sheath are exchanged over an 0.035" guidewire for a platform that will provide secure renal artery access during the therapeutic intervention. Most commonly used angioplasty and stenting devices will pass through a 6 F-sized lumen. Access options include the use of guide sheaths and guide catheters. These vary in shape and diameter with multiple configurations available to facilitate renal artery access. We prefer the use of guiding catheters (Terumo Medical Corp, Elkton, MD; Boston Scientific, Natick, MA). These catheters come in many different shapes, fit through a short 6-F sheath, and can be easily manipulated to allow easy access of the renal ostium. Guiding catheters are typically used to engage the renal ostium and perform the diagnostic and planning portion of the procedure (Figure 46–8). After the tip of the guiding catheter is positioned at or within the ostia of the renal artery, and the selective image (which is usually magnified) confirms that intervention is warranted, guidewire access to the lesion is obtained, frequently employing the "road mapping" features of contemporary digital imaging packages. It is important during all subsequent manipulations to refrain from advancing the guiding catheter beyond the orifice of the renal artery as its nontapered tip may cause intimal injury, dissection, or embolization. Typically, an 0.18" or 0.14" guidewire with a floppy, radiopaque tip is chosen. Our preferred guidewire is the 0.18" Thruway™ guidewire (Boston Scientific, Natick, MA). This guidewire has a short taper and a very floppy, radiopaque, 5 cm long tip. The guidewire also has a silicon coating to ease catheter exchanges. Generally, a 190 cm guidewire is adequate for renal interventions since a rapid-exchange or monorail platform is most often used. The guidewire is gently advanced across the lesion into the distal renal artery. Once it is in place, the guidewire and access platform are secured, and remain there until the intervention and any postintervention imaging is complete.

Transluminal angioplasty of the renal artery may be used as the sole mode of therapy for a renal artery lesion or as a means to predilate a lesion to allow for the passage of a stent. Angioplasty alone is effective in some cases of main renal artery disease (for example, fibromuscular dysplasia and nonostial atherosclerosis), but is frequently ineffective for atherosclerotic ostial renal artery disease. Angioplasty balloon size is most often chosen, based on quantitative software packages that are available on most digital angiographic systems. In general, the angioplasty balloon should be sized slightly larger than the adjacent normal artery for primary treatment and somewhat smaller for use in lesion predilation. For predilating lesions prior to transluminal stent placement, a 4 mm by 20 mm low profile angioplasty balloon is generally used to facilitate stent passage (Figure 46–9). This usually allows for a less traumatic passage of the

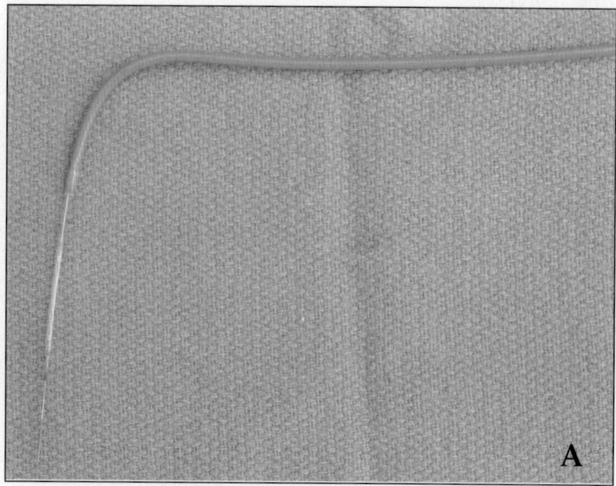

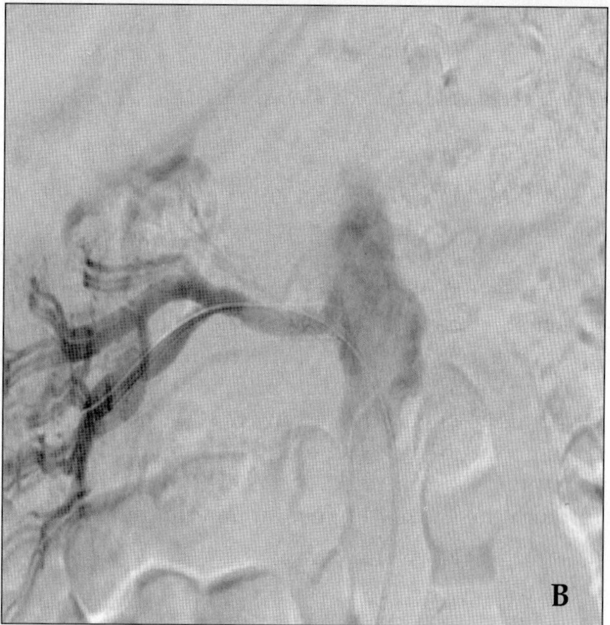

Figure 46-8. (A) Angioplasty balloon catheter extending from a guiding catheter. **(B)** Aortogram demonstrating the use of a guiding catheter for renal artery cannulation.

stent and also helps to estimate the stent diameter and length. Following complete deflation of the balloon, confirmed by intermittent fluoroscopic imaging, the balloon is removed and selective angiography repeated to assess lesion response. It is imperative to maintain guidewire access until the end of the procedure to allow for the treatment of any suboptimal results such as dissections or residual stenoses.

Stent placement may be performed as either a primary procedure or as a secondary procedure in response to suboptimal results following angioplasty. Most FMD lesions and nonostial atherosclerotic lesions respond well to angioplasty alone. However, secondary stent placement should be considered for nonostial lesions that do not respond appropriately to angioplasty. Secondary stent placement is typically performed to address elastic recoil, residual stenosis (≥30%), and myointimal flaps or

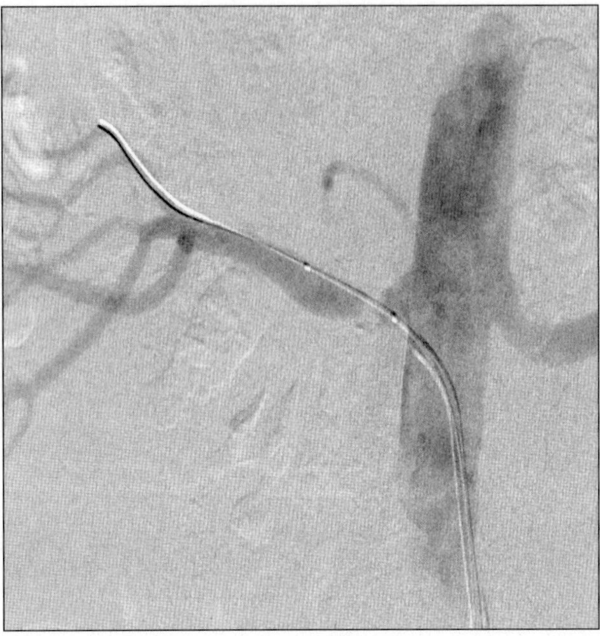

Figure 46-9. Passage of an angioplasty balloon across an in-stent restenosis. A 4 mm by 20 mm low profile balloon is commonly used to predilate the stenosis to allow passage of a larger, balloon-expandable stent.

dissections. It is our practice to employ balloon expandable stents primarily in the treatment of ostial atherosclerotic renovascular disease to take advantage of their greater radial strength and precise placement. In general, the technical aspects of stent placement parallel the performance of transluminal angioplasty. Frequent small hand injections of contrast through the guiding catheter are employed to direct the stent into position across the lesion prior to deployment. After the stent has been deployed, the guiding catheter can abut and support the stent as the balloon (used in balloon-expandable stents) is withdrawn. We prefer to perform the completion angiogram through the guiding catheter while still maintaining wire access across the stent. If aortography is also needed, a second (buddy) wire and flush catheter can be introduced through the sheath while maintaining renal access with the 0.18" wire (Figure 46–10).

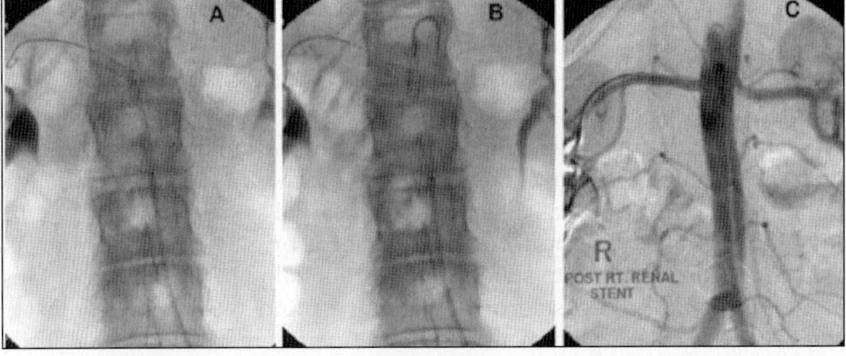

Figure 46-10. A second guidewire is introduced to allow placement of a flush catheter for arteriography while maintaining the original guidewire platform across the renal artery lesion.

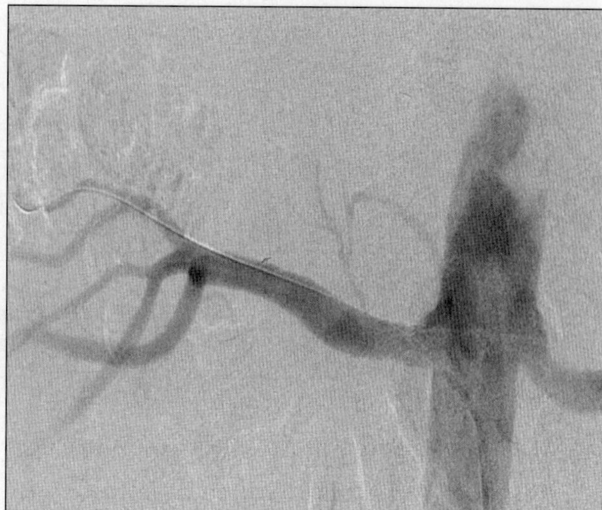

Figure 46-11. Anteroposterior view of a properly positioned right renal artery stent for ostial or proximal renal artery lesions. Note that the proximal portion of the stent extends slightly into the aortic lumen.

A slight extension of the stent of 1–2 mm into the aorta is preferred for the treatment of ostial or proximal renal artery lesions (Figure 46–11).[6] Since recurrent disease can occur that may not respond to further endovascular attempts, the shortest possible stent should be selected. A stent extending into the distal renal artery (Figure 46–12) can make later surgical options more difficult, and carries a higher failure rate.[21] Conversely, a stent placed too far into the aorta may expose the patient to the risk of future distal embolic events (Figure 46–13). In addition to bare metal stents, covered stents have also been used in the treatment of renovascular disease,[22,23] and are the subject of several on-going clinical trials.

Postoperative Care and Follow-up

Following renal artery stenting, most patients are treated with 90 days of clopidogrel (Plavix®; Bristol-Myers Squibb Co.) and/or aspirin. Aspirin therapy is then continued indefinitely if no contraindications exist. Renal artery duplex ultrasound is performed at the time of the first office visit, usually within two weeks. Renal artery duplex is then performed every four months for two years and then annually to detect any recurrent disease.[24,25]

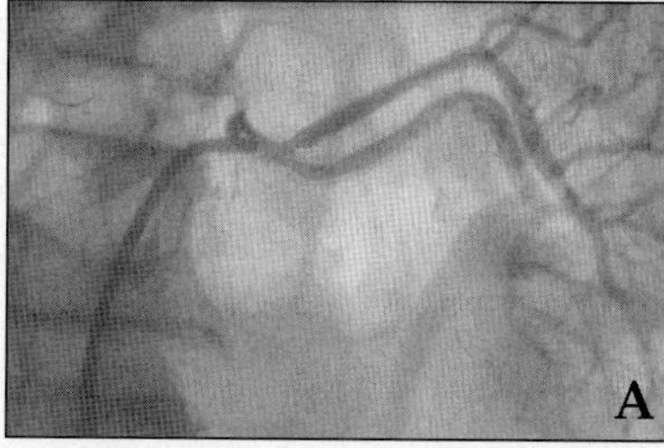

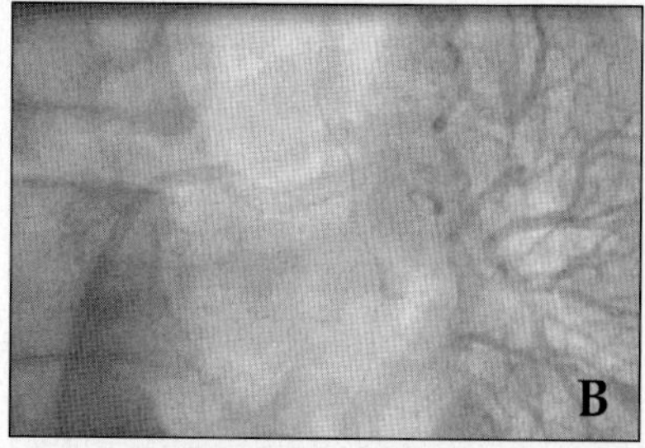

Figure 46-12. (A) and **(B)** Images depicting stent placement into the mid and distal renal artery, which can compromise subsequent open surgical interventions.

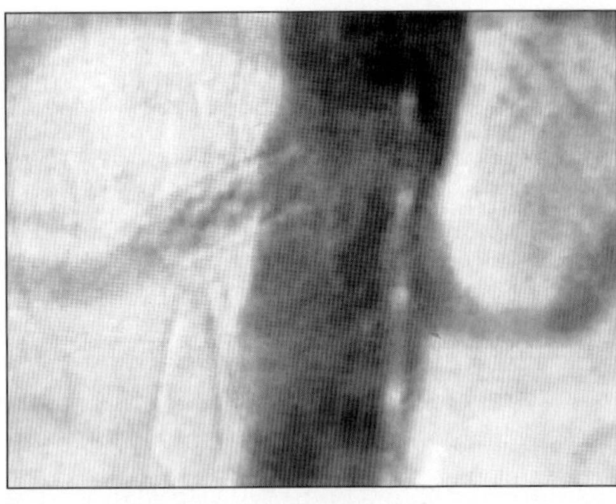

Figure 46-13. Image of an improperly placed renal artery stent with the proximal portion of the stent placed too far into the aortic lumen.

Recurrent Disease and In-stent Stenosis

Recurrent disease occurring after renal artery stenting can be a particularly challenging problem (Figure 46–14). Our experience has found repeat balloon angioplasty of these lesions to be less than optimal. Since the etiology of this lesion is most often intimal hyperplasia, repeat balloon angioplasty generally does little to improve the lesion. For recurrent lesions, initial dilatation with a "cutting" balloon is extremely useful to release fibrous scar tissue of the restenotic lesion and allow for subsequent larger diameter dilatation with a conventional angioplasty balloon.[26] The cutting balloon (Boston Scientific, Natick, MA) consists of a noncompliant balloon with four atherotomes (microsurgical blades) mounted longitudinally on its outer surface (Figure 46–15). When the cutting balloon is inflated, the atherotomes score the intimal hyperplasia within the stent. The balloon is then rotated and re-inflated to score the lesion in multiple planes. This technology has been used in coronary arteries for several years, but its use has also been studied with renal artery in-stent restenosis.[25] A larger balloon may then be used to enlarge the stent and is the usual mode of therapy. Treatment of in-stent restenosis with bare metal stents, drug eluting stents, and covered stents has also been reported, with encouraging results.[27,28]

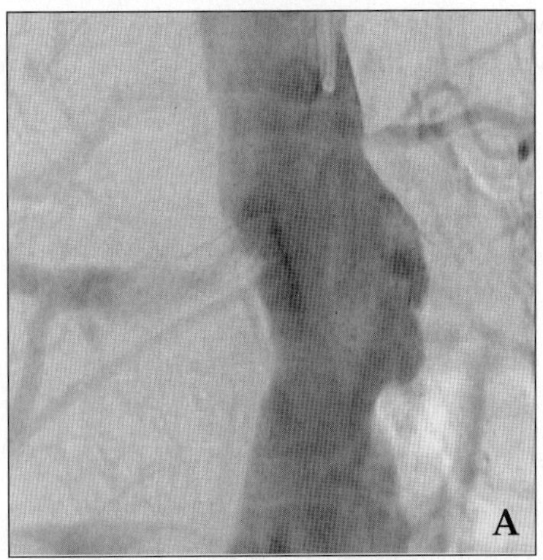
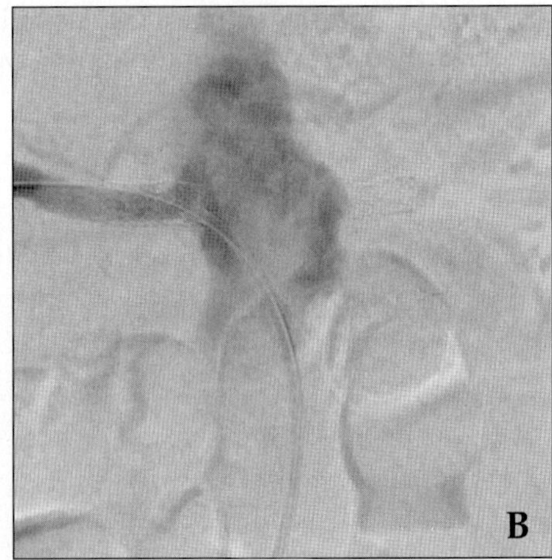

Figure 46-14. (A) In-stent stenosis. **(B)** Results of cutting balloon angioplasty on the same in-stent stenosis.

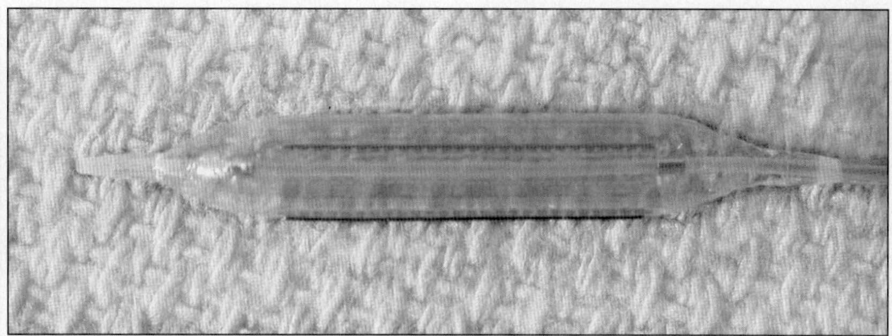

Figure 46-15. Cutting angioplasty balloon.

Results of Endovascular Treatment of Renovascular Disaese

Endovascular Therapy ad Blood Pressure Response.   Three randomized controlled studies have been completed comparing endovascular to medical treatment for renovascular hypertension. In 1998, the EMMA Study Group was the first to publish in this regard.[29] Their study, limited to patients with unilateral renal artery stenosis, was unable to demonstrate a statistically significant lowering of the blood pressure. The angioplasty group, however, demonstrated improvement in hypertension control as evidenced by a reduction in the amount of anti-hypertensive medications required.

The second prospective, randomized study comparing endovascular to medical treatment was reported by the Scottish and Newcastle Renal Artery Stenosis Collaborative Group in 1998.[30] The study found a modest improvement in blood pressure control, but only in patients with bilateral disease.

The largest prospective, randomized study reported to date was performed by the Dutch Renal Artery Stenosis Intervention Cooperative Study Group.[31] The authors concluded that angioplasty had little advantage over antihypertensive therapy.

Nordmann has subsequently performed a meta-analysis of these randomized controlled studies,[32] reviewing data from 210 patients. From these meta-analysis data, the authors concluded that balloon angioplasty has a modest but significant effect on blood pressure control.

A meta-analysis of retrospective literature was performed by Leertouwer and reported in 2000.[7] Fourteen articles involving 678 patients who were treated with renal artery stenting were combined with 10 articles involving 644 patients who were treated with angioplasty alone. Renal artery stenting demonstrated a high (98%) technical success rate. The overall hypertension cure rate was 20%, and 49% of the patients had improved blood pressure control. The restenosis rate was 17% at six to 29 months. However, when PTRA with stenting was compared to angioplasty alone, the restenosis rate was significantly lower for stenting (17% versus 26%; p<0.001).

Table 46–2 summarizes 27 contemporary case series (published between 1991 and 2001) reporting results of blood pressure response following primary stent placement for treatment of atherosclerotic renal artery stenosis.[33]

There has only been one prospective, randomized controlled study comparing endovascular treatment with open surgery repair for the treatment of renovascular hypertension.[34] Published in 1993, Weibull et al reported on 58 patients with RVH randomized to either surgery or angioplasty. An angiogram was performed at 10 days, one year, and two years after treatment. At 24 months, the primary patency rate

TABLE 46-2. RESULTS AFTER PRIMARY RENAL ARTERY STENT PLACEMENT FOR ATHEROSCLEROTIC RENAL ARTERY STENOSIS

Reference	Patients (n)	Technical Success (%)	Patient with renal dysfunction (n)	Renal Function Response (%)			Hypertension Response (%)			Restenosis (%)	Major Complicatons (%)
				Improved	Unchanged	Worsened	Cured	Improved	Failed		
Rees CR (1991)	28	96%	14	36%	36%	29%	11%	5%	36%	39%	18%
Wilms GE (1991)	10	80%	1	0%	100%	0%	30%	40%	30%	22%	18%
Kuhn FP (1991)	8	92%	n/r	n/r	n/r	n/r	22%	34%	44%	17%	13%
Joffre F (1992)	11	91%	4	50%	50%	0%	27%	64%	9%	18%	13%
Hennequin LM (1994)	15	100%	6	20%	40%	40%	7%	93%	0%	27%	19%
Raynaud AC (1994)	15	100%	7	0%	43%	57%	7%	43%	50%	13%	13%
MacLeod M (1995)	28	100%	16	25%	75%	75%	0%	40%	60%	17%	19%
van de Ven PJ (1995)	24	100%	n/r	33%	58%	8%	0%	73%	27%	13%	13%
Dorros G (1995)	76	100%	29	28%	28%	45%	6%	46%	48%	25%	11%
Henry M (1996)	55	100%	10	20%	80%	80%	18%	57%	24%	9%	3%
Iannone LA (1996)	63	99%	29	36%	46%	18%	4%	35%	61%	14%	32%
Harden PN (1997)	32	100%	32	35%	35%	29%	n/r	n/r	n/r	13%	19%
Blum U (1997)	68	100%	20	0%	100%	0%	16%	62%	22%	17%	0%
Boisclair C (1997)	33	100%	17	41%	35%	24%	6%	61%	33%	0%	21%
Rundback JH (1998)	45	94%	45	18%	53%	30%	n/r	n/r	n/r	26%	9%
Fiala LA (1998)	21	95%	9	0%	100%	0%	53%	53%	47%	65%	19%
Dorros G (1998)	163	99%	63	No change in mean SCr	1%	42%	57%	n/r	14%		
Tuttle KR (1998)	120	98%	74	16%	75%	9%	2%	46%	52%	14%	4%
Gross CM (1998)	30	100%	12	55%	27%	18%	0%	69%	31%	13%	n/r
Henry M (1999)	200	99%	48	29%	67%	2%	19%	61%	20%	11%	2%
Rodriguez-Lopez JA (1999)	108	98%	32	No change in mean SCr	13%	55%	32%	26%	12%		
van de Ven PJ (1999)	40	88%	29	17%	55%	28%	15%	43%	42%	14%	30%
Baumgartner I (2000)	64	95%	n/r	33%	42%	25%	43%	43%	57%	28%	9%
Giroux MF (2000)	30	95%	21	76%	76%	24%	53%	53%	47%	n/r	n/r
Perkovic V (2001)	148	97%	99	8%	56%	36%	n/r	n/r	n/r	29%	7%
Lederrman RJ (2001)	300	100%	111	8%	78%	14%	70%	70%	30%	21%	2%
Bush RL (2001)	73	89%	50	23%	51%	26%	n/r	n/r	n/r	n/r	9%
Totals	1808	98%	778	20%	59%	21%	10%	51%	39%	19%	9%

n/r: Not Related

SCr: Serum Creatinine

From: Costanza, MJ, Strilka RJ, Edwards MS, Benjamin ME. Endovascular Treatment of Renovascular Disease. In Rutherford RB et al. Vascular Surgery, New York; Elsevier/Mosby; 2005: 1825-1846.33

was 75% in the PTRA group versus 96% in the surgical group. Secondary patency rates were 90% in the PTRA group and 97% in the surgery group. Hypertension was cured, or improved, in approximately 90% of the patients in both groups, and the treatment response rates between the two cohorts were not statistically different. It must be noted however, that more than half of the patients who failed angioplasty crossed over to the surgical arm for revascularization. Based on these results, the authors recommend angioplasty as the treatment of choice for selected renovascular lesions contributing to renovascular hypertension with aggressive follow-up and repeat intervention (endovascular and surgical) as needed.

Endovascular Therapy and Renal Function Resiponse.   The result of endovascular treatment on renal function is uncertain. Several factors hinder an accurate assessment of the effect of renal artery angioplasty and stenting on renal function. No prospective studies have been performed to compare renal function after medical, surgical, or endovascular treatment of renal artery stenosis. Most observational series report results from a diverse group of patients whose renal function response varies widely. Most studies demonstrate short and intermediate term improvement or stabilization in serum creatinine following endovascular treatment of renovascular disease. It is still unclear whether endovascular treatment associated with immediate benefit results in improved survival or decreased adverse cardiovascular events for these patients. Future studies that incorporate direct measures of renal function, long-term follow-up, and outcome predictors are essential to resolve these issues.

Restenosis.   Restenosis continues to be a weakness of renal artery angioplasty and stenting. Despite initial technical success rates that exceeded 95%, reports by Gill et al,[35] Ramos et al,[36] Yutan et al,[37] and Lederman et al[38] have documented high rates of restenosis that ranged from 14–37%. In most cases, restenosis results from neointimal fibrous hyperplasia that is amenable to further endovascular treatment. Bax and colleagues[39] successfully treated 20 in-stent renal artery stenoses with repeat angioplasty in 18 cases and a second stent in two cases. The six- and 12-month patency after this intervention was 93% and 76%, respectively. The technical limits of repeat angioplasty and the risk of additional neointimal fibrosis with a second stent has prompted the search for alternative endovascular techniques for treating restenosis. Alternative treatments including atherectomy[40] and cutting balloon angioplasty[26] have been described in case reports.

REFERENCES

1. Cambria RP, Brewster DC, L'Italien GJ, Moncure A, Darling RC Jr, et al. The durability of different reconstructive techniques for atherosclerotic renal disease. J Vasc Surg. 1994 Jul;20(1):76–85.
2. Cherr GS, Hansen KJ, Craven TE, Edwards MS, Liguish J Jr, et al. Surgical management of atherosclerotic renovascular disease. J Vasc Surg. 2002 Feb;35(2):236–45.
3. Novick AC. Long-term results of surgical revascularization for renal artery disease. Urol Clin North Am. 2001 Nov;28(4):827–31.
4. Tegtmeyer CJ, Kellman CD, Ayers C. Percutaneous transluminal angioplasty of the renal artery. Results and long-term follow-up. Radiology. 1984 Oct;153(1):77–84.

5. Dorros G, Jaff M, Mathiak L, He T; Multicenter Registry Participants. Multicenter Palmaz stent renal artery stenosis revascularization registry report: four-year follow-up of 1,058 successful patients. Catheter Cardiovasc Interv. 2002 Feb;55(2):182–8.

6. Blum U, Krumme B, Flugel P, Gabelmann A, Lehnert T, et al. Treatment of ostial renal-artery stenosis with vascular endoprostheses after unsuccessful balloon angioplasty. N Engl J Med. 1997 Feb 13;336(7):459–65.

7. Leertouwer TC, Gussenhoven EJ, Bosch JL, van Jaarsveld BC, van Dijk LC, et al. Stent placement for renal arterial stenosis: Where do we stand? A meta-analyisis. Radiology. 2000;216:78–85.

8. Harden PN, MacLeod MJ, Rodger RS, Baxter GM, Connell JM, et al. Effect of renal-artery stenting on progression of renovascular renal failure. Lancet. 1997 Apr 19;349(9059):1133–6.

9. Rundback JH, Gray RJ, Rozenblit G, Poplausky MR, Babu S, et al. Renal artery stent placement for the management of ischemic nephropathy. J Vasc Interv Radiol. 1998 May–Jun; 9(3):413–20.

10. Bush RL, Najibi S, MacDonald MJ, Lin PH, Chaikof EL, et al. Endovascular revascularization of renal artery stenosis: technical and clinical results. J Vasc Surg. 2001 May;33(5): 1041–9.

11. Qanadli SD, Soulez G, Therasse E, Nicolet V, Turpin S, et al. Detection of renal artery stenosis: prospective comparison of captopril-enhanced Doppler sonography, captopril-enhanced scintigraphy, and MR angiography. AJR Am J Roentgenol. 2001 Nov;177(5):1123–9.

12. Hansen KJ, Tribble RW, Reavis SW, Canzanello VJ, Craven TE, Plonk GW, Dean RH. Renal duplex sonography: evaluation of clinical utility. J Vasc Surg. 1990 Sep;12(3):227–36.

13. Rudnick MR, Goldfarb S, Wexler L, Ludrook PA, Murphy MJ, et al. Nephrotoxity of ionic and nonionic contrast media in 1196 patients: a randomized trial. Iohexol Cooperative Study. Kidney Int. 1995 Jan;47(1):254–61.

14. Steinberg EP, Moore RD, Powe NR, Gopalan R, Davidoff AJ, et al. Safety and cost effectiveness of high-osmolality as compared with low-osmolality contrast material in patients undergoing cardiac angiography. N Engl J Med. 1992 Feb 13;326(7):425–30.

15. Barrett BJ, Parfrey PS, McDonald JR, Hefferton DM, Reddy ER, McManamon PJ. Nonionic low-osmolality versus ionic high-osmolality contrast material for intravenous use in patients perceived to be at high risk: randomized trial. Radiology. 1992 Apr;183(1):105–10.

16. Tepel M, van der Giet M, Schwarzfeld C, Laufer U, Liermann D, Zidek W. Prevention of radiographic-contrast-agent-induced reductions in renal function by acetylcysteine. N Engl J Med. 2000 Jul 20;343(3):180–4.

17. Hawkins IF Jr, Wilcox CS, Kerns SR, Sabatelli FW. CO2 digital angiography: a safer contrast agent for renal vascular imaging? Am J kidney Dis. 1994 Oct: 24(4):685–94.

18. Schreier DZ, Weaver FA, Frankhouse J, Papanicolaou G, Shore E, et al, A prospective study of carbon dioxide-digital subtraction vs standard contrast arteriography in the evaluation of the renal arteries. Arch Surg. 1996 May;131(5):503–7;discussion 507–8.

19. Grollman JH Jr, Marcus R. Transbrachial arteriography: techniques and complications. Cardiovasc Intervent Radiol. 1988;11(1):32–5.

20. Verschuyl EJ, Kaatee R, Beek FJ, Patel NH, Fontaine AB, Daly CP, et al. Renal artery origins: best angiographic projection angles. Radiology. 1997 Oct;205(1):115–20.

21. Wong JM, Hansen KJ, Oskin TC, Craven TE, Plonk GW, et al. Surgery after failed percutaneous renal artery angioplasty. J Vasc Surg. 1999;30:468–83.

22. Tan WA, Chough S, Saito J, Wholey MH, Eles G. Covered stent for renal artery aneurysm. Cather Cardiovasc Interv. 2001 Jan;52(1):106–9.

23. Sprouse LR 2nd, Hamilton IN Jr. The endovascular treatment of a renal arteriovenous fistula: Placement of a covered stent. J Vasc Surg. 2002 Nov;36(5):1066–8.

24. Hudspeth DA, Hansen KJ, Reavis SW, Starr SM, Appel RG, Dean RH. Renal duplex sonography after treatment of renovascular disease. J Vasc Surg. 1993 Sep;18(3):381–8.

25. Tullis MJ, Zierler RE, Glickerman DJ, Bergelin RO, Cantwell-Gab K, Strandness DE Jr. Results of percutaneous transluminal angioplasty for atherosclerotic renal artery stenosis: a follow up study with duplex ultrasonography. J Vasc Surg. 1997 Jan;25(1):46–54.

26. Munneke GJ, Engelke C, Morgan RA, Belli AM. Cutting balloon angioplasty for resistant renal artery in-stent restenosis. J Vasc Interv Radiol. 2002 Mar;13(3):327–31.
27. N'Dandu ZM, Badawi RA, White CJ, Grise MA, Reilly JP, et al. Optimal treatment of renal artery in-stent restenosis: repeat stent placement versus angioplasty alone. Catheter Cardiovasc Interv. 2008 Apr 1;71(5):701–5.
28. Zeller T, Sixt S, Rastan A, Schwarzwalder U, Muller C, Frank U, et al. Treatment of reoccurring instent restenosis following reintervention after stent-supported renal artery angioplasty. Catheter Cardiovasc Interv. 2007 Aug 1;70(2):296–300.
29. Plouin PF, Chatellier G, Darne B, Raynaud A. Blood pressure outcome of angioplasty in atherosclerotic renal artery stenosis: a randomized trial. Essai Multicentrique Medicaments vs Angioplastie (EMMA) Study Group. Hypertension. 1998 Mar;31(3):823–9.
30. Webster J, Marshall F, Abdalla M, Dominiczak A, Edwards R, Isles CG, et al. Randomized comparison of percutaneous angioplasty vs continued medical therapy for hypertension patients with athermatous renal artery stenosis. Scottish and Newcastle Renal Artery Stenosis Collaborative Group. J Hum Hypertension. 1998 May;12(5):329–35.
31. Van Jaarsveld BC, Krijnen P, Pieterman H, Derkx FH, Deinum J, et al. The effect of balloon angioplasty on hypertension in atherosclerotic renal-artery stenosis. Dutch Renal Artery Stenosis Intervention Cooperative Study Group. N Engl J Med. 2000 Apr 6;342(14):1007–14.
32. Nordmann AJ, Woo K, Parkes R, Logan AG. Balloon angioplasty or medical therapy for hypertensive patients with atherosclerotic renal artery stenosis? A meta-analysis of randomized controlled trials. Am J Med. 2003 Jan;114(1):44–50.
33. Costanza, MJ, Strilka RJ, Edwards MS, Benjamin ME. Endovascular Treatment of Renovascular Disease, in Rutherford RB et al. Vascular Surgery, 6th Ed. New York Elsevier/Saunders; 2005:1825–1846.
34. Weibull H, Bergqvist D, Bergentz S, Jonsson K, Hulthen L, Manhem P. Percutaneous transluminal renal angioplasty versus surgical reconstruction of atherosclerotic renal artery stenosis: A prospective randomized study. J Vasc Surg. 1993;18:841–52.
35. Gill KS, Fowler RC. Atherosclerotic renal arterial stenosis: clinical outcomes of stent placement for hypertension and renal failure. Radiology. 2003;226:821–826.
36. Ramos F, Kotilar C, Alvarez D, Baglivo H, Rafaelle P, Londero et al. Renal function and outcome of PTRA and stenting for atherosclerotic renal artery stenosis. Kidney International. 2003;63:276–282.
37. Yutan E, Glickerman DJ, Caps MT, Hatsukami T, Harley JD, Kohler et al. Percutaneous transluminal revascularization for renal artery stenosis: veterans affairs puget sound health care system experience. J Vasc Surg. 2001;34:685–693.
38. Lederman RJ, Mendelsohn FO, Santos R, Phillips HR, Stack RS, Crowley JJ. Primary renal artery stenting: characteristics and outcomes after 363 procedures. Am Heart J. 2001 Aug;142(2):314–23.
39. Bax L, Mali WPTM, Van de Ven PJG, Beek FJA, et al. Repeated intervention for in-stent restenosis of the renal arteries. J Vasc Interv Radiol. 2002;13:1219–1224.
40. Rao BH, Chandra KS. Renal artery in-stent restenosis: treatment with high speed rotational atherectomy. Indian Heart J. 2000;52:205–206.

47

Surgical Revascularization of Renal Artery after Complicated or Failed Percutaneous Transluminal Renal Angioplasty

Jean-Baptiste Ricco, M.D., Ph.D.
Michel Lacombe, M.D.

INTRODUCTION

Percutaneous transluminal renal angioplasty (PTRA) is now liberally used for treatment of renal artery stenosis.[1] Though the immediate outcome of PTRA is generally good, complications or failures requiring surgical revascularization occur in a nonnegligible percentage of patients.[1-7] The purpose of this retrospective study was to evaluate the effectiveness of surgical renal artery reconstruction after failed or complicated PTRA.

PATIENTS AND METHODS

This retrospective study includes a consecutive series of 45 patients (27 women and 18 men) referred to our departments after 52 unsuccessful PTRA procedures. In all patients, the indication for PTRA was severe hypertension that did not respond to optimal medical treatment. Five patients presented moderate kidney insufficiency and one patient presented severe kidney insufficiency.

In 25 patients (55%), the underlying arterial disease was fibrodysplasia classified on biopsy findings as medial in 13 patients including five with branch involvement, perimedial without branch involvement in five patients, and intimal without branch involvement in five patients. Precise classification of fibrodysplasia could not be established in two cases. In 17 cases (38%), the underlying disease was atherosclerosis. Atheromatous lesions were non ostial in all but two patients who were treated by primary stent placement. In the remaining three patients (7%), the underlying disease

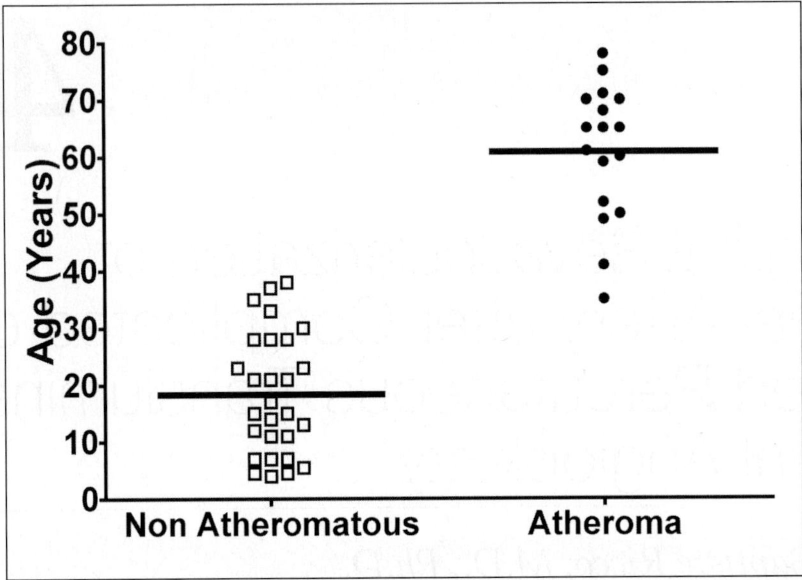

Figure 47-1. Age distribution according to the etiology of renal artery disease. Bimodal age distribution was correlated with underlying disease etiology. Young patients presented renal fibrodysplasia or Takayasu's disease (Mean age: 18±11 years), while older patients presented atheroma disease (mean age: 61±12 years). Reprinted with permission from: Lacombe M, Ricco JB. Surgical revascularization of renal artery after complicated or failed percutaneous transluminal renal angioplasty. *J Vasc Surg* 2006;44:537-44. Copyright (©) 2006 by The Society for Vascular Surgery

was Takayasu's disease. Nine patients in this series had one kidney. Mean age was 18±11 years for patients with fibrodysplasia or Takayasu disease, and 61±12 years for patients with atheromatous disease (Figure 47–1).

CRITERIA OF EFFECTIVENESS

The same criteria were used to assess the effect of PTRA and surgery on hypertension[8] and renal function.[9]

Concerning hypertension, patients were considered as cured if blood pressure was strictly normal without medication and as improved if less medication was needed to achieve normal blood pressure. Failure was defined as no change in blood pressure level or treatment requirements in comparison with preoperative data.

Concerning renal function, the response to angioplasty or surgery was defined as follows: "cured" if serum creatinine concentration was less than 1,5 mg/dL; "improved" if serum creatinine concentration decreased more than 20%; and "worsened" if serum creatinine increased more than 20%, dialysis was required, or renal-related death occurred. Patients who had a 20% or less change in serum creatinine concentration after the procedure were considered as "stable" renal function.

PTRA TECHNIQUES

The PTRA procedures in this series were performed between January 1980 and December 2003 at various outside centers. The patients underwent one to four consecutive PTRA procedures on the same renal artery (mean, 1.4 ± 0.6 per renal artery). Seven patients had bilateral PTRA that was done during the same procedure in three patients, and in separate procedures in four patients. A stent was inserted in eight arteries; five were used for primary treatment, one following arterial dissection after PTRA and two for recurrent stenosis after PTRA.

PTRA COMPLICATIONS

Major complications of PTRA (Figure 47–2) occurred in 19 arteries in 15 patients with four bilateral complications. Complications were immediate in 13 patients including arterial rupture in one patient, covered perforation in two (Figure 47–3), acute arterial thrombosis in five (Figure 47–4), and dissection in five (Figure 47–5). Complications were delayed in two patients (major worsening of renal artery stenosis in one patient (Figure 47–6) and aneurysm in one patient) (Figure 47–7).

PTRA FAILURES

Immediate or late failure occurred in a total of 33 PTRA procedures in 30 patients with three bilateral failures (Figure 47–2). Patients in whom catheterization of the renal artery failed were excluded from the study. Immediate failure (n = 16) was defined as either inability to dilate the stenosis after successful catheterization despite inflation of the balloon to a pressure of at least 10 bars, or the persistence of residual stenosis of at

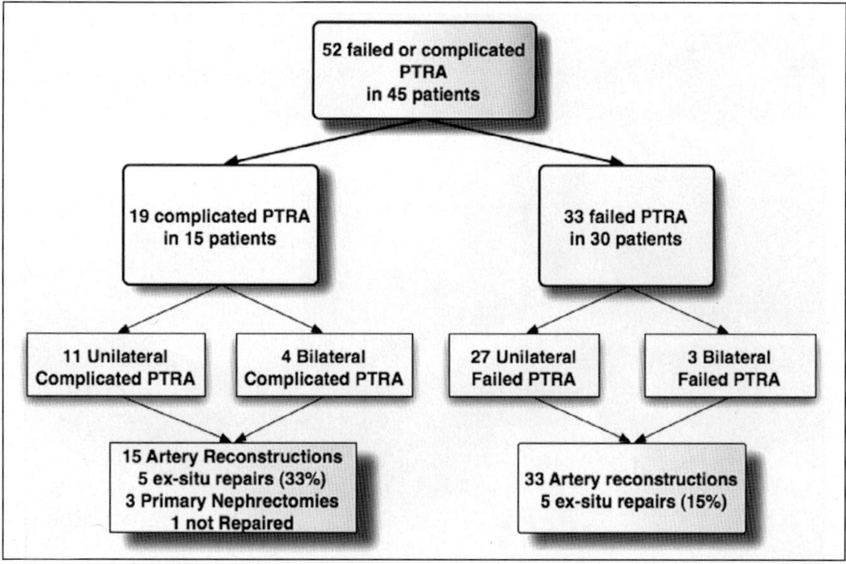

Figure 47-2. Study flowchart showing outcome of 52 percutaneous transluminal renal angioplasties (PTRA) procedures in 45 patients. A total of 48 renal artery reconstruction procedures including 10 involving extracorporeal repair were performed. Primary nephrectomy was performed in three cases. One patient had an atrophic kidney that prevented operative treatment. Reprinted with permission from: Lacombe M, Ricco JB. Surgical revascularization of renal artery after complicated or failed percutaneous transluminal renal angioplasty. *J Vasc Surg* 2006;44:537-44. Copyright (©) 2006 by The Society for Vascular Surgery

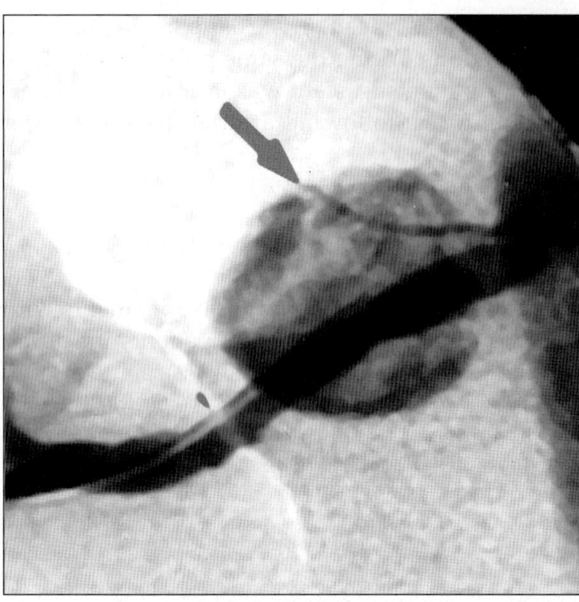

Figure 47-3. Angiography showing covered perforation of a renal artery during angioplasty. Large arrow indicates a peri-arterial hematoma. Small arrow indicates the angioplasty catheter. Reprinted with permission from: Lacombe M, Ricco JB. Surgical revascularization of renal artery after complicated or failed percutaneous transluminal renal angioplasty. *J Vasc Surg* 2006;44:537-44. Copright (©) 2006 by The Society for Vascular Surgery

least 50% of the lumen at the end of the procedure. Late failure (n = 17) was defined as restenosis greater than 50% of the vessel lumen, occurring one to 84 months (mean: 7.9 months) after angioplasty. Among the seven patients who underwent bilateral PTRA, one had bilateral complications, three had bilateral failures, and three had failure on one renal artery combined with complication on the contralateral renal artery.

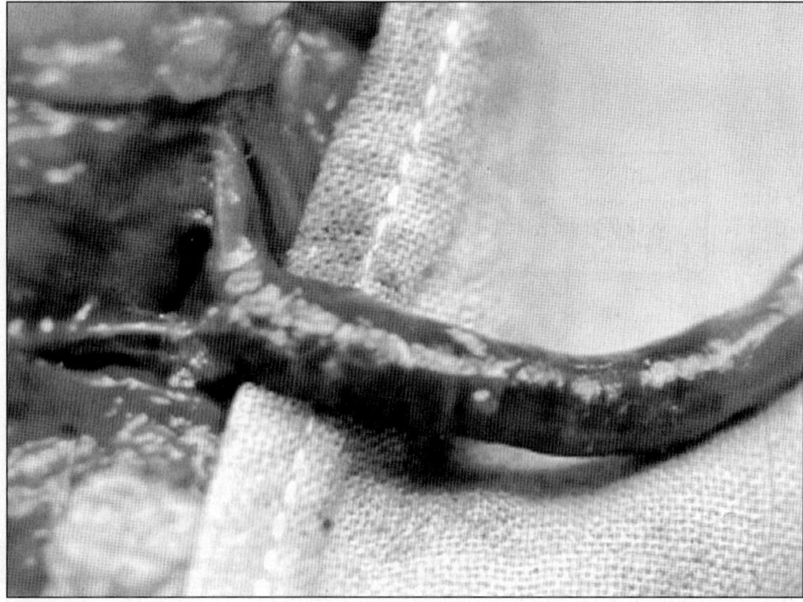

Figure 47-4. Operative view showing postangioplasty dissection of the renal artery with acute thrombosis. The patient underwent emergency surgical revascularisation. Reprinted with permission from: Lacombe M, Ricco JB. Surgical revascularization of renal artery after complicated or failed percutaneous transluminal renal angioplasty. *J Vasc Surg* 2006;44:537-44. Copyright (©) 2006 by The Society for Vascular Surgery

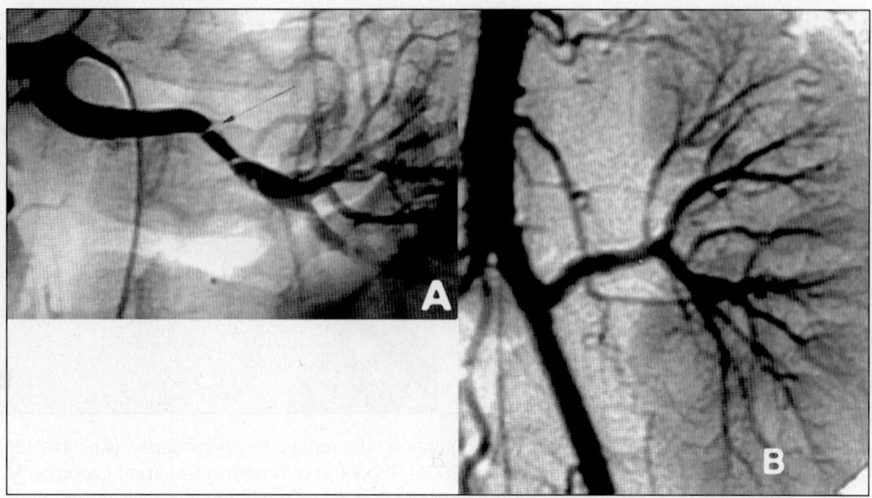

Figure 47-5. (A) Angiography showing dissection (arrow) after angioplasty of a recurrent stenosis of the left renal artery after spleno-renal anastomosis in a patient with only one kidney. **(B)** Angiography after emergency extracorporeal repair with autotransplantation of the kidney into the left iliac fossa and renal artery anastomosis to the common iliac artery. Reprinted with permission from: Lacombe M, Ricco JB. Surgical revascularization of renal artery after complicated or failed percutaneous transluminal renal angioplasty. *J Vasc Surg* 2006;44:537-44. Copyright (©) 2006 by The Society for Vascular Surgery

PTRA Effectiveness

For arterial hypertension, the response was as follows. In the nonatherosclerotic disease group including patients with fibrodysplasia and Takayasu's disease (n = 28),

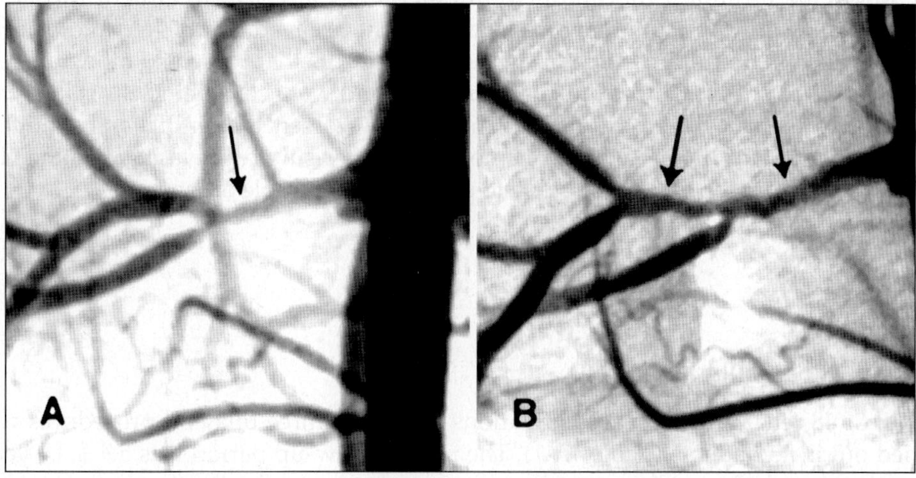

Figure 47-6. Significant aggravation of a renal artery stenosis after angioplasty in a patient with arterial fibrodysplasia. **(A)** Initial status. Right renal artery fibrodysplasia with proximal stenosis (arrow). **(B)** Final status after two angioplasties. The stenosis (arrows) has extended and involves the full length of the previously healthy superior renal artery branch. Reprinted with permission from: Lacombe M, Ricco JB. Surgical revascularization of renal artery after complicated or failed percutaneous transluminal renal angioplasty. *J Vasc Surg* 2006;44:537-44. Copyright (©) 2006 by The Society for Vascular Surgery

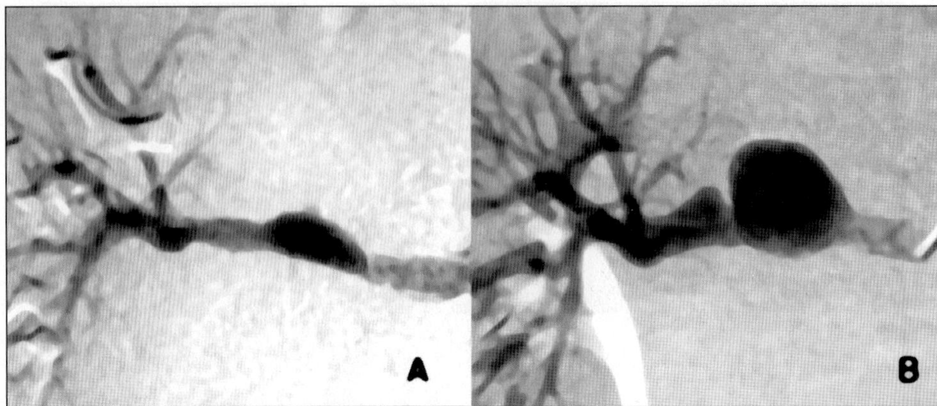

Figure 47-7. Evolution of a pseudoaneurysm occurring after a right renal artery angioplasty. **(A)** Immediate result after angioplasty in 1998. **(B)** Same artery in January 2001. Reprinted with permission from: Lacombe M, Ricco JB. Surgical revascularization of renal artery after complicated or failed percutaneous transluminal renal angioplasty. *J Vasc Surg* 2006;44:537-44. Copyright © 2006 by The Society for Vascular Surgery

there were 15 initially successful PTRA followed by normalization of blood pressure. In the remaining patients, PTRA led to either immediate failures (n = 10) or acute complications requiring emergency surgical intervention (n = 3). In the atheromatous group (n = 17), there were eight initially successful PTRA, followed by improvement in blood pressure in five patients and no change of blood pressure in three. In the remaining patients, PTRA led to immediate failure (n = 5) or acute complication requiring emergency surgical intervention (n = 4).

Concerning renal function, in the nonatheromatous group, all patients had normal renal function before PTRA. Renal function remained normal after PTRA in all but one case involving an infant that underwent emergency surgical treatment for PTRA-related dissection with acute renal insufficiency that resolved completely after surgical revascularization. In the atheromatous group, six patients that presented moderate renal insufficiency showed no improvement after PTRA and were considered as "stable," and one patient presented severe renal insufficiency that worsened after bilateral simultaneous angioplasty and finally required hemodialysis after surgical revascularization. This patient died within the first 90 days due to progressive multiple organ failure.

RESULTS

Surgical Revascularization

A total of 48 renal artery revascularizations including three bilateral procedures were carried out in 45 patients (Table 47–1). The mean follow-up period was 5.9 ± 3.6 years. No patient was lost to follow-up. All patients underwent color duplex scanning of the renal arteries and angiography within 30 days after surgical revascularization. Each patient was examined by a nephrologist and by the surgeon at one month, six months, and yearly with color duplex scanning thereafter. In cases involving arterial surgery in children, follow-up included angiography to assess the morphology of renal revascularization in function of the child's growth.

TABLE 47-1. RENAL ARTERY REVASCULARIZATION USED IN 45 PATIENTS

Renal Artery Revascularization Techniques	Arteries
Partial resection of renal artery with end-to-end anastomosis or allograft interposition	4
Bypass originating from the aorta	
• Prosthesis	11
• Arterial autograft with hypogastric artery	13
• Saphenous vein	1
Bypass originating from a splanchnic artery	
• spleno-renal	6
• hepato-renal	2
• mesenterico-renal	1
Extracorporeal surgery with hypogastric arterial autografting and kidney autotransplantation	10
Total	48

In situ revascularization was performed in 38 patients (79%). In the remaining 10 patients (21%), revascularization required extracorporeal repair with hypogastric artery grafting and reimplantation or autotransplantion of the kidney (Figure 47–5). Overall primary patency for the 48 renal revascularizations in this series was 93.5 ± 6.5% at five years. Satisfactory restoration of renal blood flow was achieved in all but three patients (6%) who presented with postoperative occlusion of the revascularized artery that occurred immediately after treatment of arterial fibrodysplasia in two patients and after treatment of atheromatous stenosis in one. These three patients presented extensive PTRA-related arterial and peri-arterial lesions that prevented repair from being performed.

In addition, permanent lesions of the kidney in the form of segmental infarcts were observed in six patients (12.5%). These lesions were caused by embolism, thrombosis, or distal dissection that occurred during PTRA since all were diagnosed prior to surgical revascularization.

Feasibility of Surgery after Failed PTRA

In all 33 patients treated after failed PTRA, surgical repair consisted of renal artery revascularization including five extracorporeal repairs (15%). Technical problems were encountered in four of 33 patients (12%) treated after failed PTRA. Operative findings showed evidence of PTRA-related renal damage after repeated angioplasty, causing lesions of the terminal branches of the renal artery that had been documented as nondiseased on pre-angioplasty arteriograms (Figure 47–6). In these patients, surgical exposure of the renal artery was impeded by the presence of peri-arterial fibrosis. In addition, three patients in this group presented PTRA-related segmental kidney infarction that compromised functional outcome.

Feasibility of Surgery after Complicated PTRA

A total of 19 patients underwent surgical repair after complicated PTRA (Figure 47–2). Treatment consisted of renal artery revascularization in 15 patients including five extracorporeal repairs (33%). In three patients, renal artery revascularization was unfeasible. Treatment in these patients consisted of three primary nephrectomies for PTRA-related complications: arterial rupture in one case, extensive dissection involving the terminal branches of the renal artery with kidney infarction in one case, and major postangioplasty renal artery fibrosis precluding any type of surgical revascularization in one case. In the remaining patient in whom PTRA caused worsening of renal artery stenosis and severe renal atrophy, renal artery repair was not attempted.

Major technical problems were encountered in 14 of the 19 patients (74%) treated after complicated PTRA. The most frequent problem involved major peri-arterial fibrosis that prevented surgical dissection of the artery in which angioplasty had been performed so that the only alternative was to perform distal anastomosis on the primary branches of the renal artery. Ex situ revascularization was required in four patients. In addition, renal anastomosis was problematic in five patients in whom the renal artery had been fragilized by arterial wall dissection during angioplasty.

Emergency surgical exploration of the renal artery (Figure 47–8) was carried out in seven of 19 patients presenting acute PTRA-related complications, including arterial dissection (n = 5 with four thromboses), thrombosis without dissection (n = 1), and arterial rupture (n = 1).

Effectiveness of Surgery According to Etiology

Improvement in blood pressure and kidney function after surgery according to our previous definitions[8,9] depended on the underlying arterial disease. Outcome was ex-

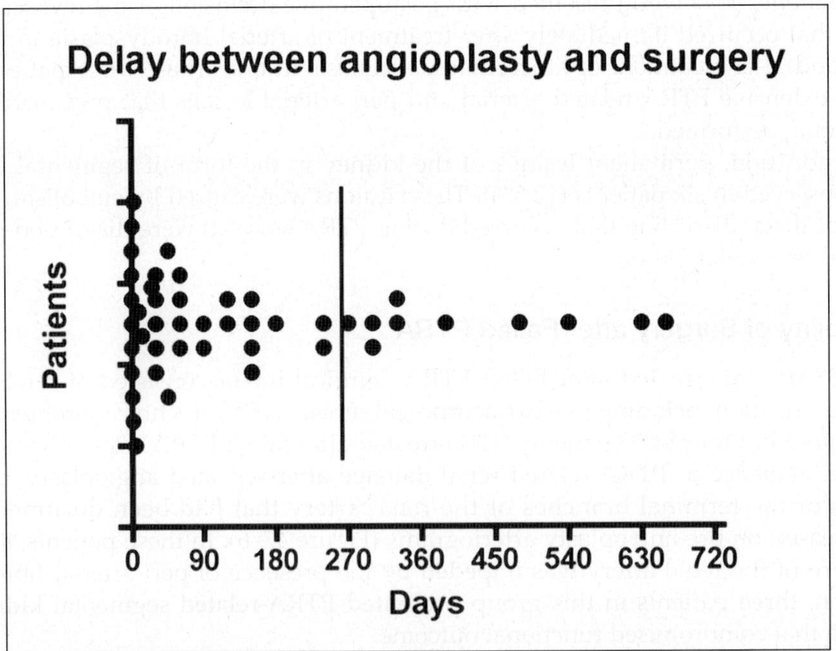

Figure 47-8. Interval between the last percutaneous transluminal renal artery angioplasty (PTRA) and open surgical treatment. The mean interval (vertical line) was 263 days. Thirteen procedures (25.5%) including seven emergency procedures were performed within the first 30 days following PTRA.Reprinted with permission from: Lacombe M, Ricco JB. Surgical revascularization of renal artery after complicated or failed percutaneous transluminal renal angioplasty. *J Vasc Surg* 2006;44:537-44. Copyright (©) 2006 by The Society for Vascular Surgery

cellent in the 25 patients with arterial fibrodysplasia. Blood pressure became normal in 21 (84%) that were considered as "cured," improved in three (12%), and remained unchanged in one patient (4%) that presented PTRA-related kidney infarcts. All patients with arterial fibrodysplasia maintained or recovered normal renal function.

Surgical revascularization was less beneficial in 17 patients with atheromatous lesions. Blood pressure improved in nine patients (53%) and remained unchanged in seven (41%). Of the eight patients who initially presented moderate kidney insufficiency, only one recovered normal renal function after surgical renal artery reconstruction and was considered as "cured." As mentioned above, one patient progressed to dialysis dependence after bilateral PTRA that was complicated by bilateral covered perforation. Despite surgery, this patient died at day 90.

DISCUSSION

Despite its many advantages, PTRA presents a number of technical limitations that can lead to failures and complications. In a review of 996 patients who underwent PTRA at major interventional radiology centers in North America and Europe, Martin[1] reported that the rate of immediate complications involving either the dilated artery or the kidney was 13%. Regarding failure, series describing PTRA showed high immediate and secondary restenosis rates consistently ranging from 15 to 25%.[1]

In an effort to reduce restenosis rates, renal artery stenting became widespread during the 1990s. However, the effectiveness of stenting proved to be limited due to the relatively high incidence of intrastent recurrences. In a 1998 review of 11 series dealing with renal artery stenting, Fiala et. al.[2] found that restenosis rates ranged from 6% to 44%. In more recent series[3-5,10] with low-profile systems, restenosis rates after stent placement have ranged from 10% to 30%. These findings suggest that stenting had limited impact on the incidence of restenosis after PTRA.

The extent of mechanical injury induced by PTRA at the angioplasty site varies with distension of the arterial layers, especially the media with hemorrhagic suffusion and even rupture of the internal elastic lamina with dissection of the artery. Dean et. al.[6] stressed the role of postangioplasty peri-arterial fibrosis. In our experience, the most extensive injuries were noted in the complicated PTRA group and appeared to be related to two mechanisms: organization of a peri-arterial hematoma due to covered perforation of the artery, and fibrous transformation of hemorrhagic suffusion in the arterial wall. The fact that some hemorrhagic areas extended well beyond the limits of the initial narrowing could explain the worsening and distal extension of the stenosis considered as late complications in four patients in our series.

In our experience, most technical problems were observed in patients treated after complicated PTRA (n = 19). Five patients (33%) in the complicated PTRA group required extracorporeal repair (33%), and three (16%) required primary (n = 2) or secondary (n = 1) nephrectomy. Fewer problems were encountered during surgical revascularization after failed PTRA (n = 33). The percentage of patients requiring extracorporeal repair was lower in patients treated after failed PTRA than complicated PTRA (12% versus 33%).

Most technical problems involved surgical dissection of the artery, and operative strategies must be tailored to each case. A great deal of patience is needed to "carve" the artery out of the fibrosis. We recommend progressing first to the division branches of the renal artery. Locating the nondissected division branches is essential so that distal anastomosis can be performed on a healthy arterial segment. In some patients, it may be impossible to dissect the arterial segment in which angioplasty was performed due to the high risk of arterial injury. The presence of dense fibrosis can be an indication for kidney autotransplantation to optimize conditions for ex situ revascularization.

Primary surgical repair of the renal artery probably would have avoided the need for nephrectomy in this series since all three indications for nephrectomy were due to PTRA-related complications (i.e., arterial rupture and extensive dissection of the artery). Similarly, primary surgical revascularization might have avoided postoperative thrombosis since all three cases in this series occurred in patients presenting extensive arterial and peri-arterial lesions following PTRA.

Therapeutic indications following unsuccessful angioplasty depend on the setting, and should be made on a case-by-case basis by a team including a nephrologist, a radiologist, and a surgeon. Emergency surgery was required in seven patients in our series (15%). Repeat angioplasty carries the risk of repeat failure and surgical revascularization can be more difficult when performed after multiple PTRA procedures. In our opinion, there is little use in repeating PTRA more than twice.

Few authors have studied the feasibility and effectiveness of surgical revascularization after unsuccessful angioplasty. Wong et. al.[7] encountered similar problems during surgical revascularization following failed or complicated angioplasty in 59% and 68% of patients, respectively. Despite these difficulties, Wong[7] and other authors[7,11-13] have documented the feasibility of surgical revascularization after unsuccessful angioplasty. The results of our experience support this conclusion since the outcome of surgical renal artery revascularization was good in most patients. Nevertheless, it must be noted that balloon angioplasty causes peri-arterial fibrosis that can impede vessel dissection and fibrous lesions of arterial layers that increase the risk of postoperative thrombosis. Because of these potential problems, conversion from in situ to extracorporeal repair should always be considered as a contingency in patients with failed or complicated PTRA.

Like Wong et. al.,[7] we observed that surgical revascularization was more difficult after stent placement. If stent removal is not possible during surgery, suture or ligation of the renal artery should include the stent to rule out the risk of stent migration into the aorta.

Dean et. al.,[6] who encountered technical difficulties in five out of 12 surgical revascularization procedures after unsuccessful angioplasty, strongly advocated more selective use of PTRA, taking into account the fact that surgical treatment is easier when performed as a primary rather than secondary procedure. We agree with this strategy. We performed 689 primary renal revascularizations with 17 postoperative occlusions (2.5%) as compared to three postoperative occlusions (6.6%) in this series. Consequently, we recommend surgical revascularization as the primary treatment for all types of arterial fibrodysplasia. Surgical revascularization may also be indicated for primary treatment in several other situations such as atheromatous stenosis associated with extensive calcification, anatomically difficult lesions like those involving the renal bifurcation or associated with aneurysm, lesions causing extensive obstruction of the renal artery, lesions associated with multiple sites in the terminal branches, and stenosis in children that is frequently associated with hypoplasia of the artery. Primary surgical treatment should also be discussed in patients with only one kidney, who accounted for 20% of the patient population (n = 9) in this series of failed or complicated PTRA.

CONCLUSIONS

This study does not question the usefulness of PTRA for the treatment of renal artery stenosis. However, our findings do suggest that indications should be carefully selected and emphasize the need for careful PTRA technique.

ACKNOWLEDGMENTS

This chapter is a summary of the study previously reported in greater detail in Lacombe M, Ricco J.-B. Surgical revascularization of renal artery after complicated or failed percutaneous transluminal renal angioplasty. *J Vasc Surg* 2006;44:537-44. Copyright (©) 2006 by The Society for Vascular Surgery.

REFERENCES

1. Martin L. Renal revascularization using percutaneous balloon angioplasty for fibromuscular dysplasia and atherosclerotic disease. In : *Modern management of renovascular hypertension and renal salvage*, KG Calligaro, MJ Dougherty, RH Dean, eds, Williams & Wilkins 1996, 125–44.
2. Fiala LA, Jackson MR, Gillespie DL, O'Donnell SD, Lukens M, Gorman P. Stenting primaire des lésions athéroscléreuses ostiales de l'artére rénale. *Ann Chir Vasc* 1998; 12: 128–33.
3. Perkovic V, Thomson KR, Mitchell PJ, Gibson RN, Atkinson N, Field PL, Becker GJ. Treatment of renovascular disease with percutaneous stent insertion : long-term outcomes. *Australas Radiol* 2001; 45: 438–43.
4. Lederman RJ, Mendelsohn FO, Santos R, Phillips HR, Stack RS, Crowley J.-J. Primary renal artery stenting : characteristics and outcomes after 363 procedures. *Am Heart J* 2001; 142: 314–23.
5. Bucek RA, Puchner S, Reiter M, Dirisamer A, Minar E, Lammer J. Long-term follow-up after renal artery stenting. *Wien Klin Wochenschr* 2003; 115: 788–792.
6. Dean RH, Callis JT, Smith BM, Meacham PW. Failed percutaneous transluminal renal angioplasty : experience with lesions requiring operative intervention. *J Vasc Surg* 1987; 6: 301–7.
7. Wong JM, Hansen KJ, Oskin TC, Craven TE, Plonk GW Jr, Ligush J Jr, Dean RH. Surgery after failed percutaneous renal artery angioplasty. *J Vasc Surg* 1999; 30: 468–83.
8. Rundbach JH, Sacks D, Kent KC, Cooper C, Jones D, Murphy T, et al. Guidelines for the reporting of renal artery revascularization in clinical trials. *J Vasc Interv Radiol* 2002;13:959–74.
9. Cambria RP, Brewster DC, L'Italien GJ, Gertler JB, Abbott WM, LaMuraglia GM, et al. Renal artery reconstruction for the preservation of renal function. *J Vasc Surg* 1996;24:371–82.
10. Nolan BW, Schermerhorn ML, Rowell E, Powell RJ, FillingerMF, Rzucidlo EM et al. Outcomes of renal artery angioplasty and stenting using low-profile systems. *J Vasc Surg* 2005;41:46–52.
11. McCann RL, Bollinger RR, Newmann GE. Surgical renal artery reconstruction after percutaneous transluminal angioplasty. *J Vasc Surg* 1988; 8: 389–94.
12. Martinez AG, Novick AC, Hayes JM. Surgical treatment of renal artery stenosis after failed percutaneous transluminal angioplasty. *J Urol* 1990; 144: 1094–6.
13. Desay TR, Meyerson SL, McKinsey JF, Schwartz LR, Bassiouny HF, Gewertz BL. Angioplasty does not affect subsequent operative renal artery revascularization. *Surgery* 2000; 128: 717–25.

48

Renal Revascularization: Conventional Surgery versus Endoluminal Catheter-based Therapy in the United States

Gilbert R. Upchurch Jr., M.D., Brian S. Knipp, M.D., Justin B. Dimick, M.D., Peter K. Henke, M.D., and James C. Stanley, M.D.

Arteriosclerotic renal artery occlusive disease accounts for 95% of reported cases of renovascular hypertension.[1] It may even be more common because most reported experiences represent surgical series that exclude many older patients who are not operative candidates. Arteriosclerotic renovascular disease most commonly presents during the sixth decade of life. Men are affected twice as often as women. Many of these patients exhibit occlusive disease of the coronary, cerebral, mesenteric, or extremity circulation.[2-5] This is particularly the case in black patients, who exhibit more severe extrarenal arteriosclerotic vascular disease.[6]

These stenoses characteristically affect the proximal third of the vessel in the form of eccentric or concentric narrowings. Nearly 80% of these lesions occur as spillover of diffuse aortic atherosclerosis. These stenotic lesions are bilateral in three-quarters of patients, and lesions affect the right and left renal arteries with equal frequency, although the left renal artery often appears more severely diseased.

Atherosclerotic renal artery stenosis, prior to the introduction of percutaneous endovascular techniques, was treated by open surgical revascularization including renal artery bypass or endarterectomy. The latter were often demanding technical procedures accompanied with modest morbidity and mortality.[7-13] In addition, these procedures were frequently undertaken in the setting of concomitant surgery for aortic aneurysms or aortoiliac occlusive disease with an associated operative mortality ranging 5% to 7%.

Catheter-based management management of arteriosclerotic renal artery occlusive disease has recently gained widespread favor, in part, because of its lesser risk to patients.[14] Although few randomized trials exist comparing percutaneous transluminal angioplasty (PTA) and conventional surgical therapy for renovascular hypertension, an early report by Weibull described similar patency and decreased mortality and morbidity rates for renal PTA compared to open renal revascularization.[15] It is well recognized that some innovations are not always uniformly adopted.[16-18] In fact, variation in the rate of adopting new treatments are largely invisible and very little data is available regarding how new technology is disseminated.[19-20] Insight into the diffusion and effect of catheter-based therapy in the management of arteriosclerotic renal artery disease is important in making accurate predictions about future practice patterns as they affect patient care.

THE INTRODUCTION OF ENDOLUMINAL TREATMENT OF ARTERIOSCLEROTIC RENAL ARTERY DISEASE

In 1978, Gruntzig and colleagues[21] were the first to report the use of PTA in the management of renovascular hypertension. The minimally invasive nature of renal artery PTA offers certain obvious advantages over conventional surgical intervention.[22-23] Most renal artery stenoses can be traversed with a guidewire and subsequently dilated with or without a stent, with minimal morbidity and mortality.[24] The ease of this therapy has led to its rapid introduction into clinical practice, often without clear guidelines as to when it should be used.[25-28] To justify PTA, the clinical significance of the renal artery stenosis should be documented prior to initiating endovascular therapy. In particular, the patient should have sustained hypertension despite simple drug therapy in the case of treatment for elevated blood pressure and adequate renal cortical reserve to recover kidney function when treatment is for renal insufficiency.

The presence of generalized clinically overt arteriosclerotic cardiovascular disease versus focal renal artery disease, as well as aortic spillover arteriosclerosis versus isolated renal artery arteriosclerosis, have an important impact on long-term clinical results. Historically, PTA without stent placement has resulted in a technical success rate of only 70% to 80%. Ostial spillover lesions, treated by PTA alone, have technical success rate of only 30% to 50%. These latter stenoses often manifest excessive recoil and many exhibit acute dissections. As a result of high early post-PTA restenosis rates, stenting of atherosclerotic lesions became appropriate in treating the vast majority of these patients.

Results following renal artery stenting for atherosclerotic disease vary depending on outcome definitions and the indication for intervention, yet many studies have very good results (Table 48–1). For example, Palmaz stents placed in 64 renal arteries in 59 patients, resulted in a two-year secondary patency rate of 92%.[29] Others have documented five-year primary and secondary patency rates of 84% and 92%, respectively.[30] In treating patients for hypertension, long-term benefits have been reported in 52% to 78% of patients. PTA with stenting for progressive ischemic nephropathy is not as effective at reversing renal failure. In these cases, benefits appear related to the degree and duration of ischemic nephropathy prior to PTA, with those having rapid onset of renal failure and a serum creatinine of less than 2 mg/dL demonstrating the best response.

Complications accompanying renal artery PTA for atherosclerosis are uncommon, with severe complications occurring in less than a few percent of cases. Intimal disrup-

TABLE 48-1. PTA WITH STENT PLACEMENT FOR ARTERIOSCLEROTIC RENOVASCULAR DISEASE

Author	Patients	Stents	Indication		Follow-up Mean (Mo)	Postprocedural Blood Pressure Response (%)*		
			Hypertension	Renal Insufficiency		Cured	Improved	Failed
Dorros-Feuer Foundation	76	92	76	48	6	6	46	48
University Hospital Freiburg, Germany	68	74	68	29	27	16	62	22
Ochsner Clinic	66	88	66		19	2	64	34
Polyclinique D'Essey	59	64	59	10	14	19	57	24
Hotel-Dieu de Montreal	33	35	33	17	13	6	61	33
University of Texas Health Center (Multicenter Study)	28	28	28	14	7	11	48	36

*Outcomes defined in reports from individual institutions.

tion occurs more often with proximal renal artery dilation where the vessel elasticity is greater and medial disruption is less likely. Medial tears are more common with distal renal artery dilation where vessel elasticity is less. Surgery following failed renal artery PTA is much more hazardous than primary surgery alone[31] because it is associated with a much higher incidence of emergent repair and nephrectomy. Furthermore, blood pressure benefits after a failed renal artery PTA that necessitates secondary operation are significantly lower: 57% after reoperation versus 89% for a primary operation.

CONVENTIONAL SURGICAL TREATMENT OF ARTERIOSCLEROTIC RENAL ARTERY DISEASE

Operative treatment of patients with renovascular occlusive disease has become relatively well defined.[1,32-38] It is important that the primary revascularization procedure be successful. This is underscored by the fact that nephrectomy accompanies nearly half of the reoperations for failed initial reconstructions.[39] Careful preoperative assessment of extrarenal occlusive disease in patients with arteriosclerotic renovascular disease is mandatory to ensure the patient's ability to undergo complex renal artery surgery. Operative details vary and are dependent on the different subgroups of renal artery disease, the involvement of the aorta, and the patients' overall cardiovascular status.

Bypass Procedures

Aortorenal bypass in adults with arteriosclerotic renal artery occlusive disease is most often performed using autologous reversed saphenous vein. Dacron or expanded polytetrafluoroethylene conduits may also be used in reconstructing these vessels. Nonanatomic bypass procedures are important in treating many patients with renovascular hypertension. The hepatic artery or iliac arteries may be used as sites of origin for bypass grafts to the renal artery, especially when originating a graft from the aorta would entail unacceptable risks.[40] Use of the splenic artery in situ for a left-sided splenorenal bypass is appropriate in adults, but only after ascertaining that this vessel and the celiac trunk are free of stenotic disease.[41-42] Splenorenal bypasses are not recommended in children because of the potential existence of a celiac artery growth arrest that may not be evident at the time of reconstruction but which may evolve later.

Endarterectomy

Endarterectomy is often performed for proximal renal artery arteriosclerotic disease.[1,43-45] The two techniques most often used are (1) transaortic renal endarterectomy through an axial aortotomy or the transected infrarenal aorta, and (2) direct renal artery endarterectomy. The extent of aortic and renal artery disease, as well as the need to perform coexistent aortic reconstructive surgery, dictates which of these procedures is most appropriate. In most cases, a linear aortotomy is begun just to the left of the superior mesenteric artery and extended in the midline to below the renal arteries. The diseased aortic intimal and medial tissues are elevated, and with gentle traction, the renal artery atheroma is extracted. This type of endarterectomy is particularly useful in treating bilateral disease or when the disease affects multiple renal arteries. Extensive plaque of the more distal renal artery, especially when involving bifurcations, may be better treated by a direct renal artery arteriotomy and endarterectomy with a patch-graft closure.

Conventional surgical treatment of renovascular hypertension affords excellent outcomes.[1,38] Differences among most individual experiences reflect variations in the prevalence of different renovascular disease categories (Table 48–2). Cures are uncommon and are a reflection of coexistent essential hypertension in older patients with arteriosclerotic disease. Arteriosclerotic renovascular hypertension occurs in two subgroups of patients: (1) those with focal renal artery disease whose only clinical manifestation of arteriosclerosis is secondary hypertension, and (2) those with clinically overt extrarenal arteriosclerosis affecting the coronary and carotid arteries, aorta, or extremity vessels. The severity and duration of hypertension, age, and gender in these two subgroups are similar, yet the surgical outcome regarding amelioration of hypertension is worse in patients with overt extrarenal arteriosclerotic disease. The open surgical treatment of ischemic nephropathy and renal failure is less likely to pro-

TABLE 48-2. ARTERIOSCLEROTIC RENOVASCULAR HYPERTENSION IN ADULTS

Institution	Patients	Operative Outcome (%)			Surgical Mortality Rate
		Cured	Improved	Failed	
Bowman Gray	152	15	75	10	1.3
University of Michigan					
Focal renal arteriosclerosis	64	33	58	6	0
Overt extrarenal arteriosclerosis	71	25	47	28	8,5
University of California,					
San Francisco	84	39	23	38	2.4
Cleveland Clinic	78	40	51	9	2
University of Lund,					
Malmo, Sweden	66	49	24	27	0.9
Hospital Aiguelongue,					
Montpellier, France	65	45	40	15	1.1
Vanderbilt University	63	50	45	5	9

Modified from Stanley JC. The evolution of surgery for renovascular occlusive disease. *Cardiovasc Surg* 1994;2:195–202.

vide excellent results.[46-47] Similar to outcomes following PTA in these patients, a rapid onset of renal insufficiency and coexistent hypertension provide the best setting for a salutary outcome. Nevertheless, open revascularization of a kidney with an occluded renal artery, unamenable to PTA, offers recovery of renal function and improvement in blood pressure control in nearly half the patients.

THE EVOLUTION AND IMPACT OF ENDOLUMINAL TREATMENT OF ARTERIOSCLEROTIC RENAL ARTERY DISEASE IN THE UNITED STATES

The Nationwide Inpatient Sample is a 20% stratified random sample of all hospital discharges in the United States.[48] Patients studied included those discharged during years 1988 to 2001 with an *International Classification of Diseases, Ninth Revision, Clinical Modification* (ICD-9-CM) code for renovascular hypertension (405.01, 405.11, or 405.91) and a concomitant code for renal artery arteriosclerosis (440.1). Patients in this population were then subdivided into two treatment groups. Group I, isolated open renal revascularization, included patients with codes for renal artery revascularization (38.1, 38.10, 38.16, 38.3, 38.30, 38.36, 38.4, 38.40, 38.46, 39.24, 55.4, 55.5, 55.51, 55.52, and 55.54), and without codes for aortoiliac revascularization (38.14, 38.34, 38.44, and 39.25) or aortic aneurysm repair. Group II patients undergoing angioplasty and stenting included those with no surgical revascularization codes and a code for catheter-based revascularization (39.50, 39.59, and 39.90). Exclusion criteria were age less than 20 years and a code for vascular trauma (902.xx).

All 10,320 patients, discharged from 1988 to 2001, were included with a diagnostic code for renovascular hypertension and renal artery arteriosclerosis. Of the 5,433 patients who underwent an intervention, 976 underwent isolated renal revascularization (561 patients undergoing combined aortic and renal revascularization were excluded), and 3,896 underwent renal artery angioplasty and stenting (Table 48–3).

Factors favoring performance of angioplasty and stenting were identified to evaluate patterns in allocation of resources. The primary outcome was in-hospital mortality. Secondary outcomes assessed to ascertain changes in resource utilization included length of stay (LOS), average hospital charge, and unfavorable discharge (to any location other than home).

Univariate analyses, using chi-squared testing, were performed to assess differences over time in rates of angioplasty and stenting, mortality, LOS, hospital charges, and unfavorable discharge. For modeling purposes, calendar years were divided into three time periods: 1988–1992, 1993–1997, and 1998–2001. Race was analyzed as a dichotomous variable: white versus nonwhite. Comorbid diseases were used as a marker of case-mix in accordance with previously established standards.[49-51] True population-based rates were obtained by using sampling weights to find the estimated number of total procedures performed each year in the United States. This estimate was then divided by the total adult population for each year to approximate true population-based rates. Multivariate analyses of predictors of catheter-based treatment, mortality, and unfavorable discharge were performed by multiple logistic regression: $P < .05$ was considered significant. SPSS Version 11.0 (Chicago, IL) was used for all statistical analyses.

The number of patients with a discharge diagnosis of renovascular hypertension and renal artery arteriosclerosis increased 46% during the period of study from 1.5 cases to 2.2/100,000 adults ($P < .001$). This may have reflected a change in coding practices or may reflect an increase in the recognition of the disease, with more frequent diagnostic catheterization procedures being performed. Isolated renal revascularization

TABLE 48-3. PATIENT DEMOGRAPHICS

Patient Characteristics	Conventional Surgical Revascularization	Angioplasty and Stenting	P-Value
Total number of patients	976	3896	
Age (years, mean ± SD)	63 ± 12	67 ± 12	<.001
Female gender	62% (605)	61% (2365)	.038
Nonwhite race	5.4% (35)	10.0% (266)	<.001
Median local annual income rank* (mean ± SD)	2.36 ± 1.07	2.60 ± 1.07	<.001
Urgent admission	18% (161)	28% (1000)	<.001
Emergent admission	9% (79)	18% (642)	<.001
Chronic renal disease	0.8% (8)	0.6% (25)	.767
Diabetes Mellitus	10% (93)	14% (539)	<.001
Chronic obstructive pulmonary disease	9% (84)	8% (296)	<.001
History of myocardial infarction	5% (46)	5% (210)	.276
Mortality	2% (21)	1% (30)	<.001
Unfavorable discharge	17% (161)	9% (346)	<.001

Median local annual income was ranked into four levels: (1) Less than $25,000; (2) $25,000 to $35,000; (3) $35,000 to $45,000; and (4) Greater than $45,000. (Modified from Knipp BS, Dimick JB, Eliason JL, et al. Diffusion of new technology for the treatment of renovascular hypertension in the United States: Surgical revascularization versus catheter-based therapy, 1988-2001. *J Vasc Surg.* 2004;40:717–723).

decreased 56%, from 0.2 to 0.09/100,000 adults ($P < .001$). During this same period, angioplasty and stenting increased 173%, from 0.4 to 1.1/100,000 adults (Figure 48–1) ($P < .001$). There was a 67% increase in interventions in general during this time period, from 0.73 to 1.22/100,000 adults ($P < .001$).

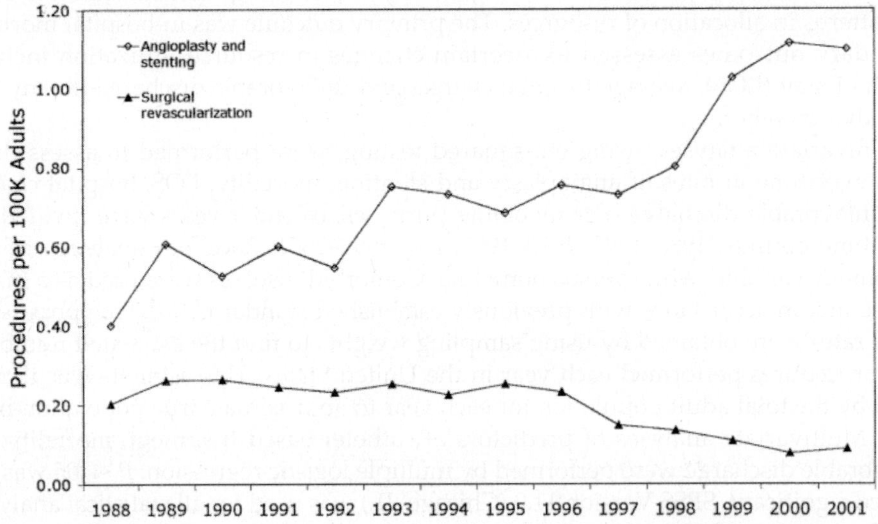

Figure 48-1. A 56% decline in isolated renal revascularization (P < .001) occurred over the 14-year study period. Angioplasty and stenting increased 173% (*P* < .001). (Modifed from Knipp BS, Dimick JB, Eliason JL, et al. Diffusion of new technology for the treatment of renovascular hypertension in the United States: Surgical revascularization versus catheter-based therapy, 1988-2001. *J Vasc Surg.* 2004;40:717–723).

PTA was more likely to be performed in patients having emergent or urgent admissions, older age, and nonwhite race when comparing isolated renal artery revascularization to catheter-based intervention, (Table 48–4) Comorbidities and gender were not significant predictors of the type of intervention. Catheter-based interventions occurred more frequently from 1993–1997 (P = .001) and 1998–2001 (P < .001) compared to 1988–1992.

In-hospital mortality did not significantly change over the 14-year period with an overall rate of 2.2% for isolated renal revascularization, and 0.8% for angioplasty and stenting (Figure 48–2). In a multivariate analysis, significant predictors of mortality included increasing age, surgical intervention, emergent admission, and nonwhite race (Table 48–5). Median income, comorbidities, gender, and time period were not significant predictors of mortality.

TABLE 48-4. MULTIVARIATE ANALYSIS OF PREDICTORS OF ANGIOPLASTY OR STENTING: COMPARISON BETWEEN ISOLATED RENAL ARTERY RECONSTRUCTION VERSUS ANGIOPLASTY AND STENTING

Independent Variable	Predictors of Angioplasty or Stenting, Odds Ratio (95% CI)	P-Value
Emergent admission	3.5 (2.7 to 4.7)	<.001
Urgent admission	2.2 (1.8 to 2.8)	<.001
Age ≥ 77*	2.5 (1.9 to 3.3)	<.001
Age 71 to 76*	1.5 (1.2 to 1.9)	.001
Nonwhite race	1.7 (1.2 to 2.4)	.003

*Compared to age ≥ 60 years. Modified from Knipp BS, Dimick JB, Eliason JL, et al. Diffusion of new technology for the treatment of renovascular hypertension in the United States: Surgical revascularization versus catheter-based therapy, 1988-2001. *J Vasc Surg.* 2004;40:717–723).

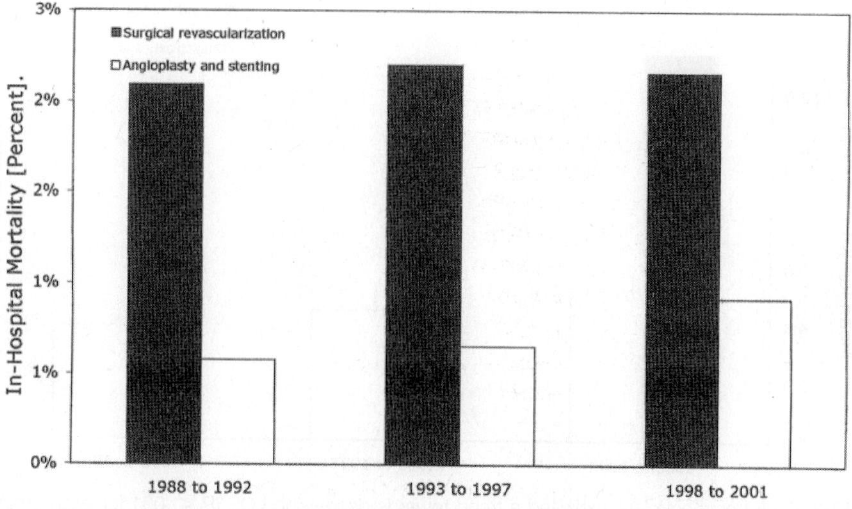

Figure 48-2. In hospital mortality versus time. By chi-square analysis, there were no significant variations in mortality over time for either treatment class. (Modified from Knipp BS, Dimick JB, Eliason JL, et al. Diffusion of new technology for the treatment of renovascular hypertension in the United States: Surgical revascularization versus catheter-based therapy, 1988-2001. *J Vasc Surg.* 2004;40:717–723).

TABLE 48-5. MULTIVARIATE ANALYSIS OF MORTALITY: INDEPENDENT PREDICTORS OF IN-HOSPITAL MORTALITY FOLLOWING INTERVENTION FOR RENOVASCULAR HYPERTENSION

Independent Variable	Risk of Mortality, Odds Ratio (95% CI)	P-Value
Age ≥ 75 years*	10.4 (2.3 to 46.0)	.002
Age 68 to 74 years*	6.5 (1.5 to 28.7)	.014
Age 60 to 67 years*	7.2 (1.6 to 32.1)	.009
Conventional renal artery surgery**	4.1 (1.9 to 8.7)	<.001
Emergent Admission	3.9 (2.1 to 7.4)	<.001
Nonwhite race	3.1 (1.5 to 6.7)	.004

*Compared to age ≥ 59 years
**Compared to angioplasty or stenting procedures
Modified from Knipp BS, Dimick JB, Eliason JL, et al. Diffusion of new technology for the treatment of renovascular hypertension in the United States: Surgical revascularization versus catheter-based therapy, 1988-2001. *J Vasc Surg.* 2004;40:717–723).

LOS decreased significantly in each treatment group ($P < .001$ for each). At all time points, LOS was shortest for catheter-based interventions ($P < .001$) (Figure 48–3). Hospital charges did not change significantly for surgical interventions over the 14-year period of study, although catheter-based charges increased 61% ($P < .001$). Nevertheless, catheter-based revascularizations had the lowest charges ($P < .001$) (Figure 48–4).

In each treatment group, rates of unfavorable discharges to any location other than home (excluding in-hospital mortality) increased significantly with time ($P = .004$) and

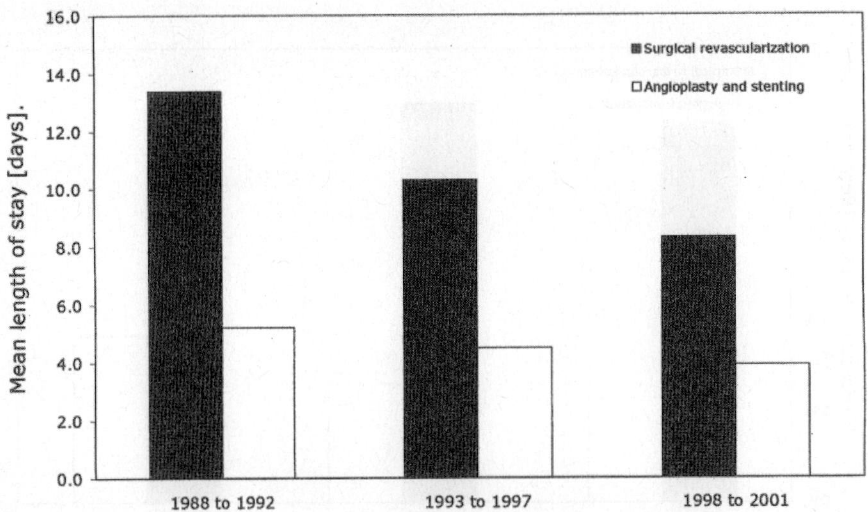

Figure 48-3. Each treatment class exhibited a trend towards decreasing LOS (P < .001 for each group). At all timepoints, isolated renal revascularization had a longer LOS than angioplasty and stenting (P < .001). (Modified from Knipp BS, Dimick JB, Eliason JL, et al. Diffusion of new technology for the treatment of renovascular hypertension in the United States: Surgical revascularization versus catheter-based therapy, 1988-2001. *J Vasc Surg.* 2004;40:717–723).

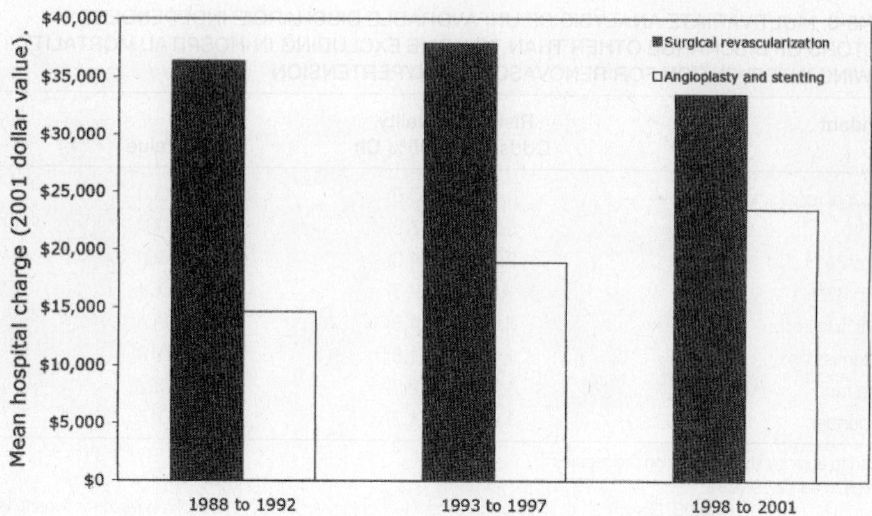

Figure 48-4. There were no significant trends in total hospital charges for isolated renal surgical repairs. Charges for angioplasty and stenting increased significantly (P < .001), approaching charges for isolated surgical renal revascularization. All costs were corrected for 4% annual inflation. (Modified from Knipp BS, Dimick JB, Eliason JL, et al. Diffusion of new technology for the treatment of renovascular hypertension in the United States: Surgical revascularization versus catheter-based therapy, 1988-2001. *J Vasc Surg.* 2004;40:717–723).

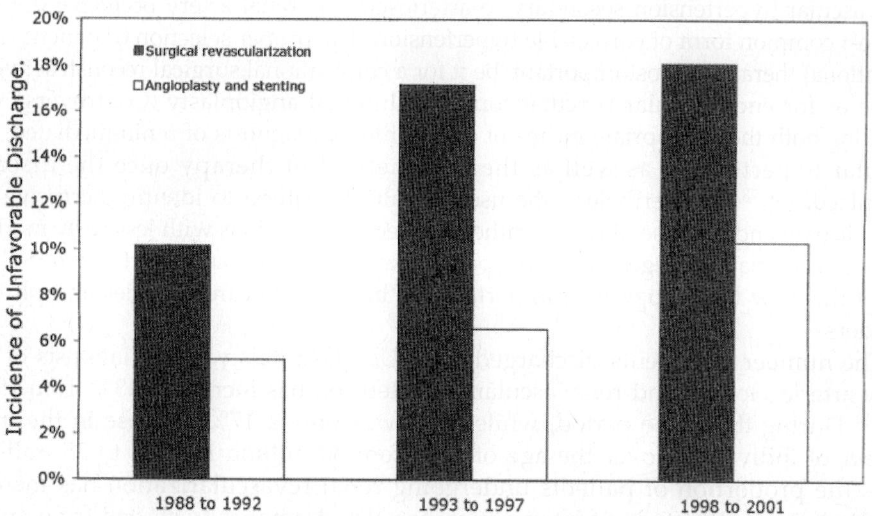

Figure 48-5. Each treatment class exhibited a significant trend towards an increased risk of unfavorable discharge (P=.004 for isolated renal revascularization and P < .001 for angioplasty and stenting). (Modified from Knipp BS, Dimick JB, Eliason JL, et al. Diffusion of new technology for the treatment of renovascular hypertension in the United States: Surgical revascularization versus catheter-based therapy, 1988-2001. *J Vasc Surg.* 2004;40:717–723).

P < .001 for isolated renal and catheter-based revascularizations, respectively (Figure 48–5). In a multivariate analysis, predictors of an unfavorable discharge included surgical intervention, increasing age, admission acuity, nonwhite race, and female gender (Table 48–6).

TABLE 48-6. MULTIVARIATE ANALYSIS OF UNFAVORABLE DISCHARGE: INDEPENDENT PREDICTORS OF DISCHARGE OTHER THAN TO HOME EXCLUDING IN-HOSPITAL MORTALITY FOLLOWING INTERVENTION FOR RENOVASCULAR HYPERTENSION

Independent Variable	Risk of Mortality, Odds Ratio (95% CI)	P-Value
Conventional renal artery surgery*	4.3 (3.2 to 5.9)	<.001
Age ≥ 75**	5.2 (3.5 to 7.6)	<.001
Age 68 to 74**	2.9 (2.0 to 4.3)	<.001
Age 60 to 67**	1.8 (1.2 to 2.8)	.004
Emergent admission	3.6 (2.7 to 4.8)	<.001
Urgent admission	1.4 (1.1 to 1.8)	.019
Nonwhite race	1.6 (1.1 to 2.3)	.022
Female gender	1.3 (1.1 to 1.7)	.014

*Compared to angioplasty and stenting procedures
**Compared to age ≥ 59 years
Modified from Knipp BS, Dimick JB, Eliason JL, et al. Diffusion of new technology for the treatment of renovascular hypertension in the United States: Surgical revascularization versus catheter-based therapy, 1988-2001. *J Vasc Surg.* 2004;40:717–723).

DISCUSSION

Renovascular hypertension secondary to arteriosclerotic renal artery occlusive disease is the most common form of correctable hypertension. The proper selection of patients for interventional therapy is most important, be it for a conventional surgical reconstructive procedure or for endovascular percutaneous transluminal angioplasty. Controversy exists regarding both the appropriate means of establishing a diagnosis of renin-mediated, renovascular hypertension as well as the best method of therapy once the disease is recognized.[22,26-28,36] Nevertheless, the use of multiple criteria to identify occlusive renal artery disease and the ease of newer catheter-based interventions with less early morbidity has caused dramatic changes in treating patients with renovascular hypertension.[14] The impact of this new technology is of importance to both health care agencies and physician providers.

The number of patients discharged from U.S. hospitals with a diagnosis of renal artery arteriosclerosis and renovascular hypertension has increased 43% from 1988 to 2001.[14] During this same period, while there was only a 17% increase in the overall number of individuals over the age of 65—from 30 million in 1988 to 35 million in 2001—the proportion of patients undergoing renal revascularization has increased 67%. Importantly, the type of intervention has also dramatically shifted from an open surgical revascularization to a catheter-based intervention. In addition, percutaneous catheter-based interventions are increasingly associated with an older population and a higher disease acuity. The association of nonwhite race to increased likelihood of catheter-based intervention may result from demographic characteristics of populations near tertiary care centers where this technology is accessible.

Hospital charges have increased in the catheter-based treatment group, reflecting the greater utilization of this technology, and are approaching inpatient charges for isolated renal revascularizations.[14] It is notable that these charges do not include radiographic studies commonly performed in follow-up of these patients. In addition, these charges do not include those accompanying late endovascular failures. This suggests that the potential exists for the cost of catheter-based therapy of renal artery arteriosclerosis to eclipse that of conventional surgical repair.

Length of stay has decreased significantly in each treatment group, despite trends toward poorer outcomes.[14] It is possible that the poorer outcomes observed in more recent years reflected increasing technical savvy and application of these technologies to sicker patients, a likelihood supported by the fact that the Romano-Charleson comorbidity index increased significantly over the time period of the study (data not shown). A confounding factor in length of stay analysis was the lack of information on length of time from admission to procedure. It was assumed that all procedures in this study occurred at admission.[52]

Conventional surgical renal revascularization procedures carry the potential for significant morbidity and mortality, especially when combined with aortic reconstructions. Mortality in this setting was 5.2% for patients treated from 1988 to 2001.[14] The mortality of isolated catheter-based intervention during that time was 0.8%, less than the 2% associated with open surgical repair.[14] Nevertheless, serious complications may be associated with angioplasty and stenting, perhaps related to the treatment of patients with more extensive renal artery pathology. Perhaps better preintervention data would be helpful in determining which patients are most likely to benefit.[28] A recent study by Sharafuddin documented the use of the resistive index as a good predictor of who would most likely benefit from angioplasty and stent placement for renal artery stenosis.[53] It is incumbent on the physician to carefully evaluate each particular patient and choose therapy appropriate for that individual.

Administrative database limitations are offset in studies such as the current one by strengths such as large patient volumes, hard clinical endpoints like mortality, and an opportunity to evaluate practice trends across all levels of practice. However, administrative databases are poor in providing long term follow-up and efficacy of therapy. For example, data regarding reintervention rates for endovascular treatment of renal artery stenosis is notoriously lacking.

Many medical specialties, particularly surgery, have witnessed an accelerating introduction of new technology over the past decade. The quick pace of change has affected vascular surgery in particular, with the increasing application of endovascular therapy for many common vascular diseases. Percutaneous angioplasty and stenting to treat peripheral occlusive disease, placement of endovascular grafts to treat abdominal aortic aneurysms, and, most recently, angioplasty and stenting for treating carotid stenosis has profoundly changed the specialty of vascular surgery.[19,29,54]

Previous studies have documented increased utilization of percutaneous angioplasty and stenting for the treatment of peripheral occlusive disease. Tunis and colleagues demonstrated that despite an increase in use of such less invasive techniques, the rate of peripheral bypass surgery increased.[19] It is not uncommon to observe an increase in the overall number of procedures being done after the dissemination of the less invasive technology, as witnessed by laparoscopic procedures becoming commonplace therapy for many nonvascular diseases. The same phenomena appear to occur in the treatment of renovascular hypertension and renal artery stenosis where there has been a moderate increase in diagnosis but an explosion in the number of procedures, primarily endovascular to treat this disease.

CONCLUSIONS

Diffusion of innovations has been widely studied by others who have provided insight into apparent variations accompanying the adoption of new technology. A new medical treatment tends to spread at varying rates depending on certain attributes of the innovation including its *relative advantage* compared to traditional treatment. Nonsurgeons and teaching hospitals, more than others, appear to have embraced this newer technology. The less invasive catheter-based treatment of renal artery stenosis with its significantly improved short-term outcomes, especially with use of stents compared to renal artery bypass and endarterectomy, is very attractive to clinicians.[55-58] Such short-term outcomes, even more so than long-term outcomes, are likely to influence the lowering of the threshold to treat a patient by endovascular means. The cost benefits in the short term may not persist in the long term, and only further follow-up of patients treated in a randomized study will define this aspect of endolumi-nal therapy of renovascular hypertension.

REFERENCES

1. Stanley JC. Surgical treatment of renovascular hypertension. *Am J Surg.* 1997;174:102–110.1.
2. Louie J, Isaacson JA, Zierler RE, Bergelin RO, Strandness DE Jr. Prevalence of carotid and lower extremity arterial disease in patients with renal artery stenosis. *Am J Hypertens.* 1994;7:436–439.
3. Missouris CG, Buckenham T, Cappuccio FP, MacGregor GA. Renal artery stenosis: a common and important problem in patients with peripheral vascular disease. *Am J Med.* 1994; 96:10–14.
4. Valentine RJ, Clagett GP, Miller GL, et al. The coronary risk of unsuspected renal artery stenosis. *J Vasc Surg.* 1993;18:433–439.
5. Valentine RJ, Martin JD, Myers SI, et al. Asymptomatic celiac and superior mesenteric artery stenoses are more prevalent among patients with unsuspected renal artery stenoses. *J Vasc Surg.* 1991;14:195–199.
6. Novick AC, Zaki S, Goldfarb D, Hodge EE. Epidemiologic and clinical comparison of renal artery stenosis in black patients and white patients. *J Vasc Surg.* 1994;20:1–5.
7. Allen BT, Rubin BG, Anderson CB, et al. Simultaneous surgical management of aortic and renovascular disease. *Am J Surg.* 1993;166:726–732.
8. Cherr GS, Hansen KJ, Craven TE, et al. Surgical management of atherosclerotic renovascular disease. *J Vasc Surg.* 2002;35:236–245.
9. Darling RC 3rd, Shah DM, Chang BB, Leather RP. Does concomitant aortic bypass and renal artery revascularization using the retroperitoneal approach increase perioperative risk? *Cardiovasc Surg.* 1995;3:421–423.
10. Erdoes LS, Berman SS, Hunter GC, Mills JL. Comparative analysis of percutaneous transluminal angioplasty and operation for renal revascularization. *Am J Kidney Diseases.* 1996;27:496–503.
11. Kulbaski MJ, Kosinski AS, Smith RB 3rd, et al. Concomitant aortic and renal artery reconstruction in patients on an intensive antihypertensive medical regimen: long-term outcome. *Ann Vasc Surg.* 1998;12:270–277.
12. Poulias GE, Skoutas B, Doundoulakis N, et al. Surgical treatment of renovascular hypertension and respective late results. A twenty years experience. *J Cardio Surg.* 1991;32:69–75.
13. van Bockel JH, van Schilfgaarde R, Felthuis W, et al. Influence of preoperative risk factors and the surgical procedure on surgical mortality in renovascular hypertension. *Am J Surg.* 1988;155:770–775.

14. Knipp BS, Dimick JB, Eliason JL, et al. Diffusion of new technology for the treatment of renovascular hypertension in the United States: Surgical revascularization versus catheter-based therapy, 1988-2001. *J Vasc Surg*. 2004;40:717–723.

15. Weibull H, Bergqvist D, Bergentz SE, et al. Percutaneous transluminal renal angioplasty versus surgical reconstruction of atherosclerotic renal artery stenosis: A prospective randomized study. *J Vasc Surg*. 1993;18:841–852.

16. Berwick DM. Disseminating innovations in health care. *JAMA*. 2003;289:1969–1975.

17. Gelijns AC, Fendrick AM. The dynamics of innovation in minimally invasive therapy. *Health Policy*. 1993;23:153–166.

18. Tunis SR, Gelband H. Health care technology in the United States. *Health Policy*. 1994;30: 335–396.

19. Tunis SR, Bass EB, Steinberg EP. The use of angioplasty, bypass surgery, and amputation in the management of peripheral vascular disease. *N Engl J Med*. 1991;325:556–562.

20. Tunis SR, Bass EB, Klag MJ, Steinberg EP. Variation in utilization of procedures for treatment of peripheral arterial disease. A look at patient characteristics. *Arch Intern Med*. 1993; 153:991–998.

21. Gr,ntzig A, Kuhlmann U, Vetter W, Lutolf U, Meier B, Siegenthaler W. Treatment of renovascular hypertension with percutaneous transluminal dilatation of a renal-artery stenosis. *Lancet*. 1978;1:801–802.

22. Ayerdi J and Hodgson WJ. Balloon angioplasty and stenting for renovascular occlusive disease. *Persp Vasc Surg Endovasc Ther*. 2004;16:25–42.

23. Leertouwer TC, Gussenhoven EJ, Bosch JL, et al. Stent placement for renal arterial stenosis: where do we stand? A meta-analysis. *Radiology*. 2000;216:78–85.

24. Kwolek CJ. Endovascular management of renal artery stenosis: current techniques and results. *Persp Vasc Surg Endovasc Ther*. 2004;16:261–279.

25. Axelrod DA, Fendrick AM, Carlos RC, et al. Percutaneous stenting of incidental unilateral renal artery stenosis: Decision analysis of costs and benefits. *J Endovasc Ther*. 2003; 10:546–556.

26. Ives NJ, Wheatley K, Stowe RL, et al. Continuing uncertainty about the value of percutaneous revascularization in atherosclerotic renovascular disease: a meta-analysis of randomized trials. *Nephrol Dial Transplant*. 2003;18:298–304.

27. Mwipatayi BP, Beningfield SJ, White LE, et al. A review of the current treatment of renal artery stenosis. *Eur J Vasc Endovasc Surg*. 2005;29:479–488.

28. Rocha-Singh KJ, Mishkel GJ, Katholi et al. Clinical predictors of improved long-term blood pressure control after successful stenting of hypertensive patients with obstructive renal artery atherosclerosis. *Catheter Cardiovasc Interv*.1999;47:167–172.

29. Henry M, Amor M, Henry I, et al. Stent placement in the renal artery: Three-year experience with the Palmaz stent. *J Vasc Intervent Radiol*. 1996;7:343–350.

30. Blum U, Krumme B, Flugel P, et al. Treatment of ostial renal artery stenoses with vascular endoprostheses after unsuccessful balloon angioplasty. *N Engl J Med*. 1997;336:459–465.

31. Wong JM, Hansen KJ, Oskin TC, et al. Surgery after failed percutaneous renal artery angioplasty. *J Vasc Surg*. 1999;30:468–482.

32. Anderson CA, Hansen KJ, Benjamin ME, et al. Renal artery fibromuscular dysplasia: results of current surgical therapy. *J Vasc Surg*. 1995;22:207–215.

33. Cambria RP, Brewster DC, L'Italien G, et al. Simultaneous aortic and renal artery reconstruction: evolution of an eighteen-year experience. *J Vasc Surg*. 1995;21:916–925.

34. Cherr GS, Hansen KJ, Craven TE, et al. Surgical management of atherosclerotic renovascular disease. *J Vasc Surg*. 2002;35:236–245.

35. Hansen KJ, Starr SM, Sands RE, et al. Contemporary surgical management of renovascular disease. *J Vasc Surg*. 1992; 16:319–330.

36. Hansen KJ, Wilson DB, and Edward MS. Surgical revascularization of atherosclerotic renovascular disease: State of the art. *Persp Vasc Surg Endovasc Ther*. 2004;16:281–298.

37. Murray SP, Kent KC, Salvatierra O, Stoney RJ. Complex branch renovascular disease: management options and late results. *J Vasc Surg*. 1994;20:338–345.

38. Stanley JC. The evolution of surgery for renovascular occlusive disease. *Cardiovasc Surg.* 1994;2:195–202.

39. Stanley JC, Whitehouse WM Jr, Zelenock GB, et al. Reoperation for complications of renal artery reconstructive surgery undertaken for treatment of renovascular hypertension. *J Vasc Surg.*1985;2:133–144.

40. Cambria RP, Brewster DC, L'Italien GJ, et al. The durability of different reconstructive tech *J Vasc Surg.* 1994;20:76–85.

41. Khauli RB, Novick AC, Ziegelbaum M. Splenorenal bypass in the treatment of renal artery stenosis: experience with 69 cases. *J Vasc Surg.* 1985;2:547–551.

42. Moncure AC, Brewster DC, Darling RC, et al. Use of the splenic and hepatic arteries for renal revascularization. *J Vasc Surg.* 1986;3:196–203.

43. Dougherty MJ, Hallett JW Jr, Naessens J, et al. Renal endarterectomy vs. bypass for combined aortic and renal reconstruction: is there a difference in clinical outcome? *Ann Vasc Surg.* 1995;9:87–94.

44. McNeil JW, String ST, Pfeiffer RB Jr. Concomitant renal endarterectomy and aortic reconstruction. *J Vasc Surg.* 1994;20:331–336.

45. Stoney RJ, Messina LM, Goldstone J, Reilly LM. Renal endarterectomy through the transected aorta: a new technique for combined aortorenal arteriosclerosis-a preliminary report. *J Vasc Surg.* 1989;9:224–233.

46. Marone LK, and Cambria RP. Revascula.rization for renal function retrieval? Which patients will benefit? *Persp Vasc Surg Endovasc Ther.* 2004;16:258–260.

47. Hansen KJ, Cherr GS, Craven TE, et al. Management of ischemic nephropathy: Dialysis-free survival after surgical repair. *J Vasc Surg.* 2000;32:472–482.

48. Nationwide Inpatient Sample (NIS). Agency for Health Care Policy and Research, Rockville, MD. Available from: URL:http://www.ahcpr.gov/data/hcup/nisbroch.htm.

49. Charlson ME, Pompei P, Ales KL, MacKenzie CR. A new method for classifying prognostic comorbidity in longitudinal studies: development and validation. *J Chronic Dis.* 1987; 40:373–383.

50. Deyo RA, Cherkin DC, Ciol MA. Adapting a clinical comorbidity index for use with ICD-9-CM administrative databases. *J Clin Epidemiol.* 1992;45:613–619.

51. Romano PS, Roos LL, Jollis JG. Adapting a clinical comorbidity index for use with ICD-9-CM administrative data: differing perspectives. *J Clin Epidemiol.* 1993;46:1075–1079.

52. Sivamurthy N, Surowiec SM, Culakova E, et al. Divergent outcomes after percutaneous therapy for symptomatic renal artery stenosis. *J Vasc Surg.* 2004;39:565–74.

53. Sharafuddin MJ, Raboi CA, Abu-Yousef M, et al. Renal artery stenosis: duplex US after angioplasty and stent placement. *Radiology.* 2001;220:168–73.

54. Finlayson SR, Birkmeyer JD, Fillinger MF, Cronenwett JL. Should endovascular surgery lower the threshold for repair of abdominal aortic aneurysms? *J Vasc Surg.* 1999;29:973–985.

55. Plouin PF, Chatellier G, Darne B, Raynaud A. Blood pressure outcome of angioplasty in atherosclerotic renal artery stenosis: A randomized trial. Essai Multicentrique Medicaments vs Angioplastie (EMMA) Study Group. *Hypertension.* 1998;31:823–829.

56. van de Ven PJ, Kaatee R, Beutler JJ, et al. Arterial stenting and balloon angioplasty in ostial atherosclerotic renovascular disease: A randomized trial. *Lancet.* 1999;353:282–286.

57. van Jaarsveld BC, Krijnen P, Pieterman H, et al. The effect of balloon angioplasty on hypertension in atherosclerotic renal-artery stenosis. Dutch Renal Artery Stenosis Intervention Cooperative Study Group. *N Engl J Med.* 2000;342:1007–1014.

58. Webster J, Marshall F, Abdalla M, et al. Randomised comparison of percutaneous angioplasty vs continued medical therapy for hypertensive patients with atheromatous renal artery stenosis. Scottish and Newcastle Renal Artery Stenosis Collaborative Group. *J Human Hypertens.* 1998;12:329–s335.

Mesenteric Ischemia

49

Management of Mesenteric Ischemia in the Elderly

Kenneth T. Piercy, M.D., Matthew S. Edwards, M.D., and David B. Wilson, M.D.

Mesenteric ischemia in the elderly may present with acute, chronic, or acute-on-chronic symptoms. All three of these conditions are interrelated and frequently diagnosed late in their course secondary to symptom complexes that overlap those of more common abdominal conditions. Acute and acute-on-chronic mesenteric ischemia (AMI) are uncommon causes of acute abdominal pain that rapidly progress to intestinal gangrene and patient death if untreated. Chronic mesenteric ischemia (CMI) is a similarly uncommon cause of chronic postprandial abdominal pain that may progress to patient death from inanition or acute mesenteric ischemia if uncorrected. This chapter provides a review of the pathophysiology, prevalence, demographics, current treatment options, and outcomes for AMI and CMI focusing on recent data published by our group and others.

PATHOPHYSIOLOGY AND PRESENTATION

Acute Mesenteric Ischemia (AMI) can be broadly classified into four etiologies: arterioembolic, arteriothrombotic, venoocclusive, and nonocclusive. AMI has a classic but nonetheless vague pattern of presentation, and can be difficult to recognize. The classic presentation consists of abdominal pain out of proportion to physical exam findings with an acute or subacute onset. Other associated symptoms frequently include nausea, anorexia, fever, expulsive activity (vomiting or diarrhea), melena, and hema-tochezia. If the diagnosis is delayed and intestinal infarction has occurred, patients may present with peritoneal signs and/or hypotension.[1]

Arterioembolic AMI accounts for roughly 50% of AMI cases with reported series ranging from 28% to 60%.[1-9] The heart is the most common source of embolic material with etiologies including inadequately anticoagulated atrial fibrillation, mural thrombus of the left ventricle, valvular disease or replacement, atrial myxoma, and paradoxical emboli. Other sources include thoracic aortic plaques and aneurysms. Thus, a high index of suspicion must be present in the evaluation of any patient presenting with acute abdominal pain and a history of cardiac arrhythmia, recent myocardial infarction, cardiomyopathy, or valvular heart disease. The superior mesenteric artery (SMA) is the most commonly affected mesenteric artery, due to its higher blood flow in comparison to the celiac and inferior mesenteric arteries (IMA). Emboli tend to lodge distal to the takeoff of the middle colic artery where the SMA narrows. This produces an angiographic pattern of a short stump of SMA ending in an abrupt occlusion (Figures 49–1 and 49–2) and the classic clinical pattern of proximal jejunal sparing at laparotomy. Synchronous embolization of other vascular beds (lower extremity, upper extremity, cerebral, and so forth) is common. A recent report by our group has described an experience in which 10 of 32 patients (31%) with arterioembolic AMI had synchronous embolization. Nine of these cases (90%) involved embolization of the lower extremities.[1]

Arteriothrombotic AMI accounts for approximately 25% of AMI cases with reported series ranging from 8.5% to 64%.[1-10] It is preceded in 20%–60% of patients by prior symptoms of CMI manifest as postprandial abdominal pain and weight loss (hence the term acute-on-chronic mesenteric ischemia).[1,2] Multiple mesenteric vessels are diseased and frequently occluded in the vast majority of cases.[1] Mesenteric atheroslcerosis tends to be ostial, thus thrombotic lesions are observed angiographically to be "flush" with the aortic takeoff (Figures 49–3 and 49–4) in contradistinction to the previously described pattern for embolic occlusions. Prior to the onset of arteriothrombotic AMI, atherosclerotic disease of the mesenteric vessels may also be asymptomatic.

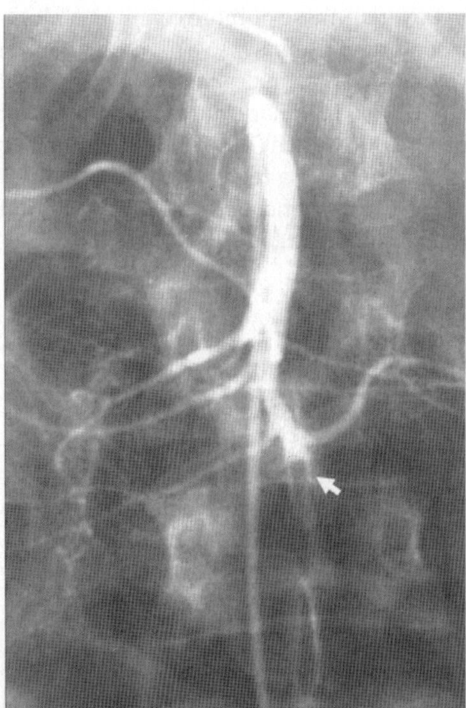

Figure 49-1. Selective angiogram revealing acute embolic occlusion of the SMA (arrow)

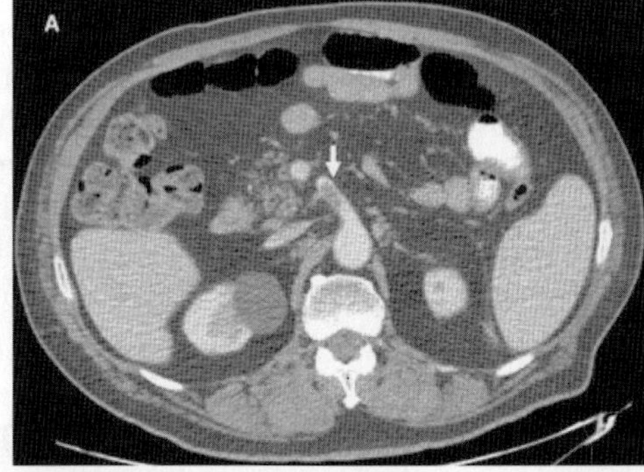

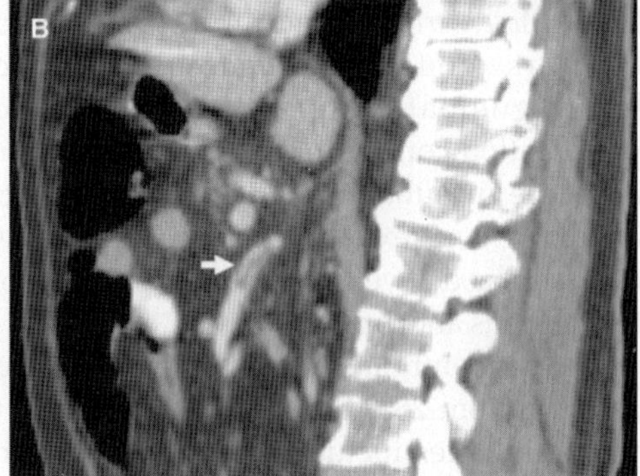

Figures 49-2. CT angiogram, transverse **A.** and sagittal **B.** views, revealing acute embolic occlusion of the SMA (arrows)

The lack of symptoms is likely due the slow progression of stenoses allowing for the development of collateral flow pathways. Stenoses of the celiac axis or SMA may be compensated for by flow through the pancreaticoduodenal arteries as well as from the IMA via the Arc of Riolan and the marginal artery systems (Figure 49–5). AMI is produced in this setting by an acute arterial occlusion that renders existing collateral flow inadequate to meet the resting metabolic demands of the viscera.

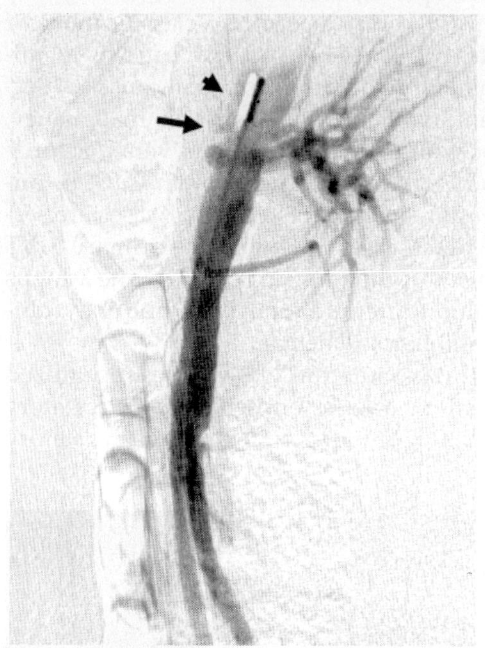

Figure 49-3. Lateral aortogram revealing thrombosis of the celiac artery (short arrow) and SMA (long arrow)

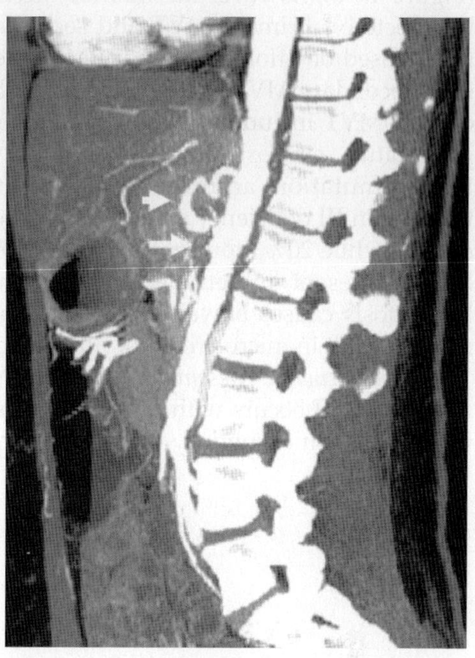

Figure 49-4. CT angiogram sagittal view revealing thrombotic occlusion of the SMA (long arrow) and atherosclerotic stenosis of the celiac artery (short arrow)

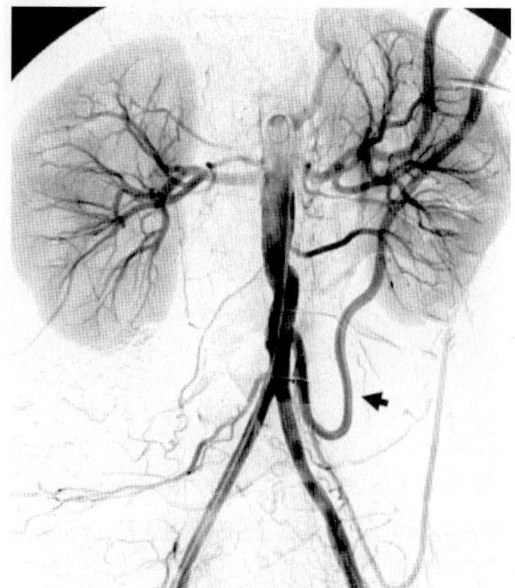

Figure 49-5. Anterioposterior aortogram of a patient with celiac artery and SMA stenoses with collateral flow via the IMA through a well developed meandering mesenteric artery (arrow)

Mesenteric Venous Thrombosis (MVT) is a rare entity representing 5%–15% of all recognized cases of AMI.[10] MVT has been increasingly recognized over the last 10–15 years due to the frequent use of infused CT scanning in the evaluation of acute abdominal pain. MVT may present differently from the other forms of AMI. Patients may complain of diffuse intermittent abdominal pain lasting several days or weeks. The pain may be of lesser severity than that seen with acute arterial occlusive mesenteric occlusion.[11] MVT involves thrombosis of the superior mesenteric vein in 95% of cases (Figure 49–6); however the inferior mesenteric, splenic, and/or portal veins may also be affected.[10] Primary MVT and secondary MVT comprise the two classifications of MVT based on etiology. Primary MVT denotes MVT when no specific cause is identified. Secondary MVT describes MVT with an identified cause. Common causes of secondary MVT include hypercoagulable and inflammatory states such as malignancy, pancreatitis, cirrhosis, hypovolemia, thrombocytopenia, polycythemia vera, Factor V Leiden mutation, antiphospholipid antibody syndrome, and protein C, S, or antithrombin III deficiency states.[12] It has been estimated that 80% of MVT cases are secondary while 20% represent primary MVT.[12] Many cases designated as primary MVT likely represent unidentified hypercoagulable and inflammatory states. The venous thrombosis causes bowel edema that can inhibit arterial blood flow, and may ultimately result in microcirculatory thrombosis and frank ischemia.

Nonobstructive Mesenteric Ischemia (NOMI) accounts for 20%–30% of recognized AMI.[10] NOMI occurs with patent major mesenteric arteries but with microcirculatory hypoperfusion secondary to vasoconstriction (Figure 49–7).[13] The microcirculatory

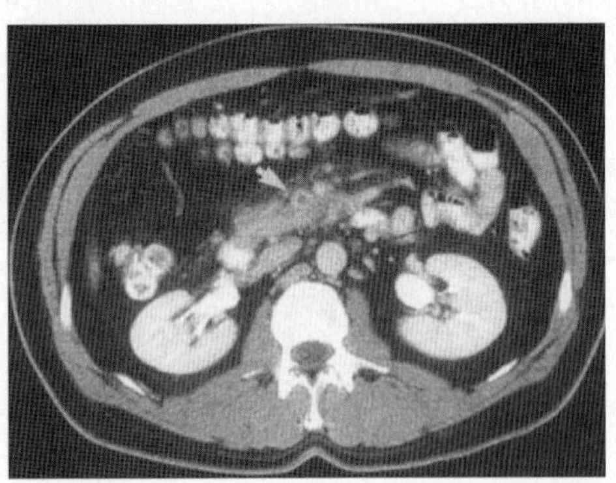

Figure 49-6. Contrast enhanced CT revealing thrombus within the superior mesenteric vein (arrow)

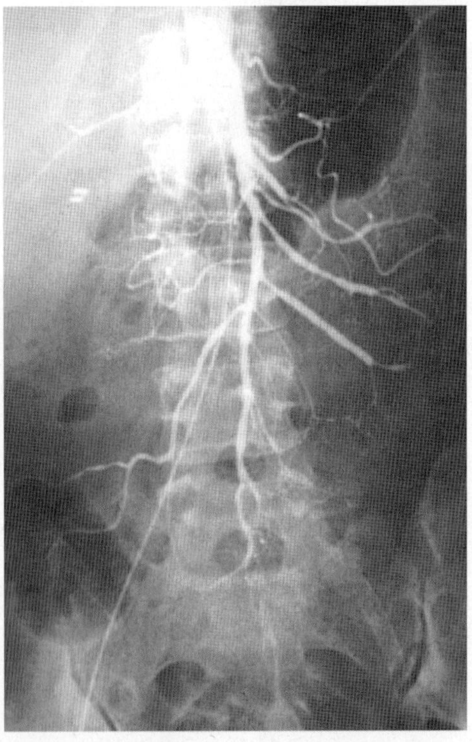

Figure 49-7. Selective angiogram revealing vasospasm of the SMA and its branches

hypoperfusion is typically secondary to low flow states of cardiogenic, septic, or hypovolemic shock, often in the setting of inotropic vasopressor administration. If this microcirculatory hypoperfusion is uncorrected, infarction may result within hours. Other etiologies include vasospasm secondary to vasoactive compounds such as cocaine, methamphetamine, and ergot alkaloids.

Chronic Mesenteric Ischemia (CMI) leads to hypoperfusion of the bowel in response to post-prandial increases in metabolic demand.[14] The two most common forms of CMI described are occlusive atherosclerotic disease of the mesenteric arteries and "Arcuate Ligament Compression Syndrome." Other conditions that may affect the mesenteric circulation resulting in chronic ischemia include neurofibromatosis, fibromuscular dysplasia, mesenteric arterial dissection, radiation exposure, and arteritidies such as Takayasu's disease.

Ninety-five percent of CMI cases are due to atherosclerotic stenoses or occlusions of the mesenteric arteries (Figure 49–8).[15] Individuals who have undergone previous bowel resection may be more likely to develop symptoms due to interruption of collateral pathways.

Patients with CMI usually have a long-term history of abdominal pain that goes undiagnosed or misdiagnosed for many years. Classic symptoms include ill-defined postprandial epigastric abdominal pain that occurs 30–45 minutes after meals and lasts for several hours. Patients may also experience nausea, vomiting, and changes in their bowel function. Symptoms of CMI are usually only present if at least two of the three (celiac, SMA, or IMA) mesenteric arteries develop critical stenoses or occlusions.[16] It is common for these patients to have undergone extensive workup (and frequently operation) for diagnoses of peptic ulcer disease, gastroesophageal reflux disease, cholelithiasis, biliary dyskinesia, and intra-abdominal adhesions. Patients may develop fear of eating due to the post-prandial pain and severely restrict their caloric intake. This results in malnutrition and weight loss. Patients exhibiting such findings are often suspected of having occult malignancies.

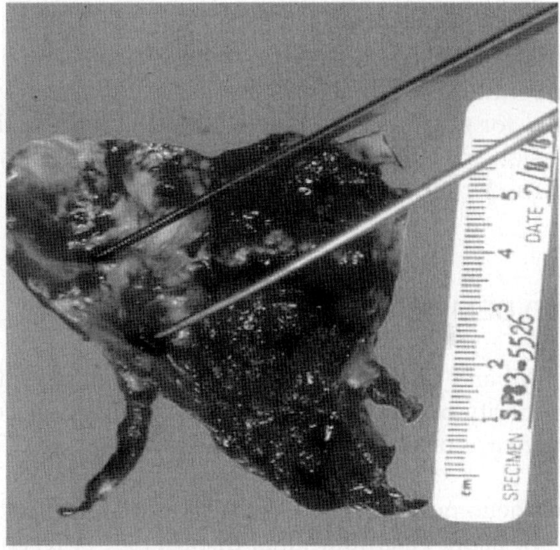

Figure 49-8. Endarterectomised aortic plaque with display of the celiac artery and SMA orifices

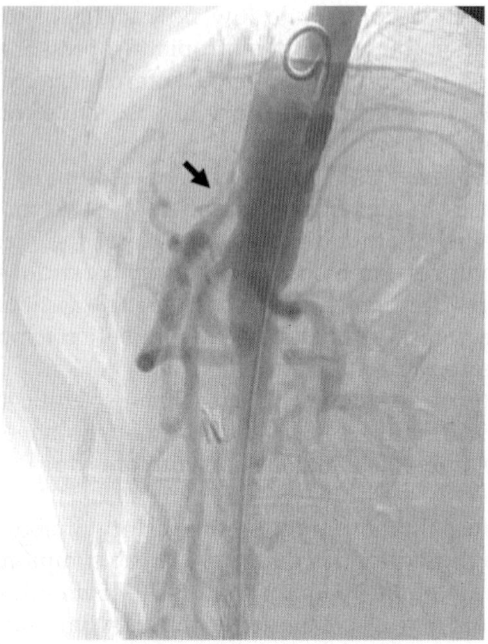

Figure 49-9. Endarterectomised aortic plaque with display of the celiac artery and SMA orifices

Arcuate ligament compression syndrome, in which the median arcuate ligament compresses the celiac axis resulting in stenosis, is a less understood entity (Figure 49–9). Patients have nonspecific postprandial complaints of nausea, vomiting, abdominal pain, and abdominal cramping. The pathophysiology of the process is poorly understood and many experts question its very existence. Some feel the symptoms may be secondary to entrapment of the celiac ganglion splanchnic nerve fibers at the aortic hiatus and are unrelated to compression of the celiac artery.[17] Recognition of this disorder also refutes the notion that two of the three main visceral arterial systems need to be affected for symptoms to manifest. Individuals with symptomatic arcuate ligament compression are predominately women and are typically much younger than patients with atherosclerotic forms of CMI.[18]

INCIDENCE AND DEMOGRAPHICS

The incidence of AMI and CMI are unknown and difficult to establish (or even estimate) due to the relative rarity of these conditions. This difficulty is compounded by the fact that these disorders are often misdiagnosed or undiagnosed in the general medical community.

AMI is a rare phenomenon estimated to account for approximately 1%–2% of hospital admissions for acute gastrointestinal disorders.[19] A recent study employing autopsy data demonstrated an incidence of 5.3–8.6 per 100,000 for AMI secondary to thromboembolic occlusion of the SMA.[20-21] Stoney et al. have observed an incidence of one in 1,000 hospital admissions at a tertiary academic medical center.[5] An overall incidence of one in every 5,000 hospital admissions has been reported for NOMI while additional autopsy data has demonstrated an incidence of 1.8 per 100,000 for MVT with intestinal infarction.[5,22] These data are obviously extremely limited by selection biases; however, they do reinforce the commonly held notion that AMI is an uncommon condition.

CMI, like AMI, is also an uncommon entity. No solid estimates of prevalence for clinically apparent CMI exist. Extrapolating the National Inpatient Sample data analyzed by Derrow et al.,[23] one can estimate that approximately 350 mesenteric revascularizations are performed each year in the United States for recognized CMI, making this condition a rarely recognized one. Potentially causative anatomic occlusive disease of the visceral vessels is much more common. Various studies of unselected autopsies have revealed some degree of mesenteric artery stenoses in 30%–80% of patients with an increasing frequency among older age groups. However, a minority (15%) of individuals in these studies have demonstrated evidence of two or more mesenteric arterial stenoses.[24-25] When encountered during autopsy, the mean degree of stenoses reported are 20%–50% for the celiac artery, 30%–40% for the SMA, and 30%–90% for the IMA with very few cases associated with evidence of antemortem gastrointestinal symptoms.[24-25] Similar findings have been made by angiographic studies among asymptomatic patients. In patients with moderate to severe stenoses of the mesenteric arteries detected during evaluation for other reasons, angiographic studies have revealed that the celiac artery was diseased in 96% of cases, while the SMA and IMA were less frequently diseased (50% and 57% of cases, respectively). Only 6% of patients later went on to develop symptoms of CMI and all who did demonstrated multiple diseased mesenteric vessels.[26]

Our group has recently published the only population-based prevalence data concerning anatomic mesenteric arterial stenosis.[27] As part of the multicenter Cardiovascular Health Study, 553 individuals over the age of 65 years agreed to undergo visceral duplex sonography. Ninety-seven participants (17.5%) demonstrated evidence of mesenteric artery stenosis. The vast majority of detected lesions (n = 83) were isolated celiac stenoses with SMA stenosis present in only 12 participants (2.2%). Multivessel disease (celiac and SMA) was observed in only seven individuals (1.3%). No participant reported any symptoms consistent with CMI during follow-up. These prevalence data are unique and support the commonly held view that CMI is a rare condition, especially when combined with the data referenced above emphasizing the necessity of multivessel involvement in the production of symptoms.[26]

Demographically, individuals presenting with AMI and CMI are strikingly similar (Tables 49–1 and 49–2). Patients presenting with AMI are typically 70 years of age or older with a female to male preponderance of 2–3:1.[13,4,20] The female to male preponderance is more pronounced among individuals with thrombotic AMI.[1] Similarly, individuals treated for CMI have an average age of 65 years and a female preponderance (3–5: 1) similar to that observed for thrombotic AMI, which is no surprise given the shared etiology.[23,28-29] Patients with AMI or CMI frequently demonstrate a myriad of preexisting comorbidities including hypertension, peripheral vascular disease, chronic pulmonary disease, coronary artery disease, carotid artery disease, diabetes, chronic renal insufficiency, congestive heart failure, and tobacco abuse.[1,3-4,20,28-29]

TABLE 49-1. ACUTE MESENTERIC ISCHEMIA: PATIENT DEMOGRAPHICS AND MEDICAL RISK FACTORS*

Variable	Thrombotic Occlusion (n = 44) [n (%)]	Embolic Occlusion (n = 32) [n (%)][n (%)]
Gender		
Male	11 (25)	12 (38)
Female	33 (75)	20 (62)
Mean age (years ± SE)	66 ± 12	70 ± 14
Race		
Caucasian	38 (87)	28 (88)
African American	5 (11)	4 (12)
Other	1 (2)	0 (0)
Coronary artery disease	27 (61)	22 (69)
Congestive heart failure	11 (25)	7 (22)
History of tobacco use	31 (70)	21 (66)
Diabetes mellitus	11 (25)	10 (31)
Chronic renal insufficiency	13 (29)	12 (38)
Hypertension	31 (70)	23 (72)
Carotid disease	13 (30)	10 (31)
Chronic obstructive pulmonary disease	31 (70)	16 (50)

*Modified from Edwards MS, Cherr GS, Craven TE, et al. Acute occlusive mesenteric ischemia: Surgical management and outcomes. *Ann Vasc Surg* 2003;17:74.

TABLE 49-2. CHRONIC MESENTERIC ISCHEMIA: PATIENT DEMOGRAPHICS AND MEDICAL RISK FACTORS*

Variable	Chronic Mesenteric Ischemia (n = 34) [n (%)]	Acute on Chronic Mesenteric Ischemia (n = 24) [n (%)]
Gender		
Male	7 (21)	6 (25)
Female	27 (79)	18 (75)
Mean age (years ± SE)	64 ± 13	63 ± 12
Race		
Caucasian	32 (94)	20 (83)
African American	2 (6)	4 (17)
Other	0 (0)	0 (0)
Coronary artery disease	16 (47)	8 (33)
Congestive heart failure	3 (9)	5 (21)
History of tobacco use	24 (71)	17 (71)
Diabetes mellitus	5 (15)	6 (25)
Chronic renal insufficiency	4 (12)	6 (25)
Hypertension	23 (68)	14 (58)
Carotid disease	11 (32)	5 (21)
Chronic pulmonary disease	16 (47)	10 (42)

* Modified from English WP, Pearce JD, Craven TE, et al. Chronic visceral ischemia: Symptom-free survival after open surgical repair. *Vasc Endovasc Surg* 2004;38:495.

DIAGNOSIS

Acute Mesenteric Ischemia

A high index of suspicion is paramount for a timely diagnosis of AMI. As previously described, abdominal pain out of proportion to physical exam findings is the classic presentation. It cannot be overstated that any patient with severe abdominal pain in the presence of advanced age, generalized atherosclerosis, arrhythmia, valvular heart disease, or hypercoagulable state should be considered to have AMI until proven otherwise. Laboratory testing such as serum amylase, arterial pH, white blood cell count, and lactic acid levels are frequently abnormal, but they are highly nonspecific and do little to confirm the presence of AMI. Early imaging studies usually performed include plain film X-rays. Suggestive findings on such studies include a thickened bowel wall and a "ground glass appearance" of the abdomen.[30] Abdominal computed tomography (CT) scanning with intravenous contrast is an extremely useful diagnostic tool in the diagnosis of AMI. CT scanning may also reveal findings of bowel wall thickening, the presence of ascites, occlusion of mesenteric vessels, or other causes of the patient's presentation. CT scanning is particularly useful in the diagnosis of MVT.[31] In centers where CT arteriography quality imaging is readily available, CT scanning can be the single test of choice in the diagnosis of AMI (Figures 49–2, 49–4, and 49–6). In other instances, prompt selective mesenteric angiography is the method of choice. Mesenteric arteriography with AP and lateral views remains the gold standard for diagnosis of AMI (Figures 49–1, 49–3, and 49–7). An additional advantage of mesenteric angiography is the potential for immediate therapeutic measures such as the installation of intra-arterial vasodilators or performance of angioplasty/stenting.

Chronic Mesenteric Ischemia

As with AMI, a high index of suspicion is also important in the diagnosis of CMI. In patients presenting with postprandial pain, aversion to food, and weight loss, CMI should be high on the differential. This is particularly true if such a history is accompanied by physical findings of an abdominal bruit, advanced age, and generalized atherosclerosis. Although highly operator dependent, and sometimes hampered by patient body habitus and bowel gas content, visceral duplex sonography is an excellent noninvasive modality for evaluating patients suspected of having CMI.[32] The IMA is often unable to be visualized; however, velocity measurements of the celiac and SMA are usually adequate to make the diagnosis given the near uniform involvement of the SMA in symptomatic patients. CT and MR arteriography offer additional noninvasive options for the diagnosis of CMI. With this being said, arteriography remains the gold standard for the diagnosis and treatment planning of CMI. Both anteroposterior and lateral projections of the aorta are required. The anteroposterior view demonstrates the visceral collateral flow patterns while the lateral view visualizes proximal mesenteric arterial stenoses or occlusions, information important in planning operative revascularization.

TREATMENT AND OUTCOMES

Acute Mesenteric Ischemia

Treatment options for AMI vary depending on etiology. However, one critical point underlies the treatment for all varieties of AMI with that point being, prompt diagnosis and restoration of perfusion are required for optimal outcome. Assessment of bowel viability and resection as needed are the obvious corollaries of this primary tenet.

In the arterial occlusive cases of AMI, emergent operative intervention should be undertaken to revascularize ischemic bowel segments. Methods of revascularization include embolectomy with balloon catheter passage via the root of the small bowel mesentery for arterioembolic AMI, and surgical bypass or endarterectomy for arteriothrombotic AMI.[1,4] In the face of necrotic bowel, the saphenous vein is the conduit of choice for bypass revascularization due to the risk of graft infection. Bypass origination from the supraceliac aorta takes advantage of a relative absence of atherosclerotic disease in that region of the aorta to simplify anastamosis.[1] This exposure may be performed via a direct approach through the lesser sac or via a left visceral mobilization. The authors prefer a subcostal incision and visceral mobilization. Following revascularization, a conservative approach to bowel resection should be undertaken in order to preserve as much bowel as possible. Our group leaves stapled bowel ends to preserve as much length as possible, and avoids the early creation of anastamoses or stomas. A second look laparotomy at 24–72 hours following the initial procedure is strongly encouraged to reassess any questionably viable segments of bowel and reestablish continuity.[1,7] The decision to perform a second-look laparotomy should be made at the time of initial operation and adhered to.

We have recently published our institution's 10-year experience with AMI involving 76 patients.[1] Surgical management consisted of exploration alone in 16 patients who had extensive intestinal infarction believed to be incompatible with survival, bowel resection alone in 18 patients, and revascularization in 43 patients including 28 who required concomitant bowel resection. Revascularization consisted of SMA embolectomy (39.5%), aorta to celiac and SMA bypass (20.9%), single vessel SMA bypass (9.3%), patch angioplasty (7.0%), endovascular angioplasty and stenting (4.7%), and a variety of other procedures. All bypass grafts were constructed in an antegrade fashion and conduit included saphenous vein in seven patients, Dacron in six patients, and PTFE in three patients. Forty-four percent of patients underwent a second-look laparotomy and additional bowel resection was required among half of these patients. Performance of a second-look laparotomy was independently associated with improved survival. Despite aggressive management, the overall results were dismal with an in-hospital mortality rate of 62%. Furthermore, many acute event survivors (31%) required long-term parenteral nutrition. These results are similar to those in excellent reports by Endean et al.[4] and Park et al.[3]

Obviously, these results leave much room for improvement. Endovascular therapy, including angioplasty and/or stenting with or without thrombolytic therapy, has been touted as a potential source of outcome improvement. Endovascular therapy certainly offers the advantage of intervention at the time of the angiographic diagnosis, and may be a quicker means of revascularization in the hands of surgeons with limited experience exposing the perivisceral aorta. Unfortunately, endovascular treatment is very limited in the treatment of mesenteric occlusions (which are common) and does not eliminate the need for assessment of bowel viability.[1] Furthermore, long-term patency data for endovascular mesenteric angioplasty/stenting are poor. As such, we still consider surgical revascularization and assessment of bowel viability the standard treatment of AMI for arteriothrombotic and arterioembolic cases of AMI.[4]

In contradistinction to the lack of progress seen with arterial occlusive AMI, treatment outcomes for MVT have improved. This improvement is primarily due to earlier diagnosis and treatment due to the widespread use of CT scanning.[33] If identified early, prior to the presence of microcirculatory thrombosis and bowel infarction, the mainstay of MVT treatment is aggressive anticoagulation therapy with heparin and close clinical observation.[6,34] Heparin anticoagulation traditionally has been continued for seven to 10 days, followed by warfarin sodium therapy for three to six months or lifelong, depending on the underlying etiology of the thrombosis.[6,35] All MVT patients should undergo extensive evaluation for hypercoagulable and inflammatory states as possible etiologies. Recent investigations have supplemented anticoagulation with thrombolytic administration, either systemically, intra-arterially, or directly into the mesenteric veins with reasonable results. However, further controlled study of these forms of therapy is required before they can be widely recommended.[35-36] Surgical intervention in MVT patients is indicated only if bowel viability is questioned, in which case, exploration should be performed with bowel resection and a second-look procedure planned as necessary.

Treatment options for NOMI emphasize prompt correction of the underlying etiology of the low flow state. Initial steps in treatment should include vigorous fluid resuscitation, invasive cardiac monitoring as needed, and minimization of inotropic/vasopressor support when possible. Catheter-directed papaverine hydrochloride (30–60 mg/h) infusion into the SMA can be used to relieve the vasoconstriction.[11] If bowel infarction is suspected, surgical exploration is performed with a second-look laparotomy planned as needed. The papaverine infusion should be continued during and following surgery to prevent a recurrence of the vasoconstriction.[6,11] The infusion can be stopped once the patient has clinically improved and a repeat angiographic study reveals no further vasoconstriction following a 30-minute SMA infusion trial of saline alone without papaverine.[8] Treatment typically requires at least 24 hours of papaverine infusion.[8] NOMI carries a significant mortality rate largely dependant on the etiology of the causative hypoperfusion state.[37]

Chronic Mesenteric Ischemia

The goal of treatment for CMI is the restoration of normal mesenteric blood flow in order to relieve symptoms of intermittent ischemia and prevent the catastrophic complication of acute-on-chronic mesenteric ischemia. Currently, there is no justification for treating asymptomatic mesenteric arterial lesions, but these patients should be closely followed for the development of CMI symptoms. Depending on the severity and time course of a patient's CMI symptoms, correction of underlying malnutrition and dehydration with parenteral nutrition may be necessary prior to intervention. Operative repairs of many configurations have been described including mesenteric artery reimplantation, mesenteric artery or transaortic endarterectomy, and bypass grafting in antegrade or retrograde configurations using autogenous and/or prosthetic conduit.[15,38-41] As previously mentioned, our group prefers a transabdominal approach through a subcostal incision and visceral mobilization. Debate exists over whether single versus multiple vessel revascularization is the best treatment. Some suggest that a higher incidence of recurrent symptoms due to graft failure exists following single vessel revascularization.[41] Our group favors the revascularization of the celiac and SMA in all CMI patients. Currently, the most popular repairs appear to involve bypass creation using prosthetic grafts (in the absence of bowel perforation or infarction) due to less extensive dissection requirements and a lower propensity for graft kinking than that seen with saphenous vein conduits.[42] Operative mortality rates of 10%, five-year survival of 65%, and five-year symptom-free survival rates of 90% have been reported.[38,43-45]

We have recently published our institutional experience with open operative treatment among 58 patients presenting with CMI (34 patients) and acute-on-chronic mesenteric ischemia (24 patients).[28] Preoperative imaging demonstrated disease of the SMA, celiac, and IMA among 100%, 89%, and 54% of patients, respectively, with 95% of patients having multiple vessel involvement (Table 49–3). Repairs included antegrade revascularization among 55 patients utilizing bypass (88%), endarterectomy/patch angioplasty (9%), or reimplantation (3%) and retrograde revascularization among three patients. The SMA and celiac arteries were revascularized in 86% and 74% of patients, respectively, and both vessels were repaired in 58%. Bypass procedures utilized prosthetic conduits in 70% of cases. Perioperative mortality was 10% among patients with CMI and 54% with acute-on-chronic AMI with similar long-term survival observed among operative survivors (Figure 49–10). Estimated five-year primary and primary assisted patency were 81% and 89%, respectively, with symptom-free survival of 57% at 5.8 years. These results are similar to those reported by Mateo et al.[44] Collectively, these findings stress the importance of recognition and treatment of CMI preemptively before AMI occurs in these patients.

Mesenteric artery angioplasty and stenting provides an alternative to open surgical intervention with the goal of reducing morbidity and mortality. The less invasive nature of endovascular therapy is intuitively appealing to patients with CMI who often have multiple comorbidities and represent less than ideal surgical candidates. Near 100% technical success rates have been reported with respectable early results in terms of symptomatic relief (75%–90%).[46-49] However, observed periprocedural mortality was significant, and the long-term durability appears to be poor, both in terms of restenosis and symptomatic recurrence.[49,50] Endovascular therapy may play a more integral role in the treatment of CMI as more long-term studies are performed, but

TABLE 49-3. CHRONIC AND ACUTE ON CHRONIC MESENTERIC ISCHEMIA: LESION DISTRIBUTION*

Vessel Involved	Chronic Mesenteric Ischemia (n=34) [n (%)]	Acute on Chronic Mesenteric Ischemia (n=22) [n (%)]
Number		
One	2 (6)	1 (5)
Two	16 (47)	10 (45)
Three	16 (47)	11 (50)
Vessel diseased		
CA	29 (85)	21 (95)
SMA	34 (100)	22 (100)
IMA	19 (56)	11 (50)
Distribution		
CA only	0	0
SMA only	2 (6)	1 (5)
IMA only	0	0
CA and SMA	13 (38)	10 (45)
SMA and IMA	3 (9)	0
CA, SMA and IMA	16 (47)	11 (50)

CA - Celiac artery, SMA - Superior mesenteric artery, IMA - Inferior mesenteric artery

* Modified from English WP, Pearce JD, Craven TE, et al. Chronic visceral ischemia: Symptom-free survival after open surgical repair. *Vasc Endovasc Surg* 2004;38:497.

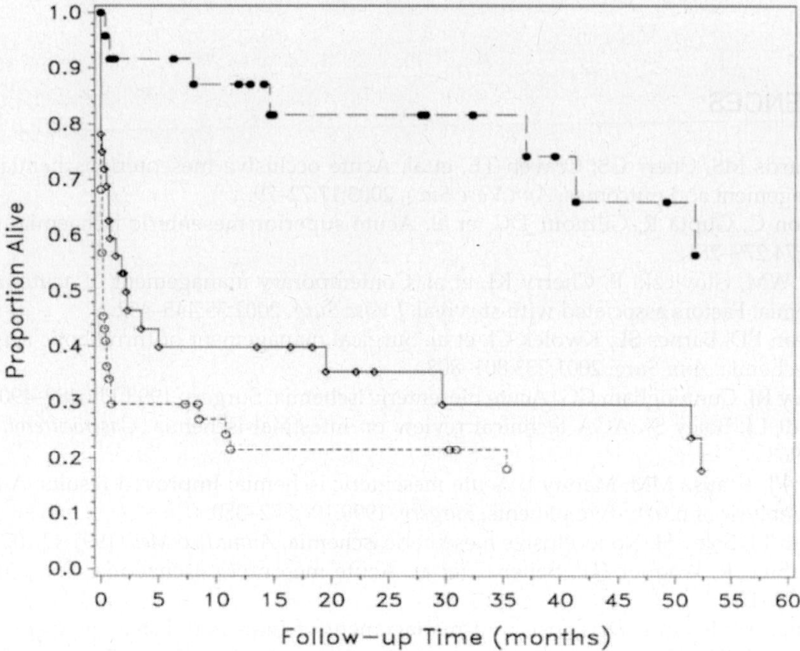

Figure 49-10. * Modified from Edwards MS, Cherr GS, Craven TE, et al. Acute occlusive mesenteric ischemia: Surgical management and outcomes. *Ann Vasc Surg.* 2003;17:76.

currently, it appears to be best utilized in individuals who are prohibitive operative risks for surgical revascularization.

Treatment of arcuate ligament compression syndrome remains controversial. The traditional therapy has been surgical division of the arcuate ligament with or without division of the celiac ganglion splanchnic nerve fibers. Reconstruction of the celiac artery is performed as needed using procedures such as reimplantation or bypass if the artery is chronically strictured.[51,52] Outcomes have been mixed. Immediate relief of symptoms has been reported to range from 85%–100%.[51,53-54] However, most of these reports describe small numbers of patients and short follow-up intervals. Three studies have provided long-term follow-up results with mean intervals of 6.3, 9, and 19.1 years. Results have been mixed with symptom recurrence in 87, 31.8, and 100% of individuals, respectively.[52-54] It is the opinion of the authors that treatment of this condition remains unproven and it should be applied only in highly selected patients.

SUMMARY

Although rare in occurrence, mesenteric ischemia can have devastating consequences if recognition and treatment are delayed. Early recognition and treatment require a high index of suspicion for AMI and CMI in the evaluation of acute and chronic abdominal pain. Currently, the prescribed treatment modalities of each are primarily surgical, especially in the case of AMI where bowel viability is an acute concern. However, endovascular therapy may become a more important treatment option as limitations are addressed.

REFERENCES

1. Edwards MS, Cherr GS, Craven TE, et al. Acute occlusive mesenteric ischemia: Surgical management and outcomes. *Ann Vasc Surg.* 2003;17:72–79.
2. Wilson C, Gupta R, Gilmour DG, et al. Acute superior mesenteric ischaemia. *Br J Surg.* 1987;74:279–281.
3. Park WM, Gloviczki P, Cherry KJ, et al. Contemporary management of acute mesenteric ischemia: Factors associated with survival. *J Vasc Surg.* 2002;35:445–452.
4. Endean ED, Barnes SL, Kwolek CJ, et al. Surgical management of thrombotic acute intestinal ischemia. *Ann Surg.* 2001;233:801–808.
5. Stoney RJ, Cunningham CG. Acute mesenteric ischemia. Surgery 1993;114:489–490.
6. Brandt LJ, Boley SJ. AGA technical review on intestinal ischemia. *Gastroenterol.* 2000;118: 954–968.
7. Levy PJ, Krausz MM, Manny J. Acute mesenteric ischemia: Improved results: A retrospective analysis of ninety-two patients. *Surgery.* 1990;107:372–380.
8. Brandt LJ, Boley SJ. Nonocclusive mesenteric ischemia. *Annu Rev Med.* 1991;42:107–117.
9. Inderbitzi R, Wagner HE, Seiler C, et al. Acute mesenteric ischaemia. *Eur J Surg.* 1992; 158:123–126.
10. Sreenarasimhaiah J. Diagnosis and management of intestinal ischaemic disorders. *BMJ.* 2003;326:1372–1376.
11. Yasuhara H. Acute mesenteric ischemia: The challenge of gastroenterology. *Surg Today.* 2005;35:185–195.
12. Abdu RA, Zakhour BJ, Dallis DJ. Mesenteric venous throumbosis 1911 to 1984. *Surgery.* 1987;101:383–388.
13. Trompeter M, Brazda T, Remy CT, et al. Non-occlusive mesenteric ischemia: Etiology, diagnosis, and interventional therapy. *Eur Radiol.* 2002;12:1179–1187.
14. Cleveland TJ, Nawaz S, Gaines PA. Mesenteric arterial ischaemia: Diagnosis and therapeutic options. *Vasc Med.* 2002;7:311–321.
15. Cunningham CG, Reilly LM, Stoney R. Chronic visceral ischemia. *Surg Clin North Am.* 1992;72:231–244.
16. Mikkelsen WP, Berne CJ. Intestinal angina. Its surgical significance. *Am J Surg.* 1957;94:262
17. Carey JP, Stemmer EA, Connolly JE. Median arcuate ligament syndrome. *Arch Surg.* 1969;99:441–446.
18. Reilly LM, Ammar AD, Stoney RJ, et al. Late results following operative repair for celiac artery compression syndrome. *J Vasc Surg.* 1985;2:79–91.
19. Schneider TA, Longo WE, Ure T, et al. Mesenteric ischemia: Acute arterial syndromes. *Dis Colon Rectum.* 1994;37:1163–1174.
20. Acosta S, ÷gren M, Sternby NH, et al. Incidence of acute thrombo-embolic occlusion of the superior mesenteric artery - A population-based study. *Eur J Vasc Endovasc Surg.* 2004;27: 45–150.
21. Acosta S, Bjârk M. Acute thrombo-embolic occlusion of the superior mesenteric artery: A prospective study in a well defined population. *Eur J Vasc Endovasc Surg.* 2003;267:179–183.
22. Acosta S, ÷gren M, Sternby NH, et al. Mesenteric venous thrombosis with transmural intestinal infarction: A population-based study. *J Vasc Surg.* 2005;41:59–63.
23. Derrow AE, Seeger JM, Dame DA, et al. The outcome in the United States after thoracobdominal aortic aneurysm repair, renal artery bypass, and mesenteric revascularization. *J Vasc Surg.* 2001;34:54–61.
24. Croft RJ, Menon FP, Marston A. Does "intestinal angina" exist? A critical study of obstructed visceral arteries. *Br J Surg* 1981;68:316–318.

25. J‰rvinen O, Laurikka J, Sisto T, et al. Atherosclerosis of the visceral arteries. *VASA*. 1995; 24:9–14.

26. Thomas JH, Blake K, Pierce GE, et al. The clinical course of asymptomatic mesenteric arterial stenosis. *J Vasc Surg*. 1998;27:840–844.

27. Hansen KJ, Wilson DB, Craven TE, et al. Mesenteric artery disease in the elderly. *J Vasc Surg*. 2004;40:45–52.

28. English WP, Pearce JD, Craven TE, et al. Chronic visceral ischemia: Symptom-free survival after open surgical repair. *Vasc Endovasc Surg*. 2004;38:493–503.

29. Moawad J, Gewertz BL. Chronic mesenteric ischemia. Clinical presentation and diagnosis. *Surg Clin N Am*. 1997;77:357–369.

30. Wolf EL, Sprayregen S, Bakal CW. Radiology in intestinal ischemia: Plain films, contrast and other imaging studies. *Surg Clin North Am*. 1992;72:104–124.

31. Bradbury MS, Kavanagh PV, Bechtold RE, et al. Mesenteric venous thrombosis: Diagnosis and noninvasive imaging. *Radiographics*. 2002;22:527–541.

32. Moneta GL. Screening for mesenteric vascular insufficiency and follow-up of mesenteric artery bypass procedures. *Semin Vasc Surg*. 2001;14:186–192.

33. Morasch MD, Ebaugh JL, Chiou AC, et al. Mesenteric venous thrombosis: A changing clinical entity. *J Vasc Surg*. 2001;34:680–684.

34. Hassan HA, Raufman JP. Mesenteric venous thrombosis. *South Med J*. 1999;92:558–562.

35. Poplausky MR, Kaufman JA, Geller SC, et al. Mesenteric venous thrombosis treated with urokinase via the superior mesenteric artery. *Gastroenterology*. 1996;110:1633–1635.

36. Train JS, Ross H, Weiss JD, et al. Mesenteric venous thrombosis: Successful treatment by intraarterial lytic therapy. *J Vasc Interv Radiol*. 1998;9:461–464.

37. Ward D, Vernava AM, Kaminski DL, et al. Improved outcome by identification of high-risk nonocclusive mesenteric ischemia, aggressive reexploration, and delayed anastomosis. *Am J Surg*. 1995;170:5777–5781.

38. Cunningham CG, Reilly LM, Rapp JH, et al. Chronic visceral ischemia. *Ann Surg*. 1991;214: 276–287.

39. Jaxheimer EC, Jewell ER, Persson AV. Chronic intestinal ischemia. *Surg Clin North Am*. 1985;64:123–130.

40. Baur GM, Millay DJ, Taylor LM, et al. Treatment of chronic visceral ischemia. *Am J Surg*. 1984;148:138–144.

41. Hollier LH, Bernatz PE, Pairolero PC, et al. Surgical management of chronic intestinal ischemia: A reappraisal. *Surgery*. 1981;90:940–946.

42. Taylor LM, Moneta GL, Porter JM. Treatment of Chronic Visceral Ischemia. In: Rutherford, ed. *Vascular Surgery 5th ed*. Denver: Saunders; 2000:1532–1541.

43. Park WM, Cherry KJ, Chua HK, et al. Current results of open revascularization for chronic mesenteric ischemia: A standard for comparison. *J Vasc Surg*. 2002;35:853–859.

44. Mateo RB, O'Hara PJ, Hertzer NR, et al. Elective surgical treatment of symptomatic chronic mesenteric occlusive disease: Early results and late outcomes. *J Vasc Surg*. 1999;29:821–832.

45. Kihara TK, Blebea J, Anderson KM, et al. Risk factors and outcomes following revascularization for chronic mesenteric ischemia. *Ann Vasc Surg*. 1999;13:37–44.

46. Maspes F, Mazzetti di Pietralata G, Gandini R, et al. Percutanious transluminal angioplasty in the treatment of chronic mesenteric ischemia: Results and 3 years of follow-up in 23 patients. *Abdom Imaging*. 1998;23:358–363.

47. Matsumoto AH, Angle JF, Spinosa DJ, et al. Percutanious transluminal angioplasty and stenting in the treatment of chronic mesenteric ischemia: Results and longterm followup. *J Am Coll Surg*. 2002;194:S22–S31.

48. Allen RC, Martin GH, Rees CR, et al. Mesenteric angioplasty in the treatment of chronic intestinal ischemia. *J Vasc Surg*. 1996;24:415–421.

49. Rose SC, Quigley TM, Raker EJ. Revascularization for chronic mesenteric ischemia: Comparison of operative arterial bypass grafting and percutaneous transluminal angioplasty. *J Vasc Interv Radiol*. 1995;6:339–349.

50. Kasirajan K, O'Hara PJ, Gray BH, et al. Chronic mesenteric ischemia: Open surgery versus percutaneous angioplasty and stenting. *J Vasc Surg*. 2001;33:63–71.

51. Takach TJ, Livesay JJ, Reul GJ, et al. Celiac compression syndrome: Tailored therapy based on intraoperative findings. *J Am Coll Surg*. 1996;183:606–610.

52. Reilly LM, Ammar AD, Stoney RJ, et al. Late results following operative repair for celiac artery compression syndrome. *J Vasc Surg*. 1985;2:79–91.

53. Geelkerken RH, van Bockel JH, de Roos WK, et al. Coeliac artery compression syndrome: The effect of decompression. *Br J Surg*. 1990;77:807–809.

54. Plate G, Eklàf B, Vang J. The celiac compression syndrome: Myth or reality? *Acta Chir Scand*. 1981;147:201–203.

50

Argument For Open Repair

William H. Pearce, M.D.

Open surgery is preferred over endovascular surgery for the treatment of mesenteric ischemia. Mesenteric ischemia is an unusual clinical problem. Because of its rarity, its diagnosis is often missed and the patient presents with catastrophic bowel infarction. The presence of intra-abdominal sepsis associated with bowel infarction may limit the utility of endovascular procedures. Bare metal stents may, in fact, become infected.[1]

Surgical revascularization has been the gold standard for the treatment of both acute and chronic mesenteric ischemia. Over the years, there has been an evolution of thinking about mesenteric ischemia and the number of vessels needed to be revascularized. In our own practice. for many years, we have used multiple visceral revascularizations as our standard procedure.[2] This procedure required a supraceliac origin of the bypass graft with distal anastomosis to the celiac and superior mesenteric arteries (SMA) (Figure 50–1). The supraceliac aorta is often chosen because of its lack of atherosclerotic plaque. However, the supraceliac aortic clamp may produce hemodynamic changes, further compromising the patient. Therefore, I have commonly preferred to use the iliac arteries as inflow when they are free of major occlusive disease (Figure 50–2).

In patients with chronic mesenteric ischemia, the therapeutic options are either endovascular repair or open surgical bypass. Endovascular treatments are attractive because of their less invasive nature. Angioplasty and stenting can be performed for both celiac and superior mesenteric artery (SMA) stenosis. However, most interventionalists have shied away from celiac artery stenting because of compression produced by the median arcuate ligament. Most stents placed in this location will occlude. In recent years, there has been a trend to perform angioplasty and stenting only for SMA stenosis in the chronic setting.[3] However, the downsides to this approach may be substantial. The SMA leaves the aorta at almost right angles to make a turn over the left renal vein. These right angles may predispose the artery to dissection. We have several patients in whom dissection has occurred in the attempt to treat total occlusions of the SMA. Dissections of the SMA make revascularization almost impossible, and clearly make a straightforward operation much more difficult. The group from Portland has recommended open revascularization of the single artery (the SMA) with excellent results.[4] We tend to agree with that position and changed our practice from multiple visceral artery revascularizations to single vessel reconstructions in most cases.

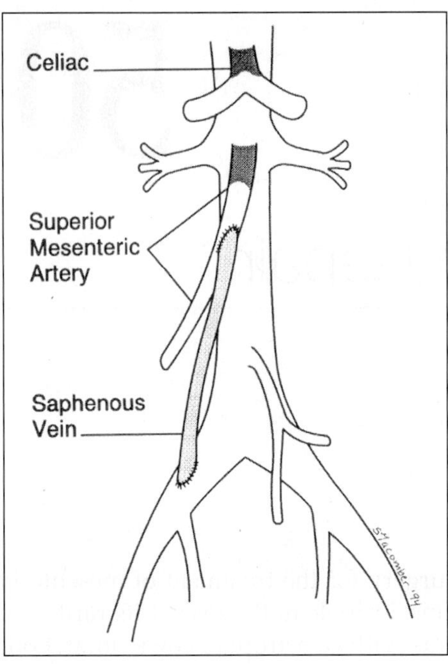

Figure 50-1. Configuration of antegrade supraceliac saphenous vein mesenteric bypass with "piggyback" technique. Note single aortic anastomosis and origin of SMA graft. From McMillan MD, McCarthy WJ, Bresticker MR, et al. Mesenteric artery bypass: Objective patency determination. *J Vasc Surg.* 1995;21:729–741. Reproduced by permission.

In patients with acute mesenteric ischemia, the situation is complicated by marginal and/or necrotic bowel. In these settings, several options are available. The first option is to perform a thrombectomy through an arteriotomy in the SMA, which if not successful, can be used as the site of the proximal anastomosis in a bypass procedure. Again, the inflow source is the iliac arteries and the conduit is autogenous saphenous vein. Recently, it has been reported that retrograde angioplasty and stenting of the SMA with patch closure can replace a venous bypass.[5] While this approach appears attractive in that it minimizes the operative procedure, it only does so in a limited

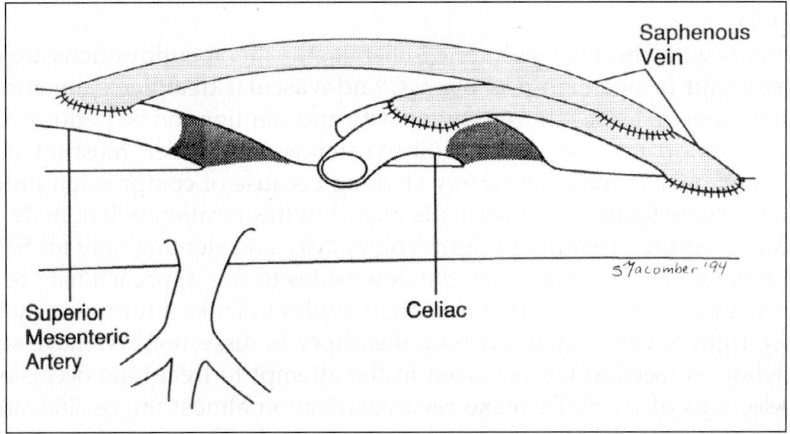

Figure 50-2. Configuration of retrograde saphenous vein bypass from iliac artery to SMA with "reversed" distal anastomosis. From McMillan MD, McCarthy WJ, Bresticker MR, et al. Mesenteric artery bypass: Objective patency determination. *J Vasc Surg.* 1995;21:729–741. Reproduced by permission.

fashion. Placing a stent in retrograde fashion in the SMA requires a lateral view of the aorta and somewhat precise placement. Performing endovascular procedures in off hours may be problematic in that the proper personnel and equipment may not be readily available. One can argue that the time it takes to obtain the radiographic images, place the stent, and patch the artery is the same time that would be required to do the bypass procedure and avoid any implant. The proponents of this endovascular approach suggest that harvesting of the vein segment for the bypass procedure is lengthy and more dangerous for the patient. The only role, in my opinion, for retrograde stenting of the SMA is in the patient with severely calcified arteries in all potential inflow locations, and in whom there is not a good venous conduit.

The endovascular revolution in vascular surgery has changed the way we have done many things. As in almost every case, endovascular procedures have a role in selected patients. However, endovascular aneurysm repair (EVAR) is not suitable for all patients with aneurysmal disease, nor is stenting of the mesenteric arteries. Preliminary results suggest good initial results with stenting of the mesenteric vessels but long term follow-up is rare.[6,7] In addition, the potential downside to patients undergoing stenting, particularly with SMA occlusion, is possible dissection of the distal SMA with disastrous consequences. Another potential downside for widespread use of mesenteric artery stenting is the stenting and ballooning of arteries in patients who do not have mesenteric ischemia. Celiac artery stenosis is common and is frequently associated with the median arcuate syndrome. Many patients have been referred for evaluation of this common CT finding. Without prior clinical experience, these patients may be subjected to unnecessary mesenteric artery stenting.

In sum, open surgery remains an important adjunct in patients with both acute and chronic mesenteric ischemia. Clamping of iliac vessels does not produce significant hemodynamic impact. Proper construction of a retrograde bypass does not adversely impact the patient, and provides excellent long-term outcome. In the setting of acute mesenteric ischemia, the use of a bypass procedure avoids any implant. Unfortunately, despite our best efforts in the treatment of patients with acute mesenteric ischemia, mortality remains high because of the reperfusion of an ischemic visceral bed and the attendant medical complications associated with this disease.

REFERENCES

1. Hogg ME, Peterson BG, Pearce WH, et al. Bare metal stent infections: Case report and review of the literature. *J Vasc Surg.* In press.
2. McMillan WD, McCarthy WJ, Bresticker MR, et al. Mesenteric artery bypass: Objective patency determination.*J Vasc Surg.* 1995;21:729–741.
3. Brown DJ, Schermerhorn ML, Powell RJ, et al. Mesenteric stenting for chronic mesenteric ischemia. *J Vasc Surg.* 2005;42:268–274.
4. Foley MI, Moneta GL, Abou-Zamzam AM Jr, et al. Revascularization of the superior mesenteric artery alone for treatment of intestinal ischemia. *J Vasc Surg.* 2000;32:37–47.
5. Wyers MC, Powell RJ, Nolan BW, Cronenwett JL. Retrograde mesenteric stenting during laparotomy for acute occlusive mesenteric ischemia. *J Vasc Surg.* 2007;45:269–275.
6. Schaefer PJ, Schaefer FK, Hinrichsen H, et al. Stent placement with the monorail technique for treatment of mesenteric artery stenosis. *J Vasc Interv Radiol.* 2006;17:637–643.
7. Landis MS, Rajan DK, Simons ME, et al. Percutaneous management of chronic mesenteric ischemia: Outcomes after intervention. *J Vasc Interv Radiol.* 2005;16:1319–1325.

51

Mesenteric Ischemia: The Case for Stents

Mark C. Wyers, M.D., and
Robert M. Zwolak, M.D., Ph.D.

Unlike renal or peripheral percutaneous intervention, angioplasty and stenting for mesenteric occlusive disease has been extremely slow to gain clinical acceptance. The most likely explanation is the fear of catastrophic acute mesenteric ischemia that might follow should the patient suffer acute arterial closure or distal embolization during or after the procedure. Indeed, almost every seasoned vascular surgeon has an anecdotal horror story related to unsuccessful or complicated attempts at percutaneous mesenteric intervention. Nevertheless, science is beginning to overtake suspicion in this arena. Experts at percutaneous intervention have published prospectively collected series with credible results during elective therapy, and more recently, a new treatment option for acute mesenteric ischemia has been introduced that involves the use of arterial stenting.

CHRONIC MESENTERIC ISCHEMIA

Involvement of the mesenteric arteries with atherosclerotic occlusive disease is an uncommon disorder that may go unrecognized for months or years before the diagnosis is established and treatment undertaken. Chronic mesenteric ischemia (CMI) accounts for less than 2% of revascularization procedures for atherosclerotic disease. CMI is unusual for an atherosclerotic disorder in that it affects women more frequently than men. Even more rare sources of CMI include fibromuscular dysplasia, polyarteritis nodosa, and median arcuate ligament syndrome. Development of duplex ultrasound to identify visceral artery stenosis and occlusion in CMI has expedited diagnosis of this disorder,[1,2] but many patients are still extremely malnourished by the time the diagnosis is established. The debilitated patient is a poor candidate for a major intra-abdominal revascularization operation. Open surgical bypass for CMI has been reported to carry mortality rates as low as 0%[3] but most reports cite mortality in the 5–8% range.[4]

Manuscripts citing 10% or higher perioperative mortality usually include concomitant surgical procedures to reconstruct the aorta, thereby adding an entire additional layer of complexity to the surgery.[5] Nevertheless, from the perspective of a skilled interventionalist, when as many as one in every 10 patients dies within 30 days of surgery, the utility of minimally invasive percutaneous techniques must be considered.

PERCUTANEOUS INTERVENTION FOR CMI

Kasirajan and colleagues from The Cleveland Clinic provided an early report of percutaneous intervention. Twenty-eight patients who underwent percutaneous revascularization for symptomatic CMI (percutaneous angioplasty, stenting, or both) between 1995 and 1997 were compared to 85 patients from the same institution treated with open surgical revascularization (bypass graft, transaortic endarterectomy, or patch angioplasty) between 1977 and 1997.[6] The cohorts were similar in terms of nonacute symptomatic status, demographics, and multiple vessel involvement. However, the percutaneous treatment patients were older (median age 72 versus 65 years) and fewer vessels per patient were treated. Eight-six percent of the percutaneous group underwent one vessel revascularization, while the surgical group underwent a 50/50 mix of single versus two-vessel treatment. The early in-hospital mortality rate was 10.7% for percutaneous revascularization versus 8.2% for open surgery (ns), and there was no statistical difference in complication rate, 18% for percutaneous therapy versus 33% for open surgery. Percutaneously treated patients had a statistically shorter hospital length of stay. They also had a higher incidence of recurrent symptoms ($p<0.001$), although there was no difference at three years in recurrent stenosis or mortality. The authors reached a conclusion favoring open surgical revascularization, although in retrospect, these data seem almost a wash.

Sivamurthy et. al. also published a retrospective nonrandomized single-center review of open versus percutaneous treatment for CMI.[7] Treatment dates spanned from January 1989 to September 2003. All patients had atherosclerosis with median two-vessel involvement. Like other reports, most were women. Open surgery in 46 patients included 43 vessels that were bypassed and 23 that underwent endarterectomy. Endoluminal treatment was undertaken in 21 patients with 22 vessels treated. In-hospital and 30-day mortality rates were 15% in the open group and 21% in endovascular patients ($p = 0.08$). Cumulative patency at six months was 83% for open surgery and 68% for endovascular. Major morbidity, median postoperative length of stay, and freedom from recurrent symptoms at six months were all statistically greater in the open group. Three-year survival by life table analysis was 62% following open surgery and 63% after percutaneous therapy. The authors reached a negative conclusion regarding endovascular therapy, but these outcomes seem equally modest, perhaps reflecting the early nature of the experience (dating back to 1989), and the low treatment volume (22 interventions in 14 years).

More recent series of endovascular treatment for CMI demonstrate substantially lower complication rates. For instance, Brown et. al. from Dartmouth reported a consecutive series of 14 patients who underwent mesenteric stenting for CMI from 2001 to 2004.[8] Mean patient age was 73, and 64% were women. In-hospital and 30-day mortality was zero, and there was no major morbidity. Mean length of stay was two days. Restenosis, diagnosed by duplex scan, occurred in eight patients (57%) during a mean follow-up period of only 13 months. Seven of eight were symptomatic, and arteriography confirmed significant restenosis. Mean time to reintervention was nine months (range two to 22 months). One patient required surgical bypass while the others were treated by repeat percutaneous intervention. All retreatments were successful, and 93% of patients were symptom-free at last recorded follow-up. The authors performed a comparison to 33 patients from the same institution who underwent open surgical mesenteric revascularization from 1990 to 2004. The stented patients had lower perioperative major morbidity (0% versus 30%, p< 0.01), while perioperative mortality failed to reach statistical significance (0% versus 9%, ns). Stented patients had shorter median length of stay (two versus 10 days, p<0.01) and shorter intensive care stay (0 versus three days, p<0.01). In conclusion, the authors confirmed a substantial rate of early restenosis associated with visceral artery stenting, but morbidity and mortality of the procedure were less than reported in earlier series.

Less morbid endovascular outcomes were also reported by Biebl et. al. from The Mayo Clinic, Jacksonville.[9] Forty-nine patients underwent surgical or endovascular treatment for CMI. The authors chose relief of symptoms as the primary endpoint with mortality, morbidity, and patency analyzed as secondary endpoints. Twenty-six patients underwent surgical revascularization, while 23 were treated endoluminally. Preoperative demographics were comparable. Immediately following intervention, freedom from CMI symptoms was 100% after surgery and 90% after percutaneous therapy (p = ns). After 25 months mean follow-up, freedom from symptoms was 89% surgical versus 75% endoluminal. Similar to most other reports, reocclusion or restenosis was higher in the endoluminal group, 25% versus 8% (p = 0.003). Symptomatic mesenteric ischemia recurred in 9% of the endoluminal patients versus none of the surgical patients. In parallel with recurrent symptoms and ischemia, 13% of endoluminal patients required reintervention while none of the surgical patients required retreatment. Surgical patients experienced significantly more early complications (42% versus 4%), longer hospital stay (11.6 days versus 1.3 days), and higher overall mortality at the end of the follow-up (31% versus 4%). Interpretation of these results is complicated by the fact that several of the surgical patients underwent simultaneous aortic reconstruction, shifting them into a much more complex clinical situation. The authors concluded that while surgical treatment has superior long-term revascularization patency and requires fewer reinterventions, it is also associated with greater mortality and morbidity than endovascular therapy. They recommended individualization when considering treatment choice, based on patient characteristics.

Atkins et. al. recently reviewed the Massachusetts General Hospital experience with elective mesenteric revascularization using percutaneous and open techniques. In order to clarify the analysis, the authors excluded patients who required simultaneous complex aneurysm repair.[10] Thirty-one patients underwent percutaneous intervention with treatment of 42 vessels. Open revascularization was performed in 49 patients, and 88 vessels were treated. Mean follow-up was shorter in the percutaneous group (15 versus 42 months). Baseline comorbidities were similar. Percutaneously treated patients had fewer vessels revascularized (1.5 versus 1.8, p = 0.001). In-hospital mortality was 3% endoluminal and 2% surgical (ns). In-hospital major morbidity was 13% endoluminal and 2% open surgical (ns). At one year, radiographic primary patency was 58% endoluminal compared to 90% open surgical (p = 0.001), while primary assisted patency was 65% endoluminal versus 96% open surgical (p<0.001). This series differs from others in its strikingly low surgical morbidity and mortality, some of which must be due to exclusion of those requiring major aortic reconstructions, and some of which must be due to excellent surgery and postoperative care. The experience also differs in terms of a higher requirement for late secondary intervention in the surgical group. Overall, 22% of open surgical patients required a second intervention during follow-up, not unlike the 16% requirement in the percutaneous group. These authors also stressed the need for individualization when considering treatment choice, based on patient anatomy and comorbidities.

A recent review of endovascular therapy for CMI was based on a MEDLINE search for English language literature including series of at least five patients. Sixteen manuscripts totaling 328 patients were identified and pooled for outcomes.[11] Technical success was claimed in 91% with clinical success in 82%, and "late" clinical success in 75%. Overall, the group had 11 deaths within 30 days (3%). Complication rate was 9%. Restenosis occurred in 84 patients (28%) at an average of 26 months follow-up. Repeat intervention was required in 79 patients (27%). Despite the latitude of self-reported single-center data, these results are very promising when considered in light of the multiply comorbid patients who require treatment for CMI. The high rate of restenosis and repeat intervention has been demonstrated in almost every series and represents a challenge for innovative clinicians. Nevertheless, having a live patient who needs re-treatment is better than not having a patient at all.

ACUTE MESENTERIC ISCHEMIA

Acute mesenteric ischemia (AMI) carries a high mortality, between 60 and 80%, based on a recent review by Oldenburg and associates.[12] AMI has a wider range of causes than CMI, including arterial embolism (~40-50% of cases), acute arterial thrombosis superimposed on preexisting atherosclerotic disease (~25%), nonocclusive mesenteric ischemia (~20%), and venous thrombosis (~10%). Treatment for AMI depends on the causative agent. Embolization is typically treated with emergent open surgical embolectomy, while the primary treatment for nonocclusive mesenteric ischemia is medical unless gangrenous bowel requires excision. Venous thrombosis is treated with heparin anticoagulation or venous thrombectomy, with excision of necrotic bowel as needed. This leaves, perhaps, the most challenging AMI cohort, terminal thrombosis of an atherosclerotic SMA. These patients are likely to have suffered CMI symptoms of malnutrition and weight loss prior to the terminal thrombosis. Successful treatment requires revascularization, meaning that some method must be undertaken to provide arterial inflow beyond the advanced atherosclerosis that typically occupies the origin and initial 3-6 centimeters of the SMA. This is done with emergent bypass graft placement, using inflow from the supraceliac aorta, the infrarenal aorta, or the iliac arteries. The operation is complex, and recovery is challenging in the very ill patient. Kougias et. al. reviewed 72 patients who underwent emergent operative intervention for acute mesenteric thrombosis or embolism in a report published in 2007.[13] Treatments included thrombectomy (31%), mesenteric bypass grafting (46%), patch angioplasty (12%), reimplantation (7%), and endarterectomy (4%). Bowel resection was required during the initial operation in 31%, and during a second look operation in 53%. Perioperative morbidity and 30-day mortality rates were 39% and 31%, respectively, excellent results for these critically ill patients. Age greater than 70 and prolonged symptom duration were independent predictors of mortality.

Percutaneous interventional treatment for AMI is rare. A few case reports have been published, but wide experience is lacking.[14-16] However, Wyers and coauthors recently reported a hybrid open/interventional approach for treatment of acute atherosclerotic SMA thrombosis.[17] Similar to a technique described in an earlier case report by Milner,[18] the Dartmouth authors described Retrograde Open Mesenteric Stenting (ROMS) of the SMA. With the diagnosis of AMI, laparotomy is typically required to explore and resect gangrenous bowel. This allows ready access to the SMA at the base of the transverse mesocolon for retrograde cannulation. Following heparin anticoagulation, the SMA is incised longitudinally, and a local thromboendarterectomy is performed if necessary. Placing a patch angioplasty then facilitates the remaining portions of the procedure. We typically use bovine pericardial patch, but saphenous vein would be suitable. A purse-string suture can be placed in the patch around the puncture site to facilitate sheath removal without having to reclamp the SMA. A 6F, 35-cm-long flexible sheath (Arrow International Inc, Reading PA) is placed through the patch into the SMA in retrograde direction, headed toward the aorta. The extra diameter provided by the patch allows angiographic evaluation of the distal mesenteric arcades through the sheath, both before and after restoration of SMA inflow. The long sheath also allows the surgeon to avoid extensive fluoroscopic exposure while working comfortably away from the image intensifier.

Once the sheath is in place, metallic retractors are removed, and the surgeon performs hand injection retrograde lateral angiography (Figure 51–1). This demonstrates the exact site of stenosis or occlusion. A simultaneous flush aortogram from a percutaneous femoral or brachial catheter may be used to profile the aorta, thereby completely outlining the lesion that must be crossed and treated to regain arterial inflow. A 0.035-inch glidewire (Terumo, Somerset, NJ or other similar) is often useful to cross the lesion, with subsequent exchange for a lower profile platform. Predilation with a 2 or 3 mm angioplasty balloon is usually necessary. This is followed by retrograde stent placement using 5, 6, or 7 mm low-profile balloon expandable stents (Figure 51–2). The leading edge of the proximal-most stent is positioned to protrude 1-2 mm into the aortic lumen. More than one stent is oftentimes required to fully treat the SMA lesion.

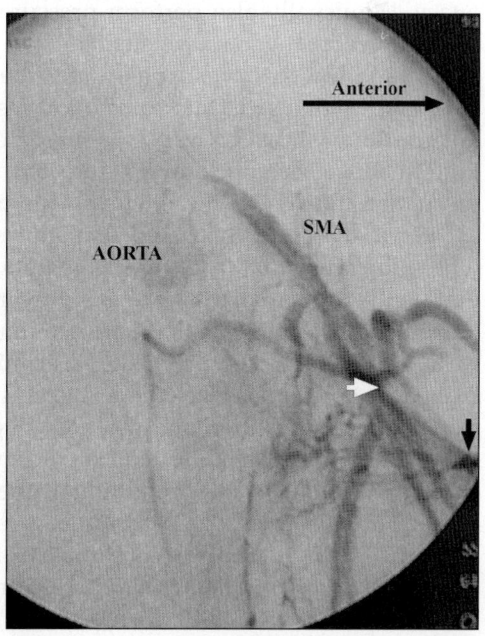

Figure 51-1. Retrograde SMA injection. Note the proximity of the sheath's point of entry (black arrow) and of the sheath's tip (white arrow) to the proximal SMA occlusion. There is no reflux of contrast into the aorta. With permission.

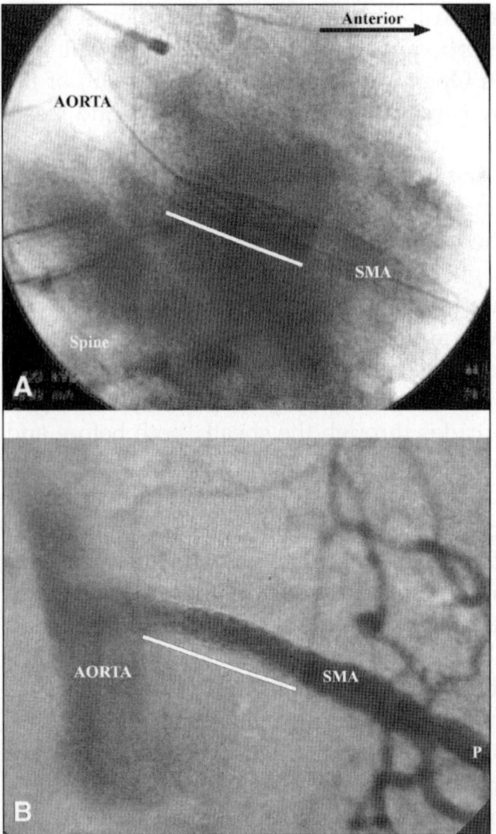

Figure 51-2. (A) Intraoperative lateral fluoroscopic image shows two stents (underscored by white line) deployed in the SMA origin with the 0.018-inch wire still in place. Note the lumbar vertebral bodies to the left. **(B)** Completion retrograde arteriogram shows free reflux of contrast into the aorta and no residual angiographic stenosis; P denotes the approximate location of the SMA patch angioplasty. With permission.

Completion arteriography is performed in multiple views to confirm technical adequacy. We usually also perform pressure measurements to confirm the absence of a residual gradient across the stented area. Completion imaging of the SMA arcades is recommended, and vasospasm may be treated with injections of papaverine or glucagon. With a satisfactory technical result achieved, the sheath is removed and the hole in the patch is sutured. The mesentery is closed over the SMA exploration site. Perforated and necrotic bowel is resected. Close attention is given to generous fluid resuscitation during the immediate postop period.

Our 2007 report compared six patients with acute thrombotic mesenteric ischemia who underwent ROMS to five patients who underwent emergent mesenteric bypass graft, and to two patients who were treated with percutaneous antegrade SMA stent placement.[17] This is a small series with no statistically significant results, but the ROMS outcomes were promising. Technical success with ROMS was 100%, even in five patients who had previous unsuccessful attempts to cross the SMA from a percutaneous antegrade approach. The ROMS group suffered only 17% in-hospital mortality compared to 80% following emergent mesenteric bypass, and 100% in the two percutaneous stent patients, although these results did not reach significance due to low "n." Five of the six ROMS patients were discharged to home after a mean hospital stay of 20 days. During one year mean follow-up, three of them died of unrelated causes, while two were alive and well, one with an asymptomatic recurrent stenosis.

In conclusion, ROMS during emergent laparotomy for AMI is a promising technique and an attractive alternative to emergent surgical bypass. This method needs to be tested by others to determine its true value in comparison to traditional methods.

CLINICAL AND DUPLEX FOLLOW-UP

Based on the available data, patients undergoing endovascular visceral revascularization for chronic or acute mesenteric ischemia are likely to develop recurrent stenosis. Close clinical follow-up would appear to be indicated, and the issue arises whether duplex ultrasound would be a valuable adjunct. The literature on this topic is meager. Fenwick et. al. reviewed their experience using color Doppler ultrasound to identify recurrent stenosis in patients who had undergone successful percutaneous mesenteric intervention, and they attempted to relate this to recurrence of symptoms or weight loss.[19] With a total "n" of five, they identified restenosis in three patients. However, all three individuals were asymptomatic when the duplex observations were made. The authors were appropriately circumspect, but this is an extremely modest report with little interpretive information. In a more robust report, Liem et. al. characterized duplex-derived flow velocities in mesenteric artery bypass graft limbs, although they did not study patients who had·undergone percutaneous mesenteric revascularization or ROMS.[20] Our experience at Dartmouth with mesenteric duplex and following interventional visceral artery therapy is promising, although still empiric-based on an anticipated high rate of restenosis. We have not identified an absolute velocity threshold that would indicate the need for prompt reintervention. However, the traditional velocity criteria for native vessels seem to provide reasonably accurate information to guide clinical decision-making. Suffice to say the entire concept of clinical and duplex follow-up after open and percutaneous visceral revascularization deserves further evidence development.

CONCLUSION

There are no randomized trials we are aware of, but as published experience accrues, percutaneous therapy for CMI may be the best option for high-surgical risk patients with advanced malnutrition and wasting. Possibly, percutaneous intervention may be the treatment of choice for all patients with anatomically suitable lesions at centers of excellence where periprocedural morbidity and mortality are low. Patients with long total occlusions still require open surgical bypass or endarterectomy. Based on the majority of reports, percutaneous treatment carries a higher rate of recurrent stenosis. Recurrence can usually be treated percutaneously, but the choice of open versus percutaneous retreatment should be considered carefully when the need arises. Acute mesenteric ischemia usually requires open laparotomy to explore the bowel. This requirement provides the opportunity for retrograde open mesenteric stenting (ROMS), a new method to revascularize the SMA. Finally, realizing that recurrent stenosis is likely, close clinical follow-up is indicated. The role of duplex ultrasound following percutaneous visceral intervention is yet to be defined.

REFERENCES

1. Moneta GL, Lee RW, Yeager RA, et al. Mesenteric duplex scanning: A blinded prospective study. *J Vasc Surg*. 1993;17:79–86.
2. Zwolak RM, Fillinger MF, Walsh DB, et al. Mesenteric and celiac duplex scanning: a validation study. *J Vasc Surg*. 1998;27:1078–1087; discussion 1088.
3. Johnston KW, Lindsay TF, Walker PM, Kalman PG. Mesenteric arterial bypass grafts: early and late results and suggested surgical approach for chronic and acute mesenteric ischemia. *Surgery*. 1995;118(1):1–7.
4. Mateo RB, O'Hara PJ, Hertzer NR, et al. Elective surgical treatment of symptomatic chronic mesenteric occlusive disease: early results and late outcomes. *J Vasc Surg*. 1999;29(5): 821–831; discussion 832.
5. McAfee MK, Cherry KJ, Jr., Naessens JM, et al. Influence of complete revascularization on chronic mesenteric ischemia. *Am J Surg*. 1992;164(3):220–224.
6. Kasirajan K, O'Hara PJ, Gray BH, et al. Chronic mesenteric ischemia: open surgery versus percutaneous angioplasty and stenting. *J Vasc Surg*. 2001;33(1):63–71.
7. Sivamurthy N, Rhodes JM, Lee D, et al. Endovascular versus open mesenteric revascularization: immediate benefits do not equate with short-term functional outcomes. *J Am Coll Surg*. 2006;202(6):859–867.
8. Brown DJ, Schermerhorn ML, Powell RJ, et al. Mesenteric stenting for chronic mesenteric ischemia. *J Vasc Surg*. 2005;42(2):268–274.
9. Biebl M, Oldenburg WA, Paz-Fumagalli R, et al. Surgical and interventional visceral revascularization for the treatment of chronic mesenteric ischemia—when to prefer which? *World J Surg*. Mar 2007;31(3):562–568.
10. Atkins MD, Kwolek CJ, LaMuraglia GM, et al. Surgical revascularization versus endovascular therapy for chronic mesenteric ischemia: a comparative experience. *J Vasc Surg*. 2007;45(6):1162–1171.
11. Kougias P, El Sayed HF, Zhou W, Lin PH. Management of chronic mesenteric ischemia. The role of endovascular therapy. *J Endovasc Ther*. 2007;14(3):395–405.
12. Oldenburg WA, Lau LL, Rodenberg TJ, et al. Acute mesenteric ischemia: a clinical review. *Arch Intern Med*. 24 2004;164(10):1054–1062.
13. Kougias P, Lau D, El Sayed HF, et al. Determinants of mortality and treatment outcome following surgical interventions for acute mesenteric ischemia. *J Vasc Surg*. 2007 July 26 [Epub ahead of print].
14. Leduc FJ, Pestieau SR, Detry O, et al. Acute mesenteric ischaemia: minimal invasive management by combined laparoscopy and percutaneous transluminal angioplasty. *Eur J Surg*. 2000;166(4):345–347.
15. Brountzos EN, Critselis A, Magoulas D, et al. Emergency endovascular treatment of a superior mesenteric artery occlusion. *Cardiovasc Intervent Radiol*. 2001;24(1):57–60.
16. Gartenschlaeger S, Bender S, Maeurer J, Schroeder RJ. Successful Percutaneous Transluminal Angioplasty and Stenting in Acute Mesenteric Ischemia. *Cardiovasc Intervent Radiol*. 2007 Jan 4. [Epub ahead of print]
17. Wyers MC, Powell RJ, Nolan BW, Cronenwett JL. Retrograde mesenteric stenting during laparotomy for acute occlusive mesenteric ischemia. *J Vasc Surg*. 2007;45(2):269–275.
18. Milner R, Woo EY, Carpenter JP. Superior mesenteric artery angioplasty and stenting via a retrograde approach in a patient with bowel ischemia—a case report. *Vasc Endovascular Surg*. 2004;38(1):89–91.
19. Fenwick JL, Wright IA, Buckenham TM. Endovascular repair of chronic mesenteric occlusive disease: the role of duplex surveillance. *ANZ J Surg*. 2007;77(1–2):60–63.
20. Liem TK, Segall JA, Wei W, et al. Duplex scan characteristics of bypass grafts to mesenteric arteries. *J Vasc Surg*. 2007;45(5):922–927; discussion 927–928.

Index